THE
VETERINARY
CARE
of the
HORSE

THE VETERINARY CARE
of the
HORSE

Sue Devereux BA BVSc MRCVS

Edited by Karen Coumbe
MA VetMB CertEP MRCVS

J. A. ALLEN

© *Sue Devereux 2006*

First edition published in Great Britain by J.A.Allen in 1992.
This second edition published in 2006.

ISBN-10: 0 85131 924 6
ISBN-13: 978 0 85131 924 7

J. A. Allen
Clerkenwell House
Clerkenwell Green
London EC1R 0HT

J. A. Allen is an imprint of Robert Hale Ltd

British Library Cataloguing in Publication Data
A catalogue record for this book is available from the British Library

Design by Judy Linard
Illustrated by Maggie Raynor and Sue Devereux
Edited by Jane Lake
Printed by Kyodo Printing Co (S'pore) Pte Ltd, Singapore

CONTENTS

ACKNOWLEDGEMENTS

I would like to thank everyone who helped with the production of this book. Special thanks must go to Liz Morrison who was my co-author and inspiration for the first edition of The Veterinary Care of the Horse. I am also grateful to Karen Coumbe MA VetMB CertEP MRCVS for her work as veterinary editor and to Karen, Alex Thiemann MA VetMB CertEP MRCVS and Margrit Coates MNFSH MBRCP for the valuable chapters they contributed.

The people listed below have helped in a number of ways, either by supplying photographs or diagrams, the figure numbers of which are listed after their names, or allowing me to photograph their horses.

Liz Atkinson and Princess

Helen Bridges

Julia Brooks DO (Hons) MSc

Jill Carpenter MA VetMB MSc CertVR FRCVS –
15.12, 24.6, 24.9, 24.10, 24.11, 24.13

Dr Mary Carroll MD FRCP

Lucy Challis and Lily

Caroline Champion and Sula

Margrit Coates MNFSH MBRCP

Hilary Cotter

Felicity Craddock, Nutty, Tico and Charm

E. Crozier-Cole

R. S. Cull BVetMed MRCVS

Sandra Dunn

Equilibrium Products – 18.7, 18.20. 22.6

Emmanuel Engeli DVM MRCVS DipACVS
DipECVS – 5.3

Peter Goody BSc MSc(Ed) PhD

Ted Greaves, National Sweet Itch Centre: 18.11

Louise Hartgill – 19.25, 19.26, 19.27a–e, 19.29,
19.30a, 19.32

Alex and Andrew Harris

Lady Herries

Mark Hillyer BVSc DipECVS PhD CertEP
CertEM (Int Med) CertES (Soft Tissue)
MRCVS – 17.5

Kay Humphries – 12.9, 12.10, 12.11, 12.12a and b,
12.13, 12.14, 12.15, 12.17a and b, 12.18

Belinda Inwood and Posy

Jackson Arenas and Lincoln University: 22.4

Ruth Jacobson and Casper

Jan Jarvis

Derek Knottenbelt BVM&S DVM&S MRCVS –
18.15a and b, 18.36, 18.41, 21.8, 21.14, 21.15,
21.17, 21.22, 21.23, 21.26, 21.28

J. G. Lane BVetMed DESTS FRCVS – 15.17,
15.20

Deborah Lucas MSc CBiol MIBiol RNutr

T. S. Mair BVSc PhD DipECEIM DEIM DESTS
MRCVS – 15.22, 15.23

Merial Animal Health – 2.14, 2.16, 2.19, 2.20, 18.16

John R. B. Mould BA BVSc DVOphthal MRCVS – 21.13a

Michael J. Murray DVM MS Dipl ACVIM – 17.3a and b

David Nicholls AWCF RJF – 6.22, 6.29, 6.36, 6.41b, 6.49a and b, 6.51

Mark Oliver DipWCF

Virginia Phillimore

Andrew Poynton FWCF – 6.47, 6.50a, b and c,

Anthony Pusey DO FE Cert

Jonathon Pycock BVetMed PhD DESM MRCVS – 19.18

Jim Ravenscroft AWCF

Tony Rose (Advanced EDT)

Roxy, Sporty and Joan

Karen Rowsell and Mabel

Dietrich von Schweinitz BSc DVM MRCVS – 5.7a and b

Heather Scott Parsons – 7.1b, 15.1c, 15.15, 15.18, 16.1, 17.1, 21.27

Jane Sleeman

Luisa Smith BVMS MRCVS – 7.3a and b

Carol Soormally

Annie Standen

Sarah Stoneham BVSc Cert ESM MRCVS – 8.17, 11.8, 19.22

Amanda Sutton MSc Vet Phys MCSP Grad Dip Phys

Frank Taylor BVSc PhD MRCVS – 11.7a and b, 15.6, 15.8, 17.15, 17.18

The Donkey Sanctuary – 8.19, 17.19, 23.1, 23.2, 23.3, 23.4, 23.5, 23.6, 23.7

Alex Thiemann MA VetMB CertEP MRCVS

John Thompson – 12.9, 12.10, 12.11, 12.12a and b, 12.13, 12.14, 12.15, 12.17a and b, 12.18

Penny Unwin

Wendy Vere MRCVS MA VetMB

Clodagh and Jason Wallace

Martin Walls C/EqD BAEDT – 2.7, 2.9, 2.10

Tammy Weal

Matt Webb

Whitsbury Manor Stud

Elaine Woolley

Alan Wright BVSc MRCVS – 18.2a and b, 18.8d, 18.12a, 18.13, 18.18a, 18.28a, 18.38b, 18.43

Tina Yarrow

All other photographs by Karen Coumbe and the author.

Thank you also to everyone at J. A. Allen who provided encouragement at every stage, especially my editor Jane Lake, also Caroline Burt and Cassie Campbell. Thank you to Maggie Raynor for her illustrations and to Judy Linard for the excellent design and cover. Finally, the biggest thank you is to my children Alex and Laura who were so supportive and tolerant of the time I spent writing and researching this book.

PREFACE

Welcome to the second edition of *The Veterinary Care of the Horse*. Since the first edition was published in 1992, many new developments have occurred in the equine veterinary world. Our understanding of the diseases that affect horses is increasing all the time and we have a wide range of new and sophisticated equipment to help us make a diagnosis. New diseases have emerged and more treatment options are available.

The aim of this book is to bring you up-to-date with these developments while still presenting the information in the easy-to-read format that was popular with the first edition. Horse owners are now requesting more information and so the subjects have been covered in greater depth and a broader range of topics has been included.

I am delighted to welcome the guest authors Karen Coumbe MA VetMB CertEP MRCVS, Alex Thiemann MA VetMB CertEP MRCVS and Margrit Coates MNFSH MBRCP and thank them for their valuable contributions to the book.

As always it is important to remember that the symptoms of any disease can vary from horse to horse. This book is in no way intended to replace advice from your own veterinary surgeon who will make a diagnosis and recommend the most suitable treatment for each individual patient.

I hope you enjoy this edition of *The Veterinary Care of the Horse*. The aim is to help everyone involved with horses to understand the vet's approach and provide the best of care for their horses.

Sue Devereux BA BVSc MRCVS

1

THE HEALTHY HORSE

It is important to be familiar with the signs of good health, so that any illness or abnormality can be detected in the early stages. A healthy horse or pony should have:

- a bright, alert attitude, with pricked ears and an interest in the surroundings
- a good appetite
- a shiny coat with healthy skin that is loose and supple
- clear, bright eyes with no discharge
- clean nostrils (a small amount of watery discharge is normal)
- good condition without being fat
- droppings that are passed regularly and are not loose or too firm
- a body temperature of between 37 and 38 °C (98.5-100.5 °F)
- a pulse of 28–42 beats per minute
- a respiration rate of 8–16 breaths per minute (the horse's breathing movements should be smooth and gentle)
- salmon-pink mucous membranes (some horses have areas of black pigmentation).

It is important to know what is normal for your own horse. For example, horses will often have an increased pulse and respiratory rate if they are excited or anxious. They may also pass loose droppings when they are excited at a competition, but under these circumstances it is not a sign of illness. If you have any doubts about your horse's health, the best person to consult is your vet.

PREVENTIVE MEDICINE

Preventive medicine includes the procedures that should be routinely carried out to keep the horse in good health and protect it from disease.

These procedures include:
- vaccination against equine influenza and tetanus and, depending on the risks of your particular situation, vaccination against equine herpesvirus (EHV-1, EHV-4) and strangles may also be recommended

- a worming programme
- regular dental checks
- a hoof care and shoeing programme.

In addition, every horse should be checked regularly throughout the day. Horses and ponies out at grass should be inspected at least twice daily.

Planning ahead

Missing any of these important procedures can prevent the horse from working and be an expensive oversight. If a vaccination is given late, the whole course may need to be started again. It is therefore advisable to plan your worming programme and book visits for vaccination, dentistry and shoeing in advance. Mark the dates in a diary or on a calendar.

Do not forget retired horses, brood mares and companion animals as they require the same consideration and veterinary care. They are at risk even if they rarely leave the field.

Sharing the cost

Whether you keep your horse at home or in a livery yard, it is more cost effective to arrange a shared visit from the vet. The travelling costs of the vet can then be divided between a number of owners. Another economic option is to take your horse to the vet since you will not have to pay a call-out fee. If your horse is examined at an equine hospital there will be more help and equipment to carry out any investigations and treatments required.

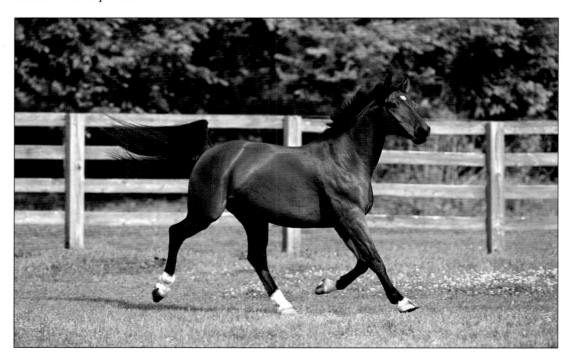

2

PREVENTIVE MEDICINE

VACCINATION

Vaccines are available to protect horses and donkeys against a number of diseases including tetanus, equine influenza virus, equine herpesvirus (EHV) and strangles. There is also a vaccine that is given to pregnant mares to protect their foals against diarrhoea caused by equine rotavirus.

Equine influenza and tetanus vaccination programme

All horses should be vaccinated against tetanus and equine influenza. The recommended programme which complies with both the Jockey Club and International Equestrian Federation (Fédération Equestre Internationale [FEI]) rules is as follows.

PRIMARY COURSE

Two injections of a combined influenza and tetanus vaccine are given between 21–92 days apart. The vaccine manufacturers recommend that the interval between the first two injections is 4–6 weeks.

SIX-MONTH BOOSTER

A booster vaccination against influenza and tetanus is given between 150 and 215 days (approximately 5–7 months) after the second injection of the primary course.

ANNUAL BOOSTERS

Subsequent boosters should be given at intervals of no more than 12 months. The first annual booster is usually for equine influenza only, as adequate protection against tetanus will be provided by the primary course. Protection against tetanus is given in alternate years or with some vaccines and veterinary recommendation every third year.

The FEI requirement for equine influenza vaccination was changed on 1 January 2005 and boosters are now required at 6-month intervals. It is likely that other disciplines' ruling bodies may follow this. Other horses at high risk of exposure to the virus such as racehorses and those that regularly attend shows and competitions may be boosted against equine influenza every 6 months.

Only healthy horses should be vaccinated. If your horse is coughing or off colour, you should inform the vet before the vaccine is given.

Exercise following vaccination

Wherever possible, vaccinations should be given at a time when the horse is going to have a couple of days off. This is because although the majority of horses appear to suffer no ill effects from the vaccine, some are definitely below par for a few days or experience soreness at the site of injection. Occasionally a horse develops a temperature and is quite unwell, so it is not advisable to vaccinate in the midst of a busy competition schedule.

For horses that are in work, the following guidelines are suggested.

- Do not travel long distances or tire the horse immediately before or after a vaccination.
- Following a vaccination, the horse should be allowed a few easy days. Ridden walking exercise and turning out can be continued as normal, but the horse should not be worked hard enough to make it sweat or become tired.
- If the horse does seem unwell following vaccination, contact your vet and do not work it at all.

Pregnant Mares

Pregnant mares should be given an influenza and tetanus booster 4–6 weeks prior to foaling to give the foal maximum protection. Antibodies are passed to the foal in the colostrum and will protect it for approximately the first 5 months of life. This is known as 'passive immunity'.

Foal immunization

It is recommended that foals from vaccinated mares begin their primary vaccination course at 5 months of age. Most are protected by the maternal antibodies until this age. There is no point in vaccinating the foal before the passive immunity wanes, as the antibodies can prevent the vaccine stimulating an immune response.

If the mare is not vaccinated, then the foal may start its vaccination programme from 3 months of age. Tetanus antitoxin is often administered to foals at birth and should also be given if they have a wound before their vaccination programme is complete. Tetanus antitoxin is not a vaccine, but it gives immediate protection against tetanus for a few days.

Equine herpesvirus (EHV) vaccination programme

There is a vaccine available which gives protection against EHV-1 and EHV-4. Pregnant mares are vaccinated during the 5th, 7th and 9th months of pregnancy to reduce the risk of infectious abortion caused by herpesvirus.

Foals may be vaccinated from 5 months of age. Following the primary course when the first and second injections are given 4–6 weeks apart, boosters are recommended every 6 months. Immunity following vaccination and natural infection is relatively short-lived, but vaccination is considered to be beneficial.

Vaccination against strangles

A new vaccine developed to protect horses against strangles became available in the UK in September 2004. It is injected into the mucosa on the inside of the horse's upper lip. The primary course is 2 injections given 4 weeks apart. Foals can be vaccinated from 4 months of age. Whenever possible, all the horses kept together in a group should be vaccinated at the same time.

Horses in high-risk situations (e.g. new horses regularly being introduced into the group, horses that regularly attend competitions or horses close to an outbreak of strangles) should be given boosters every 3 months. Those in medium-risk situations (e.g. occasional outings to shows or lessons) should be vaccinated every 6 months. Horses that are kept in a group that do not attend shows or otherwise travel where they may mix with other horses are generally low risk and may not need vaccinating. Your vet is the best person to ask for advice.

IF AN OUTBREAK OCCURS

If an outbreak of strangles occurs in the vicinity, any horse that has not had a booster within 3 months should be re-vaccinated. Provided the last injection was less than 6 months ago, a single dose is sufficient. Only healthy horses should be vaccinated so the vaccine should not be given if the horse is thought to be developing the disease. Thus it is not advisable to vaccinate horses that have had been in contact with an infected horse.

PRECAUTIONS

Pregnant or lactating mares should not be vaccinated and this vaccine should not be administered at the same time as other vaccines. Some horses experience temporary swelling of the upper lip and muzzle or develop a slight temperature on the day of vaccination.

Vaccination against equine rotavirus

Pregnant mares are vaccinated in the 8th, 9th and 10th months of pregnancy. Antibodies produced are passed to the foals in the colostrum and help to protect them against the diarrhoea and illness caused by rotavirus.

Vaccination certificates and passports

A record of all vaccines administered is included in equine passports and vaccination certificates. These must be kept up-to-date. If an equine influenza booster is overlooked and given more than 12 months after the last injection, it may be necessary to begin the whole programme again.

DENTISTRY

It is normal for horses to have sharp and ridged grinding teeth (molars). This design of dentition has evolved because the horse is a herbivore. In the wild, the horse spends up to sixteen hours a day with its head down chewing coarse grass material which contains abrasive silicates that continually wear the teeth. To compensate for this, the permanent teeth of the horse continue to erupt for most of its life at a rate of 2–3 mm ($\frac{1}{10}$ in) a year.

Many of the problems we see today are the result of domestication. The mouth and dentition of the horse were not designed to accommodate a bit or to have a diet composed mainly of concentrate feeds with relatively little forage fed at head height or above in mangers and haynets. Equine dentistry seeks to promote health and accommodate man's influence on the horse, thus preventing any pain or discomfort.

The dental formula of the horse

The dental formula is used to describe the number of teeth present in each side (i.e. the left or right side) of the mouth. 'I' refers to incisor teeth, 'C' to canines, 'P' to premolars and 'M' to molars. The number of teeth in the top jaw is placed above the number of teeth in the lower jaw. This is then multiplied by 2 for the total number of teeth in the horse's mouth.

DECIDUOUS OR TEMPORARY (BABY) TEETH

(I $\frac{3}{3}$, P $\frac{3}{3}$) x 2 = 24 teeth

The young horse, therefore, has 3 incisors and 3 premolars in each side of the upper and lower jaws, a total of 24 teeth.

PERMANENT TEETH

The full complement of adult teeth is normally present by the time the horse is 5 years of age. The number varies between 36 and 44, depending on whether canine and wolf teeth are present. Male horses normally have four permanent canine teeth but in mares these are usually absent. The first premolar tooth, known as a wolf tooth, is not consistently present. The dental formula of the adult horse is therefore variable.

(I $\frac{3}{3}$, C $\frac{1}{1}$ or $\frac{0}{0}$, P $\frac{3\text{-}4}{3\text{-}4}$, M $\frac{3}{3}$) x 2 = 36–44 teeth

There is now a new and more accurate system for identifying teeth individually, similar to that used by human dentists, where each tooth has an individual number to enable specific identification. This is illustrated in the equine dental chart shown in Figure 2.1.

NAME OF EQUINE DENTAL TECHNICIAN

QUALIFICATIONS
ADDRESS
CONTACT TELEPHONE NUMBER

Client: .... Date: ....

Horse: .... Age: ....

Address: ....

.... Telephone: ....

Comments: ....

....

MOLAR TABLE ANGLES BEFORE DENTAL WORK

FAR SIDE............... NEAR SIDE...............

GUM LINE

GUM LINE

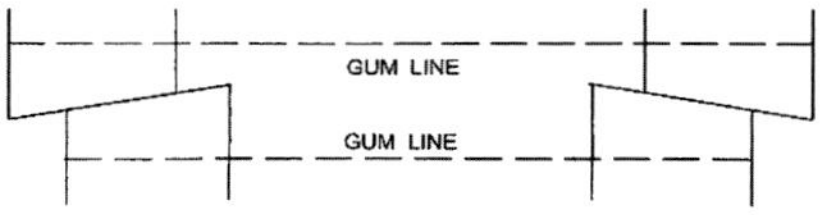

MOLAR TABLE ANGLES AFTER DENTAL WORK

FAR SIDE............... NEAR SIDE...............

INCISOR TABLE ANGLES

BEFORE............... AFTER...............

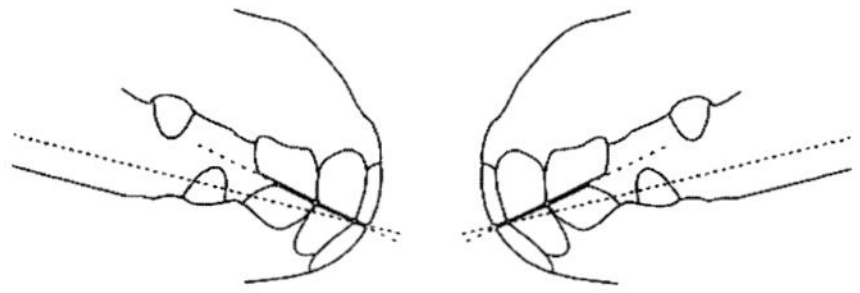

LATERAL EXCURSION & OCCLUSION

BEFORE............... AFTER...............

ANTERIOR / POSTERIOR MOVEMENT

BEFORE............... AFTER...............

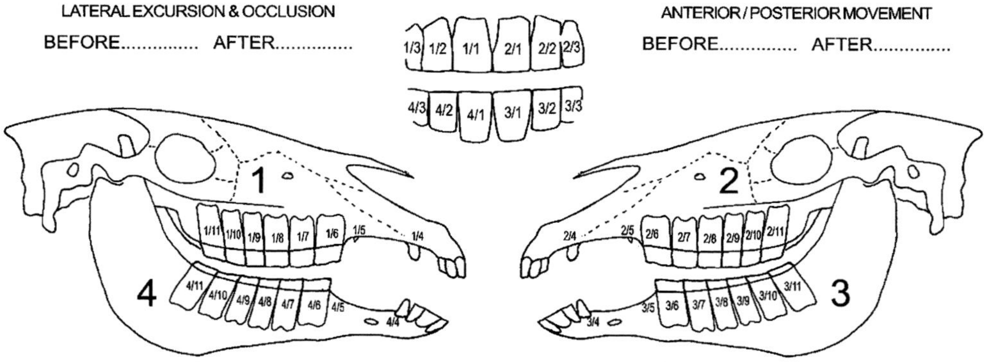

1/3 1/2 1/1 2/1 2/2 2/3

4/3 4/2 4/1 3/1 3/2 3/3

1

2

1/11 1/10 1/9 1/8 1/7 1/6 1/5 1/4

2/4 2/5 2/6 2/7 2/8 2/9 2/10 2/11

4

4/11 4/10 4/9 4/8 4/7 4/6 4/5 4/4

2/4 3/11

3/5 3/6 3/7 3/8 3/9 3/10

3

3/4

INCISORS	CANINES	WOLF TEETH	MOLARS	
CAPS	NONE	EXTRACT	FLOAT	A - ABCESSED
FRAGMENTS	MALE	NORMAL	BITSEAT	B - BURR
EXTRACT	FEMALE	LINGUAL	BALANCE	C - CUT
REALIGN	CUT	ANTERIOR	CAPS	D - DECAY
CUT	BUFF	ABERRANT	FRAGMENT	E - EXTRACT
FLOAT	REMOVE TARTAR	FRAGMENT	STEPPED	F - FLOAT
FILE	NORMAL	UNERUPTED	WAVE	M - MISSING
BURR	BLIND	BLIND	SHEAR	R - REPEL
OVERJET	ELEVATE	OTHER	HOOKS	S - SUPERNUMARY
OVERBITE	OTHER		RAMPS	T - TARTAR
UNDERJET			RIMS	U - UNERUPTED
UNDERBITE			CUT / EXTRACT	X - CAP
TARTAR			DECAY	
OTHER			ATR	
CHARGES	CHARGES	CHARGES	CHARGES	

Call back date: .... Reason: .... Total charges: ....

Figure 2.1 Equine dental evaluation and maintenance chart

Functions of the teeth

The **incisor** teeth are used to crop and tear off forage and also for defence. The **canine** teeth are primarily used for defence. The **premolars** and **molars**, collectively known as the **cheek teeth** are used to grind down the food into small particles so that it can be swallowed.

Signs of dental problems

These include:

- loss of condition
- failure to gain weight despite good nutrition
- eating more slowly than usual or than other horses
- dropping food
- quidding – boluses of partially chewed forage are dropped from the mouth or accumulate between the teeth and the cheeks
- head tossing while eating
- the presence of unchewed grain in the droppings
- roughage pieces longer than normal in the droppings
- tenderness of the cheeks overlying the teeth
- tenderness around the temporomandibular joint (TMJ) on palpation
- bad breath
- excessive salivation or drooling
- putting the hay in the water bucket to make it softer and easier to chew
- facial swellings
- discharging sinuses
- foul-smelling nasal discharge
- recurrent choke
- some types of colic, e.g. impactions.

Performance problems caused by dental issues

These include:

- reluctance to come onto the bit
- head tilting or tossing when ridden
- stiffness on one or both reins
- opening the mouth when asked for collection
- difficulty in turning
- reluctance to take the correct lead
- stiffness and pain in the horse's back and neck
- rearing
- unexplained change in performance or behaviour.

Routine dental inspection

Routine dental inspection every 6–12 months is recommended so that problems can be identified and dealt with *before* they cause discomfort and suffering. This can be done by your vet or a qualified and experienced equine dental technician (EDT).

PREPARING FOR THE INSPECTION

- Put the horse in a stable with plenty of head room. The roof should not be too low or supported by low beams in case the horse throws his head up during the examination.
- Use a headcollar with a loose or adjustable noseband. If the noseband is too tight it prevents the horse's mouth opening fully.
- Have a bucket of clean water and a towel ready.
- If possible, do not feed the horse just before the procedure or the mouth will need to be flushed out to remove the food material.

THE DENTAL EXAMINATION

The examination begins with assessment of the horse's body condition and facial symmetry. The temporomandibular joint (TMJ) and the cheeks are palpated for any tenderness and the owner will be asked if the horse has experienced any problems. The

vet or EDT will then part the horse's lips to check the incisors for abnormal wear. The soft tissues of the mouth including the tongue, cheeks, bars and corners of the mouth will be checked for injury caused by the bit or sharp teeth (Figure 2.2). A full-mouth speculum or Haussman's gag and a powerful light source are necessary for detailed evaluation of the cheek teeth (Figures 2.3 and 2.4). If sharp edges are present, the outside edges of the upper teeth are lightly rasped to remove the sharp points before the gag is opened fully. This is because when the gag is open, the cheeks of the horse are stretched over the sharp points and this is ·mely uncomfortable. Both the teeth and the ɩcent cheek tissues are inspected visually and palpated. The range of motion of the jaw and the grind of the teeth is checked.

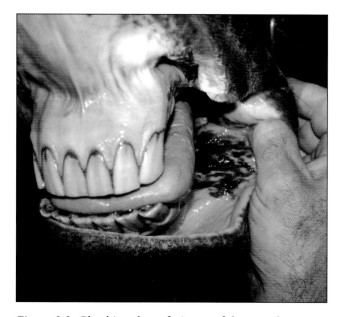

Figure 2.2 Checking the soft tissues of the mouth

The findings are recorded on a dental chart (see Figure 2.1). This also has information on the treatment given and recommendations for future examination intervals and treatment.

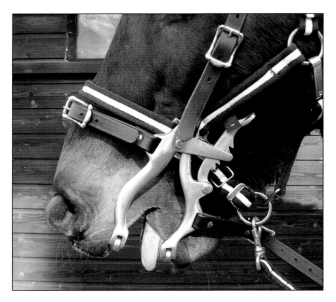

Figure 2.3 Haussman's gag

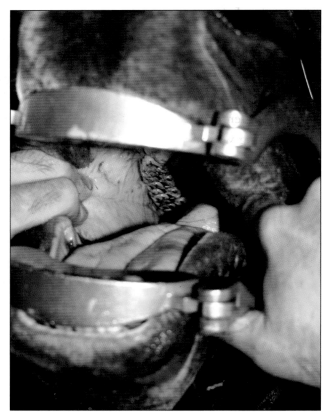

Figure 2.4 A gag and a bright light are necessary for detailed evaluation of the cheek teeth

The dental programme

It is recommended that foals are checked at or shortly after birth to ensure that their incisors meet normally and they do not have a parrot mouth. This is a condition where the lower jaw is shorter than the upper jaw and the incisors do not meet (Figure 2.5). Thereafter, youngsters should be inspected annually to check for sharp points and to ensure that the permanent teeth are erupting normally and that the temporary ones are being shed. Removal of retained deciduous teeth and minor corrections should be performed as appropriate. Wolf teeth that are likely to cause a problem may be removed before the horse comes into work.

Once a horse is in work, the teeth should initially be inspected every 6 months. It may then be possible to extend the period to 9 or 12 months if no problems are encountered.

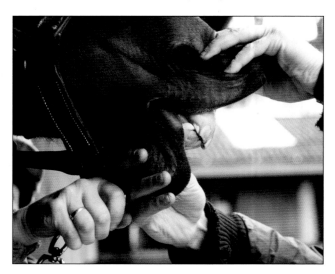

Figure 2.5 Parrot mouth

How do I find a good dental technician?

Equine dentistry is now regulated. The increase in number of skilled equine dental technicians has significantly improved the welfare of the horse over the last few years. All members of the British Association of Equine Dental Technicians (BAEDT) have passed an examination set by the British Equine Veterinary Association (BEVA) and the British Veterinary Dental Association (BVDA). A list of these dental technicians can be found on the following web sites:

- British Association of Equine Dental Technicians (www.equinedentistry.org.uk)
- British Equine Veterinary Association (www.beva.org.uk)
- British Veterinary Dental Association (www.BVDA.co.uk).

BEVA also runs both basic and advanced training courses for vets and many practices now undertake equine dentistry to a high standard. Alternatively, your vet may be able to recommend an experienced local EDT with the above qualifications.

Common dental problems

Some of the most common dental problems are described below.

SHARP POINTS CAUSING ULCERATION

The upper jaw of the horse is slightly wider than the lower jaw, and so the upper and lower teeth are not completely in alignment. The horse grinds the food with a mainly side-to-side motion of the jaw and over a period of time, sharp enamel points normally develop on the outer edge of the upper cheek teeth and the inner edge of the lower cheek teeth. These can be razor-sharp and cause lacerations and ulcers on the insides of the cheeks and the edge of the tongue (Figures 2.6 and 2.7). They can be a source of great discomfort. A tightly applied noseband in this situation compounds the horse's misery.

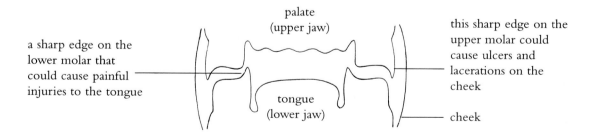

Figure 2.6 The development of sharp edges on the horse's teeth; as the top jaw is wider than the lower jaw, sharp edges may develop on the outside edge of the upper molars and the inside edge of the lower molars

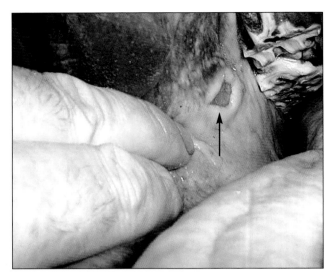

Figure 2.7 A painful ulcer on the horse's cheek

Treatment

The sharp points are removed from the teeth by a procedure known as 'rasping' or 'floating'. The vet or EDT will have a number of dental rasps (also known as floats) of various shapes and lengths so that all of the teeth can be reached and none of the sharp edges is missed. The aim of rasping is to remove sharp points and maintain the normal conformation of the teeth so that the horse can chew in comfort with a normal action. Any slightly tall teeth can be reduced in height and any developing hooks removed. Each tooth is examined again at the end of the procedure to check that nothing has been missed.

Sedation

Most horses tolerate the examination and rasping of teeth. However, fractious horses and those requiring a lot of work or procedures likely to be painful should be sedated and given routine analgesia by the vet. The safety of the horse and the people assisting must be considered when the horse is wearing a full-mouth speculum; unpredicted sudden movements by the horse can cause serious injury to the people nearby.

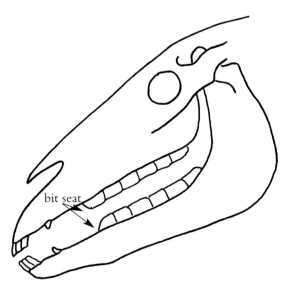

Figure 2.8 The front upper and lower premolars may be rounded off to produce a 'bit seat'

BIT SEATS

When a contact is taken up with the reins, the bit pushes the soft tissues of the mouth against the second premolar teeth. This occurs particularly with a snaffle bit. To minimize any discomfort, the upper and lower second premolars are often rounded and smoothed off. This procedure is called a 'bit seat' (Figure 2.8)

WOLF TEETH

The first premolars or wolf teeth are not present in every horse. They vary in size and position; the usual site is in the upper jaw, just in front of the second premolar teeth (Figure 2.9). However, they may develop in the interdental space, 2–3 cm ($\frac{3}{4}$–$1\frac{1}{4}$ in) in front of the second premolar. Less commonly they occur in the lower jaw. Wolf teeth erupt when the horse is between 6–18 months of age. Sometimes they do not come through the gum but can be felt as bumps underneath it. These are known as 'blind' wolf teeth.

In some cases, wolf teeth cause no problems, but they can cause bitting problems and discomfort in ridden or driven horses. They should be removed if there is any suspicion they are causing a problem. Removal is necessary if a bit seat is to be performed. The length of the roots and difficulty of extraction is variable but this is a routine procedure that can be done under sedation in the standing horse. Following extraction, the horse should not be ridden for up to two weeks (or occasionally longer) while the gum heals and any bruising subsides.

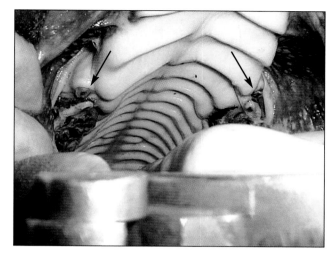

Figure 2.9 The usual site and position of wolf teeth

CANINE TEETH

Canine teeth erupt in male horses (and occasionally in mares) when they are between 4 and 6 years old.

Long, sharp canines can cause injury to the horse's tongue and to people's hands. In some cases they reduce the space available for the tongue, causing discomfort. These horses benefit from reduction in height of the canines and smoothing of the tooth surface. Tartar tends to accumulate on these teeth and should be regularly removed as it can cause gum inflammation.

TWO-YEAR-OLD 'BUMPS'

Horses between $2\frac{1}{2}$ and 4 years of age may develop non-painful bony swellings on the underside of their lower jaw. These are associated with development of the erupting permanent teeth and are considered to be normal. The swelling usually subsides over a period of time.

ABNORMALITIES OF TOOTH HEIGHT

The grinding surfaces of the teeth are known as the 'tables'. In the ideal situation, the permanent teeth will erupt normally and the tables remain at the correct heights and angles. However, problems such as retained deciduous teeth (caps) or asymmetrical loss of the deciduous teeth can alter the normal grinding action and consequent wear of the permanent teeth. Unless this is corrected, the teeth will not meet properly and the problem will become progressively worse over time. Any source of oral discomfort can alter the chewing action and lead to table height abnormalities.

Tall teeth and abnormalities of wear

When the horse chews, the upper and lower molar teeth opposite each other usually wear down evenly. However, if the tooth or part of it does not contact the opposing molar, then

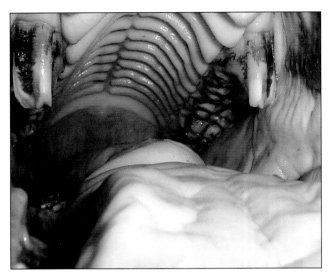

Figure 2.10 Severe overgrowth of the 2nd premolars (upper 6s) in the upper jaw

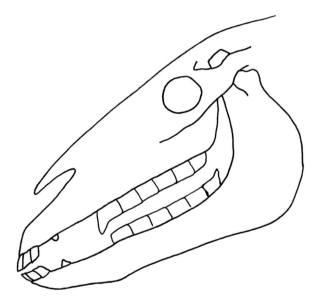

Figure 2.11 Common sites for dental overgrowths which prohibit normal movements of the jaw

all or part of the tooth will become abnormally tall (long). Common sites for these dental overgrowths (sometimes called hooks) are:

- opposite a missing tooth; the unopposed tooth will erupt into the space left by the absent tooth
- the front part of the second premolar in the upper jaw (upper 6 hook) (Figure 2.10)
- the very back of the last molar tooth in the lower jaw (lower 11 hook)

These overgrown teeth have a significant effect on performance horses. When the horse is asked to flex its neck and come onto the bit, the lower jaw glides forward in relation to the upper teeth. Hooks on the front upper cheek teeth and the back lower molars make this impossible unless the horse opens its mouth (Figure 2.11). Unfortunately some riders will then use nosebands to prevent the mouth from opening without understanding the problem. This can cause pain in the horse's TMJ, neck and back. Hooks on the second premolar can also cause pain in the soft tissues of the mouth caused by pressure from the bit.

Routine inspection and rasping will prevent these problems developing. Once the hooks are present, they can be removed with power instruments or special molar cutters, for which the horse needs to be sedated. Small hooks can often be rasped down with hand instruments. Following the procedure, it may take up to six weeks for the TMJ pain to subside and for the action of the jaw to return to normal.

It is not uncommon to see hooks that have grown so long that they have penetrated the soft tissues of the opposite jaw causing wounds to the gum. The condition is particularly common in elderly Shetland ponies who have not received routine dental care. These ponies can be presented in an emaciated state after a long period of unnoticed suffering.

Step mouth

This is the name given to an abrupt variation in height of the adjacent teeth (Figure 2.12). It arises owing to missing teeth in the opposite jaw or abnormalities of eruption. Regular and appropriate rasping can correct the problem. Where a tooth is missing, the opposite tooth must be reduced every 6–12 months.

Shear mouth

This is the name given to the condition where the grinding surfaces of the molars are abnormally slanted. The angle of the grinding surface or tables is normally 15 degrees to the horizontal. In a horse with shear mouth, the inside edge of the lower cheek teeth and the outer edge of the upper cheek teeth grow abnormally long and the grinding surfaces become steeper than normal (up to 45 degrees). This can be the consequence of any condition which causes pain and prevents normal side-to-side chewing. It also occurs in horses with abnormally narrow mandibles. The chewing action becomes more of an up-and-down movement. High concentrate diets with little forage may contribute to the development of this condition.

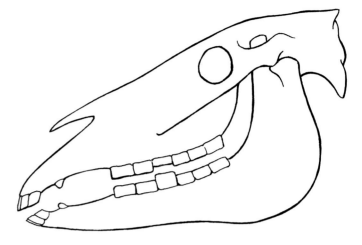

Figure 2.12 Step mouth

Wave mouth

In this condition, the surfaces of the molar teeth form an undulating 'wave' pattern (Figure 2.13) This is due to abnormal wear. Correction is easiest if identified early. The teeth that have grown too long are reduced in height and the opposite, shorter, teeth, which then have

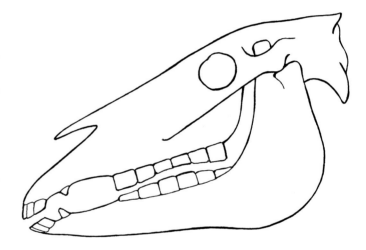

Figure 2.13 Wave mouth

nothing to grind against, will grow to meet them. This may have to be done in stages. A wave mouth should be treated conservatively in older horses as radical reduction of the taller teeth may prevent the teeth from ever meeting again as there may be insufficient tooth left to erupt from the opposite jaw and provide a grinding surface.

Exaggerated transverse ridges

The molar teeth have transverse ridges of enamel on the grinding surfaces that efficiently crush and shear roughage into small pieces. However, in some horses these ridges become overdeveloped and those of the upper and lower jaws interlock when the horse is ridden. This prevents the forward movement of the lower jaw when the horse is asked to flex during ridden exercise. Correction involves reducing the ridges sufficiently so that normal movement of the jaw is restored.

Incisor reduction

In some horses, especially those on concentrate diets or stabled for long hours, the incisor teeth are not worn down sufficiently by grazing. Over the years they become longer so that by the time the horse is 10 years or older, they are long enough to prevent the molar teeth from meeting properly. This is remedied by reducing the height of the incisors with hand or power tools. The procedure should only be done by an experienced practitioner as removal of too much tooth can create other problems. If the incisors are very long, they are lowered in two stages to allow the jaw muscles to accommodate the new range of movement.

THE GERIATRIC HORSE

If a horse lives to old age, it is likely to suffer from tooth loss and table height irregularities. The teeth get worn down to the roots and become very smooth as the roots contain no hard enamel ridges. Chewing of forage becomes more difficult and so they can be more susceptible to choke and intestinal impactions. To reduce the likelihood of this, the diet should be altered so that the nutritional needs are met by specially formulated concentrate rations which can be soaked if necessary. If the horse is managing to eat well, care should be taken not to loosen the remaining teeth by over-zealous rasping. Very loose teeth and those associated with an unpleasant smell are removed. In these situations, antibiotics are given to treat accompanying infection

MISSING TEETH

Whenever a tooth is missing for any reason, the opposite tooth or teeth will become over-long and should be regularly reduced in height. The teeth next to the space tend to move into it so that narrow gaps may develop between adjacent teeth. This can lead to pockets of food being trapped between teeth which may cause quidding, inflammation of the gums and discomfort to the horse. Sometimes this can be helped by carefully widening the gap with power tools so the food is no longer trapped. Regularly cleaning out the pockets of food is beneficial where this is possible. Rasping of the opposite teeth to prevent them growing into the space will stop food being forced into these gaps.

Equine dentistry and the law

Procedures such as the use of power tools for corrective dentistry and the extraction of wolf teeth or loose teeth should only be carried out by those with training and experience in the use of the required instrumentation. At the time of writing The Royal College of Veterinary Surgeons (RCVS) and The Department for Environment, Food and Rural Affairs (DEFRA) are amending the Veterinary Surgeons' Act 1966 so that the above procedures can legally be carried out by qualified EDTs who have passed the BEVA/BVDA dental examination. In many cases the horse will require sedation and medication and so the vet and EDT will work together as it is against the law for anyone other than a vet to administer sedatives and analgesics. More advanced dentistry must be performed by the vet.

Tetanus protection

Horses with sharp teeth and those undergoing dental procedures are likely to sustain abrasions inside their mouths. It is therefore essential that they are protected against tetanus. If the horse is not vaccinated against tetanus, then tetanus antitoxin should be administered by the vet at the same time as the dentistry is performed.

Pain relief

If the horse has had its mouth held open for a period of time by a gag or experienced any tissue trauma during the dental procedures, it may be sore for a few days afterwards. The administration of non-steroidal anti-inflammatory drugs such as phenylbutazone or flunixin can relieve the discomfort and so encourages the horse to adopt a normal chewing action. If the gag is in place for a lengthy procedure, it may be closed every twenty minutes to allow the jaw to relax.

Horses can also be sore if too much tooth is removed at one time and the pulp is exposed. Care should be taken to avoid this as it may also lead to infection within the tooth at a later date.

Dental extractions

If cheek teeth are diseased, this may present as:

- discharging sinuses from the lower jaw or side of the face
- nasal discharge
- facial swelling and pain
- difficulty eating
- performance problems
- an accompanying sinusitis in some cases.

These are investigated using imaging techniques such as radiography, nuclear scintigraphy, computed tomography (CT) and magnetic resonance imaging (MRI). The most common reasons for extraction include extensive dental disease or tooth fracture with concurrent infection. Wherever possible, extractions are performed orally in the standing horse. However, some teeth can only be removed using a surgical approach under general anaesthesia. Following cheek tooth extraction, the cavity is sealed with dental wax to prevent the hole filling up with food material. If the diseased tooth had its roots in the maxillary sinus, this is flushed regularly for a few days following surgery. Horses require regular, lifelong dental care following extraction of a permanent tooth and post-operative complications are not uncommon.

Summary

Routine maintenance is the key to your horse having a comfortable, healthy and functional mouth. Early detection of any developing problems and appropriate remedial action should improve both your horse's performance and its overall wellbeing. Horses are like humans in that routine maintenance increases the probability of long-term dental health into old age. Unlike humans though, once work has been done, change occurs rapidly and thus maintenance is essential.

WORM CONTROL

Worms can cause a variety of clinical signs from loss of condition to death of the horse. Adopting an effective worming programme is an essential part of horse care. The actual programme will vary depending on the individual horse and its environment, and so the best person to ask for specific advice is your own veterinary surgeon. There is a move now towards regular diagnostic testing and treating the individual horse only when necessary, rather than adhering to a routine worming programme. This prevents the horse from being treated unnecessarily and helps to slow down the development of resistance of the worms to the treatments we have available. The veterinary name for a worm treatment is **anthelmintic**.

Worms commonly causing problems for the horse
SMALL STRONGYLES (SMALL REDWORM)

There are many different types of small strongyle. One important group, called cyathostomes has over 50 different species.

Size and colour 0.5-2.5 cm($\frac{2}{10}$ –1 in) long; red or white in colour (Figure 2.14).

Life cycle The adult worms live in the caecum and colon of the horse where they cause ulceration and inflammation of the gut wall. They lay eggs in large numbers which are passed out in the droppings. The larvae hatch and develop in the faeces, then migrate onto the pasture. In warm, moist conditions, they can develop to the infective stage in as little as 1–3 weeks. During spring and summer, the number of larvae on the pasture increases rapidly. If ingested by a horse, the larvae burrow into the wall of the large intestine. Here they develop further and may emerge into the gut lumen to mature into egg-laying adult worms. This cycle usually takes between 6 and 12 weeks. In the autumn, however, some of the ingested larvae enter a state of arrested development and remain in the wall of the large intestine where they encyst until late winter or early spring of the following year when they emerge in large numbers. Larvae that are not ingested can survive on the pasture during mild winters in the UK.

Clinical signs In late autumn and early winter, large numbers of adult worms, together with the burrowing larvae, can cause symptoms which include weight loss, loose droppings and colic (Figure 2.15). Emergence of large numbers of encysted larvae in the late winter and early spring can cause loss of condition, severe watery diarrhoea, colic, inappetance and death. Young animals are often more severely affected than adults, as

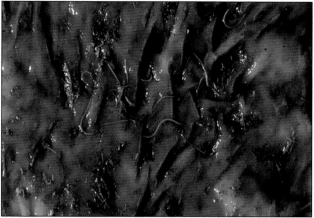

Figure 2.14 Small strongyles

Figure 2.15 Typical picture of an unthrifty pony with a high worm burden

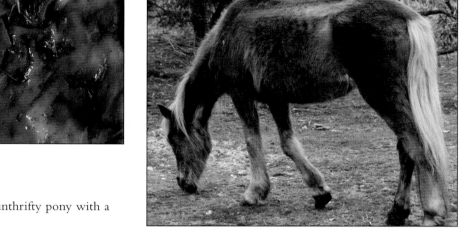

horses may develop some resistance to worms with age. The disease is known as **cyathostomosis**.

Treatment of cyathostomosis

Treatment is likely to include:

- larvicidal anthelmintics to eliminate the encysted larvae, but no drug is 100% effective at eliminating the early larval stages. Moxidectin is one of the most effective treatments; another strategy is to give a 5-day course of fenbendazole with ivermectin on the 6th day and repeating this 3 times at 10-day intervals
- fluid replacement – by mouth, stomach tube or intravenously as necessary
- codeine phosphate to control the diarrhoea
- corticosteroids to reduce the inflammation of the gut.

Treatment of young animals not showing signs but sharing the same grazing has to be done with care. Removal of adult worms from the gut lumen may stimulate large numbers of larvae to emerge from the gut wall at once and actually trigger the onset of severe and possibly fatal diarrhoea. These horses should be closely monitored after being wormed and treated at once if diarrhoea develops. Only 40% of severely affected animals recover over a 2–3 month period.

LARGE STRONGYLES (LARGE REDWORM) e.g. *Strongylus vulgaris*

Adult size and colour 1.4 – 2.5 cm ($\frac{6}{10}$ –1 in), red in colour (Figure 2.16).

Life Cycle The adult worms of *St. vulgaris* live in the large intestine, attached to the gut

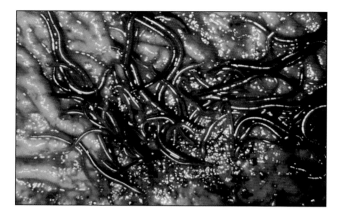

Figure 2.16 Large strongyles

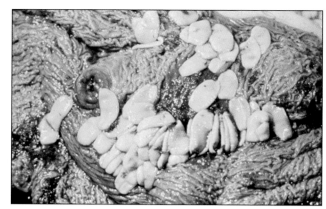

Figure 2.17 Tapeworms

wall. Here they cause damage leading to blood and protein loss. They also release chemicals which affect the normal movement of the gut. The adult worms lay eggs which pass out on to the pasture in the faeces. Infective larvae develop from the eggs and when these are ingested, they burrow through the gut wall, into the intestinal arteries. They cause inflammation within the blood vessels and the formation of blood clots which can cause loss of the normal blood supply to sections of the intestine, causing severe colic and death (see figure 17.10). Some species of large strongyle larvae migrate to the liver and the abdominal cavity where they may cause hepatitis and peritonitis. The larvae then return to the large intestine where they develop into adult worms. In warm, moist conditions, the whole life cycle can occur in six months. Infective larvae can survive on the pasture over winter.

Clinical signs Anaemia, anorexia, weight loss, reduction of growth rate, rough coat with delayed shedding in spring, pot-bellied appearance, diarrhoea, oedema, poor performance, colic and death. 1–3 year olds are particularly susceptible

Treatment and prevention Disease caused by the large strongyles can be effectively prevented and treated with the use of a suitable worming programme. In recent years, modern medications have reduced the incidence of these worms significantly. When disease does occur, supportive treatment is given as necessary. Surgery is sometimes required to remove a severely diseased section of gut that has lost its blood supply. If the damage is widespread, euthanasia may be necessary.

TAPEWORMS – *Anoplocephala perfoliata*

Adult size and colour Up to 8 cm x 1.2 cm (3 in x $\frac{1}{2}$ in), yellow/green/grey in colour (Figure 2.17)

Life Cycle The adult tapeworms live in the ileo-caecal area (where the small and large intestine join) of the intestine of the horse. Here they cause inflammation of the gut wall and are thought to release chemicals which decrease the normal movement of the gut. The mature tapeworms release segments full of eggs which are passed in the droppings onto the pasture. Here they are eaten by an intermediate host, the oribatid (forage) mite and the eggs hatch and the larvae begin to develop inside the mite. The horse will ingest these mites while grazing and the larvae develop into adults over the next 6–10 weeks. This life-cycle takes approximately 5–6 months.

Clinical signs Tapeworms may cause no symptoms at all. However, large numbers in the ileo-caecal area can lead to symptoms of ill thrift, weight loss, diarrhoea and spasmodic colic, especially in young animals. Tapeworm-infected horses are more likely to experience spasmodic colic than uninfected horses. Very heavy parasite burdens can cause impaction of the ileum, which may result in intussusception or ileal or caecal rupture.

Treatment Tapeworms are effectively controlled by dosing with a suitable anthelmintic twice a year. Where they cause intestinal obstruction, surgery or euthanasia is indicated.

ASCARID WORMS (ROUNDWORMS) – *Parascaris equorum*

Adult size and colour These large white worms can grow up to 50 cm (1 ft 8 in) in length.

Life Cycle The adult worms are commonly found in the small intestine of foals, yearlings and young horses up to 3 years of age. They produce large numbers of eggs which pass out onto the pasture. Larvae develop inside the eggs which are sticky and can stick to the udder and teats of mares. When ingested by a foal, the larvae hatch and burrow through the small intestine wall. They enter the bloodstream and are carried to the liver and then the lungs where they develop further. The larvae in the lungs are then coughed up and swallowed. On reaching the small intestine they develop into adult worms. This life cycle takes approximately 3 months. The eggs can survive on the pasture for several years.

Clinical signs Poor coat, reduced growth rate, coughing, nasal discharge, diarrhoea, colic, bowel obstruction and rupture, peritonitis.

Treatment Surgery is sometimes necessary to relieve an impaction caused by large numbers of these worms (Figure 2.18). The adult worms are readily controlled by appropriate worming treatments. The prevention of a build up of large numbers is achieved by regular dosing of foals.

THREADWORM – *Strongyloides westeri*

This is a very small worm that can cause diarrhoea in young foals aged between 2 weeks and 4 months.

Colour and size 2–9 mm ($\frac{1}{10} - \frac{4}{10}$ in), translucent, white.

Life cycle Infective larvae pass to the foal in the mare's milk. They are swallowed and on reaching the small intestine, they develop into egg-laying adults within 8–15 days. The eggs pass out in the faeces

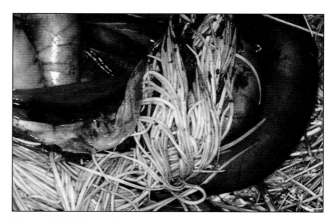

Figure 2.18 Roundworms seen at post mortem

and can develop into infective larvae within 24 hours in warm, damp conditions. The larvae are also capable of completing their life cycle in the environment, thus increasing the numbers that can infect the foal. The foal may eat the larvae or they can penetrate the skin and migrate through the liver and lungs. They are then coughed up and swallowed. Once in the small intestine, the larvae develop into adults.

In adult horses, the larvae penetrate the tissues and do not continue their development to adults. When the mare starts to produce milk after foaling, the larvae migrate to the udder and infect the foal.

Clinical signs Heavy infections result in yellowish diarrhoea which may contain blood. Severely affected foals lose weight and can become dehydrated. Large numbers of larvae migrating through the lungs occasionally cause respiratory signs.

Diagnosis This is made on the clinical signs and the presence of large numbers of eggs in the faeces.

Treatment For advice on treating such young foals, consult your vet.

Control Treating the mares with ivermectin just before they foal will reduce the numbers of larvae in the milk. This is only necessary on studs where these parasites reach high numbers and are a problem. In these situations, the foals may be routinely wormed at an early age (1–2 weeks) but the vet should be consulted as not all treatments are appropriate for young foals.

BOTS – *Gasterophilus intestinalis and Gasterophilus nasalis*

Adult size and colour The adult is an insect that looks rather like a bumble bee (Figure 2.19).

Life cycle In the summer months the adult insects hover round the horses and lay their eggs on the horse's legs, chest, shoulders, mane and under their throats. The adult flies usually live for only a few days. The cream-coloured eggs are firmly attached to the horse's coat. The

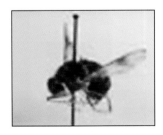

Figure 2.19 Adult bot fly

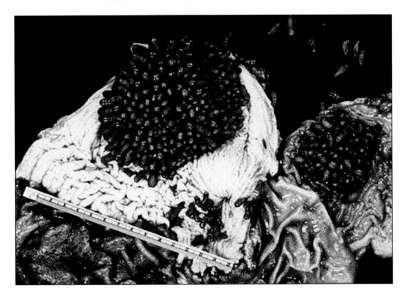

Figure 2.20 Bots in a horse's stomach

larvae begin to develop inside the egg and are ready to hatch after a few days. Some do not hatch until they are eaten or licked by the horse. The larvae then penetrate the mucosa of the tongue and mouth and migrate towards the pharynx and then to the horse's stomach. Here they attach to the stomach lining (Figure 2.20) and cause inflammation and ulceration. After approximately 9 months the large red or yellow larvae are passed in the faeces the following spring and summer. Following a period of 6 weeks pupation, the adult fly emerges.

Clinical signs Some horses are very bothered by the adult flies and will run round the field to escape them. Bots rarely cause clinical signs in the horse unless they are present in very large numbers when they occasionally cause significant gastric ulceration, perforation and death.

Control Where possible, eggs should be removed from horses on a daily basis. The horse should be treated with a suitable anthelmintic to kill the larvae present in the mouth and stomach in November.

Gasterophilus percorum has recently been found in the UK for the first time. It differs from the other bot species by laying eggs on the pasture. These are eaten by the horse, and the larvae attach to the soft palate. Symptoms include coughing and difficulty eating. It is possible that this parasite which is common in some parts of Europe may be seen more commonly in the UK in future, possibly the result of global warming.

LUNGWORM – *Dictyocaulus arnfieldi*

Adult size and colour Slender white worms up to 8 cm (3 in) long.

Life cycle The adult worms live in the bronchi of infected donkeys. They lay eggs which are coughed up and swallowed, then pass out of the donkey in the droppings. The larvae hatch and if swallowed by a horse or donkey will migrate from the intestine to the lungs via the bloodstream or lymphatic vessels. Here they mature into adults in the bronchi. In a donkey, the adults will lay eggs, but in many horses the cycle is not completed and no eggs are laid by the adults.

Clinical signs The donkey is able to tolerate the parasite without any symptoms in most cases. Occasionally, there may be an increased respiratory rate. Horses with lungworm usually cough, especially during exercise and may have an increased respiratory rate and a nasal discharge. Worms may be visible in the bronchi on endoscopy.

Treatment and control This is achieved by regular dosing of donkeys and horses grazed together with a suitable anthelmintic.

Diagnosis of worm infestation

Diagnosis is usually made on the clinical signs, the grazing and worming history and the following laboratory tests.

FAECAL EGG COUNT

A fresh sample of the horse's droppings is mixed with saline and examined under the

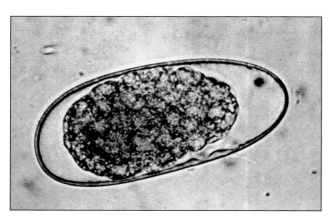

Figure 2.21 Strongyle egg as seen under the microscope

microscope for worm eggs. The eggs from different species of worm have a different appearance and can be identified and counted. The result is given as the number of eggs per gram (EPG) of faeces. It is used for strongyles and ascarids. (Figure 2.21.)

Dung samples can also be examined for tapeworm eggs using a different method.

A negative worm egg count does not exclude the presence of worms. For example, if the horse has just been treated with an anthelmintic, there may be very few adults left to produce eggs. However, the horse may still be infected with large numbers of larvae unless a larvicidal drug was used. A low positive worm egg count (less than 200 epg) is thought to be acceptable and does not justify treatment, since a few worms will help to boost the horse's immunity to infection.

BLOOD TESTS

When large numbers of worms or larvae are present, the following results may be seen on blood tests:

- anaemia due to blood loss
- raised neutrophils and eosinophils as a response to the parasites
- elevated levels of $\beta1$ globulin where strongyle larvae are present
- low plasma albumin
- raised plasma fibrinogen as a response to the inflammation and tissue damage
- a blood test which detects antibodies to the tapeworm and gives information about the level of tapeworm infection is now available.

TRACHEAL WASH

When a horse has lungworm, adult worms, larvae or eggs may be recovered from a tracheal wash sample.

IDENTIFICATION OF WORMS IN THE GUT AT SURGERY OR POST MORTEM EXAMINATION

This can be the unfortunate result of worms being allowed to develop and multiply unchecked.

Treatment and prevention

There are many considerations that affect one's choice of worming programme. The decision will be influenced by factors which include the following.

- The grazing history of the pasture. Those that are heavily grazed by a number of horses and never have the droppings removed are likely to harbour a high parasite burden.

- Stocking density – the ideal is 1–2 horses per acre.
- Age range of the horses grazing together – young or very old horses are more likely to have high worm burdens and be a source of pasture contamination.
- Worming history of all the horses.
- Level of co-operation between individual owners with shared grazing. For an effective worm control programme, all the horses that graze together should be treated with the same preparation at the same time or tested together and treated individually as appropriate.
- Veterinary advice received after consideration of the above.

For example, the programme for horses in a livery yard without a strict worm-control policy where there is limited grazing and regular introduction of new horses is likely to be very different from one designed for a couple of privately owned horses living on a farm with plenty of fields available.

Worms can be controlled by a combination of:
- good pasture management
- regular testing of the droppings for eggs and larvae
- blood testing to detect tapeworms
- strategic use of wormers appropriate for the situation.

PASTURE MANAGEMENT
Removal of droppings
Regular removal of droppings is very effective at reducing the number of eggs and infective larvae on the pasture. Daily removal is the best policy, but once or twice weekly is still effective. Manual removal is time-consuming but the usual method for small establishments. There is now a range of machinery available to pick up the droppings from larger areas.

Dropping removal has the added benefit of increasing the grazing area. Untended horse paddocks have rough areas of long, sour grass where the horses pass their droppings. The larval contamination of the rough areas is much higher than that of the rest of the field and fortunately the horses avoid eating the sour grass. They prefer to graze the rest of the field which will be much closer cropped. Removal of the droppings can reduce the size of the rough areas.

If good pasture hygiene is combined with regular monitoring of worm egg counts, it is often possible to reduce the number of worming treatments given in a year.

Harrowing
Harrowing the pasture in warm dry periods of weather scatters the droppings so the larvae dry out and die quickly. If harrowing is done in warm damp conditions, it simply spreads the infective larvae into the grazing area.

Stocking density and mixed grazing

The fields should not be overgrazed because the horses are then more likely to eat contaminated grass from the rough areas. Where horses are grazed with sheep or cattle, the ruminants eat the rough areas and clear the eggs and larvae without becoming infected.

Pasture rotation

Resting pastures is effective at reducing contamination, but strongyle larvae can survive over winter and ascarid eggs can remain viable for years. If clean pasture becomes available, it is very important to dose every animal effectively before allowing them onto the grass. They should be stabled for 2–3 days to allow any eggs already present in their intestines to be passed in the droppings rather than contaminating the new pasture.

Introducing a new horse

It is a good idea to have a worm egg count and a blood test for tapeworms done for each new horse as it arrives. If your vet recommends treatment, these horses should be wormed with a larvicidal preparation or tapeworm treatment as appropriate and kept off the pasture for 3 days to prevent eggs already laid and still present in the horse's gut from contaminating the pasture.

WHICH WORMER SHOULD I USE AND WHEN SHOULD I USE IT?

There is a wide choice of worming preparations or anthelmintics on the market. No treatment kills every type of worm. The choice depends on whether it is being used to treat a specific problem or as part of a routine control programme.

There is no single anthelmintic strategy that can be recommended for every situation. In order to choose the most suitable combination of worming products and time of administration, one needs to know the level of risk to your horse from the different types of worm. **Your vet is the best person to ask for advice as he/she will be familiar with your situation and also be aware of any local problems of resistance to a particular medication.**

The wormers currently available and their efficacy against the most harmful types of worm are listed in Table 1. Each type also has a different time interval that is recommended between treatments. This is generally based upon the time that elapses before the worm egg output begins to rise again. The dosing intervals for the main classes of anthelmintic are given in Table 2.

ANTHELMINTIC RESISTANCE

In the UK, there is widely recognized resistance of small strongyles to the class of wormers called benzimidazoles. The more frequently the various wormers are used, the greater the

Table 1 Table showing the efficacy of available drugs against various parasites

Drug	Trade name	Paste or Granules	Large redworm A L	Small redworm A L	Ascarids	Tapeworm	Bots	Lungworm	Worming Interval	Foal age at first worming
Moxidectin	Equest	P	+ +	+ +	+	-	+	+	13 weeks (1)	4 months
Ivermectin	Eqvalan Panomec Vectin Eraquell Noromectin Furexel	P P P P P P	+ + + + + + + + + + + +	+ (+) + (+) + (+) + (+) + (+) + (+) (2)	+ + + + + +	- - - - - -	+ + + + + +	+ + + + + +	8–10 weeks	6–8 weeks
Pyrantel embonate	Strongid-P Strongid Caramel Pyratape-P Embotape	P and G P P P	+ - + - + - + -	+ - + - + - + -	+ + + +	effective with double dose	- - - -	- - - -	4–6 weeks	4 weeks
Praziquantal	Equitape	P	- -	- -	-	+	-	-	6 months	8 weeks (3)
Ivermectin + Praziquantal	Equimax Eqvalan Duo Furexel Combi	P P P	+ + + + + +	+ (+) + (+) + (+)	+ + +	+ + +	+ + +	+ + +	6 months 6 months 6 months	2 weeks 5 months 5 months
Mebendazole	Telmin	P and G	+ -	+ -	+	-	-	increased dose for 5 days (4)	6 weeks	No restriction (5)
Fenbendazole (benzimidazole) (R) (6)	Panacur Panacur Equine Guard Zerofen	P and G Suspension G	+ +★ + + +★	+ +★ ★ 8 x dose or 1 dose for 5 days for larvae 5 day course + +★	+ + +	- -	- - -	+ (8)	6 weeks (7) 6–12 months 6 weeks	4 weeks 4 weeks 4 weeks

A: adult worms; L: larvae P: paste; G: granules
+ effective   (+) limited effect   – no effect   +★ effective against migrating and encysted larvae at 8x standard dose or standard dose daily for 5 days
(R) Some small redworms are resistant to this drug

1   Moxidectin has a persistent effect and prevents re-infection by small strongyles for 2 weeks after dosing.
2   Ivermectin does not eliminate 3rd stage inhibited larvae in the gut wall.
3   Praziquantal is not licensed for use in mares during pregnancy and lactation. Note: as the tapeworm life cycle takes 5–6 months, foals are unlikely to need treatment for tapeworm before this age.
4   The higher dose rate to treat lungworm should not be used for the first 4 months after service in brood mares.
5   No age restriction but foals are unlikely to need worming before 2 weeks of age.
6   Also some effect on killing the eggs.
7   The worming interval is 6 weeks for a single dose. The 5-day course or 8x standard dose may be given once or twice a year as necessary.
8   Fenbendazole not licensed for lungworm but effective at increased dose.

likelihood of the worms becoming resistant to them. It is therefore important to use the drugs as sparingly as possible.

WORMING INTERVAL

There are three ways of using worming preparations:

1   interval dosing
2   strategic (seasonal) dosing
3   targeted strategic dosing.

Interval dosing

This is when worming treatments are used at the regular intervals recommended by the manufacturers throughout the spring and summer grazing season or throughout the year.

Table 2 Summary of the dosing intervals for equine anthelmintics

Benzimidazoles	6 weeks
Pyrantel embonate	4–6 weeks
Ivermectin	8–10 weeks
Moxidectin	13 weeks
Praziquantal	6 months

While this protects the individual horse, it may result in unnecessary treatments being given. This is not only expensive, but it can speed up the development of parasite resistance.

Strategic seasonal dosing

Horses are routinely dosed in the spring, in the middle of the grazing season, and again in the autumn in order to prevent the build up of large numbers of larvae on the pasture. It is a rather hit-and-miss method, especially when the horses are of mixed ages and new horses are regularly introduced. Also, unusually warm weather in the early spring or autumn can lead to early or late peaks in the pasture larval burden.

Targeted strategic dosing

The horses are dosed at specific times of the year to minimize pasture contamination with larvae, but this is combined with regular worm egg counts. Only those horses with egg counts of more than 200 eggs per gram are treated. This programme must include larvicidal treatments as the build-up of larvae in a state of arrested development in the large intestine will not be detected and should be prevented. This is usually given in November and in high risk situations may be repeated in February. The need for tapeworm treatment can be identified with a blood test. The advantages of this method are:

- susceptible horses are identified
- unnecessary treatments are avoided
- there is less contamination of the environment from drug residues in the droppings
- it reduces the risk of worm resistance to the drugs.

FREQUENCY OF WORM EGG COUNTS

By using the wormers only when needed, the development of resistance to them will be delayed. Worm egg counts are recommended at regular intervals throughout the grazing season in the first year of instituting a strategic dosing policy. It would be sensible to test the droppings before the programme is started and then again following the first worming treatment at the time the manufacturer of the drug selected recommends repeat treatment. If the egg count is low or negative, discuss when to test again with your vet. This will depend on the factors such as the age of the horses, the time of year and the pasture management. Once your level of risk has been assessed and the egg count monitored, routine testing can be done 2–4 times a year. If benzimidazole wormers are used, a faecal egg count reduction test should be done to check for worm resistance. This is done by testing dung samples before dosing and again 10–14 days later. If significant numbers of eggs are still present, then your vet should be consulted and a different treatment will be recommended. A reduction of 85% or above is considered acceptable. Blood samples to test for the presence of tapeworm should be done annually.

WHICH ANTHELMINTIC?

The choice of anthelmintic depends on which parasites your horse is exposed to. This can be established by regular diagnostic testing and discussions with your vet.

Should I use one wormer continuously or change it regularly?

In the past, the following strategies have been used:

a   using one wormer continuously

b   using one class of wormer for one year and a different one the following year

c   using different classes of wormer within one year.

Each method has its advantages and disadvantages and yet again no policy will suit every situation. As no wormer is effective against all worms, a combination of treatments based on the test results is the most usual.

General rules for worming horses

- Every horse in the field should be wormed with the same product at the same time unless worm egg counts/tapeworm blood tests show that individuals do not require treatment.
- It is essential that each horse receives the correct dose based on bodyweight.
- A record should be kept of the product used and the date given.
- The efficacy of the programme should be monitored by regular diagnostic testing.

- New horses should be tested and then given a larvicidal drug and kept in for 3 days before being allowed onto the pasture.
- Foals can be wormed with some preparations from 2 weeks of age but this should only be done on veterinary advice.
- Mares should be wormed when they return from stud and one month before foaling as part of their treatment programme.

COMMON REASONS FOR FAILURE OF ANTHELMINTIC PROGRAMMES

1   The dosing interval is too long. It is important to remember that different classes of anthelmintic suppress the output of worm eggs for different lengths of time.
2   Failure to treat or check all animals at the same time. A single horse that misses a treatment can release millions of eggs onto the pasture each day and put all the others at risk.
3   A horse has not received an adequate dose. This may be because the body-weight was underestimated or the horse rejected the feed or spat out the paste unnoticed. Under dosing does not kill the worms and it may encourage the development of resistance. Special weigh tapes are available to help you estimate your horse's weight, or ask your vet for advice.
4   Anthelmintic resistance – this can be checked for by measuring egg output on the day of dosing and 10–14 days later.
5   Horses may have been purchased with arrested larvae in their gut lining. The use of a larvicidal drug does not guarantee that all of these will be removed.

REMEMBER, THE FIRST RULE IS TO ASSESS THE RISK

Consider:
- your grazing situation
- the age of the horses
- use diagnostic tests
- talk to your vet.

PRACTICAL CONSIDERATIONS

Paste or granules?

Both treatments are equally effective. Paste is usually administered directly into the mouth by syringe and the granules are mixed in with the feed.

To administer a **paste**:
1   adjust the syringe to give the required dose for the horse's weight
2   put a headcollar on the horse and make sure there is no food in its mouth
3   remove the cap and push the nozzle gently into the side of the horse's mouth at the corner of the lips (Figure 2.22)

4 direct the syringe backwards and push the plunger to deposit the paste onto the tongue

5 hold the horse's head up for a few seconds to prevent it spitting out the dose

6 check that none of the dose has been wasted.

Advantages Paste is usually quick and easy to administer.

Disadvantages Some horses object to the treatment and the whole procedure becomes a struggle. If any of the dose is wasted, the amount must be estimated and a replacement amount given. This situation may be avoided by mixing the paste in the feed.

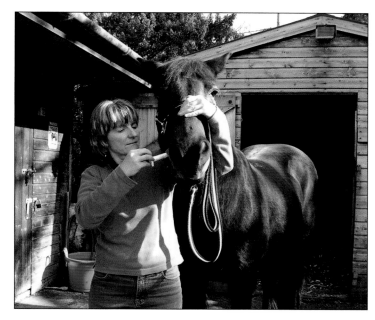

Figure 2.22 Administering an oral paste

To administer **granules**, mix them into the feed. Molasses or carrots may be added to increase palatability.

Advantages Granules are often slightly cheaper than paste.

Disadvantages Feeding must be supervised to ensure the whole dose is consumed. If the horse rejects the feed, the treatment is wasted.

Tip If you know the horse is a fussy feeder, try mixing the wormer with a small amount of a palatable mix and feed it first when the horse is hungry. Once it has been eaten, the horse can then be given the rest of his feed to enjoy.

> **Warning**
> Moxidectin and ivermectin can have severe adverse effects on dogs and cats. Keep syringes safely and make sure these animals have no access to feeds containing the paste or the droppings of the horse for 3 days after worming. Wherever possible, administer the paste directly into the horse's mouth.

CARE OF THE HORSE'S FEET

Looking after your horse's feet is a very important part of the animal's routine care and management programme. This subject is discussed in detail in Chapter 6.

3

THE ILL OR INJURED HORSE

SIGNS OF ILL HEALTH

Sometimes the signs of ill health or injury are very obvious. On other occasions, the symptoms can be subtle. Early recognition of a problem and prompt attention can make a big difference to the eventual outcome. Some of the 'warning signs' that something is wrong are discussed below.

Depression and withdrawal
When a horse is not feeling well, the first outward sign is often a change of demeanour. It may be just a little quieter and less responsive than usual or very obviously depressed. These horses will often stand on their own in the field, away from the other horses.

Change of breathing rate and pattern
The respiratory rate will increase with exercise, excitement, pain, a high temperature and with respiratory disease. Depending on the nature of the disease, breathing may become fast and shallow or there may be a double expiratory effort.

Temperature
The horse's temperature will increase slightly after it has worked hard or in hot weather. A significant rise in temperature, i.e. above 39 °C or 102 °F, is usually due to viral or bacterial infection. A very low temperature may indicate a state of shock.

Increased pulse rate
A raised pulse rate can be due to anxiety, fear, excitement, exercise, a high temperature or pain.

Nasal discharge
A small trickle of watery nasal discharge is normal. If it is profuse, thick or coloured, the horse may be suffering from an allergy or infection.

Loss of appetite

Some horses seem to eat anything whilst others are very fussy. If a normally greedy horse refuses to eat, it is a sure sign that there is something wrong.

Reduced number of droppings, constipation and diarrhoea

With horses that are stabled overnight, you should be familiar with the usual number and consistency of droppings passed. Many horses and ponies will have loose droppings if they are anxious, excited or have just been moved onto lush, new pasture. If a stabled horse passes fewer droppings overnight that are firmer than normal, the animal should be observed carefully as it might be developing an impaction or obstruction.

Urine

The colour of a horse's urine varies from yellow to a light brown. It is normal for it to be cloudy, especially at the end of urination. Very dark reddish brown urine is abnormal and the cause should be investigated. Horses often urinate if put into a box with fresh straw. This is the best time to collect a sample and observe if there is any abnormality.

Dehydration

If you gently pinch together a fold of the horse's skin, it should go back to its normal position almost immediately. If there is a delay of a few seconds, the horse is likely to be dehydrated. This may occur if the horse is not drinking enough or has lost an abnormal amount of fluid, e.g. through severe exertion and sweating or diarrhoea.

Sweating

Horses sweat if they are worked and also if they are excited or nervous. Sweating at rest can be a sign of pain or disease.

Mucous membranes

The mucous membranes of the horse should be salmon pink in colour. These can be examined on the gums and around the eye. If they are very pale, or have a yellow or purple/blue tinge, the horse has a serious problem. Some horses have black pigment on their gums; this is nothing to worry about.

Unusual stance

It is often possible to see at a glance that something is wrong with a horse from their stance. For example, horses with severe foot pain will often point the foot or intermittently lift it off the ground.

Lying down more than usual

Horses and ponies may lie down more than normal if they are feeling unwell or experiencing pain. Examples include the pony suffering from laminitis or the horse with abdominal pain.

Lameness

Lameness is a sign of pain and should never be ignored. It is important to check the horse over thoroughly to try to find the cause. A tiny puncture that penetrates a joint or tendon sheath, for example, may look insignificant but could have serious consequences if left untreated for any length of time.

Heat

Heat in a limb or any part of the horse's body is a sign of inflammation. Heat may be the first sign of a problem developing in a horse's leg and should be treated as significant.

Swelling

Swelling is a warning sign that all is not well. It may occur as a result of an injury, fly bites, an abscess developing or systemic disease.

Trauma

Any cut or other injury is likely to heal best if given prompt attention. Vets are sometimes asked to treat wounds that have gone unnoticed for days because the horse has only been observed from a distance.

Change of temperament

Many horses experience chronic pain that goes unrecognized because it does not make them obviously lame. Examples include back pain or bilateral forelimb or hind limb pain. This will affect their willingness and ability to work. They may become withdrawn and grumpy. Some start to resent grooming and are less cooperative than usual for the farrier.

If your horse or pony appears to be off colour, it is a good idea to check its temperature and pulse rate. It is helpful if you know what is normal for your animal.

BASIC HEALTH CHECKS FOR YOUR HORSE

How to take a horse's temperature

- Unless the horse or pony is familiar with the procedure, it should be held by an assistant.
- If using a digital thermometer, switch it on. If you have a mercury thermometer, shake it vigorously until the mercury is below the start of the temperature scale.

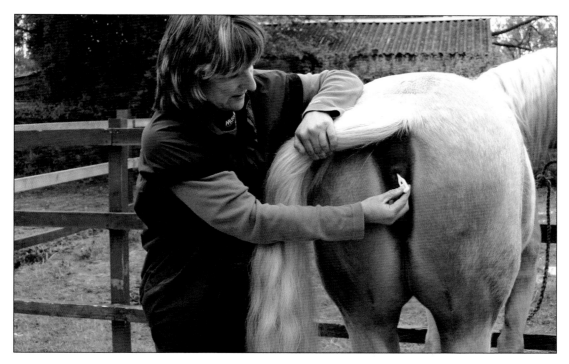

Figure 3.1 Taking a horse's temperature

- Lubricate the bulb with petroleum jelly, e.g. Vaseline, or saliva.
- Run your hand over the horse's quarters and lift the tail.
- Stand close to the horse and to one side to avoid being kicked (Figure 3.1). Gently slide the thermometer into the anus until about two thirds of it is inside the rectum.
- Tilt the thermometer so the end of it lies against the rectal wall. This ensures it is measuring the horse's temperature and not that of the droppings.
- Wait a full minute or until the digital thermometer beeps.
- Withdraw the thermometer and wipe it clean.
- Read the temperature.
- Switch a digital thermometer off or shake down the mercury of a glass thermometer.
- Clean the thermometer with cold water and disinfectant before returning it to its case.
- Store the thermometer in a cool place.

Remember The normal temperature of a horse is 38 °C (100.5 °F). However, many healthy horses have a temperature as low as 37 °C (98.5 °F). Temperatures up to 38.5 °C (101.5 °F) are acceptable on hot days or after exercise.

How to take a horse's pulse

The easiest place to take a pulse is where the facial artery passes under the lower jaw (Figures 3.2 and 3.3). The horse must be standing still and not eating or the pulse will be difficult to find.

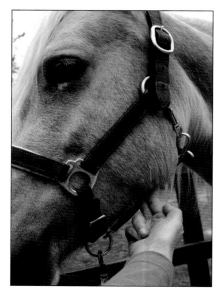

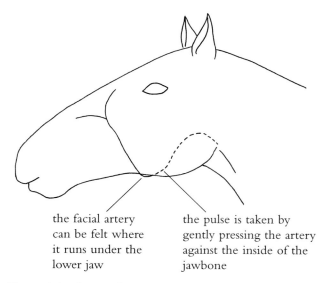

the facial artery can be felt where it runs under the lower jaw

the pulse is taken by gently pressing the artery against the inside of the jawbone

Figure 3.2 Taking a horse's pulse

Figure 3.3 The site for taking a horse's pulse

- Run your fingers along the lower border of the mandible. The artery can be felt as a tubular structure.
- Apply *light* pressure with the flat of your first three fingers.
- Feel the pulse under your fingers.
- Count the number of beats in a 15-second period.
- Multiply this by 4 to obtain the horse's pulse rate.

Tip Practise this immediately after exercise when the pulse is faster and more easily felt.

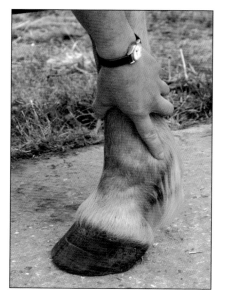

Figure 3.4 Taking the digital pulse

TAKING THE DIGITAL PULSE

If the horse is standing quietly, another place to take the pulse is where the digital artery runs over the sesamoid bones, just above the fetlock joint (Figure 3.4). This can be more difficult to locate unless the horse has a foot problem such as an abscess or laminitis. A strong or 'bounding' digital pulse in both front feet is common in horses and ponies with laminitis.

FEELING THE PULSE ON THE CHEST WALL OVER THE HEART

In thin or fit, fine-skinned animals it is often possible to take the pulse by feeling the heart beat through the chest wall. Place your hand on the chest wall, just behind the elbow.

Remember The resting pulse should be between 28 and 42 beats per minute.

How to measure your horse's respiratory rate

This should be done when the horse is resting and relaxed. Stand quietly and watch the movement of the flanks for one minute. The flanks and chest wall move up and outwards as the horse breathes in. They will move down and in as the horse exhales. If the horse has allergic respiratory disease, breathing out may occur in two stages as the abdominal wall is used to squeeze air from the lungs. Each time the horse breathes in and out is counted as one respiratory cycle.

Tip In cold weather you can see their breath as they breathe out.

Remember The resting respiratory rate of a normal horse is between 8 and 16 breaths per minute.

How to take a urine sample

Most horses will urinate if put into a stable with a fresh straw bed. If a urine sample is required, your vet may provide you with a sterile pot. Otherwise, you can collect it into a clean container that has been thoroughly washed and dried. Take special care to ensure there are no traces of any sugary substance. Stand quietly in the stable and as the horse starts to pass urine, move slowly and quietly so you can collect a sample at arm's length. It is a good idea to wear disposable gloves to protect your hands.

FIRST AID

The management of the injured horse can be divided into two key areas:
- immediate first aid
- ongoing treatment of the injuries.

The first-aid kit

Every horse owner or yard should have a first-aid kit which contains the materials most likely to be needed to treat an injury. It should be kept in a clean tin or plastic box with a secure lid, preferably in a relatively dust-free area such as a cupboard. Items must be replaced as they are used and so it is helpful to keep a list of contents attached to the inside of the lid. It is also a good idea to have a list of useful telephone numbers, e.g. vet, horse transporters etc., and to take the first-aid kit with you when you and your horses are travelling anywhere.

CONTENTS OF THE FIRST-AID KIT
- Clean bowl or bucket.

- Clean towel.
- Large roll of cotton wool.
- Round-ended curved scissors for trimming hair from wound edges.
- Anti-bacterial scrub, e.g. Hibiscrub® or Pevidine®.
- Pack of sterile saline.
- Ready-to-use poultice, e.g. Animalintex®, Poultex®.
- Wound gel, e.g. Derma Gel® or Intrasite Gel®.
- Non-stick dressings, e.g. Melolin®, Rondopad®.
- Gamgee® and large scissors for cutting it to size.
- A selection of bandages including:
    - stretch cotton bandages, e.g. Knit-firm®, K-band® and crepe bandages, which should mould to the shape of the limb and are useful for holding dressings in place and providing light support
    - adhesive bandages, e.g. Elastoplast®
    - elastic conforming self-adhesive bandages, e.g. Vetrap®, Co-plus®
    - tubular bandages, e.g. Tubigrip®
    - synthetic orthopaedic bandage, e.g. Soffban®
    - a set of stable bandages.
- A roll of electrical insulating tape 2 cm ($\frac{3}{4}$, in) wide.
- A roll of black PVC tape or silver carpet tape 7.5 or 10 cm (3 or 4 in) wide.
- A gentian violet or antibiotic spray.
- Petroleum jelly, e.g. Vaseline®.
- Wound gel, cream or ointment, e.g. aloe vera-containing preparations.
- Small pair of tweezers.
- Thermometer.
- Paper and pen or pencil.
- A bright torch for inspecting wounds in poor light (and spare batteries).

ADDITIONAL USEFUL ITEMS

- A length of baler twine.
- Rope halter.
- Hoof pick.
- Shoe removal kit, i.e. buffer, hammer, pincers, pliers.
- Wire cutters.
- Pen knife.

Prescribed medicines

In certain circumstances, your vet may prescribe particular medicines that cannot be obtained over the counter for your first-aid kit. This may happen, for example, if your horse has a recurrent problem. If the vet feels confident in your ability to detect the early signs and that immediate treatment is beneficial, sufficient medication may be left with you so that treatment can begin while a visit is being arranged.

Never be tempted to use prescribed medicines on another horse without speaking to your vet first.

WOUND MANAGEMENT

The healing of a wound is influenced by the way it is managed *immediately* after an accident occurs. Whether you decide to call the vet straight away or to treat the injury yourself, a systematic approach should be adopted.

Immediate action

- If possible, move the horse to a safe place so that it is not likely to injure itself further or cause injury to others.
- Control any bleeding.
- Assess the injury and call the vet if necessary.
- Protect the wound from contamination and further injury.
- Assess whether the horse is shocked.
- Clean the wound.
- Prevent or control infection.
- Prevent or reduce swelling.

The above procedures are very important and are worth considering in more detail.

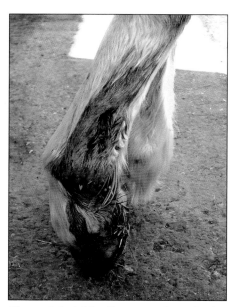

MOVING THE HORSE
If the horse can be moved safely, it should be taken away from ditches, water, wire, fences and traffic. If the horse cannot be moved, then drivers, pedestrians and other riders should be warned that there is an accident ahead. When a traffic accident occurs, the police should be notified.

THE CONTROL OF BLEEDING
Any wound which is bleeding profusely looks very alarming (Figure 3.5), but **do not panic**. First, assess the flow of blood. A cut vein results in a constant, steady flow of blood. A cut artery emits a pulsed jet of blood in time with the heartbeat. Significant blood loss is only likely to occur if haemorrhage from a large vein

Figure 3.5 A bleeding wound can look very alarming

or artery is left uncontrolled. The average Thoroughbred horse has more than 50 litres (88 pt) of blood, so a relatively large volume has to be lost for it to be critical.

The methods used to control bleeding all rely on applying pressure at the site of the injury (a tourniquet is not generally recommended). Although stopping the bleeding is your first priority, **try not to contaminate the wound further.** Wherever possible, wash your hands and use clean materials.

- Ideally a sterile, non-stick dressing pad should be placed on top of the wound and covered with a layer of Gamgee®. If you are out on a ride and these are not to hand, a clean T-shirt or vest can be used in an emergency. Apply pressure with your thumb or hand, depending on the size of the wound.
- If the wound is on a limb and the bleeding does not stop within a few minutes or the horse is agitated, these dressings can be bandaged firmly in place with self-adhesive conforming bandages. The amount of pressure required depends on the severity of the injury and which blood vessels are damaged.
- If the blood soaks through the dressings, use more padding and increase the pressure. Pressure bandages should not be left on for more than a couple of hours. If the wound is still bleeding, call your vet.
- Where the wound is on a site that cannot easily be bandaged, place a non-stick dressing onto the wound with a pad of cotton wool or Gamgee® on top and hold it firmly in place. The bleeding usually stops after a few minutes. If not, re-apply the pressure.
- If there is an obvious foreign body in the wound, pressure may be applied around it but not directly onto it.

If the bleeding continues, the vet will clamp the bleeding vessels with artery forceps wherever possible.

ASSESSING THE INJURY

Many small cuts and grazes can be cleaned and treated without calling the vet.

When to call the vet

Always call the vet if:

- the wound is large or deep.
- the wound is more than 2.5 cm (1 in) long and goes through the whole skin thickness (Figure 3.6)
- the bleeding cannot be controlled
- the horse is in a lot of pain

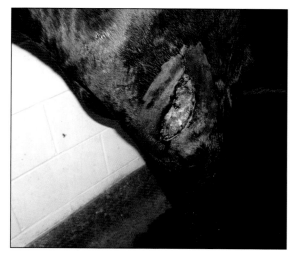

Figure 3.6 A wound requiring veterinary attention

- the lameness is more severe than you would expect from the appearance of the wound
- you suspect a foreign body is present
- you think a vital structure such as a joint or tendon sheath has been penetrated
- the horse shows signs of shock
- tetanus injections are not up-to-date
- you are uncertain how to proceed.

When you telephone your vet, try to give accurate directions and also a contact telephone number. Listen carefully to any instructions given over the phone.

Eight things to do while waiting for the vet

1   Keep the horse warm.
2   Apply essential first aid.
3   Clean the wound if it is dirty. Apply a moist hydrogel product and cover lower limb wounds with a dressing.
4   If applicable, arrange transport for the horse.
5   Boil water and leave it to cool in a clean container.
6   Have a bridle or headcollar ready.
7   Carry out any instructions given by the vet.
8   Check the vaccination and insurance status of the patient.

Protecting the wound

Once bleeding is under control, take steps to minimize further contamination or damage. Straw, wood shavings, dust, mud and flies all introduce **infection**, which delays healing.

- If the horse has to be walked through a muddy gateway or transported in a vehicle, bandage a non-stick dressing and a pad of Gamgee® over wounds below the knee or hock first.
- Stand the horse on a clean, hard surface while preparing to treat the wound.
- **Do not apply any topical medication, e.g. wound powder, spray or ointment** at this stage, especially if the wound is likely to be sutured (stitched). The one exception is a clear hydrogel preparation, e.g. Derma Gel® or Intrasite® which helps to rehydrate devitalized tissue and to assist healing. Other preparations will interfere with the vet's inspection of the wound and can actually delay healing.

Managing a shocked horse

Following an accident, a horse may show signs of shock. These include:

- trembling
- fast, shallow breathing
- rapid and/or weak pulse

- pale mucous membranes
- a low body temperature
- anxiety or depression.

Consult your vet immediately. Shock usually indicates a serious injury or severe pain. While waiting for the vet to arrive, move the horse to a warm stable with a deep, dry bed. Put on a warm rug if the horse is cold.

Cleaning the wound
STEP 1

Thorough cleaning of any wound is essential. It should be done in an area of good light with a clean floor so wood shavings, straw or mud do not enter the wound. If the bleeding is under control, gently hose off any dirt before the vet arrives. If the injury is on a limb, begin hosing below the wound. Gradually work upwards while quietly reassuring the horse. Try to ensure that dirty water from around the wound does not run onto the damaged tissue. Continue hosing until the wound is clean and protect it with a non-stick dressing, Gamgee® pad and a firm support bandage until the vet arrives. This will minimize any swelling.

Not every horse will tolerate hosing or even gentle cleaning if it is anxious or in a lot of pain. In this case, do what you can to protect the wound from contamination while waiting for the vet. Do not risk being injured yourself while attempting to help the horse. In these cases, the vet is likely to administer a sedative so the horse can be treated efficiently and safely.

STEP 2

The following points should be followed if you decide at this stage to treat the wound yourself.

- Wash your hands.
- Use curved round-ended scissors to trim away any hair overhanging the wound edges, taking care not to let it fall into the wound. The wound can be covered with a wound gel, e.g. Intrasite® or K–Y Jelly® while this is being done. This prevents tiny pieces of hair adhering to the injured tissue.
- Now clean the skin around the wound with warm water and a diluted antiseptic scrub, e.g. Hibiscrub®. If this is not available, a saline solution made from 500 ml (just under a pint) of cooled boiled water with a level teaspoonful of salt dissolved in it can be used. Use moistened cotton wool or gauze swabs. Alternatively, antiseptic-impregnated moist wipes are useful for this. Try to avoid dirty water running onto the injured tissue.
- Clean the wound with cooled boiled water and diluted Hibiscrub® or sterile saline. If the wound is large and very dirty, begin at the centre of the wound and work

outwards. Discard each swab or wipe as soon as it has been used – *never* put it back into the bowl of washing solution. Do not use strong, undiluted antiseptics on the wound as they can cause further damage to the exposed tissues.

- Forceps or tweezers can be used to remove any foreign material.
- Little pieces of dirt can be flushed from wounds using a 35 ml syringe containing sterile saline or diluted Hibiscrub® with a 19 gauge needle attached. This also helps to remove bacteria attached to the wound surface. If the wound is relatively clean, this is the best method of cleaning as swabbing can sometimes cause further trauma to the tissues and also spread bacteria.

If the wound is contaminated with mud that cannot be removed by washing, the cleaning procedure can be continued by:

- using a cleansing wound gel, e.g. Derma Gel® or Intrasite®
- application of a ready-to-use poultice, e.g. Animalintex®.

You may decide to call the vet at this stage if the wound is still very dirty or it is more extensive than originally thought. The vet will trim away any dead or badly damaged tissue and give the wound a thorough clean. This is known as 'debriding' the wound.

Has a joint or tendon sheath been penetrated?

If there is a puncture wound near a joint or tendon sheath, it is best to call the vet immediately. Sometimes, clear, straw-coloured synovial fluid can be seen escaping from the wound. However, it is not always easy to decide whether these structures have been penetrated and special diagnostic techniques may be required.

In some cases the horse will be lamer than expected for a small wound. Again, immediate veterinary attention is essential. If these injuries are not dealt with at once, the horse can remain permanently lame and may have to be destroyed.

The control of infection

The risk of infection is reduced by:

- immediate treatment
- thorough cleaning
- maintaining cleanliness with appropriate dressings
- the use of antibiotics either topically (applied directly onto the wound) or systemically (a course is given by injection or by mouth) which must be prescribed by your vet
- rapid diagnosis and treatment of severe injuries such as joint penetrations.

The control of swelling and pain

Excessive soft tissue swelling should be prevented where possible as it:

- impedes the circulation of blood through the damaged tissues

- makes the tissues more difficult to suture
- puts strain on the suture line which can cause the wound to split open and break down.

After cleaning and treatment, the swelling can be prevented or reduced by:
- bandaging
- light walking exercise in hand
- administration of non-steroidal anti-inflammatory drugs, e.g. phenylbutazone which is also an analgesic; reducing the pain encourages the horse to use the injured leg.

Your vet will make recommendations taking into account the site and nature of the wound and the individual horse's reaction to the injury.

WOUND HEALING

The stages of healing

Any damage to living tissue – whether a cut, a bruise or a sprain – results in **inflammation**. Inflammation is a vital part of the repair process and it starts immediately an injury has been sustained. The blood supply to the area is increased and white blood cells migrate from the blood into the tissue. They ingest dead tissue, bacteria and foreign material. With open wounds, a scab forms on the surface and this protects the healing tissues underneath.

After a few days, the inflammatory exudate is replaced by proliferating **granulation tissue** which fills in any tissue defects (Figures 3.7a and 3.7b). It consists of collagen fibres and capillaries. The dividing epithelial cells at the skin edges migrate across this bed of healthy tissue to close the wound.

When the skin is broken, its normal tension causes the wound edges to pull apart immediately after the injury occurs. Within 3–4 days, most wounds undergo a degree of

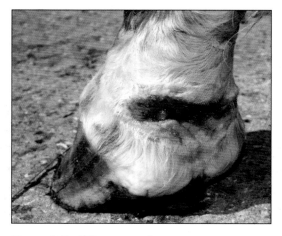

Figure 3.7a Wire cut to the pastern

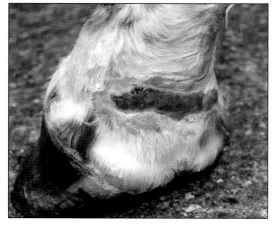

Figure 3.7b The same wound after the tissue defect has filled with granulation tissue

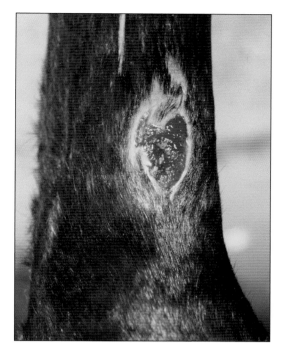

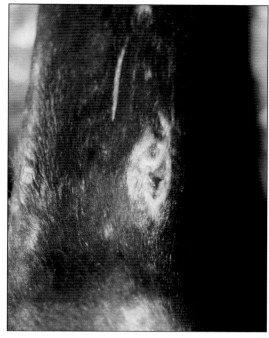

Figure 3.8a A healthy granulating wound

Figure 3.8b The same wound at a later stage of healing

contraction and the skin edges are drawn closer together. The growth of new skin is a very slow process. It proceeds at an approximate rate of 0.5–2 mm (up to $\frac{1}{10}$ in) a day (Figures 3.8a and 3.8b). For this reason, some wounds benefit from being sutured by a vet with surgical stitches or staples.

Suturing

Suturing a wound can result in rapid healing with the smallest possible scar. Closing the skin edges minimizes the amount of new tissue required to heal the defect. This is known as **first intention healing**. The repaired covering of skin stops the development of proud flesh.

Even if skin has been lost and the wound can only be partially sutured, the healing time is greatly reduced. *Do not apply any wound powder, spray, cream or ointment apart from a moist wound gel if the wound is likely to be sutured.*

Wounds cannot be sutured if:
- there is extensive skin loss
- the wound is contaminated by grit, hair or other foreign material
- the skin is not viable due to crushing or loss of blood supply
- bacterial infection is present
- there is a deep puncture with dirt trapped in the deeper tissues
- the wound is more than eight hours old.

There are occasional exceptions to these guidelines. A large, contaminated wound may be cleaned and treated with antibiotics for a few days before being surgically debrided and sutured. Additionally, if a horse is too shocked for sedation to be safe and will not allow the wound to be treated, there are occasions when it can be successfully sutured the following day provided it is kept clean and protected.

Suturing is therefore done at the discretion of the vet, following close inspection of the wound. If all is well, sutures are removed 10–14 days later. However, sutured wounds sometimes pull apart and are said to have '**broken down**'. This is usually due to foreign material or infection in the wound. The skin edges are no longer in apposition and healing proceeds by granulation. This is **second intention healing**.

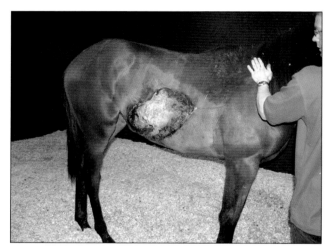

Figure 3.9 Wounds on the trunk are difficult to bandage but often heal well if they are kept clean

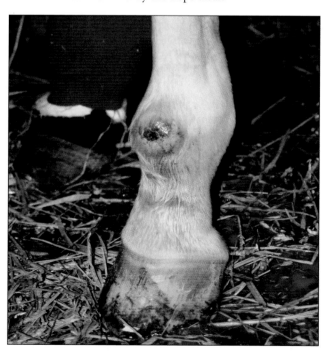

Healing of open wounds that cannot be sutured

Problems can arise with wounds that cannot be sutured or have broken down. Wounds on the head and trunk are difficult to bandage. However, these often heal well without being covered if they are kept very clean (Figure 3.9). Sticky plaster-type dressings with absorbent, non-stick pads in the centre can be useful in these situations. If necessary, your vet will apply a whole body bandage. Clean paper or cardboard is the most suitable bedding if a wound has to be left uncovered.

Open wounds below the knee and hock heal slowly owing to:

- poor blood supply
- low temperature
- minimal wound contraction as the skin is bound to the underlying tissues
- susceptibility to contamination and infection
- swelling
- proud flesh.

These problems can be minimized by appropriate use of bandages and dressings, but wounds on the lower limb frequently take longer to heal than wounds elsewhere on the body (Figure 3.10).

Figure 3.10 This leg wound failed to heal because of the difficulty of protecting it from repeated injury

Wound dressings

Excessive use of creams, powders and ointments can impair healing of wounds other than minor scratches and grazes. During the early stages of the healing of open wounds, the following dressing materials may be useful.

FIRST LAYER

- A wound gel, e.g. Derma Gel® or Intrasite® can be put directly into the wound and covered by an absorbent non-stick pad such as Melolin® or Rondopad®. This may be secured in place with a soft orthopaedic bandage such as Soffban®. The gel helps to keep the wound moist and healthy and provides the right environment for the white blood cells to clear up any dead tissue or foreign material.

SECOND LAYER

- Layers of cotton wool or Gamgee® are wrapped around the limb. These keep the first layer in place and absorb exudates including blood, serum and pus. Sufficient padding must be used to absorb the discharges between dressing changes otherwise bacteria from the environment may be drawn through a wet bandage towards the wound.
- Several layers of cotton wool or at least one layer of Gamgee® must be used to reduce the risk of pressure injuries from the securing bandage.
- A conforming type of bandage, e.g. K-band® or Knit-firm® is used to keep the dressings in place and provide compression which reduces swelling and the risk of proud flesh.

THIRD LAYER

- An elastic, conforming self-adhesive bandage such as Vetrap® or Co-plus® may be applied as a top layer to secure and protect the dressings underneath. Alternatively, an adhesive bandage such as Elastoplast® or a stable bandage may be used. Bandaging techniques are described on pages 79–84.

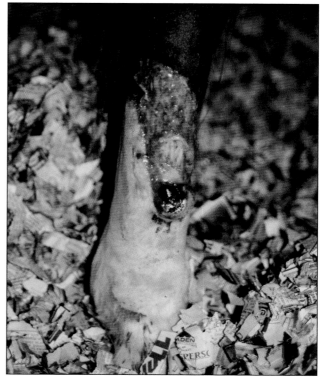

Managing proud flesh

When granulation tissue grows above the level of the skin, it is called '**proud flesh**' or '**exuberant granulation tissue**'. It is usually knobbly, pink and shiny in appearance (Figure 3.11). It may have a yellowish tinge and it bleeds very easily if knocked.

Figure 3.11 Proud flesh

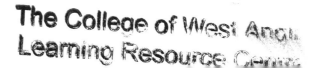

Sometimes the tissue can bulge out of the wound and look like a pink cauliflower. This acts as a physical barrier to the healing of the skin which will not grow over a mound of proud flesh. The skin cannot close until the proud flesh has been removed.

The most common sites for proud flesh are on the limbs from the hock and knee downwards.

There are several methods of managing proud flesh, and so **veterinary advice is essential.** They include the following.

- **Surgical removal** This is carried out by the vet and is necessary whenever there is a large mound of proud flesh. Local anaesthesia is not required as there are no nerve endings in the granulation tissue. The proud flesh is trimmed to just below the skin level. With a fractious horse, sedation may be necessary for this procedure. The tissue bleeds freely and the haemorrhage is controlled with a firm bandage.

- **Application of a topical corticosteroid** The cream or ointment is applied under a non-stick dressing and a firm bandage. This method is suitable when there is only a small ridge of proud flesh protruding above the skin. However, corticosteroids can also inhibit the growth of epithelial cells at the skin edges and long-term use can prevent the wound from healing. Corticosteroid and antibiotic combinations are often used.

- **Application of caustic substances, e.g. copper sulphate** Copper sulphate crystals destroy proud flesh but they also damage the delicate epithelial cells at the wound margin. The skin should be protected with a coat of Vaseline® before the fine crystals are applied to the proud flesh. These are bandaged in place with a firm bandage over a non-stick dressing and an absorbent pad. The vet will advise you when to remove the bandage.

- **Immobilization** Proud flesh often forms at sites where there is a considerable amount of movement. Firm bandaging can help to control the amount of granulation tissue but sometimes this is not enough. In cases where proud flesh keeps forming below the knee or hock, a cast may be applied.

- **Skin grafting** Where there is a large area of lost skin or a recurrent problem with exuberant granulation tissue, a skin graft may assist healing. Small pieces of skin are removed from the horse's neck, flank or thigh. They are embedded at intervals in a healthy bed of granulation tissue. Not all of the grafts will take successfully, but those that survive produce a hormone called epithelial growth factor. This stimulates the division of epithelial cells and inhibits the growth of proud flesh.

- **Laser therapy** Low intensity lasers can be used to stimulate wound and skin healing. An experienced operator is essential as incorrect use can encourage the growth of proud flesh.

- **Leaving the wound uncovered** Opinions vary on whether some wounds benefit from being left completely open and exposed to the air. To a certain extent it depends on the site, the type of injury, the stage of healing and also the individual horse's healing response.

With sites such as the head and trunk which are difficult to bandage, wounds are frequently left uncovered. The management of the horse should be altered to reduce contamination of these injuries by bedding or hay. The most suitable bedding is clean paper or cardboard and, with head wounds, the hay should be soaked and fed from the floor.

All lower limb wounds need to be covered if possible until the defect has filled in with healthy granulation tissue. If healing is proceeding satisfactorily, it is advisable to leave the dressings on for several days at a time. Where proud flesh keeps developing, the vet may suggest leaving the wound uncovered for part of the day once healing is nearly complete. The wound must be kept as clean as possible. This can be achieved by:

- keeping the horse in a box with non-slip matting and no bedding while the wound is uncovered
- skipping out the box every couple of hours
- soaking hay which can be fed from a net to reduce the amount of dust; any uneaten hay should be removed regularly from the floor
- covering the wound with a light dressing before returning the horse to its usual stable to urinate or spend the night
- **not turning the horse out with the wound unprotected** into muddy or dusty fields or where it is likely to be bothered by flies.

The important thing to remember is that no two wounds are the same and they may change from day to day. If you are concerned by lack of progress or worried by any changes, contact your vet.

Treating minor cuts and grazes

Small, superficial cuts and grazes usually heal well if left open, provided they are not contaminated by mud or bedding. The following steps should be taken:

- clean the wound thoroughly with an antiseptic wash, e.g. diluted Hibiscrub®
- apply a moist wound gel or antiseptic cream or spray
- re-examine the wound twice daily
- check for secondary bacterial infection which can develop unnoticed beneath a crust of wound dressing and exudate; this will not occur if the wound is regularly cleaned, thus preventing a build up of debris.

WHICH TOPICAL PREPARATION SHALL I USE?

The type of topical treatment for minor cuts and grazes is a matter of personal choice or availability. In the summer, a preparation with an insect repellent is useful but few such products remain available due to health and safety reasons. It is best to keep a moist wound gel product in the stables to use as the first choice in encouraging healthy wound healing.

Aerosols and sprays are convenient to use and are useful for small grazes and scratches. If the horse dislikes the noise, spray the preparation onto cotton wool first. Never spray near the eyes.

Creams and ointments can be useful for applying to skin lesions. There are many available and they contain a variety of substances to assist healing. Your vet will recommend the most appropriate one for a specific condition.

Wound powder is puffed onto the wound from a small plastic container. It is easy to apply and adheres well to a moist surface. Do not use it near a horse's eyes. When treating a head injury, puff the powder onto a piece of cotton wool before applying it to the wound. Some preparations can slow the healing in certain situations.

Warning

However big or small the wound, the tetanus status of the horse or pony should be checked. If they are not already protected, tetanus antitoxin and a course of vaccinations should be administered.

PUNCTURE WOUNDS

Puncture wounds occur when small, sharp objects, e.g. nails or thorns, pierce the skin. The object may penetrate to quite a depth and deposit bacteria and foreign material deep in the tissues. Cleaning the wound properly is difficult because the wound is often deep with only a small skin opening. There is a tendency for the wound to close, leaving dirt trapped within the tissue. This can lead to infection, an abscess or a discharging sinus.

Treatment

It is advisable to contact the vet as the risk of infection is high and antibiotics are often required. The vet may explore the wound and remove any trapped dirt. If you decide to treat the wound yourself, the following steps should be taken:

- remove any visible foreign material
- apply a poultice if the site is suitable
- where poulticing is not possible, foment the wound for 15 minutes, 2–3 times daily (see page 78)
- keep the wound open so that it can continue to drain
- check that the horse's tetanus vaccination is up to date.

HAEMATOMAS

A haematoma is an accumulation of blood that collects under the skin like a giant blood blister. It can develop from:

- a kick
- a blow, e.g. if a horse hits a jump (Figure 3.12)
- intramuscular injections given into the brisket (Figure 3.13)
- a surgical incision.

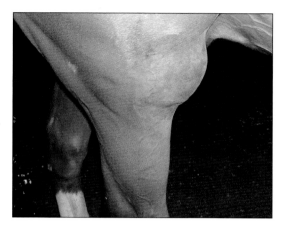

Figure 3.12 This haematoma formed after the horse hit its stifle on a cross-country fence

Figure 3.13 This haematoma formed on the brisket after an intramuscular injection

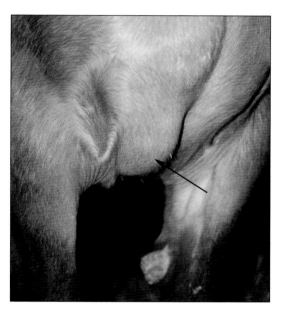

Blood leaks from the damaged blood vessels and accumulates under the skin forming a swelling. If the bleeding continues, the swelling will continue to enlarge over several days. The size can be variable, ranging from a few centimetres in diameter to the size of a football. It may be hard and tender at first, becoming soft and painless as it begins to resolve. The swelling tends to move downwards on the horse's body over a period of a few days.

The diagnosis is usually made on the clinical signs. A sample of fluid may be aspirated from the swelling and analysed to differentiate it from an abscess. Diagnostic ultrasound is also helpful in confirming that the swelling is a haematoma.

Treatment

In many cases, small haematomas resolve within 1–2 weeks without treatment. However, the following may hasten resolution of a haematoma.

- Cold treatment, e.g. cold hosing or ice packs for 48 hours after the injury occurs reduces the bleeding and inflammation.
- Non-steroidal anti-inflammatory drugs, e.g. phenylbutazone, help to reduce the pain

and swelling. Topical anti-inflammatory treatments are sometimes used.

- Once the bleeding has stopped, physiotherapy may help to disperse the fluid and reduce the formation of fibrous scar tissue.
- When the bleeding has stopped, the vet may drain the haematoma but this carries a small risk of introducing infection.

The prognosis is generally good. Occasionally a haematoma becomes infected and is then treated as an abscess which must be drained.

ABSCESSES

An abscess is a collection of pus in the tissues, which can develop anywhere on the body. Abscesses can form under the skin as a result of penetrating wounds which introduce bacteria or in lymph nodes following infections such as strangles. They can also occur in joints due to direct injury or from circulating bacteria in the blood of septicaemic foals.

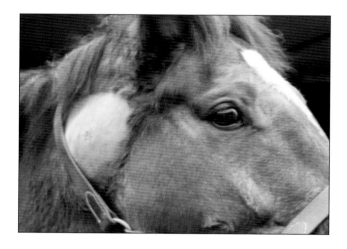

Clinical signs
Abscesses are discrete swellings which are usually hot and painful to touch. Initially they are hard, but as they enlarge and 'ripen', the overlying skin becomes thinner and eventually bursts to release the pus (Figures 3.14 and 3.15a and b).

Treatment
The best way to treat an abscess is to apply warmth

Figure 3.14 A 'ripe' abscess

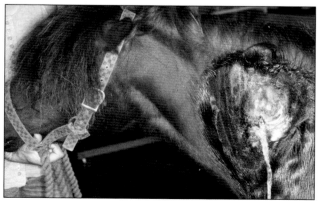

Figure 3.15a An incision has been made to drain the abscess which formed following an intramuscular injection

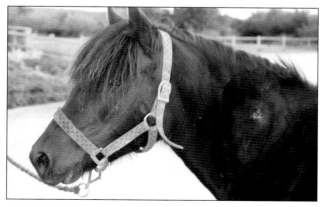

Figure 3.15b The same pony when the abscess had almost healed

with a poultice or hot compress. This increases the blood supply and speeds up the maturing process. When the abscess 'points', an area of the overlying skin becomes very thin and may feel softer than the rest of the abscess. It can often be depressed quite easily. At this stage it may burst naturally or be lanced with a scalpel by the vet. The cavity can then be flushed out with an antiseptic solution, e.g. diluted hydrogen peroxide or chlorhexidine (Hibiscrub®).

Once an abscess has formed, antibiotics are not usually of benefit unless the animal is very unwell with a high temperature. The antibiotics do not penetrate the fibrous tissue capsule of the abscess sufficiently to deal with the infection, but they may delay the ripening of the abscess and slow down healing.

Complications

Occasionally, abscesses do not respond to medical management alone and surgery is needed to remove any diseased tissue before the wound will heal. In cases where the abscess is close to major nerves, the dead tissue is dissected out as far as possible. Sterile maggots (larvae of the common greenbottle, *Lucilia sericata*) have been successfully used to continue treatment of the wound. These maggots selectively feed on the necrotic tissue. They are applied to the wound and kept in place under a gauze dressing soaked in saline. The wound is redressed and fresh maggots applied every 3 days until the unhealthy tissue is replaced by granulation tissue.

CELLULITIS

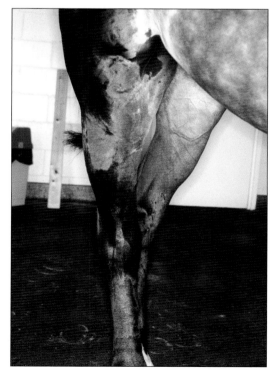

Cellulitis is the name given to diffuse tissue swelling that is caused by bacterial infection of the skin and subcutaneous tissues. It is caused by a number of different types of bacteria, the commonest are *Streptococcus spp* and *Staphyloccus spp*. It can occur anywhere on the body but the hind limbs are most often affected. This is sometimes known as lymphadenitis or lymphangitis when the lymph nodes or lymph vessels of the lymphatic system are involved.

Clinical signs
- The horse usually presents with a diffusely swollen limb which is hot, firm and painful to touch (Figure 3.16).
- There is a variable degree of lameness. It may be severe and acute in onset.
- The swelling may extend upwards above the hock or the knee.

Figure 3.16 Cellulitis of a hind limb following a suspected snake bite

- In severe cases, serum may ooze from the skin.
- The horse may have a temperature and feel very unwell.

Cause

Cellulitis is caused by bacteria entering the body through tiny nicks or abrasions in the skin. This occurs especially around the pastern, fetlock and lower cannon regions. The lesions are sometimes too small to be readily visible, but may be felt if the distal limb is carefully palpated.

Treatment

Treatment includes:

- clipping and cleaning the skin around the site of the wound with an antibacterial scrub if it is weeping; this can be very painful for the horse and sedation is sometimes necessary
- broad-spectrum antibiotics
- non-steroidal anti-inflammatory drugs to reduce the pain and swelling
- gentle exercise in hand several times a day
- a light dressing to prevent the bedding sticking to the limb
- a support dressing applied to the opposite limb.

Prognosis

The prognosis is reasonable if the infection is treated straight away with the appropriate antibiotic. Most cases make good progress within 48 hours. If treatment is delayed, fibrous tissue may be laid down, resulting in permanent thickening of the affected limb (Figure 3.17).

POULTICING A WOUND

Hot poultices are applied to:

- dirty wounds
- infected wounds
- puncture wounds on the limbs or the foot
- abscesses, to encourage them to burst.

The warmth increases the blood supply to the injured area. The white blood cells help clear away bacteria and other debris. Poultices also draw fluid from the wound and are useful for drawing out infection and small dirt particles.

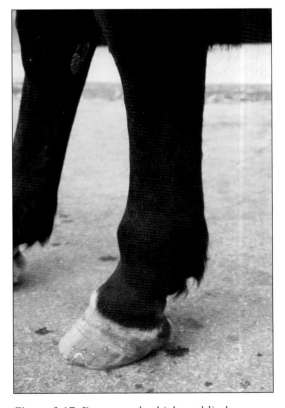

Figure 3.17 Permanently thickened limb

There are 3 potential problems:

1 the poultice should not be so hot that it burns the horse; test the temperature of the poultice on the back of your hand before applying it
2 The securing bandage *must not be too tight*; its purpose is simply to hold the poultice in place – remember that wet bandages can shrink and tighten as they dry
3 a wet poultice applied for too long may actually slow wound healing.

Types of poultice

The following are the most common types of poultice.

READY-TO-USE POULTICES, E.G. ANIMALINTEX®, POULTEX®

These consist of a thick layer of padding impregnated with boric acid. One side of the dressing has a polythene backing. The dressing is cut to size and immersed in clean, hot water. It is then squeezed to remove most of the water and placed on top of the wound with the plastic side facing outwards. A piece of aluminium foil laid on top of the poultice will help to retain the heat. This is covered with a piece of padding such as cotton wool or Gamgee® and bandaged in place.

These poultices can also be applied as a **cold** dressing to reduce swelling and inflammation from a kick or a blow. They are suitable for applying to soft tissue injuries on the limbs and also to foot injuries. They can be particularly useful for softening very hard soles overnight, making it easier for the vet to locate and drain a foot abscess.

KAOLIN AND MAGNESIUM SULPHATE PASTE

These materials are useful for foot abscesses but should not be used on an open wound. They are warmed and applied to the foot under a layer of Gamgee®. A bandage is used to keep the dressings securely in place.

BRAN AND EPSOM SALTS

This type of poultice is also used for foot injuries. A handful of Epsom salts is added to a scoop of bran. Sufficient boiling water is added to make a crumbly (not wet) mixture and the poultice is applied when the mixture has cooled sufficiently.

The 10 steps for poulticing a foot (Figures 3.18a–e)

1 Prepare all the materials you will need, i.e:
   - a poultice
   - a bucket of clean hand-hot water
   - scissors
   - Gamgee® or disposable baby nappy
   - aluminium foil

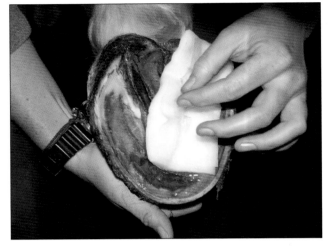

a

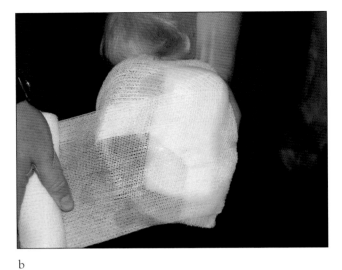

b

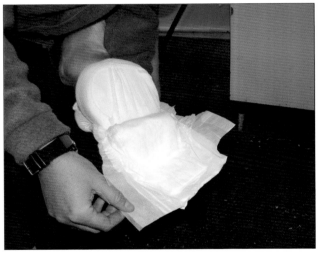

c

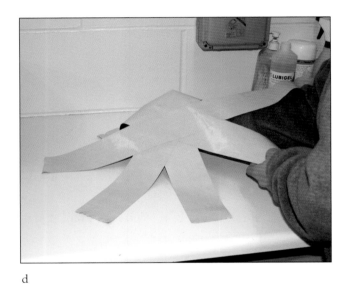

d

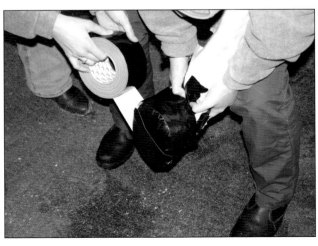

e

Figures 3.18a–e Steps in applying a poultice: a) place the poultice over the wound; b) secure the dressing with a conforming cotton bandage; c) a disposable nappy is useful for holding the dressings in place; d) pre-cut lengths of waterproof tape are applied to the sole in a star shape; e) tough waterproof tape is used to secure the dressings

- a conforming bandage
- a self-adhesive conforming bandage, e.g. Vetrap® or adhesive bandage, e.g. Elastoplast®
- 7.5 or 10 cm (3 or 4 in) black PVC tape or heavy duty tickitape.

2   Clean the *whole foot* thoroughly and dry it as much as possible.

3   Stand the horse on a clean, dry surface.

4   Cut the materials to size.

5   Apply the poultice and aluminium foil.

6   Pack the foot (see below).

7   Secure the dressings in place with a cotton conforming bandage.

8   Apply a layer of Vetrap® or Elastoplast® for extra security.

9   Finally, cut strips of heavy duty tape to reinforce the dressing and make it waterproof or use a protective boot, e.g. an Equiboot.

10 Keep the horse stabled on a thick, clean bed.

Tips for applying poultices
PACKING THE FOOT

Use layers of Gamgee® on top of the poultice to pack the concavity of the foot. Then apply another layer which extends just beyond the sole to cover the weight-bearing edge of the hoof wall. Secure these in place with a conforming bandage. The packing has 3 functions:

1   it keeps the poultice firmly in contact with the wound, ensuring maximum efficiency

2   the pressure on the sole forces pus out of the hole when the foot bears weight

3   the padding under the hoof wall reduces the wear on the covering bandage, especially if the horse is shod.

Alternatively, a disposable nappy can be used as an outer layer to hold the dressings onto the foot (see Figure 3.18c).

SECURING THE DRESSINGS

The easiest way to secure the dressings is to use a self-adhesive conforming bandage, e.g. Vetrap® or Co-plus®.

Completely wrap the sole and wall of the hoof. Bring the bandage up over the heels as this helps to prevent everything from slipping off. Make sure that the bandage is not too tight over the coronary band.

Adhesive bandages such as Elastoplast® do not stick well to damp hooves and should not be applied directly to the bulbs of the heels or the coronet as the horse will become sore. They may be applied as described for self-adhesive bandages if used on top of a stretch cotton conforming bandage to prevent direct contact with the heel and coronary band.

To make the dressing waterproof and stop urine and droppings from being absorbed by the dressings, a plastic bag or suitable 7.5 or 10 cm (3 or 4 in) tape can be used. Several pieces of the tape should be pre-cut so they are long enough to go across the sole and extend up the hoof wall to the coronary band. These are laid across the bottom of the foot until the whole of the sole is covered. It may help to prepare several lengths of tape and arrange them in a star shape first (see Figure 3.18d). A length of tape can now be wound around the hoof wall to secure the strips in place. For extra strength, a layer of tape can be wrapped around the lowest part of the hoof wall and turned in under the sole. This reinforces the dressing on the weight-bearing part of the foot (see Figure 3.18e).

CHANGING THE POULTICE

Poultices are normally changed once or twice daily. They are rarely recommended for use for longer than 3 days. After this time the tissues become very soggy and healing may be delayed.

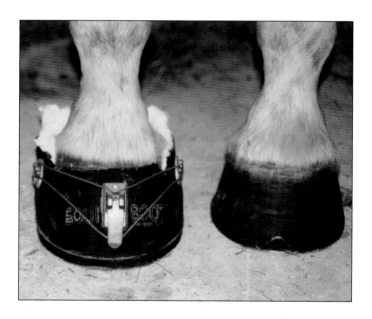

Using a protective boot

An Equiboot (Figure 3.19) is just one of many boots available for holding hoof dressings in place. These types of boot come in many different shapes and sizes. The problem is that horses' feet are also very variable in size and shape. A boot that is comfortable for one horse can rub and make another very sore, especially around the heels. If you find a boot that is comfortable for your horse it can reduce the cost of treatment as the dressing materials are expensive.

Figure 3.19 An Equiboot

Hot fomentation

This is a method of applying heat to an area that cannot be poulticed. It is usually done for 20 minutes, 2 or 3 times a day and is particularly useful for encouraging abscesses to burst, e.g. for a strangles abscess.

- Half fill a bucket with hand-hot water.
- Add a double handful of Epsom salts.
- Immerse a small towel in the water.
- Squeeze out the excess, fold the towel in four and apply to the abscess.
- Repeat these steps every few minutes.
- Top the bucket up with boiling water to keep the temperature warm.

Commercially available packs that can be warmed in hot water or the microwave are another way of applying heat.

Hot tubbing

This is useful for punctures and bruises to the sole of the foot.

- Pick out the hoof and scrub it clean.
- Add a handful of Epsom salts to a bowl or half-filled bucket of warm water. The temperature should be similar to that of a warm bath.
- Place the hoof in the bucket and keep it immersed for 10–15 minutes (Figure 3.20).
- Add more hot water as the temperature cools. Take care not to scald the horse.
- Perform the procedure twice daily.
- Dry the leg thoroughly afterwards.

BANDAGING

Bandaging is a skill which is acquired with practice. Bandages can be used to provide:

- warmth
- support
- compression (controls bleeding and swelling, inhibits proud flesh)
- protection (from contamination, bacterial infection, drying out and further injury)
- pain relief
- immobilization.

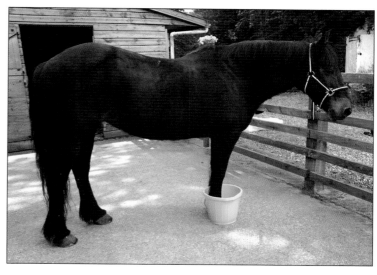

Figure 3.20 Tubbing a foot

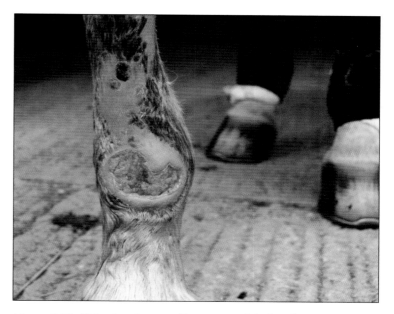

Figure 3.21 Skin slough caused by an overtight bandage

A correctly applied bandage gives light, even pressure. It is firm enough to hold dressings in place but does not restrict the circulation. Overtight bandages can cause pressure sores, skin sloughs (Figure 3.21) and tendon damage. Loose bandages are ineffective and can be dangerous.

Important points to remember

- Bandages should always be applied over a layer of padding, e.g. Gamgee® or cotton wool. This helps to distribute the pressure evenly.
- Any lumps or creases in the padding must be smoothed out.
- Overlapping half the width of the bandage with each turn helps to ensure even pressure.
- The ties and Velcro® fastenings should be laid flat and be *no tighter than the bandage*. Knots must be tied at the *side* of the limb to avoid pressing on the tendons at the front and back of the limb.
- For extra security, the ends of the ties may be covered by a strip of electrical insulating tape or adhesive bandage. This should completely encircle the limb and stick to itself.
- If the horse bears less weight than normal on the injured limb, put a support bandage on the opposite leg and, if necessary, all three other limbs.

Applying a support bandage

To apply a support bandage to the lower limb of a horse, follow these steps (Figures 3.22a–c).

1 Make sure the leg is clean.
2 Cover the wound with a non-stick dressing.
3 Use orthopaedic padding eg Soffban® to hold the dressing in place.
4 Wrap Gamgee® or cotton wool around the limb from just below the knee or hock to the coronary band. Cotton wool is easiest to use as it conforms well to the shape of the limb; a minimum of two layers should be applied. With Gamgee®, it is sometimes easier to cut a separate piece for the pastern area as it does not mould so well to the limb. A single layer of thick Gamgee® is sufficient with an overlapped double thickness layer protecting the tendons at the back of the leg.
5 Now use a conforming cotton bandage to keep the padding in place. Unwind it in the same direction as the overlap of the padding. Start halfway down the cannon bone, and spiral the bandage once around the limb. Now work down the limb to the lower pastern, then back up to just below the knee or hock and finally down to the starting point. Overlap half the width of the bandage each time and make sure the pressure is light and even. The pressure should be firm enough to provide the limb with support without restricting the blood supply. Secure the end of the bandage with electrical insulating tape. The padding should protrude from the top and bottom of the bandage.
6 The top layer can be either a self-adhesive conforming bandage or an adhesive bandage applied in the same way. Alternatively a stable bandage may be used.
7 Check the bandage twice daily to ensure it is comfortable and secure. Redo the bandage once daily (or as necessary).

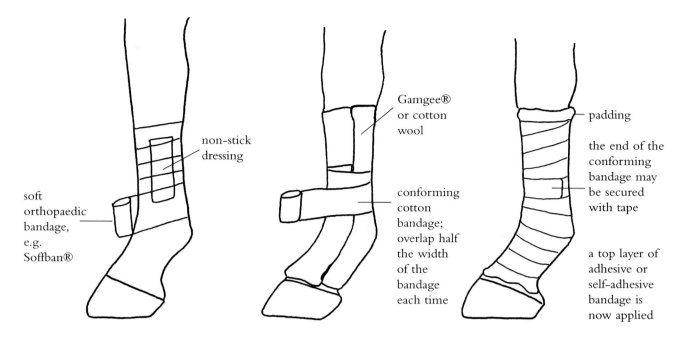

soft orthopaedic bandage, e.g. Soffban®

non-stick dressing

Gamgee® or cotton wool

conforming cotton bandage; overlap half the width of the bandage each time

padding

the end of the conforming bandage may be secured with tape

a top layer of adhesive or self-adhesive bandage is now applied

Figure 3.22a–c Bandaging the lower limb with a support bandage

Signs that a bandage is too tight

These include:

- swelling above or below the bandage
- signs of discomfort from the horse, e.g. repeated lifting of the leg or biting the dressing
- areas of skin that are sore to touch
- swelling that develops within 20 minutes of the bandage being removed.

Using a pressure bandage

A pressure bandage is used for short periods of time to control bleeding. It is applied over a layer of padding and should be left in place for a maximum of 2 hours. The bandage is applied with more tension than a support bandage.

Bandaging a heel or coronary band wound

Follow these 8 steps.

1 Cut a non-stick dressing and a piece of Gamgee® to a size that covers the wound.

2 Attach the free end of a roll of insulating tape to the hoof wall. The hoof wall must be clean and dry. Wind the tape round the hoof, passing below the heels to secure the lower edge of the dressing.

3 Pass the tape round the hoof wall again. This time bring it up over the dressing then back down onto the hoof wall.

4 Repeat 2 or 3 times until the dressing is secure.

5 Avoid direct contact between the tape and the coronary band.

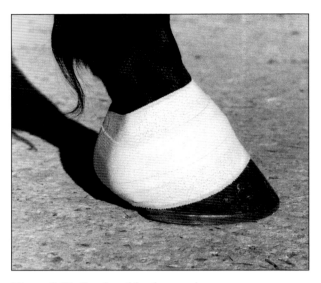

Figure 3.23 Bandaged heel wound

6   Wind a short length of conforming cotton or crepe bandage twice round the bulbs of the heels and the coronet.

7   Use self-adhesive or adhesive bandage to hold the dressing in place (Figure 3.23).

8   Either 7.5 or 10 cm (3 or 4 in) PVC tape can be used on top to make the dressing waterproof.

Bandaging the foot

Follow the instructions in the poulticing section on pages 77–78. Disposable nappies make a useful dressing that can be taped in place if no other materials are immediately available.

Bandaging the knee and hock

These are awkward sites to bandage as the constant movement tends to loosen the bandage. It can then slip down the leg and cause undesirable ridges of pressure. If bandaging of this area is necessary, your vet will demonstrate the technique which avoids pressure on the bony prominences such as the point of the hock and the accessory carpal bone at the back of the knee (Figures 3.24a and b and 3.25).

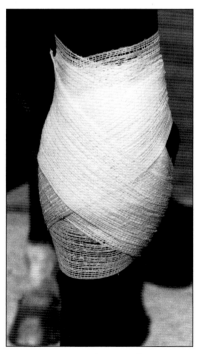

Figure 3.24a A figure-of-eight bandage applied to a horse's knee

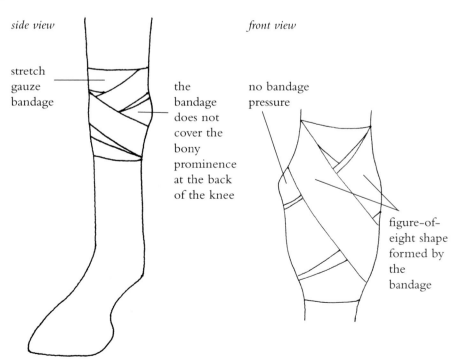

side view

stretch gauze bandage

the bandage does not cover the bony prominence at the back of the knee

front view

no bandage pressure

figure-of-eight shape formed by the bandage

Figure 3.24b Bandaging the knee with a figure-of-eight bandage

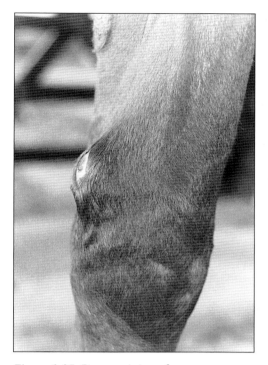

Figure 3.25 Pressure injury from an incorrectly applied knee bandage

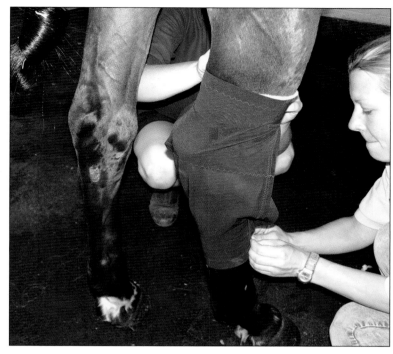

Figure 3.26 Applying a Pressage® bandage

Proprietary zip-up elasticated stockings, e.g. Pressage®, are available for securing hock and knee dressings in place. If one of the sizes fits your horse, these can be a great help. A stable bandage is usually applied below it to prevent any swelling of the lower limb and to ensure it does not slip down (Figure 3.26).

Tubular bandages, e.g. Tubigrip®, are useful for retaining dressings on these difficult parts of the body (Figures 3.27a and b). The tubular bandage can be secured to the hair above the knee or hock with an adhesive bandage such as Elastoplast®. This should be done with care as repeated applications and removal can make the skin sore. Provided it stays clean, the tubular

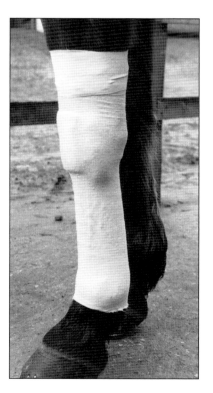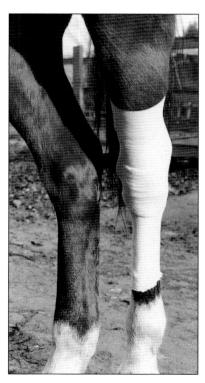

Figure 3.27a and b A tubular bandage secured with Elastoplast can be used to hold dressings on awkward areas in place: a) knee dressing; b) hock dressing

bandage does not need to be removed each time the dressing is changed. The lower edge of the bandage is simply rolled up to allow cleaning and inspection of the wound. A stable bandage is used to secure the lower end of the tubular dressing.

Robert Jones dressing

This is a very thick and solid support dressing used by vets for a number of purposes which include:

- limb support
- stabilization of certain fractures
- controlling swelling
- protecting a limb following surgery.

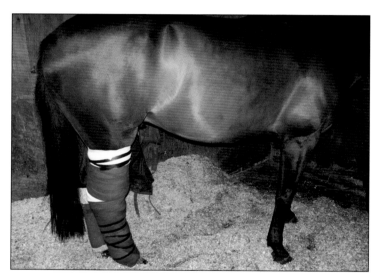

Figure 3.28 A Robert Jones dressing

It may be applied to the whole of a limb or just the lower half. Any wounds are covered with a non-stick dressing which is held in place with orthopaedic padding, e.g. Soffban®. A thick layer of cotton wool is wrapped round the limb and then compressed and secured in place with a wide conforming bandage such as K-Band®. This is repeated several times until the dressing is 6–8 cm ($2\frac{1}{2}$–3 in) thick. A top layer of adhesive bandage, such as Elastoplast®, or self-adhesive bandage is then applied (Figure 3.28).

How to stop a horse removing bandages

This problem can be overcome in a number of ways.

COMFORT

Check that the bandage is not too tight. The horse may chew at it if he is in discomfort from either the bandage or the injury.

WEARING A BIB

A bib is a plastic device which can be secured to the headcollar (Figure 3.29). It

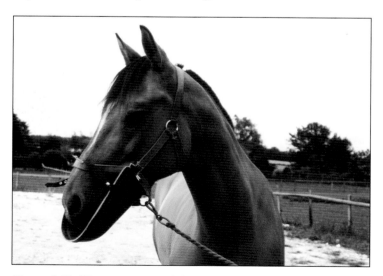

Figure 3.29 Horse wearing a bib

prevents the horse chewing its bandages or rugs. Apart from the restriction of wearing a headcollar for prolonged periods, it is relatively comfortable. The horse can still eat, drink and pull hay from a net. The comfort of the headcollar should be checked as some horses become sore around the poll with prolonged use especially if the headcollar is made from hard nylon.

WEARING A CRADLE

A cradle consists of several rounded rods of wood which are strapped around the horse's neck (Figure 3.30). It allows some movement but restricts flexion. The horse is unable to reach down to remove the bandages.

WEARING A MUZZLE

A muzzle effectively stops a horse from removing its bandages but will also prevent it from eating (Figure 3.31). Make sure the horse has learned to drink with the muzzle in place before leaving it on for any length of time. Muzzles are not designed for long-term use and should only be fitted as a temporary measure.

APPLICATION OF UNPLEASANT-TASTING SUBSTANCES

A harmless but unpleasant-tasting substance can be smeared over the surface of the outer bandage. A number of these are available and can be purchased from tack shops. They are, however, messy and do not always work.

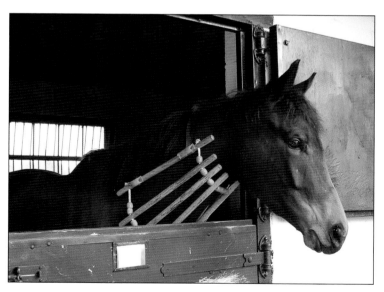

Figure 3.30 Horse wearing a cradle

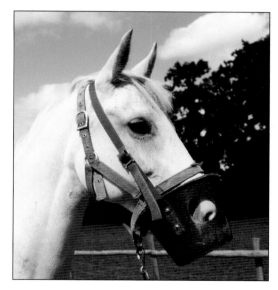

Figure 3.31 Horse wearing a muzzle

EXAMINATION OF THE LAME OR POOR PERFORMANCE HORSE

There are many causes of lameness and this chapter outlines the procedures that may be used in order to make a diagnosis.

DEFINITION OF LAMENESS

The 'normal' conformation and action of horses varies considerably. Lameness can be defined as any change in the horse's usual way of moving. It is therefore helpful to be familiar with each individual horse's action.

Whether slight or severe, lameness is usually a sign of pain. The horse should not be worked until the problem has been investigated and the cause identified and treated.

WHEN TO CALL THE VET

The following guidelines are suggested to help you decide when to call the vet. **Immediate** attention must be given to horses which are:

* unable to bear any weight on a limb
* unable to move
* trembling and sweating due to pain.

Immediate attention must also be given to those which have:

* a nasty wound
* synovial fluid leaking from a wound

- severe swelling of a limb
- a puncture wound in the foot
- suspected ligament or tendon injuries
- signs of laminitis.

In other cases it may be reasonable to wait a day or two to see if the condition resolves before seeking veterinary advice. In the meantime it is essential to:

- rest the horse
- control the horse's exercise, i.e. confine it to a stable or small turnout area to prevent further injury
- check very thoroughly for wounds and swellings on the legs
- search for flint or nail penetrations of the feet
- note any changes; if the lameness becomes worse or does not improve, call the vet.

Never ignore a slight lameness or swelling because the horse has a competition in the near future. No occasion is worth the gamble of turning a minor problem into a more serious injury.

THE VET'S VISIT

Preparation for the vet's visit
In advance of the vet's arrival:

- bring the horse in
- make sure the stable is clean
- have a headcollar and bridle ready
- pick out the hooves and clean the legs
- think carefully about the history of the case and write it down.

Steps of the examination
The cause of a particular lameness is sometimes obvious to both the owner and the vet, but on other occasions a considerable amount of diagnostic work is required to pinpoint the site of pain. Indeed, some lameness may be impossible to diagnose precisely. The examination procedure will vary with the individual situation. The vet will undertake some of the following steps.

TAKING THE HISTORY
Patient details

- Age, breed and sex of the horse.
- What is its actual and intended use?

This information is important as some orthopaedic problems tend to occur more in certain breeds or in young animals. Degenerative conditions are more likely in older animals. The type of work the horse does is also important as the different disciplines, e.g. racing and dressage, tend to put strain on different parts of the body. For example, sore shins often cause forelimb lameness in two-year-old racehorses in training, whereas older racehorses frequently experience knee and fetlock pain or tendon strains. The advanced dressage horse is more likely to experience hock pain or back pain due to the rider sitting deep and asking for collection.

It may be helpful if you consider the answers to the following questions in advance of the vet's visit.

Timing
- When did the horse first go lame?
- Did the lameness occur suddenly or was there a slight problem before? Many horses are able to cope with a degree of pain for some time and then suddenly go very lame with only a slight worsening of the injury.
- Is it a recurrent problem or is this the first time?
- Has the horse recently been purchased and is its previous history known?
- Has the farrier reported any recent problems with shoeing the horse? Horses that are experiencing hind limb pain often find lifting their hind limbs for shoeing uncomfortable.

Possible causes
- What was the horse doing when the problem was first noticed?
- Has the horse fallen or experienced any other trauma?
- When was the horse last shod?

Exercise routine
- How fit is the horse?
- What sort of exercise routine has been followed?
- When is the lameness most marked? Is there anything that consistently makes it worse?
- Does the lameness improve or become worse with exercise?
- Does it improve with rest?
- Is the lameness more obvious on a hard or soft surface? Foot problems are likely to be worse on hard going whereas soft tissue injuries, e.g. proximal suspensory or tendon problems may be exacerbated on soft going.
- Is it more obvious on a circle?
- Does the horse stumble?

Swellings and Heat
- Has any swelling or heat been detected? If either have been present, do they increase or decrease with exercise?

Stance
- Has the horse changed the way it stands at rest?
- Does the horse consistently rest or point one limb?
- Does the horse frequently shift its weight from one foot to the other?
- Is the horse lying down any more than usual or experiencing difficulty in getting up?

Management

It is important to know if the lameness is associated with any change in routine or management. For example, if there has been a change of:
- rider
- training programme
- saddle
- bit
- shoeing
- amount of turnout
- diet.

Previous treatment

Finally, it is important to know if the horse has been given any treatment and whether it appeared to help.

EXAMINATION AT REST

In the stable

Most vets will discuss the history while in the stable with the horse. This ensures there is plenty of opportunity to see the horse at rest in his own stable and observe any subtle signs of discomfort, as in the examples below, that may otherwise be missed.
- Pointing one limb – this is when one forelimb is intermittently or continually held slightly extended in front of the other limb, often with the heel slightly raised from the ground.
- Some horses will dig holes in their bedding and stand with their toes in the hole and their heels raised up on the bedding. This is often suggestive of heel pain.
- Constant shifting of the weight from one leg to the other. This can indicate bilateral foot pain or soft tissue injuries.
- Standing with the hind limbs brought forward under the body and both forelimbs extended with the weight back on the heels is highly suggestive of laminitis, especially if the horse is constantly shifting its weight.
- An occasional awkward step when the horse experiences acute pain.

Outside

Next the horse is led out of the stable and assessed while standing square on a hard, level surface. The horse should be standing on all four limbs. The vet will look at the following.

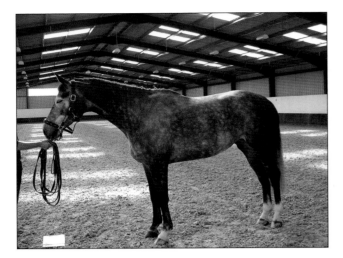

Figure 4.1 Assessing the horse from a distance

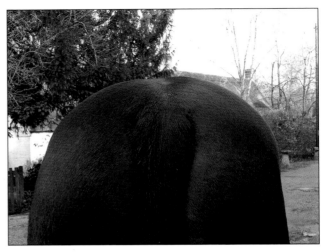

Figure 4.2 Checking the bony landmarks of the pelvis: this pelvis is asymmetrical

- Conformation: this may be important as certain types of conformation are associated with specific lameness.
- Stance.
- Condition.
- Symmetry: this is assessed from a distance and close up (Figure 4.1). In particular, the vet will be looking for any swelling or muscle wasting including:
  - abnormal distension of a joint capsule
  - any bony enlargement
  - the presence of a haematoma or oedema
  - swelling due to cellulitis or bruising
  - muscle swelling
  - muscle wasting; if this is due to a low-grade lameness, it may take months to develop
  - the presence of any scar tissue
  - the symmetry of bony landmarks of the pelvis, i.e. tuber sacrale, tuber coxae and tuber ischii (Figure 4.2).

ASSESSMENT OF FOOT SHAPE AND BALANCE

At this stage each foot is assessed for:

- size
- shape
- toe and heel length
- lateral/medial balance
- heel height – are the bulbs of the heels on each hoof the same height and how close to the ground are they?

- hoof-pastern axis
- coronary band swellings or sensitivity
- any obvious cracks or other defects
- the condition of the frog.

A slight variation in the size of the front feet is not always indicative of a problem but significant asymmetry of the front feet is a potential cause for concern (Figure 4.3). This is because one foot will contract at the heels and become smaller if the gait of the horse is altered over a period of time with reduced weight bearing on the limb for any reason.

The foot is then lifted and thoroughly cleaned so that the solar (ground) surface can be assessed. The fit of the shoes and any abnormal wear patterns can be seen. The conformation of the sole is noted. This is usually slightly concave in the front feet and more obviously concave in the back ones. A thin layer of horn may then be scraped from the sole to check for bruises and punctures. Hoof testers are then applied at regular intervals from the heel on each side to the toe to test for any regions of abnormal sensitivity (Figure 4.4). Horses with thin soles are naturally sensitive so the response is usually compared with that of the opposite limb. If the vet is concerned that there may be an abscess or an area of bruising under the shoe, then it will be removed for closer inspection. Hoof testers are also applied to the frog and across the heels. Another test for foot pain if white line lesions or nail bind is suspected is to tap the shoe at regular intervals and over each nail with the hoof testers or a hammer.

The vet will feel the lateral cartilages of the feet which should be pliable and spring back into position after being squeezed against the pastern. The digital pulse of each limb will be noted.

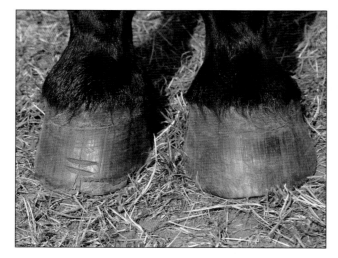

Figure 4.3 Asymmetric front feet: the horse's right forefoot is significantly smaller and more upright than the left forefoot

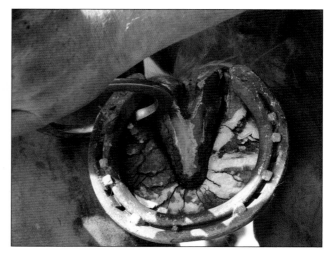

Figure 4.4 Hoof testers are used to check for abnormal sensitivity

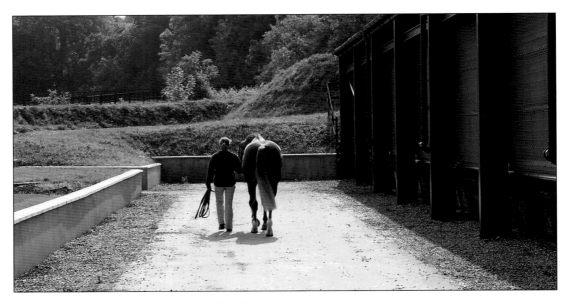

Figure 4.5 Examination in hand on a hard level surface

ASSESSMENT IN HAND

Unless the source of the pain is obvious, the horse is walked and trotted up on a hard, flat surface wherever possible (Figure 4.5). If it is necessary to use the road, the horse should always wear a bridle for maximum control.

The handler should stay slightly in front and to one side of the horse in order not to obscure the vet's view. Placid or lazy animals should be driven on from behind, as pulling on the reins or holding them too short can prevent the slight head movements which aid identification of the lame limb. The horse is observed:

- walking away from and towards the vet
- turning
- trotting away from and towards the vet
- from the side at walk and trot
- turning in a tight circle
- walking backwards.

The vet will look for the following **signs of lameness**.

Head nodding

Horses with forelimb lameness lift their heads up as the lame limb contacts the ground. The head drops as the sound limb takes the weight. If the horse is very lame, the horse may visibly tighten its neck and shoulder muscles as the head and neck are lifted. This is easiest to see at trot.

With hind limb lameness there is not likely to be a head nod unless the lameness is severe. In these cases, the horse will attempt to shift its weight forwards and lower its head at trot when the lame limb contacts the ground. For example, if the horse is very lame on its left hind, it may lower its head as the left hind contacts the ground. Since the horse moves its limbs in diagonal pairs at trot, if viewed only from the front, this could easily be mistaken for a left forelimb lameness.

Symmetry of gluteal rise

Viewed from behind, the gluteal muscles on either side of the horse's rump should rise and fall equally. With hind limb lameness, the hip on the painful side rises more than the hip on the sound side. Essentially the pelvis lifts up when the lame leg contacts the ground and sinks when the sound leg hits the ground

Symmetry of gait

The horse will be viewed from all angles to check if the strides are of the same length. A horse with slight lameness may only show a very subtle shortening of stride of the lame limb. However, horses with bilateral forelimb or hind limb pain may shorten the stride of both limbs equally so the gait becomes short and choppy but remains symmetrical. A loss of impulsion is a common finding with bilateral hind limb lameness. On other occasions, particularly with subtle hind limb lameness, the horse will not demonstrate obvious lameness but alter its gait in order to reduce the level of discomfort experienced. For example, a horse with sacroiliac pain will often swing the hind limb on the affected side outwards in a circular fashion as it brings the leg forward to avoid flexing the limb.

Alteration in the height of the foot flight arc

A horse that is bilaterally lame behind may not look obviously lame but shorten its stride and reduce the height of its foot flight arc. This may be heard as toe dragging on a hard surface or seen as the surface being scuffed in a school.

Foot placement

The horse should place its feet squarely on the ground with each stride. This alters with poor hoof balance or if the horse's foot is being placed in such a way as to alleviate pain in a particular part of the foot or higher up the limb.

Difference in sound

With some subtle lameness, it is not always easy to see a change of gait, but this may be heard when the horse is trotting on a hard surface. The lame limb is placed more gently on the ground and thus more quietly than the sound limb.

Observation of the horse turning

This is an important part of the examination. Horses with localized foot pain will sometimes flinch as the weight is taken unevenly on the affected area. Horses with hind limb pain often find turning uncomfortable.

Turning the horse in a small circle gives the vet additional information. While this is being done the vet will look at the horse's ability to flex his head and neck laterally and to cross one hind limb in front of the other (Figure 4.6).

Walking backwards

The horse is asked to walk backwards for a few strides and is then walked forwards. The horse should reverse in a straight line by moving the legs in diagonal pairs and without any sign of discomfort. This test can be useful for detecting conditions such as shivering and stringhalt (see pages 303 and 304), and also neurological conditions such as wobbler syndrome (see page 306). Horses with back pain may tense their back muscles and look uncomfortable or swish their tails when asked to reverse (Figure 4.7).

Observation of tail carriage and assessment of tail tone

Some horses with hind limb pain or muscle tension in their quarters will carry the tail towards the affected side. In certain neurological conditions the horse will have reduced tail tone and so when lifted by the vet it has a 'floppy' feel to it.

FLEXION TESTS

A flexion test may be performed after the trotting up. This test can be helpful in identifying the lame limb if the lameness is only slight. It involves picking up the horse's limb and holding it flexed for a period of up to one minute (Figure 4.8.) The horse is then asked to move straight into trot. A positive response to flexion will show as an increase in the level of lameness. The vet will look for:

- a more pronounced nod of the head or shortening of the stride with a forelimb lameness
- increased asymmetry of the gluteal rise, further shortening of the stride or decrease in foot flight arc with a hind limb lameness.

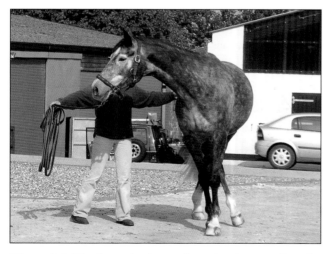

Figure 4.6 The horse is observed turning in a small circle

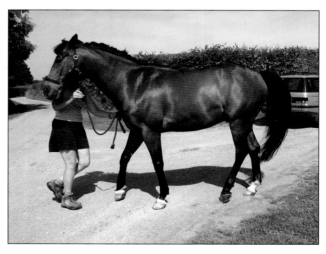

Figure 4.7 Horses with back pain might look uncomfortable and swish their tails when asked to walk backwards

The sound limb is always flexed first because the test may occasionally cause the sore limb to be more uncomfortable for a few minutes, making assessment of the other limb impossible.

It is important to recognize the limitations of a flexion test. One cannot always localize the pain to a particular area by performing a flexion test. In the forelimb, it is possible to flex the fetlock and knee independently, but owing to the arrangement of the muscles and ligaments in the hind limb it is impossible to flex the hock without also flexing the stifle and the fetlock joints. Also, flexion puts different stresses on different parts of the joint. For example, flexion of the fetlock of the forelimb raises the intra-articular pressure if the joint capsule is distended, which may cause pain, but it also places the extensor tendons under tension, so the results need to be interpreted with care, even by an experienced veterinary surgeon.

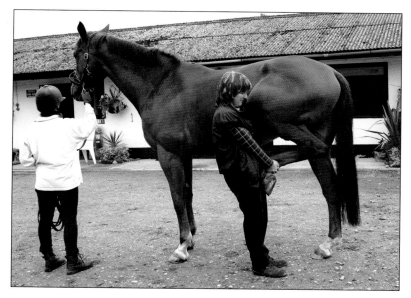

Figure 4.8 Flexion test

Finally, one also has to be careful to check that a positive response is relevant to the lameness being investigated as many horses have multiple sites of pain. The results often have to be considered together with the results of nerve blocks.

PALPATING THE HORSE

The next step of the examination is for the vet to examine the area of suspicion closely and to feel the horse for any indication of pain, heat, swelling or muscle tension. Very often the whole of the horse is palpated to make sure that nothing is overlooked. This is important as the injury causing the lameness may have developed as a result of the horse compensating for a less obvious problem elsewhere. Racehorses, for example, often have problems in the diagonally opposite pair of limbs. Forelimb injuries such as tendon strains may show up more in one leg but tend to occur bilaterally.

The horse is systematically and methodically palpated all over. Each limb is palpated while bearing weight and also while raised from the ground so the tendons and ligaments can be individually felt. The knee, fetlock and pastern joints are gently rotated to see if this causes pain. The vet will also feel for any grating of bone against bone – known as crepitus. This can be heard or felt in cases of osteoarthritis or if a fracture is present. The neck and back are carefully checked. Back pain can be the primary complaint but it is often secondary to pain elsewhere in the body

RANGE OF MOVEMENT

While the limb is raised from the ground, the vet will compare the range of movement of the various joints with that of the opposite limb and from experience with what is expected of a horse of that type and age. Reduced movement may occur in a horse with advanced osteoarthritis of a joint and resultant fibrous thickening of the joint capsule. An acute joint sprain is likely to be extremely sensitive to even gentle passive movement. These tests must be carried out with sensitivity and care as horses vary considerably in their tolerance to pain. The minimum of force should be used.

EXAMINATION ON A CIRCLE

Some types of lameness are only visible or are more obvious on a circle, for example when the horse experiences pain in both front feet. Ideally the horse should be lunged on a hard and a soft surface if the facilities are available (Figure 4.9). This is because some types of lameness will show up more on a particular surface. Foot problems are often more obvious on a hard surface, whereas some soft tissue injuries tend to show up more on a soft surface. The temperament of the horse must be taken into consideration because the lungeing of an excitable horse on a hard slippery surface is inadvisable. Although lungeing allows the horse to balance itself naturally and move more freely, in cases involving excitable horses, leading the horse around may be more appropriate.

The horse should be walked and trotted in a relaxed fashion on a 15–20 m circle. Excessive chasing of the horse or excitement can mask subtle lameness. Some types of discomfort are only momentarily obvious as the horse makes a downward transition. The size of the circle can then be gradually reduced.

Whether the lameness is more obvious when the affected limb is on the inside or outside of the circle can give the vet valuable information.

However, the results have to be interpreted with care and experience. A horse that is not used to being schooled and that is not particularly athletic will find trotting in a circle on a hard surface difficult and will look very awkward. This should not be interpreted as lameness.

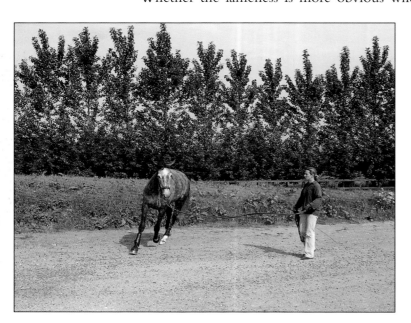

Figure 4.9 Lungeing on a hard surface

RIDDEN EXAMINATION

On occasions the lameness will only be seen when a horse is ridden. A talented and experienced rider is often able to 'feel' a slight resistance before it can be seen. In these situations the vet will see the horse under saddle and check the fit of the tack at the same time. The lameness may be accentuated when the horse is ridden owing to:

- the weight of the rider
- more advanced manoeuvres being performed
- badly fitting tack
- poor riding.

ADDITIONAL TESTS

Assessing the horse on a slope

Some types of lameness and neurological problems are most easily appreciated when the horse is walking uphill or downhill. In these cases the vet will assess the horse on a slope.

Rectal examination

On occasions a rectal examination will be performed. If, for instance, a pelvic fracture is suspected then the vet will palpate the bones making up the pelvis from within the rectum. The horse may be walked along or gently rocked from side to side to help determine if there is a fracture.

Auscultation

A stethoscope is sometimes used to listen for crepitus while a limb is being manipulated. If the humerus or femur is fractured it may not be immediately obvious as the bone is held together by the large and powerful overlying muscles. The horse will be severely lame or even non-weight-bearing on the affected limb and this technique can aid prompt diagnosis.

Sway test

If the vet is suspicious that the horse may be a wobbler, the sway test is used to check for hind limb weakness. The horse is asked to walk forwards and the vet will hold its tail to one side and gradually increase the pull. A normal horse will resist this but a horse with wobbler syndrome is easily pulled to one side.

Dental inspection

If a horse is uncomfortable in its mouth and constantly trying to evade a contact, this may lead to tension and ultimately pain in the temporomandibular joint, the neck and back. Lameness can develop as a result.

LABORATORY TESTS

Blood tests may be taken to check the overall health of the horse or specifically to check muscle enzymes to see if any muscle damage has occurred. Conditions such as exertional rhabdomyolysis (azoturia) can make a horse appear stiff and slightly sore or suddenly and acutely lame. Muscle enzyme levels can be helpful in confirming the diagnosis.

Other laboratory tests are sometimes performed including a muscle biopsy to check for diseases such as equine polysaccharide storage myopathy (EPSSM) or equine motor neuron disease.

NERVE BLOCKS

Nerve blocks are often used to confirm a diagnosis or to localize the problem when the source of lameness is not obvious. Injection of a small amount of local anaesthetic around a sensory nerve will cause the area it supplies to become numb. If the horse becomes sound following the injection, then the source of the lameness is in the area that has been desensitized. The usual procedure is to start at the foot and work upwards. Local anaesthetic may be injected:

• around a specific nerve
• into a joint space or other synovial structure such as a tendon sheath
• locally, e.g. around a splint or the origin of the suspensory ligament.

DIAGNOSTIC IMAGING

The following diagnostic imaging techniques may be used to give further information about the source of the lameness.

• Radiography (X-rays).
• Ultrasonography.
• Scintigraphy (bone scan).
• Magnetic resonance imaging (MRI).
• Thermography.

FURTHER INVESTIGATIONS

On occasions, arthroscopy is used as a diagnostic tool. This procedure allows direct inspection of joint surfaces.

Making a diagnosis

In most cases, the cause of lameness can be identified and a diagnosis made. The horse can then be given the most appropriate treatment. However, one has to accept that there are occasions when a diagnosis remains elusive despite a thorough clinical examination and extensive investigations. The horse may have multiple sites of pain, making interpretation of nerve blocks difficult and not every part of the limb can be desensitized by nerve blocks. Lesions may be present without radiographic changes and not visible on a bone scan. The lameness may be too low grade and intermittent to pinpoint. Horses undoubtedly experience 'referred pain' but our understanding of this is limited at the present time.

5

DIAGNOSTIC PROCEDURES AND IMAGING TECHNIQUES

NERVE BLOCKS

Injection of a small amount of local anaesthetic around a sensory nerve causes the area it supplies to become numb (in the same way that we may have a nerve block when we visit the dentist). Nerve blocks are useful for:
- minor surgical procedures
- assisting examination of sensitive areas, e.g. the eye
- localizing or confirming the site of pain contributing to a lameness.

Diagnosis of lameness

When the cause of lameness is not obvious from the clinical examination, nerve blocks may help the vet to reach a diagnosis. Since a horse cannot tell you exactly where it hurts, reducing or abolishing the pain with a nerve block can provide useful information as to the site and cause of the lameness. The horse must be sufficiently lame for a difference in gait to be readily appreciable following the nerve block.

There are 3 types of nerve block.

1 **Perineural** The local anaesthetic is injected around a specific nerve. If the block is successful, all structures supplied by that nerve are desensitized.

2 **Intrasynovial** The local anaesthetic is injected into a joint space, tendon sheath or bursa that is thought to be a site of pain.

3 **Local infiltration** The anaesthetic is injected around or into a region of suspicion, e.g. a splint, the origin or insertion of a particular ligament, or between the dorsal spinal processes of the thoracic or lumbar vertebrae

The procedure

When the source of the pain is not known, the usual procedure is to start at the foot and

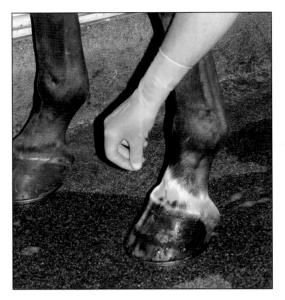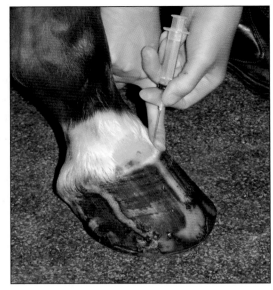

Figure 5.1a and b Injection into coffin joint: a) the needle is inserted in preparation for the injection; b) the injection is completed

work upwards once the lame limb has been identified. The procedure can take a considerable amount of time. It should be done in a clean, quiet environment.

PREPARATION

The area of interest on the horse must be clean and dry. For perineural injections it is not always necessary to clip the hair although this may make it easier if the horse has a long or thick coat. When an injection is made into a synovial structure, the site is usually clipped and always scrubbed with antiseptic to reduce the risk of infection being introduced (Figures 5.1a and b).

RESTRAINT

The horse needs to be adequately restrained by an experienced handler. This is to prevent injury to the vet, handler and the horse. It reduces the risk of sudden movements which could result in damage to the articular cartilage or cause the needle to break. Some horses will stand in a headcollar, others require a bridle or the use of a twitch. On occasions it may be necessary to lightly sedate the horse if it is too excited or very intolerant of the procedure. The sedative wears off while the block is still effective.

Following the injection, the site is lightly massaged and the horse may be gently walked around to assist spread of the local anaesthetic around the nerve or within the synovial structure. The block may take between 10–30 minutes to be fully effective. With some nerve blocks, skin sensation can be tested by assessing the horse's response to deep pressure after 5–10 minutes to check whether it is working.

ASSESSING THE RESULT

If the horse becomes sound or is significantly improved, then the cause of the lameness is very likely to be within the last region of the limb to be blocked. However, interpretation of the results is not always that simple for the following reasons.

- Many horses have multiple sites of pain contributing to their overall lameness. Taking the pain away from the most obvious site may cause the degree of lameness in that limb to improve but not be abolished. Alternatively, the horse may now show lameness in a different leg.

- Very severe pain may not be eliminated. For example, horses with pedal bone fractures, unrelieved foot abscesses or laminitis do not always respond to local anaesthesia of the foot.

- Joint pain can arise from many sources. These include the synovial membrane, the fibrous joint capsule and associated ligaments, the periosteum and subchondral bone. These structures are not reliably blocked by intra-articular anaesthesia and so the horse may remain lame after local anaesthetic has been injected into the affected joint. Subchondral bone pain, in particular, is difficult to eliminate.

- Local anaesthetic may diffuse from the site of injection to numb other nerves or nearby structures, giving a misleading result.

- Occasionally the pain is localized to a particular region, but it is not possible to identify the source, despite follow up with diagnostic imaging techniques. One example is the equine foot. The nerve blocks are not specific enough to pinpoint individual structures. The use of magnetic resonance imaging is currently improving our understanding of foot pain.

Possible complications

These are rare but include:
- local inflammation over the injection site, causing transient pain and lameness
- inflammation of the synovial membrane following a nerve block; this is known as 'joint flare' and usually settles down after a couple of days
- introduction of infection into a joint; this is an uncommon but potentially serious complication.

Contraindications for nerve blocks

- The horse may be intolerant of the procedure making it too dangerous.
- Nerve blocks are not used if a fracture is suspected as it may cause the horse to take weight on the limb with catastrophic results.
- There is no point in performing nerve blocks if the horse is not lame enough for a difference to be appreciated after the block has been performed.

RADIOLOGY

Radiology is routinely used as part of an equine lameness investigation. X-rays are usually taken if bony changes are suspected. The types of changes that show up on radiographs include:
- new bone production
- increase or decrease in bone density
- fractures.

They also show up:
- soft tissue swelling
- mineralization of soft tissues
- the presence of gas within tissues.

Different injuries have a characteristic appearance on radiographs. Careful examination of the radiograph provides the vet with information on the cause of lameness and the stage of the disease. Radiographs are helpful with the diagnosis of many conditions including:
- degenerative joint disease
- traumatic injuries to bone
- infection of joints and bone
- fractures
- bone cysts
- osteochondrosis
- tumours.

Radiation safety

When radiographs are taken, it is essential that no one is exposed to the primary beam. X-ray machines are fitted with a device called a light beam diaphragm so a beam of light shows exactly where the X-rays are going. This is an important safety feature and it also aids accurate positioning of the horse.

Lead aprons and gloves must be worn to protect the body from small amounts of scatter radiation. Anyone not directly involved in assisting the vet should move out of the area. *Pregnant women and those under eighteen years of age must not assist with the procedure.*

The procedure

Radiographs may be taken with a portable machine brought to your yard or at a veterinary hospital. In some cases, a very powerful machine is required and the horse will be taken to a specialist centre.

There are several advantages of attending a veterinary hospital. The radiographs are developed immediately so if the horse has moved or the exposure is incorrect, further views can be taken straight away. Once the lesion has been identified, additional views may be necessary from a variety of different angles.

Requirements for taking radiographs

If the X-ray machine is brought to your yard, the vet will require the following.

- A power point.
- A darkened stable so that the light beam can be seen.
- A smooth, flat surface with plenty of room available for manoeuvring the X-ray machine around the patient.
- An experienced handler.
- A second assistant to position the limb and the X-ray plate.
- The part of the horse being examined must be clean and dry. Mud, kaolin and water all show up on radiographs and may render the films useless.
- Foot X-rays require special preparation. It is usually necessary for the shoes to be removed. The feet must be picked out and scrubbed with a stiff brush to remove every trace of dirt.

The above preparations should be made before the vet arrives. Sometimes the horse will be lightly sedated for the procedure as restless, nervous horses could easily injure themselves or damage the equipment. Sedation may be required for accurate positioning of the patient and the X-ray plate, particularly if high exposures are being used.

Summary

Radiology is used as an aid to diagnosis and it may also be useful for giving a prognosis. It has a value in ruling out the possibility of bony injury in cases with severe soft tissue injury. However, it does not provide all the answers. A horse may be lame for some time before any changes are visible on the radiographs. A 40% change in bone density must occur before it can be seen on the X-ray. Any radiographic changes have to be assessed with care as they may be due to an old injury and not be the cause of the current lameness. Thus a combination of thorough clinical examination and experience in interpreting the images is essential.

ULTRASONOGRAPHY

What is diagnostic ultrasound?

Ultrasound machines produce high frequency sound waves. A hand-held transducer (the probe) is placed against the tissue being examined and the sound waves pass through the tissues until they meet another tissue of different density. At the interface between two tissues, the waves are reflected back and used to create an image on the screen. The

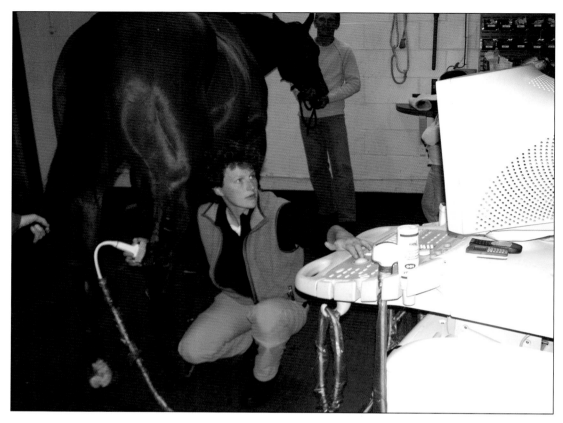

Figure 5.2 Ultrasound is used to help diagnose soft tissue injuries

reflected sound waves are known as '**echoes**' and tissues that reflect sound are described as '**echogenic**'. Bone is highly reflective and appears as a bright white line on the screen. If the sound waves pass readily through less dense tissues and there is little reflection, these appear as black (**anechoic**) areas on the screen. The soft tissues of the body have a characteristic appearance with many shades of grey between the extremes of black and white at each end of the scale.

The ultrasound frequencies used for diagnostic imaging of tissues ranges from 2 to 10 MHz. The higher frequencies give better image quality but have less penetrating power, whereas the lower frequency sound waves can reach the deeper tissues but the picture is not so good. Modern ultrasound machines have different probes which are interchangeable. Ultrasound first became popular in the 1980s for scanning the reproductive tracts of mares and this was quickly followed by its use for examination of tendons and ligaments. Today, ultrasound is widely used for examination of most parts of the body. Essentially, radiography looks at bones and ultrasound at soft tissues, but the two techniques overlap. (Figure 5.2.)

Uses of ultrasonography
Ultrasonography is used:
- to assess the severity and extent of tendon and ligament injuries

- to assess tendon and ligament damage when swelling of the area makes identification of these structures by palpation difficult
- to monitor healing of tendon and ligament injuries
- to detect inflammation of a tendon sheath or joint capsule – there is usually more synovial fluid than normal and the sheath or capsule may appear thickened
- to detect adhesions between tendons or within a tendon sheath
- for assessment of bone surfaces, cartilage and joint capsules
- for detection of bone fragments and fractures
- for detection of foreign bodies and abscesses within tissues
- to detect areas of fibrosis within muscles.

Other uses of ultrasonography include:
- monitoring the reproductive cycle of mares for breeding purposes
- identification of reproductive problems
- monitoring foetal development
- investigation of heart disease
- evaluating the eye
- investigation of respiratory disease especially in foals
- imaging the abdomen: for example, distended loops of intestine may be seen with a bowel obstruction; liver biopsy is often performed using ultrasound to aid identification of the organ and accurate biopsy of the tissue
- investigation of bladder problems.

Preparation of the patient

In order for good images to be obtained, there must be excellent contact between the ultrasound probe and the skin of the horse. Dirt, scurf, scabs, hair and air all spoil the quality of the image. The hair is clipped with a fine blade and the area is then washed with an antiseptic scrub and rinsed carefully with water. Horses with greasy skin and a coarse hair coat may require a further close shave. An acoustic coupling gel is then applied to aid contact between the probe and the skin and time is allowed for it to soak in properly. With fine-coated animals it is sometimes possible to obtain diagnostic images without clipping the hair.

For investigation of tendon and ligament injuries, it is important that the horse is bearing weight on the limb during the examination for meaningful images to be obtained. Fractious patients are sedated for the procedure in the interests of safety of the person carrying out the examination, the expensive equipment and the horse itself. In ideal circumstances, the horse will be examined in stocks in a room with subdued lighting.

The procedure

The region of interest is thoroughly and systematically examined. A standard system has been developed for evaluation of the lower limb between the knee or hock and the fetlock.

In the forelimb, it is divided into seven regions and each of these is scanned in two planes. The transverse scan detects any change in cross-sectional size, shape or echogenicity of the tendons and ligaments. The longitudinal scan shows the alignment of the tendon fibrils. In this way, the extent and severity of a lesion can be seen (see figures 7.3a and b).

The following measurements are made.

- The site of the lesion.
- The length of the lesion.
- The cross-sectional area of the tendon or of a core lesion within it. The injured tendon is usually enlarged in cross sectional area. As healing progresses, the diameter of the whole tendon and of any discrete lesions visible within it reduce.
- The shape of the tendon. This may be altered if the lesion is restricted to one side of the ligament or tendon.
- Any changes in the expected pattern of echogenicity showing if the tissue is more or less dense than expected. Recently damaged tendons and ligaments generally appear darker (less white) than normal due to disruption of the fibrils as a result of inflammation and bleeding within the tissue. As healing progresses, the tissue regains a more homogeneous appearance. If dense scar tissue forms or bone is deposited within the tissue during healing, it will eventually appear whiter than it was originally on the image.
- Assessment of the alignment of the collagen fibrils in longitudinal images. These are normally parallel and homogeneous in appearance. Where there is disruption as a result of injury, the image initially appears darker and the fibres are no longer parallel. As healing begins, the fibres will be randomly orientated and at this stage the tendon is prone to re-injury. As healing progresses, the scar tissue remodels and the longitudinal alignment improves. Assessment of this is important when advising on a programme of controlled exercise.

With tendon and ligament injuries below the knee or hock, the opposite limb is usually scanned at the same time. Very often both show evidence of wear and tear even if the injury is only clinically apparent in one limb. The images are compared with each other and with reference, i.e. 'normal', scans obtained from uninjured horses of similar type and size. The images are recorded in a variety of ways (Polaroid® film, video, computer disc). These are stored for future reference and comparison.

Interpretation of the images

Producing quality images requires good technique as poor technique can make it look as though a lesion is present in normal tissue. Vets sometimes refer to these 'false' lesions as 'artefacts'. Interpretation requires detailed anatomical knowledge and experience. There are various systems of grading the severity of changes seen on the ultrasound images and these can be helpful in giving a prognosis for recovery or otherwise.

The timing of the examination

An injured tendon should not be examined by ultrasound until at least 72 hours after the injury occurs. This is because the initial swelling either can obscure the extent of fibre disruption or make the injury appear more severe than it is. Also, the destructive enzymes released may still be causing further fibre damage. Usually the tendon is scanned again one month later and then at intervals to monitor the healing. It should be rescanned before an increase in the controlled exercise programme is recommended. If at any stage the serial ultrasound examinations reveal signs of re-injury which are not clinically apparent, the exercise regime is reduced.

Limitations of ultrasonography

- When a tendon is re-injured, it can be very difficult on the first examination to determine which of the changes in appearance are due to the original injury and which are due to the new one.

- The healing of the suspensory ligament can be difficult to assess with serial ultrasound examinations as this ligament contains variable amounts of muscle tissue which look darker on the scan and could be confused with a lesion.

- Only the surface of bones can be assessed as the ultrasound is reflected and does not penetrate the deeper tissue.

SCINTIGRAPHY (BONE SCAN)

What is scintigraphy?

Scintigraphy is a tool that the vet can use to assist with the diagnosis of lameness or an internal problem. A radioactive label is attached either to a drug or to white blood cells which are attracted to the area being investigated.

In lameness cases, the scintigraphy performed is called a bone scan. The radioactive substance injected (technetium) attaches to binding sites that are exposed when the bone is actively remodelling or soft tissue is becoming mineralized. The increased metabolism of calcium and activity of osteoblasts (bone forming cells) results in a higher concentration of radioactive material at these sites. Thus radioactivity is highest at areas of increased bone activity, such as a hairline fracture.

How is it performed?

The radioactive substance is injected intravenously and the radioactivity of the tissues is measured at different times after injection. Usually the horse is sedated to minimize movement whilst the scan is being performed. Gamma rays emitted by the radioactive material are detected and measured by a gamma camera. The distribution of radioactivity is analysed by sophisticated computer software that can make corrections for any movement of the horse. Increased radioactivity is seen where there is increased blood flow to an area or there is increased activity of the bone.

The scan can be divided into 3 phases.

Phase 1 The **vascular phase** lasts 1–2 minutes after injection while the substance is still in the blood vessels. It can be used to evaluate the blood flow to a specific area.

Phase 2 The **soft tissue phase** occurs 3–10 minutes after injection when the drug has left the blood vessels and is within the extracellular fluid of the soft tissues. It is used to evaluate blood flow to the soft tissues, e.g. the synovial membrane or capsule of a joint. It can sometimes detect tendon sheath, tendon and ligament injuries not visible on ultrasound or radiographs.

Phase 3 The **bone phase** is 2–4 hours following injection. Increased blood flow and activity of bone forming cells is detected and this is the most commonly studied part of the bone scan (Figure 5.3).

Scintigraphy is a specialist procedure that is always carried out in an equine hospital with dedicated facilities. The horse is admitted and will not be discharged until the radioactivity has reduced to a safe level.

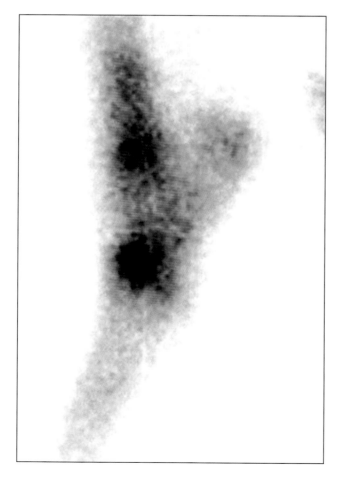

Reading the images

Interpretation of the images requires experience. The images from an injured limb are always compared with those of the opposite limb. They are also compared with others obtained from the same area of an uninjured horse of similar type and age as it is possible for both limbs to be abnormal.

Figure 5.3 Scintigraphy image showing a hot spot in the distal hock joints (with increased uptake of technetium)

What is it used for?

Scintigraphy is particularly useful for the following.

- Detecting problems in areas difficult to X-ray, e.g. the lumbar spine, or areas that can only be X-rayed under general anaesthesia, e.g. the sacroiliac and hip joints.
- Determining whether bony changes seen on radiographs are active or settled.
- Locating sites of increased bone activity in horses that are dangerous to nerve block or where nerve blocks have not eliminated the pain completely.
- Localizing sites of increased tissue uptake of the radioactive material where pain is evident but radiographic changes are negative or equivocal, e.g. some cases of dental disease.
- Aiding diagnosis in horses that have multiple causes of lameness because much or all of the patient's skeleton can be examined during the procedure.
- Investigating horses that are not lame but show reduced or uncharacteristically poor performance.
- Detecting stress fractures early enough to prevent subsequent catastrophic fracture at a time when radiographic changes are not apparent.

The bone phase may be used to detect or confirm the presence of:

- degenerative joint disease
- stress fractures
- fractures
- infection of bone
- neoplasia (cancer)
- enthesopathy (bone formation at the site of attachment of ligaments and tendons)
- periosteal reactions, e.g. sore shins
- damaged skeletal muscle in horses that have 'tied up'.

The timing of bone scans

Scintigraphy is a useful tool for early detection of bone activity that may not show up on radiographs for several weeks. However, it is possible for an injury to be missed if the bone scan is performed too quickly after the injury occurs. It generally takes at least 24–48 hours before a fracture will show up as it takes this long for the bone-forming cells at the site to become active enough to increase the uptake of radioactive tracer above that of the surrounding bone. In some fractures, e.g. pelvic fractures, this can take up to 10 days.

Limitations of bone scans

- The bone phase of the scan will detect *areas* with increased bone activity but will not differentiate the cause of the problem owing to lack of anatomical detail. Thus the procedure needs to be combined with other diagnostic modalities.

- Images obtained from old horses and in cold weather may be poor because of reduced blood supply to the distal limbs. The limbs are usually bandaged and the horse exercised prior to scintigraphy in these cases.
- The radioactive material is removed by the kidneys and excreted in urine. Some views of the pelvis, hips and stifles are obscured by superimposition of the bladder. Diuretics may be administered at the same time to minimize this by reducing the size of the bladder.
- Nerve blocks including intra-articular analgesia can affect the scans as the local inflammation caused will result in increased uptake of the radioactive material and may interfere with the interpretation of the images.
- The patient needs to be hospitalized for a minimum of 24–36 hours following the procedure while the radiation reduces to a safe level.

Summary

Thus bone scans can provide very useful information if used at the appropriate time in conjunction with careful clinical examination and other diagnostic techniques. However, it may be uninformative in cases of low-grade back pain or poor performance.

MAGNETIC RESONANCE IMAGING (MRI)

What is magnetic resonance imaging (MRI)?

Magnetic resonance imaging (MRI) is a sophisticated, non-invasive imaging technique. This is a relatively new form of scan for use on the horse, even though it has been used for people for some time. Recent developments have enabled it to be applied to the horse, but size constraints mean that it is currently only suitable for the head and the limbs from the hock and knee down.

Three dimensional images and two dimensional slices through the tissues are acquired. It is the only imaging technique that enables both soft tissues and bone to be examined at the same time. In some conditions, pathological changes can be identified earlier or at a more subtle stage than with other imaging techniques such as bone scans or X-rays. It has enormous potential for improving the diagnosis and understanding of equine lameness.

What does it involve?

- There are two types of equine MRI systems in use in the UK at the time of writing. The superior machine involves superconducting magnets, which are expensive to purchase and maintain. Such scanners are generally designed for human use and require the horse to undergo general anaesthesia for the procedure.
- The other option is MRI in the standing horse (Figures 5.4 and 5.5), which has the

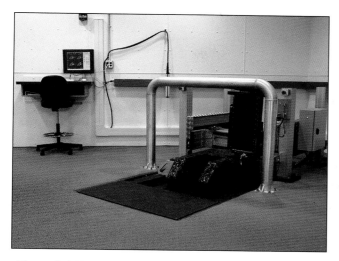

Figure 5.4 Equine standing MRI scanner

advantage of avoiding the risks of general anaesthesia although the horse will still require heavy sedation. Such equipment is considerably cheaper to purchase and maintain, but the images produced are not always of the same quality.

- The values and limitations of the different systems are still being investigated and compared.

- All equipment used must be of non-ferrous (non-iron-containing) material as the superconducting magnets attract this. The shoes and any nails in the hoof are removed.

- The part of the horse being examined must be clean and free from debris. Feet are scrubbed prior to the procedure.

- The images obtained are examined and stored (Figure 5.6). The image of one limb is compared with that of the opposite limb and also with images taken of normal horses. A large number of images are recorded from the area of interest and these take time to analyse. Do not expect an instant answer as evaluation of an MRI scan may take several hours.

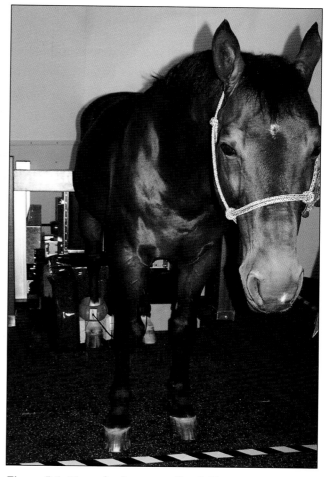

Figure 5.5 Horse having a standing MRI scan

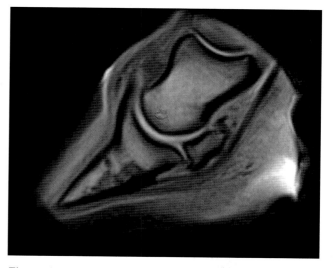

Figure 5.6 MRI image of a horse's foot

What is it used for?

- To aid diagnosis when the pain has been localized to a specific area but no radiographic or ultrasonographic changes are visible.
- It can detect pathological changes in:
    - ligaments
    - tendons
    - joint capsules
    - articular cartilage
    - muscle
    - menisci
    - bone.
- It is especially helpful in detecting lesions within the hoof capsule of the foot where other imaging techniques are limited. The findings usually need interpretation together with the use of other diagnostic techniques such as nerve blocks. With the use of MRI, several sources of palmar foot pain (pain at the back of the foot) have now been identified.
- It can localize flexor tendon injuries within the digital sheath that are not detectable with ultrasound because of the position of the ergot.
- The equine head and particularly the brain may be scanned under general anaesthesia if a horse:
    - is suffering from seizures
    - is showing particular neurological signs
    - has a suspected tumour
    - has experienced head trauma.

The disadvantages

These include the following.

- The cost of the equipment.
- The necessity for general anaesthesia in cases where standing MRI is not used.
- The equipment can be noisy to operate so this needs to be considered when handling animals.
- A specialist staff is required.
- Reading the images is time consuming and requires a great deal of experience.
- The images are occasionally disappointing if movement occurs, e.g. as a result of blood flow through vessels or respiratory movements of the horse.
- The lower neck, body and upper limbs cannot be imaged.

Summary

MRI is particularly good at detecting pathological changes in tissues before they are visible on radiographs or ultrasound. The use of this technique is improving our understanding of the causes of equine lameness generally and foot pain in particular.

THERMOGRAPHY

What is thermography?

Thermography is a non-invasive imaging technique where infrared radiation emitted from the skin surface of a horse is detected by a special camera. This produces an image of the horse that is made up of several colours, each of which represents a particular temperature on the skin surface.

Normal thermographic patterns for the horse have been established. The variations that occur in body temperature of a normal horse are bilaterally symmetrical. When tissue is injured or diseased, the thermographic image reflects any change in blood flow. 'Hot-spots' which have an increased blood flow are usually associated with inflammation. Where the local tissue perfusion decreases due to loss of blood supply, 'cold-spots' are recorded.

What is it used for?

Thermography may be used to detect:
- areas of superficial inflammation with an increased blood supply, e.g.
    - tendonitis
    - suspensory desmitis
    - plantar ligament desmitis
    - laminitis, corns, abscesses, bruises and fractures of the foot
    - bucked shins, stress fractures of the radius and tibia
    - developing osteoarthritis
    - muscle strains.

Thermography can be useful for detecting injuries in tendons and ligaments up to two weeks before they can be detected by clinical examination. Thus it is a very good tool for routine screening of performance horses at risk from these injuries. It may also help localize an injury in a horse that is not amenable to nerve blocking.

Other uses include:
- detection of areas of reduced blood supply, e.g. where there is muscle spasm with reduced muscle activity: cooler-than-normal images are a common finding in horses with chronic muscle pain
- assessment of the extent of an injury
- seeing if a painful area has associated inflammation
- monitoring the blood supply to the foot of the good leg to detect early laminitic changes if a horse has a serious injury and is not bearing weight on the opposite limb
- monitoring the response of the horse to therapy, i.e. resolution of inflammation or restoration of normal blood supply to 'cool' regions (Figures 5.7a and b)

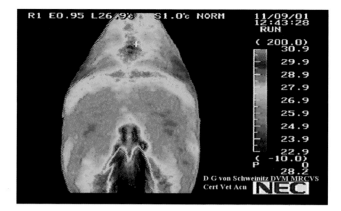 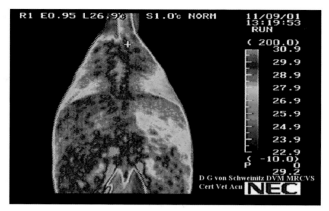

Figure 5.7a and b Thermographic images: a) (left) this image shows abnormal cold zones (due to dysfunction of the sympathetic nerves) over the back and hindquarters of an endurance horse that bucked when ridden in the six months prior to the image being taken; b) (right) during treatment with acupuncture, the thermogram demonstrates significant warming due to normalization of the sympathetic nerves and, following several treatments, the horse was ridden with no recurrence of the bucking

- as a useful tool for checking saddle fit; when the saddle is scanned after a horse has been ridden, the temperature gradient should be bilaterally symmetrical with no particularly warm or cold spots.

The procedure
REQUIREMENTS
- The horse must be clean and dry.
- It should not be exposed to sunshine or wear boots, bandages or rugs just before the examination.
- The horse should have an even coat length.

The procedure is carried out in a room with a constant temperature below 30 °C with no direct sunlight or draughts. The horse usually stands in stocks in the designated room for 15–60 minutes prior to the procedure to acclimatize to the room temperature and is not handled during this time. Sedatives are avoided as these can affect the circulation (and thus the image obtained).

The whole body is usually imaged unless a localized and specific problem is being investigated. In some cases, further images will be taken for comparison following exercise. Images of one side of the body are compared with the other and also with images obtained from uninjured horses. In general, a change of 1 °C is considered to be significant.

Limitations of the procedure
- The equipment is expensive.
- The technique takes time and is not practical in every situation.

- The technique may localize a lesion but it does not give any detailed information about the nature of the injury.

Thus thermography is a useful tool but should be used in addition to other forms of diagnostic imaging.

ARTHROSCOPY

What is arthroscopy?

In this procedure, a narrow-diameter rigid endoscope (known as an arthroscope) is inserted into a joint space through a small surgical incision (Figure 5.8). The joint is then distended with a balanced electrolyte solution. This allows visual inspection of:

- the articular cartilage
- the synovial membrane
- ligaments and menisci within the joint.

What is it used for?

It is an important tool for both diagnosis and treatment of joint lesions. The technique is especially useful for evaluation of joints which have no radiographic

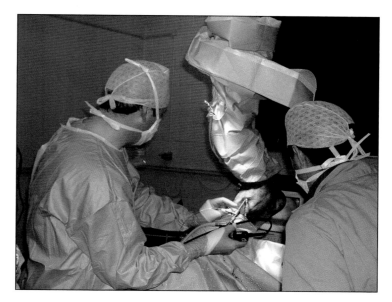

Figure 5.8 Arthroscopy of the hock joint

changes but the lameness is reduced or abolished following intra-articular analgesia. Once a lesion has been identified, surgical instruments are introduced via a second incision.

Procedures performed include:

- joint lavage – the joint is flushed to remove harmful inflammatory mediators and debris from breakdown of articular cartilage and subchondral bone
- debridement of articular cartilage defects, exposed subchondral bone and meniscal tears
- fracture repair or removal of bone fragments, e.g.
    - surgical removal of osteochondral bone fragments of traumatic or developmental origin
    - surgical removal of chip fractures of the carpus and apical fragments of the proximal sesamoid bones and the proximal dorsal aspect of the proximal phalanx
    - lag screw fixation of carpal slab fractures
    - placement of screws for fixation of metacarpal or metatarsal condylar fractures

- treatment of septic (infectious) arthritis
- surgical removal of inflamed, thickened or infected synovial membrane
- arthrodesis (see page 225).

Advantages over open joint surgery (arthrotomy)

Arthroscopy gives better visualization of the articular surface because:

- of magnification of the image
- the villi of the synovial membrane remain suspended in fluid
- more of the joint surface can be seen.

In addition:

- the small incisions are less traumatic and the horse is less likely to be lame following surgery
- there is less scarring
- there is less likelihood of wound breakdown following surgery
- lesions such as tearing of the intercarpal ligaments can only be diagnosed with this technique.

Disadvantages of arthroscopy

- The procedure requires general anaesthesia.
- The equipment is very expensive.
- Considerable training and experience are required to perform such procedures.

Aftercare

This depends on which joint was affected and the severity of the damage. Where possible the wound is bandaged. Antibiotics and non-steroidal anti-inflammatory medication are routinely administered. Intra-articular hyaluronan or polysulphated glycosaminoglycan (PSGAG) may be used following surgery and a course of intramuscular PSGAG may be given.

Possible complications

These include:

- infection
- persistent synovial effusion
- bleeding into the joint.

Tenoscopy

The arthroscope can also be used to examine synovial tendon sheaths. This is known as tenoscopy. It is valuable for diagnosis and treatment of problems in the:

- digital flexor tendon sheath

- the tarsal sheath
- the carpal sheath

Bursoscopy

This procedure allows inspection and treatment of:

- the bicipital bursa
- the navicular bursa
- the calcaneal bursa.

It is most commonly used for treating infection of these structures.

6

CONDITIONS OF THE HORSE'S FOOT

THE HORSE'S FOOT

Anatomy of the foot

The horse's foot consists of the protective hoof and all the structures contained within it. The hoof is modified skin. The wall, sole, frog and periople are derived from the epidermis; the underlying sensitive laminae and the sensitive tissues of the sole, frog, periople and coronet are derived from the dermis.

External structures

The periople, the hoof wall, the sole and the frog make up the external structures of the foot (Figure 6.1).

PERIOPLE

The periople is a band of soft, pale grey horn which extends a variable distance down the hoof wall. It bridges the junction between the skin and the hoof wall. It is widest at the heels where it merges with the frog. It has the important function of restricting evaporation of moisture from the horn.

HOOF WALL

The hoof wall extends from the coronary band to the ground surface. It is divided into the **toe**, the **quarters** and the **heels**. The wall is thickest at the toe, where most protection is needed, becoming thinner and more elastic at the heels which expand when the foot bears weight. It is reflected forwards from the heels to form the **bars**, which can be seen when the foot is viewed from the ground surface (Figures 6.2a and b).

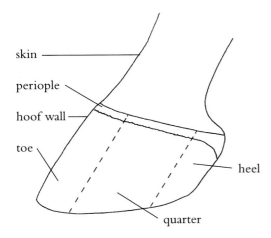

Figure 6.1 External structures of the hoof

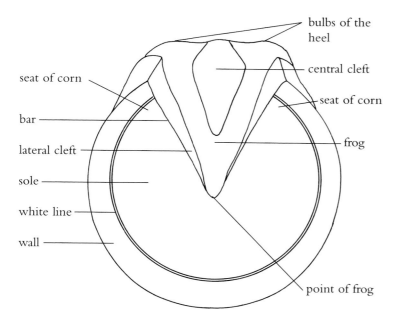

- bulbs of the heel
- central cleft
- seat of corn
- seat of corn
- bar
- frog
- lateral cleft
- sole
- white line
- wall
- point of frog

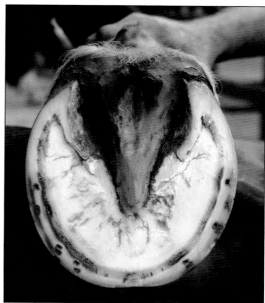

Figure 6.2a and b Ground surface of a front foot

When the horse stands on a hard surface, its weight is taken by the hoof wall and the outer rim of the sole. However, the weight is not evenly distributed around the hoof wall. Most is taken by the heels and at the junction between the toe and the quarter on either side of the hoof. In an unshod horse, the bars and the frog may also take some of the weight. On a soft surface, the sole helps to support the horse's weight.

The internal surface of the hoof wall has approximately **600 horny** or **insensitive laminae**. These interdigitate with the sensitive laminae on the surface of the **pedal bone**. This interlinking of the sensitive and insensitive laminae holds the pedal bone firmly in position.

Hoof growth

The hoof wall grows down from the **coronary band** at the rate of 6–10 mm ($\frac{2}{10}$–$\frac{4}{10}$ in) a month. It grows fastest at the toe. It takes approximately 6 months for the horn produced at the coronet to reach the ground at the heels and 9–12 months to reach the toe.

Hoof rings

The wall is normally smooth, but variation of growth rate due to diseases such as laminitis and dietary changes can cause horizontal rings to develop on the surface of the hoof (Figure 6.3).

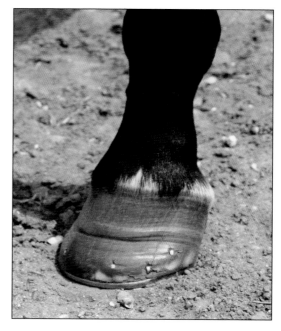

Figure 6.3 Hoof ring due to nutritional change

THE SOLE

The function of the sole is to protect the underlying sensitive structures and to help support the weight of the horse. Its concave shape ensures that on a firm surface, only the outer rim bears the horse's weight.

The thickness and concavity of the sole vary between individual horses. Some have very thin, flat soles that are more prone to puncture wounds and bruising than those with thick, concave soles. A thin-soled horse will be more sensitive and sore when moving on stony ground.

The area of sole in the angle between the outer hoof wall and the bars is known as the **seat of corn**. The junction between the sole and the hoof wall is called the **white line**. This narrow ring of soft, unpigmented horn is a useful landmark for the farrier. It shows the thickness of the hoof wall and indicates the position of the sensitive tissues which lie immediately inside it.

THE FROG

The frog is a triangular pad of soft, elastic horn which has a central cleft and deeper clefts on each side. In the unshod horse standing on a firm surface it may or may not contact the ground and support some of the horse's weight, depending on the conformation of the sole. It does help to support the weight of horses working on soft surfaces.

The frog and sole are composed of horn which is softer than that of the wall and constantly flakes away. Any ragged pieces of frog should be trimmed to prevent them trapping dirt and harbouring bacteria.

Internal structures

The internal structures of the foot (Figure 6.4) include the:

- pedal bone
- navicular bone
- distal end of the second phalanx
- coffin joint
- navicular bursa
- cartilages of the foot
- insertions of the deep digital flexor tendon and the common digital extensor tendon
- digital cushion
- sensitive laminae
- ligaments, blood vessels and nerves.

The **coffin joint** or **distal interphalangeal joint** extends between the **pedal bone (distal phalanx) (P3), the second phalanx (P2)** and the **navicular bone**. The **deep digital flexor tendon** passes over the navicular bone and attaches to the pedal bone. The **navicular bursa**, a fluid-filled sac, cushions the movement of the deep digital flexor

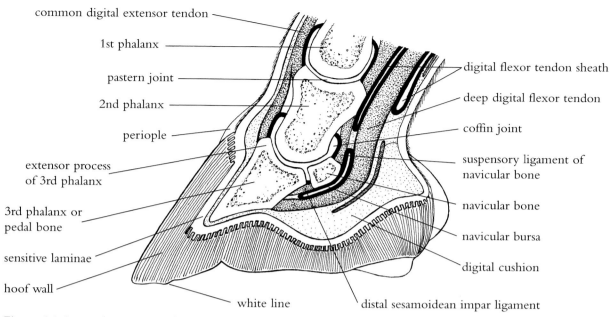

common digital extensor tendon

1st phalanx

pastern joint

2nd phalanx

periople

extensor process
of 3rd phalanx

3rd phalanx or
pedal bone

sensitive laminae

hoof wall

white line

digital flexor tendon sheath

deep digital flexor tendon

coffin joint

suspensory ligament of
navicular bone

navicular bone

navicular bursa

digital cushion

distal sesamoidean impar ligament

Figure 6.4 Internal structures of the foot

tendon over the navicular bone. The **common digital extensor tendon** attaches to the extensor process on the front of the pedal bone.

The **cartilages** of the foot (Figure 6.5) are attached to either side of the pedal bone. They project above the coronet and are easily palpated. They are normally springy, but may become hard and unyielding due to deposition of bone (**sidebone**).

The **digital cushion**, consisting of fibrous, elastic and fatty tissue, occupies the space between the frog and the cartilages towards the back of the foot. It has the important function of absorbing concussion.

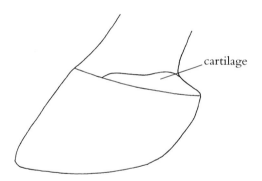

cartilage

Figure 6.5 The position of the lateral cartilages of the foot

Routine care of the feet

As the horse's feet are by far the commonest cause of lameness, regular care helps to prevent problems developing.

DAILY HOOF CARE

- The feet should be picked out at least once a day and certainly before and after exercise. Special attention should be paid to thorough cleaning of the clefts of the frog.
- The shoes should be inspected for risen clenches and any movement away from the hoof wall.
- The bedding of stabled horses should be kept clean and dry to prevent diseases such as thrush.

- Horses and ponies at grass should have a well-drained area to stand on so the hoof does not become excessively soft and crumbly.

TRIMMING

Trimming is required every 4–6 weeks. The farrier uses his skill to maintain or restore the correct hoof conformation. Without regular trimming, the hoof wall may become split and misshapen.

SHOEING

Shoeing is necessary to prevent excessive wear of the feet when horses work on hard surfaces.

The principles of trimming and shoeing

Correct trimming and shoeing is essential for long-term soundness of the working horse. Most horses are reshod every 4–6 weeks. If they are left for any longer the following problems may arise.

- The foot will become unbalanced because the hoof wall grows faster at the toe than the heels. The wall at the heels may be worn by the shoe as the heels expand and contract; hence more horn is usually removed from the toe when shod horses are trimmed.
- The hoof wall may grow over the outside edge of the shoe at the heels; the shoe then presses on the sole at the seat of corn causing bruising and lameness (Figure 6.6).
- The clenches begin to rise and can cause brushing injuries.
- If a loose shoe is wrenched off, the nails may tear away large chunks of hoof wall, making subsequent shoeing difficult (Figure 6.7).
- The horse may suffer serious injury by treading on the nails of a twisted or cast shoe.

Unshod horses and youngsters still require trimming every 4–6 weeks. This allows any potential problems to be dealt with promptly.

Assessment of foot balance

- The farrier will assess the horse in motion and standing square. He will observe:
- the horse's conformation and action
- how the hoof contacts the ground
- any abnormal wear on the shoes
- whether there are any signs of lameness
- the shape and balance of the hoof including the:
  - hoof-pastern axis and balance between the front and back of the foot (dorsopalmar balance)
  - the mediolateral balance
  - whether the front feet are a matching pair.

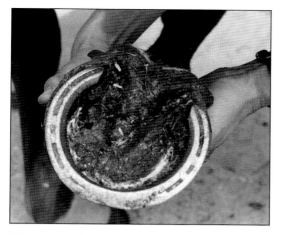

Figure 6.6 This shoe has moved off the hoof wall at the heels and is pressing on the sole

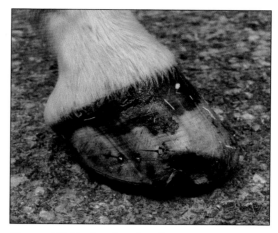

Figure 6.7 Broken hoof wall

HOOF–PASTERN AXIS AND DORSOPALMAR BALANCE

This is observed from the side view of the foot. In a balanced foot:

- a line drawn along the dorsal surface of the hoof wall should be parallel with an imaginary line drawn through the centre of the first phalanx or along the dorsal aspect of the pastern; this is the hoof-pastern axis (Figure 6.8)
- the hoof wall at the toe should be parallel to the hoof wall at the heel
- a vertical line drawn through the centre of the cannon bone should reach the ground at the back of the weight-bearing part of the heel
- when viewed from the ground surface, the width of the forefeet should approximately equal the length of the foot.

Radiographic views

On a lateral view of the foot:

- the front of the pedal bone and the anterior hoof wall should be parallel
- the hoof-pastern axis should be straight
- the lower border of the pedal bone should form a 2–10 degree angle with the ground surface, with the caudal (back) part of the pedal bone being slightly higher than the front.

Dorsopalmar imbalance may be caused by:

- incorrect or infrequent trimming
- leaving the shoes on too long
- using shoes that are too short at the heels

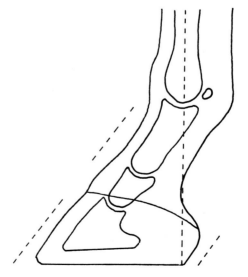

Figure 6.8 Normal hoof-pastern axis in a well-balanced foot

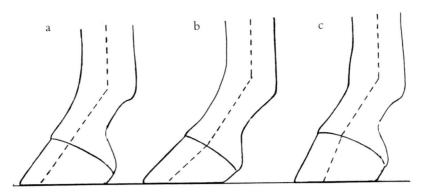

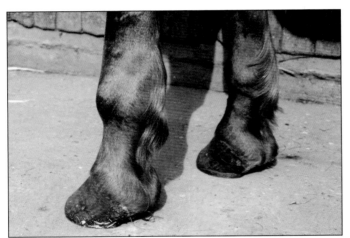

Figure 6.9 Side view of foot to show a) normal, b) broken-back and c) broken-forward hoof-pastern axes

Figure 6.10 Broken-back hoof-pastern axis

- there may be a genetic predisposition to this conformation in some Thoroughbreds.

The most common imbalance is a broken-back hoof-pastern axis with long toes and low heels (see page 147) (Figures 6.9 and 6.10).

MEDIOLATERAL BALANCE

When the hoof is viewed from the front:

- a line drawn across the coronary band should be parallel to the ground (Figure 6.11)
- a vertical line drawn down the centre of the cannon and pastern bones should divide the foot into two equal halves
- when the foot is lifted and viewed from the above the heels, imaginary lines drawn down the centre of the limb and across the heels should form 90 degree angles (Figure 6.12).

Radiographic views

When radiographs are taken from the front of the foot to check the mediolateral balance:

- the lower surface of the pedal bone should be parallel to the ground
- the coffin joint should be parallel to the ground and the joint space should be even from side to side.

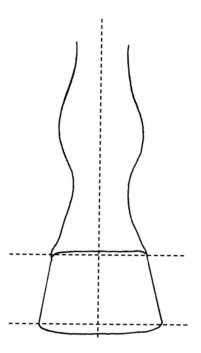

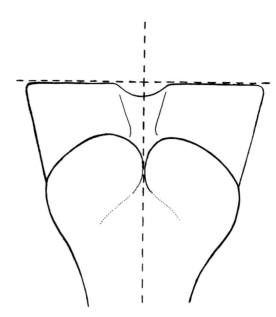

Figure 6.11 A foot with normal mediolateral balance

Figure 6.12 Checking the hoof balance: the foot is lifted and viewed from directly above the heels

Mediolateral imbalance may be caused by:

- poor trimming technique
- poor conformation which puts more stress on one side of the foot causing it to grow more slowly than the other side
- the use of road studs or nails on one side of the foot.

The effects of mediolateral imbalance include:

- hoof distortion and pain from laminar tearing
- sheared heels
- thrush
- sore heels
- quarter or heel cracks
- sidebone
- pedal osteitis
- inflammation and osteoarthritis of the fetlock, pastern and coffin joints.

Correcting a hoof imbalance requires skill and experience and will take time. The conformation and gait of the horse need to be taken into consideration. It is not always possible to achieve perfect foot balance in every horse and inappropriate attempts to achieve it can cause a sound horse to become lame.

Helping the farrier

Shoeing horses is a skilled and physically demanding job that requires dedication and patience. There are many ways in which you can help your farrier and so build up a good relationship.

- Book the correct number of horses.
- Give advance warning if a particular horse is likely to be difficult and require extra time.
- Have the horses in and ready with clean legs and feet when the farrier arrives.
- Provide a swept, hard and non-slip standing area with good light and protection from bad weather.
- Train youngsters to allow their legs to be handled and lifted.
- If a horse cannot be tied up safely, ensure that someone is available to hold it.
- Do not apply any hoof dressing before the farrier arrives.

Accidents associated with shoeing

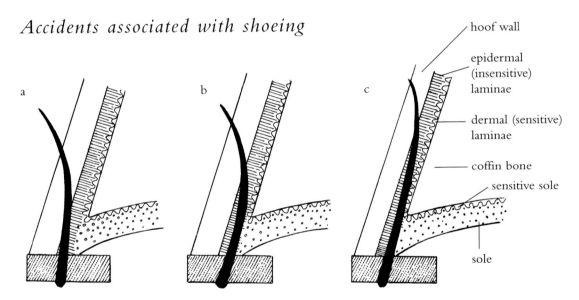

Figure 6.13 Nail positions: a) good nail; b) close nail; c) nail prick

NAIL BIND

Occasionally a nail is driven too close to the sensitive laminae when the shoe is nailed onto the foot (Figure 6.13b). This can cause pressure on the sensitive tissues. It may cause immediate lameness but the symptoms may not develop for a couple of hours or until the horse is worked (Figure 6.14).

The problem nail can be located by applying hoof testers or gentle tapping with a hammer. The horse flinches in pain and withdraws its foot when the painful site is reached.

If the nail is removed, the horse may become sound immediately. Sometimes the horse needs to be rested or have the foot poulticed for a couple of days to allow the inflammation to subside and the lameness to resolve.

NAIL PRICK

If the nail actually penetrates the sensitive structures, this is known as 'nail prick' (Figure 6.13c). The horse will often jump and pull its foot away as the accident happens. Lameness usually occurs immediately. At rest, the horse will often point the foot, paw the ground or keep lifting the affected foot.

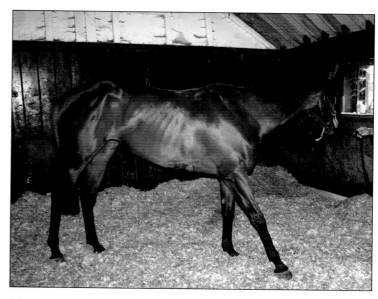

Figure 6.14 A horse with nail bind

Treatment

- The offending nail should be removed at once.
- There may be a little blood as it is removed from the foot.
- The hole should be flushed with an antiseptic such as povidone-iodine (Pevidine®) or hydrogen peroxide, or the foot can be tubbed or poulticed.
- The hole should be plugged to prevent contamination with soil and droppings.
- The horse should be kept in and observed for increased lameness over the next couple of days.
- If lameness develops or persists, the farrier or vet will remove the shoe and open a drainage hole to release any pus.
- The injury is now treated as a puncture wound (see pages 70 and 129)
- The tetanus vaccination status of the horse must be checked. If there is any uncertainty, tetanus antitoxin is administered.

If the problem is not recognized immediately, the horse is likely to become severely lame as an abscess develops. The infection can track up the white line and may cause pus to discharge from the coronary band.

SUPERFICIAL PUNCTURE WOUNDS, PUS IN THE FOOT, UNDERRUN SOLE

Hoof punctures are the commonest cause of lameness in the horse. They can lead to infection where pus and gas build up under pressure within the rigid hoof, thus causing severe pain.

Causes

- Penetration of the sole or white line by a sharp object such as a flint or a nail.
- Infection of a deep bruise.
- Accidental pricking of the sensitive tissues by the farrier.

Clinical signs

These include some or all of the following.

- Lameness. This may be slight to start with but can quickly progress and become severe. The horse may point the limb and avoid taking any weight on the affected part of the foot. For example, if the infection is near the heel, the horse will walk on its toe. Sometimes the horse will refuse to bear any weight on the affected limb (Figure 6.15).
- The horse is often found in some distress. When the pain is really severe, the horse may sweat, tremble and have fast, shallow respirations.
- Increased heat in the foot.
- An abnormally strong digital pulse on the affected limb.
- Swelling of the lower limb.
- Sensitivity to pressure from hoof testers.
- Loss of appetite.

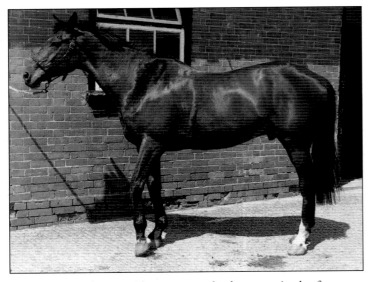

Figure 6.15 A horse with a punctured sole or pus in the foot may be reluctant to bear weight on the affected limb

As the pressure builds up inside the foot, the pus is forced along the path of least resistance. Where there is no drainage hole, it runs under the sole and up the white line. An area of the coronary band may become swollen and tender before bursting to release the pus.

If you suspect your horse has pus in the foot:

- contact the vet or farrier at once
- clean the foot and look for any obvious wound
- check the horse's tetanus vaccine is up to date
- apply a poultice and keep the horse stabled on a clean, dry bed.

Diagnosis

The diagnosis is made on the clinical signs and by examination of the sole of the foot. The site of penetration may be obvious. If not, hoof testers can be used gently to locate the most painful area. Paring a thin layer of horn from the sole with a hoof knife often reveals a small black mark in the sensitive area of the foot. Gentle pressure from the hoof testers may force black material from the lesion, confirming that this is the infected area. When the wound is on or close to the white line, it is necessary to remove the shoe.

Treatment

The aim of treatment is to drain the abscess and prevent reinfection.

DRAINAGE OF THE ABSCESS

A small area of the sole is removed to allow the escape of pus which may forcefully spurt from the wound (Figure 6.16). This often brings immediate

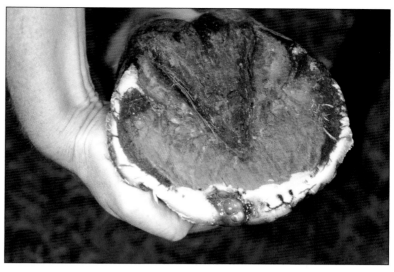

Figure 6.16 A draining abscess; bubbles of gas are released with the pus

relief. If the horn is very hard, it is sometimes necessary to poultice the foot overnight to make locating and draining the abscess easier. With a deep-seated abscess, more than one examination may be required before the infection is located. Occasionally a horse will not tolerate any attempt to drain the abscess and light sedation or nerve blocks are required.

ELIMINATING THE INFECTION

The *whole* foot should be thoroughly cleaned.

- Scrub off any mud, droppings or bedding material.
- Tub the foot in a bucket with warm water and Epsom salts (magnesium sulphate – approximately 1 tablespoon to 5 litres [8 pt] of water) to draw out the infection.
- Irrigate the hole with a dilute solution of an oxidizing agent such as hydrogen peroxide to discourage the growth of anaerobic bacteria. A syringe can be used for this procedure.
- Poultice or bandage the foot (see pages 74–78). The wound should be protected from contamination by using suitable dressings or a special boot.

Tubbing and/or poulticing is recommended once or twice daily until there is no more discharge (Figure 6.17). Poultices are not normally applied for longer than 3 days except following veterinary advice as they make the tissues very soggy and may slow healing.

ANTIBIOTICS

Oral or injectable antibiotics are rarely necessary and they may not penetrate into the damaged hoof tissues. In some cases they can *prolong* the period of lameness if administered before drainage is established.

They are likely to be prescribed:

- with deep penetrations of the foot

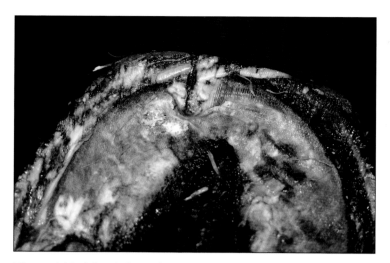

Figure 6.17 After 3 days of poulticing, all the pus has drained from this foot

- where drainage has been established but the swelling of the leg increases
- to help prevent infection of fresh wounds that are detected and treated before any pus has formed.

Antibiotic solutions that treat anaerobic infections are sometimes used to flush the foot cavity.

PAINKILLERS

A non-steroidal anti-inflammatory drug, e.g. phenylbutazone is frequently given for the first 24 hours to alleviate the pain.

TETANUS PROTECTION

Horses with foot wounds are at high risk of developing tetanus. If there is any doubt about the horse's vaccination status, tetanus antitoxin is given. This is not a vaccine but it affords immediate protection for a short period of time while the full vaccination programme is started.

Recovery

When there is no more discharge, the hoof should be covered with a dry dressing and inspected regularly until new horn has begun to grow over the sensitive tissues. Occasionally granulation tissue may form at the site of the opened abscess and treatment may be required to remove it. Once the area appears clean and healthy the horse can be shod with a protective pad to protect the healing area from further injury.

Prognosis

The prognosis for uncomplicated puncture wounds and abscesses is good.

DEEP PENETRATIONS OF THE FOOT

Deep penetrations of the foot are potentially serious and the vet should always be consulted.

Warning

If the foreign body, e.g. a nail or metal spike is still in the foot, it is very important for the vet to know the angle and depth of penetration. This can be established by taking an X-ray *before* the object is removed. If there is no danger of the foreign body penetrating any deeper, leave it where it is. If on the other hand, the horse is likely to drive it deeper into the tissues by taking weight on the foot, it must be removed. Make a note of the angle of penetration and the length of the foreign body that was inside the foot, then protect the foot with a clean dressing.

Shallow penetrations of the foot are unlikely to result in complications. The risks associated with deep penetrations vary with the location of the injury (Figures 6.18a and b). Deep penetrations in the front third of the foot may result in fracture or infection of the pedal bone. Injuries to the back two thirds of the foot put the following structures at risk:

- the coffin joint
- the navicular bone
- the navicular bursa
- the deep digital flexor tendon and its sheath.

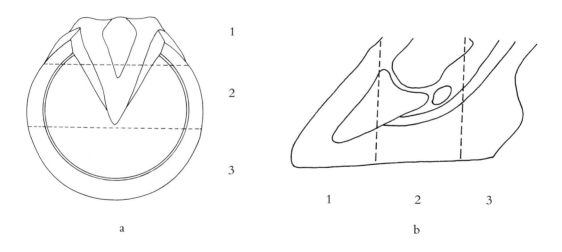

Figures 6.18a and b Foot divided into 3 regions: a) ground surface of the foot; b) section through the foot

Clinical signs and diagnosis

If the foreign body is still in place then the diagnosis is straightforward. In other cases, it can be difficult to establish the extent of the injury without further investigations. There may be no obvious signs shortly after the accident occurs. Penetrations of the frog are particularly difficult to locate as the elastic nature of the horn means that the puncture hole seals leaving very little trace of the injury. Sometimes increased warmth of the foot and an obvious digital pulse are detected. Lameness is variable to start with but quickly becomes severe if vital structures are damaged and become infected. The degree of lower limb swelling is variable depending on which structures are damaged.

As with superficial penetrations, the site of entry may be found with the aid of hoof testers and scraping away the superficial layers of horn.

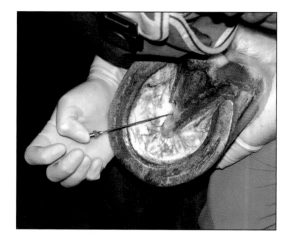

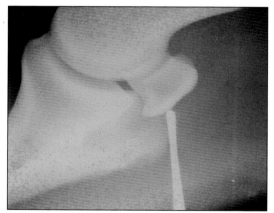

RADIOGRAPHIC EXAMINATION

Special radiographic techniques are often used to help with the diagnosis. Once the entry hole has been found, a sterile metal probe (Figures 6.19 and 6.20) or a fluid which shows up on the X-rays (contrast medium) may be introduced into the hole before the X-rays are taken. These assist the vet in determining the extent and potential seriousness of the injury. However, both of these techniques incur the risk of introducing infection and there is a risk of accidental penetration of synovial structures with a probe. Another diagnostic technique is to inject the coffin joint, navicular bursa or digital sheath with a contrast medium using a sterile technique and then X-ray it to see if the contrast agent leaks out into the penetrating tract (Figure 6.21).

Damage to bone may not show up on the radiographs until 10–14 days after the injury occurs and repeat examinations may be required.

Figure 6.19 Determining the depth of a frog penetration with a sterile metal probe

Figure 6.20 On an X-ray, the metal probe shows that the navicular bursa is likely to have been penetrated

EXAMINATION OF SYNOVIAL FLUID

If penetration of the coffin joint or navicular bursa is suspected, fluid will be aspirated and examined. An elevated white cell count and increased protein level is indicative of infection. The samples can also be cultured to identify specific bacteria and their sensitivity to different antibiotics.

Treatment

Treatment depends on which structures have been damaged. It is likely to include:

- broad spectrum antibiotics
- non-steroidal anti-inflammatory drugs to alleviate the inflammation and pain
- tetanus antitoxin
- surgery to remove any infected or damaged tissue

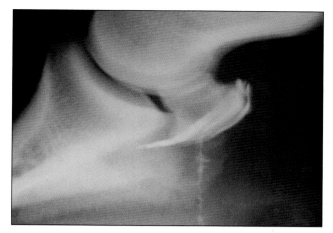

Figure 6.21 Leaking contrast medium confirms penetration of the navicular bursa

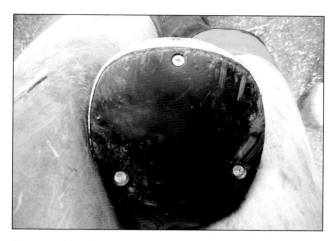

Figure 6.22 A hospital plate is used to protect the sole

- flushing of infected synovial structures.

Following these emergency treatments, the sole is protected by bandaging. Once the wound begins to heal, a special shoe with a removable metal plate, known as a hospital plate (Figure 6.22), can be used to protect the sole.

Prognosis

The prognosis depends on which structures are damaged and how quickly the horse is given the necessary treatment. Deep punctures that do not damage vital structures carry a good prognosis. Deep penetrations in the frog region have a guarded prognosis.

POOR HORN QUALITY

In some horses the hoof wall and sole is relatively thin and the growth rate is unusually slow. Despite regular trimming and shoeing, the walls tend to crack and so securing a shoe becomes increasingly difficult. The nails are then driven too close to cracks and previous nail holes, further weakening the wall.

Causes

- Genetic predisposition. Some horses suffer with weak hoof walls throughout their lives.
- Poor nutrition. The diet should provide an adequate supply of important nutrients such as biotin and methionine and the correct calcium/phosphorus balance.
- Unhealthy environment. Standing for long periods in soiled, wet bedding weakens the hooves and encourages infection.

- Very dry conditions. Under these conditions the hoof wall loses moisture and becomes less flexible so cracks develop.
- Very wet conditions. If a horse is kept in a very wet environment, the hooves become very soft and tend to spread out and flatten. Soft soles are susceptible to bruising.
- Inadequate hoof care. Regular trimming is necessary to maintain hoof balance and shape. Long or unbalanced feet are likely to develop hoof wall cracks.
- Persistent bacterial and fungal infection of the horn. Once established, these micro-organisms continually weaken the horn especially where there are cracks, and hoof wall and white line lesions.
- Lack of exercise. Exercise influences the blood supply to the sensitive laminae. Moisture diffuses from the blood and lymph vessels in the sensitive laminae outwards to the insensitive laminae and the hoof wall. The circulation may be reduced without sufficient exercise.

Treatment and Prevention
FEED A BALANCED DIET

If in any doubt about your horse's diet, consult your vet or a nutritionist. Problems often arise with horses and ponies that are 'good doers' and look well on poor pasture and little else. These animals benefit from a balanced vitamin and mineral supplement. There are many commercially produced supplements available, a number of which specifically address the nutritional needs of horses with poor quality hoof horn, e.g. Life Data Farrier's Formula® or Equi Life Formula Feet™. These supplements contain biotin, methionine and zinc amongst other ingredients.

Alfalfa is a good source of available dietary calcium. Bran should be avoided as it is high in phosphorus and reduces the availability of dietary calcium to the horse.

HAVE THE FEET REGULARLY TRIMMED AND SHOD

The importance of regular trimming has already been discussed. Shoes that are allowed to become loose are at risk of being pulled off, causing further damage to the hoof wall. If the hoof wall is too weak for conventional shoeing, glue-on shoes often provide a temporary solution while the damaged area grows out. Because no nails are used, the stress on the hoof wall is considerably reduced (Figure 6.23).

ENSURE THE HORN DOES NOT BECOME EXCESSIVELY DRY

Approximately 15–20% of the outer hoof wall and 45% of the inner hoof wall is water. This needs to remain fairly constant for the horn to maintain its strength and

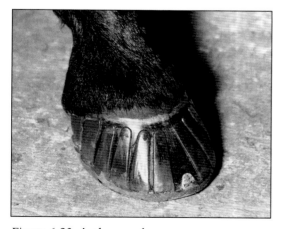

Figure 6.23 A glue-on shoe

elasticity. Where the horn is too dry it becomes brittle and cracked; if it is too moist it becomes soft and crumbly. A balance has to be established between evaporation and absorption of moisture from the hoof surface and the diffusion of moisture from blood vessels in the underlying sensitive tissues. This is effectively controlled by the waxy periople and the hard outer layer of the hoof wall under normal conditions.

The value of hoof oil and other dressings is the subject of much debate. In some situations they are helpful. If the horn is very dry, application of a lanolin-based hoof dressing may be beneficial. The best person to advise you on this is your farrier who is familiar with your horse and the environment in which it is kept.

AVOID VERY WET ENVIRONMENTS

If at all possible, remove horses from very wet pastures during the winter. Keep bedding material clean and dry.

TREAT INFECTED HORN WITH A TOPICAL HOOF DISINFECTANT

Encouraging results have been reported from a study where diseased horn was treated with a hoof disinfectant consisting of an iodine preparation in tea tree oil (Life Data Laboratories). Some horses improved within 3 weeks and the horn quality of all the horses in the study was considerably improved after 12 weeks

TRY TO KEEP THE HORSE IN WORK

Regular exercise is important for the normal function and blood supply of the foot. It is well known that long hours of stabling or box rest can lead to foot problems. If the horse has weak and damaged hoof walls, regular light exercise in a suitable environment is beneficial. Road work, hard ground and deep mud should be avoided if possible until sufficient good quality horn has grown for the shoe to be nailed on securely.

APPLICATION OF MILD BLISTERS TO THE CORONARY BAND

In some horses, daily massaging of the coronary band with mildly irritant substances, e.g. Cornucrescine® increases the local blood supply and is reported to improve the growth rate of the horn.

PROMPT TREATMENT OF CRACKS AND OTHER HOOF WALL DEFECTS

As soon as cracks begin to develop, consult your farrier. Prompt remedial action may prevent a more serious problem developing.

HOOF WALL CRACKS

Hoof wall cracks are splits in the hoof wall. They are described according to:

- location, i.e. toe, quarter or heel
- depth, i.e. superficial or full wall thickness
- site of origin, i.e. ground surface or coronary band
- orientation, i.e. vertical or horizontal
- length
- whether or not they are infected.

Grass cracks are vertical cracks that begin at the ground surface and extend upwards. They occur when hooves spread and split due to inadequate or infrequent trimming (Figures 6.24 and 6.25).

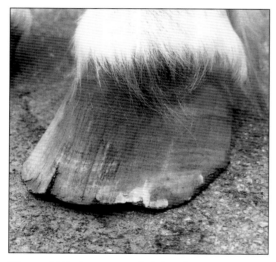

Figure 6.24 A grass crack is just beginning to develop

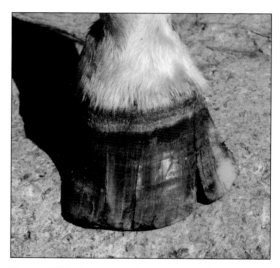

Figure 6.25 A more serious grass crack

Sand cracks are also vertical. They begin at the coronary band and extend downwards. They usually occur as a result of injury to the coronary band. If the tissues of the coronary band recover and start to produce normal horn again, the crack will grow out over a period of time. Serious injury to a local area of the coronary band results in a permanent crack down the whole length of the wall (Figure 6.26).

Quarter cracks are full thickness cracks at the quarters of the foot (Figure 6.27).

Horizontal cracks extend horizontally round the hoof wall. They are caused by an injury to the coronary band or a blow to the hoof wall.

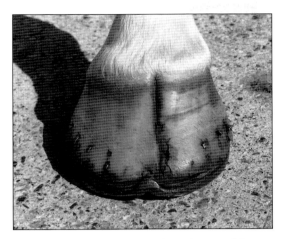

Figure 6.26 Permanent sand crack caused by a coronary band injury

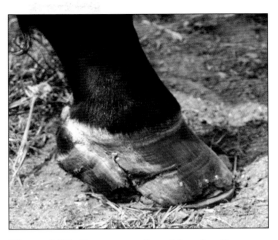

Figure 6.27 Quarter crack and hoof wall deformity due to an injury

Superficial cracks only involve the outer hoof wall and do not reach the laminae.

Deep cracks involve the full thickness of the hoof wall. These often result in lameness due to infection or pinching of the underlying sensitive tissues.

Causes

These include:

- injury to the coronary band or hoof wall as a result of trauma or infection
- irregular hoof trimming so the feet become overgrown and split (Figure 6.28)
- hoof imbalance causing uneven stresses in the hoof wall as the horse moves
- poor hoof conformation, e.g. long toe, low heel or underrun heels
- limb conformation, e.g. if the horse has toe-out conformation, the medial hoof wall is subjected to increased stress and may develop quarter cracks; toe-in conformation predisposes to lateral quarter cracks
- inappropriate shoeing, e.g. shoeing too short predisposes to quarter cracks
- poor hoof quality
- poor diet or inappropriate nutrition, e.g. excess selenium can produce hoof problems
- too much exercise on hard or rough ground
- very wet or very dry conditions; alternating wet and dry conditions
- hoof deformity.

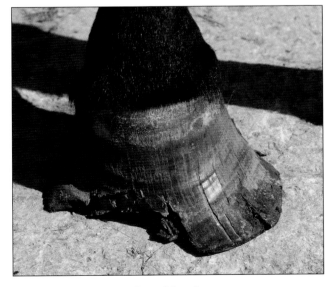

Figure 6.28 A very neglected hoof

Clinical signs

Superficial cracks do not cause any problems. Horizontal cracks rarely result in lameness. With full thickness cracks, the outer hoof wall becomes unstable and the sensitive tissues are pinched and bruised between the edges of the crack. Infection may enter the sensitive tissues resulting in pain and lameness. Blood or black pus may seep from the crack especially after exercise. The lameness may be gradual or sudden in onset. Heel and quarter cracks are the most likely to cause lameness as the wall is thinner in this region of the hoof. Quarter cracks in particular are associated with acute and severe lameness.

Diagnosis

Diagnosis is made on the appearance of the crack and the response to hoof testers applied over or close to it. Local nerve blocks may help to rule out other causes of lameness if there is any uncertainty about the origin of the pain.

Treatment

Once cracks have formed, they do not 'heal' as the outer hoof wall consists of non-living material. The aim of treatment is to prevent them becoming infected or more extensive, so they grow out with time. Depending on the use of the horse, the exercise programme may have to be modified to prevent excessive strain on the hoof wall.

SUPERFICIAL CRACKS

Restoration of hoof balance, regular trimming and appropriate shoeing is usually sufficient to prevent these from developing into a more serious problem. A full bar shoe with clips on either side of the crack minimizes any movement of the hoof wall and stabilizes the foot.

The farrier may use a burr to create a horizontal line at the upper limit of a grass crack to discourage it extending upwards to the coronary band. This should go through the hoof wall to the depth of the white line. Application of a hoof disinfectant (e.g. Life Data Hoof Disinfectant™) will help prevent bacterial and fungal infection of the exposed horn within the cracks.

DEEP, INFECTED CRACKS

All of the dead and infected material must be removed before any attempt is made to repair the defect. The farrier or vet may use a motorized tool to widen the crack and expose infection that is hidden underneath the horn. The infection is treated by thorough cleaning and applications of hoof antiseptics such as iodine for at least 48 hours. Poulticing may be necessary for a couple of days and painkillers are sometimes used in the early stages of treatment. Once the infection has resolved and the hoof is dry, there are a number of ways in which the defect can be closed.

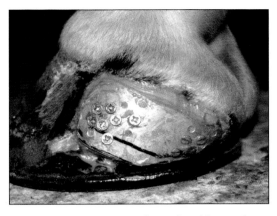

Figure 6.29 Quarter crack repair with metal plate

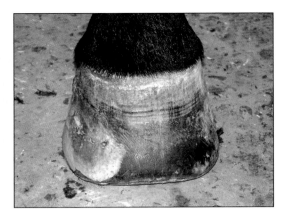

Figure 6.30 Hoof repair with acrylic material

STABILIZING THE DEFECT

This can be achieved by:

- drilling holes on either side of the crack and lacing it up with thick metal wire; the remaining defect is then filled with acrylic or fibreglass
- the use of short screws drilled into the hoof wall on either side of the crack and wire sutures across the crack
- screwing a metal plate across the defect (Figure 6.29)
- glue-on plastic patches
- repair with acrylic materials that bond to the hoof wall (Figure 6.30); these may be impregnated with antibiotics
- repair with glue.

Severe heel cracks are sometimes treated by removing the hoof wall behind the crack and applying a heart bar shoe to provide support while the new hoof wall grows down. All horses with deep hoof wall cracks should be protected against tetanus.

SUBSEQUENT TRIMMING AND SHOEING

Horses with severe cracks are shod with heart bar shoes to give maximum support and stability to the hoof wall. If the crack is at the toe, squaring the toe of the shoe brings the point of breakover back from the dorsal hoof wall and reduces the stress on this part of the hoof wall. The crack should be closely monitored during subsequent shoeings. Painkillers are used for the minimum period as the absence of pain and lameness is one method of assessing the continued success of the treatment. Every effort should be made to correct any faults of hoof conformation which predisposed the horse to the condition.

Prognosis

The prognosis is generally good.

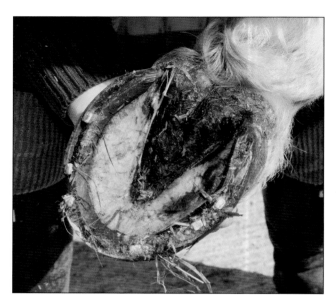

Figure 6.31 Thrush infection of the frog

CRACKED HEELS

Some horses are prone to developing painful cracks in the bulbs of the heels. These may be prevented by regular application of a lanolin-containing ointment or other barrier cream in susceptible horses (see Mud Fever on page 522 for more information).

THRUSH

Thrush is a bacterial infection which affects the frog. The horn decomposes and forms black, necrotic material which collects in the clefts and has a characteristic and unpleasant smell. If left untreated the infection may spread into the underlying sensitive tissues and cause lameness (Figure 6.31).

Causes

The infection is caused by various bacteria that damage the horn including *Fusobacterium necrophorum*. A number of factors predispose to the development of the condition:

- poor stable hygiene with dirty, wet bedding
- continually wet pastures
- lack of daily hoof care
- shoeing with pads which trap moisture and dirt underneath them
- poor hoof conformation
- inadequate trimming
- deep frog clefts
- sheared heels
- contracted heels.

Clinical signs

- An unpleasant odour.
- Black discharge in the frog clefts.
- There may be tenderness when the area is probed with a hoof pick if the horn has been eroded and sensitive tissue exposed.
- Lameness. Recent infections rarely cause lameness but well-established infection with erosion of the horn and infection of the underlying tissues can cause severe lameness.

Treatment

- The foot is thoroughly cleaned and inspected.
- Any predisposing factors should be identified and removed if possible.
- The horse should be stabled with clean, dry bedding.
- The feet should be picked out twice daily.
- The frog is trimmed to remove any loose pieces of horn which could conceal pockets of dirt or infection. All diseased tissue is removed together with areas of the frog that have been undermined by bacterial infection.
- Where infection has entered the sensitive tissues of the foot it may need tubbing with Epsom salts and protecting with a dry bandage. Occasionally antibiotics are necessary in these cases. The tetanus vaccination status of the horse should be checked.
- If the sensitive tissues are not involved, trimming and topical treatment of the frog is all that is required, together with improved hygiene.

Topical treatments include:
- an antibiotic (oxytetracycline) spray
- a mixture containing phenol, iodine and 10% formalin
- copper sulphate solution
- a large number of preparations are now advertised for treating thrush.

Prognosis

The prognosis is good if the condition is treated early and the underlying cause can be removed. In horses with contracted heels and deep, narrow frog clefts it can be very difficult to clear up. Long-term corrective trimming and shoeing by the farrier may be required to improve the hoof conformation.

Prevention

The condition is easily prevented in most horses by regular hoof care and good stable hygiene. This is especially important in horses confined to their boxes for long periods.

CANKER

Canker is a disease that affects the epidermal (outer) tissues of the foot. The frog, bars, heels and sole of the foot are most commonly affected. It is caused by infection with bacteria including *Fusobacterium necrophorum* and *Bacteroides spp*. Horses living in damp conditions or kept on dirty, wet beds appear to be particularly at risk. It is most commonly seen in heavy horses.

Clinical signs

- The horn of the frog has an abnormally ragged appearance with loose, detached fronds of horn.
- The infection can spread from the frog to the bars, heels and sole. Occasionally the wall is involved.
- Tissue that resembles granulation tissue and bleeds easily may grow out from the affected areas.
- The foot has a very unpleasant odour.
- There is a variable degree of lameness depending on the extent and depth of the infection. When the deeper, sensitive structures of the foot are involved, the resultant inflammation causes pain and lameness.

Diagnosis

The diagnosis is made on the clinical signs. It may be confused with thrush.

Treatment

This involves the following.

- Removal of the diseased tissue, which may be performed under sedation or general anaesthesia and may need to be repeated.
- Topical treatment with metronidazole, an antibiotic effective against anaerobic bacteria; the dressings are usually changed daily for the first two weeks.
- Keeping the foot clean and dry – often under a hospital plate. This is a special shoe with a screw-on plate to protect the solar surface of the foot. Dressings can be applied underneath the plate.
- Long-term treatment over several weeks may be required.

Prognosis

The prognosis is reasonable if the condition is identified and treated early in the course of the disease, but there is a high rate of recurrence in some animals.

SHEARED HEELS

Sheared heels is a condition where there is instability of the tissues between the two heel bulbs so they move independently of one another.

Causes

The condition may be caused by:

- conformational faults causing mediolateral foot imbalance
- incorrect trimming so one heel and quarter is left longer than the other.

Horses with long-toe, low-heel conformation seem to be susceptible.

The longer side of the hoof is subjected to greater forces during weight bearing and this creates a shearing force between the two heel bulbs.

Clinical signs

- When viewed from behind, one heel bulb is higher than the other. The medial heel is usually displaced upwards (Figure 6.32).
- The hoof wall on the displaced side is often straight and upright while the hoof wall on the opposite side may be longer with an obvious flare.
- The coronary band is higher on the affected side.
- The central cleft of the frog may become deep and narrow, predisposing the horse to thrush.
- The horse is not invariably lame. When the condition does cause lameness it is usually mild to moderate and is due to heel soreness or a severe thrush infection.
- It is possible to have instability between the heel bulbs in a more normal shaped foot.

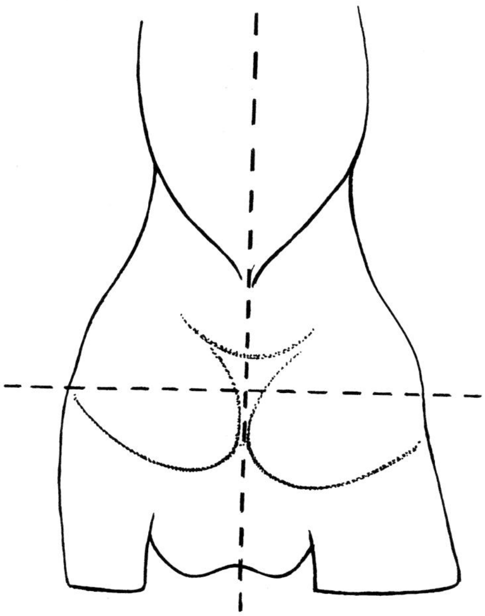

Diagnosis

The diagnosis is made on the appearance of the foot. Instability between the two heels can be observed if the heels move apart when they are grasped and twisted in opposite directions. This manipulation is often painful. The heels of a normal foot cannot be moved independently of one another.

When the horse is observed at walk, the medial heel often contacts the ground first and is displaced upwards as the foot bears weight.

Figure 6.32 Sheared heels: the heel bulb on the left is higher than the heel bulb on the right and it has a straighter and more upright hoof wall

Treatment

This involves the following.
- Correction of any mediolateral foot imbalance.
- Shortening the toe of horses with long-toe, low-heel conformation.
- Shoeing the foot with a bar shoe to provide stability to the heel region.
- The shoe should be set slightly wide on the upright medial side and any flare of the hoof wall on the lateral side should be removed.
- If the distortion is severe, it may take several trims over a period of months to correct it. The wall on the affected (displaced) side is sometimes trimmed so that it does not quite reach the bar shoe between the heel and the quarter. Over a period of time the heel may be forced back into alignment due to the body-weight of the horse.

Prognosis

The prognosis is good if the condition is detected and dealt with before severe instability occurs. Some affected horses require permanent heel support.

CONTRACTED HEELS

Causes

If a horse is lame for any period of time and takes less weight than normal on a particular limb, the foot and in particular the heels may become contracted. Other causes of heel contraction include the following.

- Dry, brittle horn. Without adequate moisture content the heels cannot expand normally when the foot bears weight.
- Lack of exercise is a contributory factor as the blood flow to the hoof is reduced and the moisture content of the horn decreases.
- Long-toe, low-heel conformation. As the foot becomes longer, the heels often move closer together.
- Incorrect shoeing, e.g. using a shoe that is too small or placing nails too far back on the hoof both restrict heel expansion.
- Long-term use of a full bar shoe, e.g. in a horse with a pedal bone fracture, often leads to contracted heels. Similarly a cast or restricting glue-on shoe can produce similar signs.

Clinical signs

The foot becomes narrower at the heel and the frog appears narrow and shrunken (Figure 6.33). The increased pressure on the sensitive tissues underneath may cause heel pain and lameness. The condition develops slowly over a period of time.

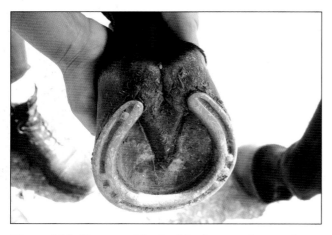

Figure 6.33 Contracted heels: this photograph was taken just before the horse was re-shod

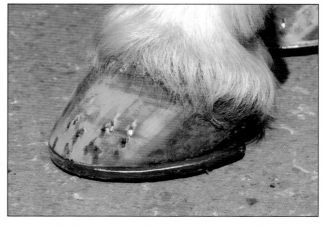

Figure 6.34 This foot has been shod wide and long to support the foot and allow the contracted heels to expand

Treatment

- Any underlying condition causing lameness should be diagnosed and treated.
- The foot should be trimmed to address any conformational defects, e.g. shortening of long toes.
- In the past, vertical grooves made in the hoof wall between the quarters and the heels were believed to encourage expansion of the foot. The value of this procedure is now questioned.
- The foot should be shod to encourage expansion of the heels, i.e. the foot should be shod wide and long (the shoe is fitted so that it is wider than the hoof wall at the quarters and heels and extends further backwards than the weight-bearing surface of the heels) (Figure 6.34).
- Increasing the level of exercise is beneficial.
- If the exercise cannot be increased, a dry, brittle foot may be soaked in wet bandages to increase its water content and encourage expansion. Topical preparations are available to seal the hoof and reduce evaporation of moisture.

BRUISED SOLES AND CORNS

Bruised soles are a common problem in horses with thin soles and flat feet. A bruise occurs when blood vessels underneath the sole are damaged. When the bruise occurs in the angle formed between the wall at the heels and the bars, it is known as a **corn**. Corns usually occur on the inner heel of the front feet (Figure 6.35).

Causes

Bruising can be caused by:

- the horse treading on a stone or other sharp object
- working on hard, rough ground
- wedging of a stone between the shoe and the sole
- pressure on the sole from shoes that are too small or incorrectly fitted
- shoes that have been left on for too long and press on the sole.

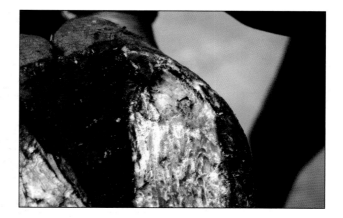

Figure 6.35 Bruising at the medial seat of corn

A number of factors predispose a horse to bruising. These include:

- thin or soft soles
- flat soles
- long-toe, low-heel conformation

- over-trimming of the hoof wall
- foot imbalance.

Clinical signs

Horses show variable degrees of lameness.

- Thin-soled horses may suddenly become acutely lame after stepping on a stone.
- Others show lameness for a couple of strides then continue normally.
- Some show temporary lameness at the time but come out of the stable lame the following day.
- Horses with mild bruising may only be lame on hard or uneven ground.
- If the bruising affects more than one foot, the horse may appear stiff or short-striding all round especially on hard ground. It may be reluctant to jump.

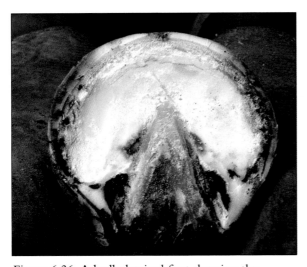

Figure 6.36 A badly bruised foot showing the discolouration on the bars

Horses with a corn may be continually or intermittently lame. The lameness is often worse when the horse turns or works on a circle.

Other symptoms include:

- withdrawal of the foot when hoof testers are applied to the affected area
- increased warmth in the foot
- increased digital pulse
- discolouration of the horn may be seen in unpigmented feet with bruising (Figure 6.36).

Bruises and corns can become infected. In these cases the lameness is usually much more severe and increases until the abscess is relieved.

Treatment

The first step is to identify and remove the cause of the problem. If the shoe is suspected as the cause or the problem is underneath it, then it is removed. In most other cases, the horse is usually more comfortable with the shoe left on. Treatment includes:

- box rest on a clean, deep bed
- poulticing the foot for a couple of days or regular tubbing to decrease the inflammation
- non-steroidal anti-inflammatory drugs to reduce the pain and inflammation
- light paring of the horn over the bruise or corn may alleviate the pressure and lameness; in a horse that repeatedly suffers from corns, the horn at the seat of corn should be pared lower than the hoof wall to avoid pressure from the shoe

- once the tubbing is finished the sole can be hardened by a phenol, formalin and iodine mixture before the horse is turned out or recommences work.

A number of shoeing systems are used to protect horses' feet from bruising. These include:
- the use of various types of protective pad
- wide web shoes that are seated-out to protect a larger area of the sole (Figure 6.37)
- the use of a bar shoe to distribute the pressure more widely over the heels.

If a bruise or corn becomes infected, it must be drained and treated as a foot abscess. A severe bruise can take up to 6 weeks to resolve. The horse must not be worked until it is sound.

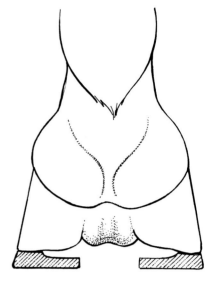

Figure 6.37 A wide web shoe protects the sole without applying pressure to it

Prognosis

The prognosis is good if the horse has good feet and the bruise was caused by stepping on a stone. However, if the horse has poor hoof conformation and is regularly worked on rough ground, recurrence is likely. Those with thin, flat soles and long-toe, low-heel conformation are the most susceptible. Chronic bruising can potentially lead to pedal bone changes such as osteitis.

LONG TOES AND LOW HEELS

Long toes and low, underrun heels are common faults of hoof conformation seen in the shod horse (Figure 6.38). They develop when the correct foot balance is not maintained by regular trimming and shoeing. As soon as the foot is trimmed and shod, there is a natural tendency for an imbalance to develop because the hoof grows faster at the toe than at the heels. There is minimal wear of the hoof wall at the toe whereas the wall at the heels experiences some wear from the shoe as the heels expand and contract.

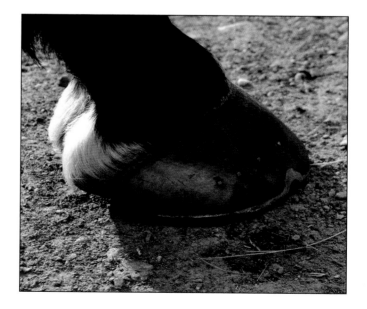

Figure 6.38 Long toe and underrun heels

Causes

- Infrequent trimming and leaving the shoes on too long.
- Trimming the heels too short and/or leaving the toe too long.
- Some Thoroughbreds have a genetic predisposition.

Clinical signs

- The toes become abnormally long and the heels too low.
- The hoof–pastern axis is broken back (see Figures 6.9 and 6.10).
- The angle between the anterior hoof wall and the ground surface gradually decreases as the toes lengthen.
- The angle of the hoof wall at the heel becomes progressively less than the angle of the hoof wall at the toe (Figure 6.39). When there is a discrepancy of more than 5 degrees the heels are said to be underrun. The altered hoof angle affects the normal blood flow through the hoof.
- The weight of the horse is shifted backwards and may cause the horn tubules of the heels to be crushed and collapse forwards.
- The front feet gradually lose their round shape and become more oval when viewed from the ground surface.
- As the hoof elongates, the heels become contracted.
- Lameness may result from:
  - increased tension on the deep digital flexor tendon and the navicular ligaments; horses with this type of conformation are susceptible to developing navicular syndrome and they often have heel pain
  - strain of the superficial digital flexor tendon
  - tearing of the laminae at the toe because the long toe and altered hoof angle increase the breakover time and impose increased strain on this area.

Breakover is the phase of the stride that starts when the heel begins to lift from the ground and ends when the toe leaves the ground. During breakover, the hoof rolls about

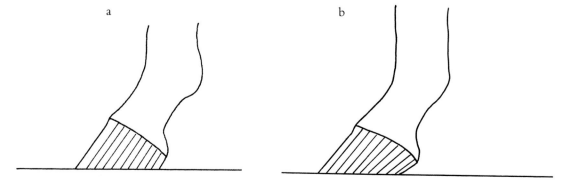

Figure 6.39 Underrun heels: a) normal hoof with parallel alignment of hoof tubules; b) underrun heel

45 degrees. The **point of breakover** is the furthest-forward part of the foot or shoe that is in contact with the ground when the heel begins to lift.

Long toes in the hind limbs may lead to hock and back pain. Radiographs of affected hind feet sometimes reveal that the orientation of the pedal bone within the foot is abnormal. The lower border of the pedal bone may become parallel with the ground surface or even tilted so that the toe of the pedal bone is higher than the heel area (rather than the normal 2–10 degree angle with the ground surface, and the back of the pedal bone slightly higher than the front).

Treatment

- The toe is trimmed as short as possible and the minimum amount is removed from the heels.
- Where the heels are very collapsed and underrun, they require some trimming in order to move the weight-bearing surface backwards on the foot. The hoof-pastern axis of these horses is sometimes improved by the use of a wedge pad or raised-heel shoe to elevate the heel. Alternatively the heel can be artificially built up with specialist materials. This also decreases the strain on the deep digital flexor tendon.
- Raising the heels can also correct the pedal bone alignment.
- A shoe is selected that best fits the requirements of the individual horse. Where the sole has become longer and narrower over a period of time, it is helpful to select a shoe with a squared toe, e.g. a Natural Balance® shoe that brings the point of breakover back from the tip of the toe.
- In every case the shoe should provide adequate support at the heels. Normal shoes with extended heels, and egg bar or heart bar shoes are commonly used. There are an increased number of purpose-designed shoes to help improve such problems.

Prognosis

With regular trimming and shoeing, this type of conformation can be successfully managed. In cases where the heels are severely underrun, the hoof changes may be irreversible.

LAMINITIS

Laminitis is a condition that affects the horse's feet, causing pain and lameness.

In a normal, healthy horse, the pedal bone (distal phalanx) is held securely in position within the hoof capsule by a complicated arrangement of interdigitating laminae. On the inner surface of the hoof wall, approximately 600 leaf-like projections – the insensitive laminae – interdigitate with the sensitive laminae on the surface of the pedal bone. Each of these laminae has 100–200 microscopic secondary

a   *normal position of the pedal bone*   b   *rotated pedal bone*

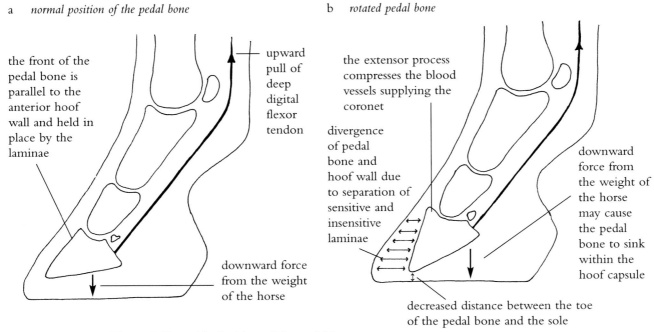

the front of the pedal bone is parallel to the anterior hoof wall and held in place by the laminae

upward pull of deep digital flexor tendon

downward force from the weight of the horse

the extensor process compresses the blood vessels supplying the coronet

divergence of pedal bone and hoof wall due to separation of sensitive and insensitive laminae

downward force from the weight of the horse may cause the pedal bone to sink within the hoof capsule

decreased distance between the toe of the pedal bone and the sole

Figure 6.40a and b Position of the pedal bone

laminae which further increase the surface area for attachment. **Laminitis** means inflammation of the laminae and when it occurs this attachment is disrupted and the laminae tear apart. The breakdown occurs at the innermost layer of the hoof wall, known as the **basement membrane**. Unless immediate steps are taken to halt the progress of the disease, the weight of the horse pushing down plus the upward pull of the deep digital flexor tendon on the pedal bone and the mechanical forces of movement may cause the pedal bone to rotate and/or sink within the foot (Figure 6.40). The sensitive tissue that produces the horn is damaged and distorted. Important arteries and veins are crushed, together with the soft tissues and this leads to severe and often unrelenting foot pain. The pedal bone may prolapse through the sole of the foot (Figures 6.41a and b).

The disease can be divided into 3 stages:

1   the **developmental phase** – this is the time when changes in the laminae begin but the horse does not yet experience foot pain

2   the **acute phase** starts as soon as the pain begins and continues until the pedal bone starts to move within the hoof capsule

3   the **chronic phase** includes all the possible subsequent outcomes from mild ongoing lameness to severe pain and penetration of the pedal bone through the sole of the foot.

The important thing to remember is that by the time the horse or pony is showing signs of lameness, damage has already occurred within the laminae and prompt action should be taken to minimize the progress of the disease.

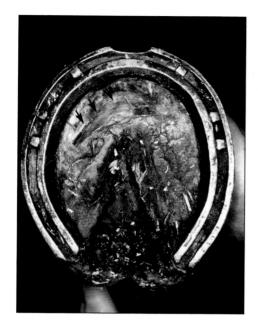
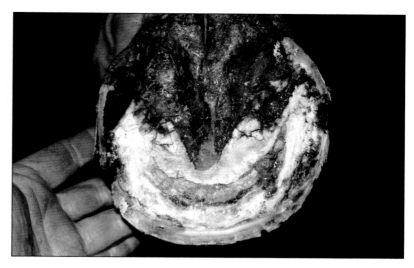

Figure 6.41a and b Pedal bone prolapsing through the sole of the foot:
a) prolapsed pedal bone; b) the pedal bone has penetrated the sole
(right), and a crescent-shaped area of imminent prolapse can be seen

Causes

Although our understanding of the disease is increasing all the time and a great deal of research is being carried out, the exact sequence of events is still unclear. There are 3 proposed mechanisms.

1 CHANGES OF THE BLOOD FLOW TO AND FROM THE FOOT

Originally, laminitis was considered to occur owing to a reduction of the blood supply to the sensitive laminae as a result of constriction of the blood vessels and an increased tendency for clotting. This causes the tissues to die due to receiving inadequate oxygen and nutrients to meet their needs. It is now thought to be rather more complicated than this and a variety of changes occur within the foot that may contribute to the development of laminitis.

2 ACTIVATION OF ENZYMES

Another theory is that the basement membrane between the hoof wall and the pedal bone is destroyed by enzymes called **metalloproteinases** (**MMPs**). In the normal hoof, controlled activity of these enzymes allows the horn of the hoof wall to grow downwards. It is thought that certain 'trigger factors' cause these enzymes to become overactive and destroy the attachment altogether. As this occurs, the capillaries within the laminae are destroyed so the blood is unable to perfuse the foot. The blood is shunted from small arteries supplying the foot directly to the veins draining it. The resistance to flow through the damaged capillary beds accounts for the bounding digital pulse.

3 TRAUMATIC AND MECHANICAL FACTORS EXPERIENCED DURING EXERCISE AND WEIGHT BEARING

These factors must play a part in cases where laminitis develops in a limb that is taking most of the weight owing to severe lameness in the opposite limb. They probably play a part in all cases of laminitis once they have been initiated by either (1) or (2) above.

It is possible that all of these factors are involved in the development of laminitis.

WHAT ARE THE TRIGGER FACTORS?

The exact nature of the trigger factors is still not clear. If a horse eats too much carbohydrate (e.g. lush grass containing lots of sugars), the capacity of the small intestine to digest it is exceeded and it spills over into the large intestine. Here it is rapidly fermented by bacteria including *Lactobacillus spp* and *Streptococcus bovis* which produce lactic acid. The proliferation of these bacteria and the increased acidity upsets the normal balance of micro-organisms in the hind gut. Some of the normal gut bacteria die and release endotoxins (poisons that are part of the bacterial cell membrane and are harmless until released when the bacteria die), while the *S. bovis* may release exotoxins (poisons released by the live bacteria). A combination of increased gut permeability (leakiness) due to the acidity and the release of chemicals by the bacteria may result in damaging trigger factors entering the circulation and reaching the laminae.

One theory is that chemicals known as 'amines' produced by lactobacilli and *S. bovis* in an acidic environment pass from the hind gut into the circulation where they cause constriction of the blood vessels entering or leaving the feet. This leads to painful oedema and laminar damage due to the capillary beds being starved of oxygen and nutrients.

Whatever the trigger, however, the laminae need to be exposed to it for a period of time before laminitis occurs. Some researchers consider that the blood vessels to the feet are dilated (open) rather than constricted during the developmental stage of laminitis. This is supported by the fact that cold therapy applied to the feet can actually *prevent* the development of laminitis in some situations (see page 159). The situation is rather confusing and more research needs to be carried out before we fully understand this disease process.

Predisposing factors

A number of different predisposing factors are known to lead to the development of laminitis. Animals that have suffered previous attacks are particularly susceptible.

- **Access to lush grass** In the process of photosynthesis, plants use energy from the sunlight to manufacture sugars from carbon dioxide and water. Many grasses produce and store high levels of carbohydrates called **fructans**. Fructans are used by plants as an energy source for growing and metabolism. These build up to high levels during the day when photosynthesis occurs. In the spring and autumn when the temperature is often cool but there are long hours of bright sunshine, fructans may accumulate to dangerously high levels. This is because cold temperatures cause growth and metabolism to slow down so the fructans are not used up by the plant. It has been demonstrated experimentally that fructans eaten in large enough quantities trigger laminitis. The horse does not have digestive enzymes to break down the fructans in the small intestine so they pass through the small intestine undigested and into the hind gut of the horse. Here they are fermented by bacteria including lactobacilli and *Streptococcus bovis* and the sequence of events discussed above may lead to laminitis.

- **Grain overload** If a horse or pony is overfed or breaks into a feed store and eats a large amount of concentrates, the carbohydrate which is normally digested in the small intestine, spills over into the large intestine. Here it is rapidly fermented by the lactobacilli and *Streptococcus bovis,* producing large amounts of lactic acid.

- **Obese animals** are particularly susceptible. The combination of excessive rations and limited exercise causes horses to deposit large amounts of fat on the crest of the neck, over the shoulders and loins, at the head of the tail and inside the abdomen. When large deposits of fat build up within the horse's abdomen, these begin to secrete hormones and cortisol which alter the horse's metabolism. Affected horses and ponies have high blood levels of insulin and glucose even after fasting. They become resistant to insulin which is secreted by the pancreas. Insulin normally lowers the blood sugar by encouraging its uptake into tissues such as muscle and the liver. Insulin resistance is also associated with reduced blood supply to the feet, possibly due to the effects of increased levels of cortisol and glucose on the blood vessels. This condition is sometimes known as obesity dependent laminitis (ODL), equine metabolic syndrome or peripheral Cushing's disease. Ponies and cobs are particularly susceptible. Unfortunately, the disease is self-perpetuating as the altered metabolism means that these animals put on weight with low calorie intakes that would not maintain a normal animal.

- **Any severe infection leading to toxaemia** can result in laminitis, e.g. endometritis due to retained placenta, a serious colic, gut inflammation, diarrhoea, pneumonia, pleurisy.

- **Toxins** from bacteria, fungi, ingested plants or chemicals may lead to laminitis.

- **Excessive weight-bearing on one limb,** e.g. due to a severe strain or fracture of the opposite limb, can lead to the development of laminitis in the uninjured, supporting leg. The pedal bone in these animals often sinks rather than rotates.

- **Administration of corticosteroids** can cause laminitis in some animals. This sometimes happens following systemic treatment for skin disease or local injection into a joint. The mechanisms by which corticosteroids cause laminitis are not fully understood. They may increase the permeability of the gut, cause contraction of the blood vessels supplying the feet, affect the action of insulin or have a direct effect on the laminae of the feet.

- **Cushing's disease** Animals affected by this disease have high circulating levels of cortisol, glucose and insulin and are prone to developing laminitis, especially in the autumn. The hormone imbalance upsets the glucose uptake by the laminae. The laminae need glucose for their metabolism and without treatment horses with Cushing's disease eventually develop laminitis.

- **Stress**, e.g. frequent travelling of overweight show animals, being sold or the loss of a companion, can precipitate an attack of laminitis. Chronic stress increases circulating cortisol and adrenaline. Glucose consumption in the skin and feet is reduced so that the vital organs (heart, brain and lungs) receive it preferentially. Sustained reduction of glucose supply to the feet is harmful.
- **Concussion** from too much work on hard going can cause laminitis as a result of mechanical and traumatic stresses on the laminae.
- **Chronic liver or kidney disease** can predispose to laminitis because these organs become less efficient at breaking down and eliminating toxins.

Clinical signs

Any number from one to all four feet may be involved. However, the two front feet are most commonly affected.

- **Stance** Many laminitic animals develop a characteristic stance. The forelimbs are extended forwards and most of the weight is taken on the heels to relieve the pressure at the toe. The hind limbs may be positioned forwards under the body so they can take more of the horse's weight (Figures 6.42a and b). When all four feet are involved, the horse may spend long periods of time lying down. In these animals the feet are often positioned close together under the body when they stand.

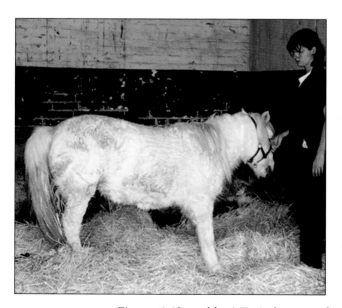 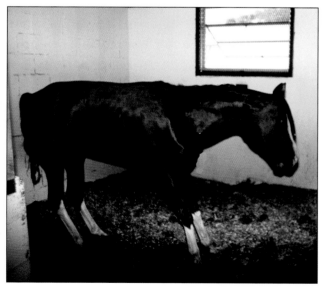

Figures 6.42a and b a) Typical stance of a pony with laminitis; b) A pony with a very severe case of laminitis

- **Reluctance to walk and variable degrees of lameness** Affected horses and ponies are often extremely reluctant to move. When they do, they bring the hind limbs well forward under the body and land carefully on the heels of the front feet, so the gait is very stilted or 'pottery'. They sometimes appear to lean backwards and the lameness is often much worse on turning. It is also accentuated on hard or uneven ground. Very mild cases may appear slightly stiff rather than lame or the lameness may only be observed on uneven ground or when the animal is turning.

- **Frequent shifting of weight from one foot to another** If one observes these animals at rest they frequently shift their weight between the feet in an attempt to relieve the constant discomfort. They may resist or refuse to lift a foot when asked because of the increased discomfort of taking more weight on the opposite limb.

- **Increased or bounding digital pulses** If the digital pulse is taken at the point where the digital artery crosses the sesamoid bones, it is often stronger than normal and described as 'bounding'.

- **Reaction to hoof testers** Most horses and ponies with laminitis will flinch when hoof testers are applied to the sole in front of the point of the frog.

- **If the pain is very severe**, the pulse and respiration rates increase and some animals have a temperature. They may seem very anxious and tremble and sweat.

- **Heat** may be felt in the hoof wall during the acute stage of the disease.

- **Coronary band depression** An abnormal depression may be palpated on the coronary band at the front of the foot if the pedal bone has started to move. Palpation may cause some discomfort in the early stages. If the bone completely sinks, the depression will extend the whole length of the coronet (Figure 6.43)

- **A coronary band discharge of serum** may occur. In severe cases, haemorrhage and serum from the inflamed laminae may build up sufficient pressure within the foot to escape at the coronary band.

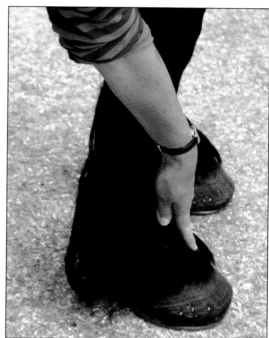

Figure 6.43 Feeling for a coronary band depression

- **Change in hoof wall conformation** As a result of recent studies, our understanding of the reasons why the hoof wall becomes deformed has increased. Originally it was thought that when the pedal bone rotates, its extensor process compresses the horn-producing tissues of the coronet at the front of the foot. This slows down the rate of new horn production at the toe. The result is laminitic growth rings which are wider at the heel than the toe. The hoof changes shape, developing high heels and a long toe with a concave anterior hoof wall (Figure 6.44). Another theory suggests that

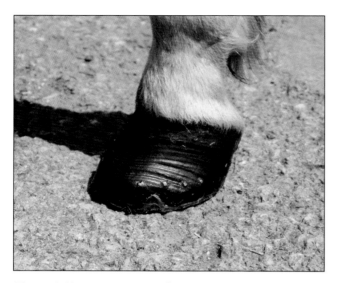

Figure 6.44 Laminitic growth rings are wider at the heel than at the toe

the change in growth rate of the hoof wall begins in the developmental stage of laminitis, before the pain begins. A faster growth rate at the heel causes the horn tubules to be distorted forwards. This causes distortion of the sensitive laminae, resulting in pain. The forward distortion of the hoof capsule results in the anterior hoof wall being lifted away from the underlying sensitive laminae starting closest to the ground and gradually working upwards. The result is a concave anterior hoof wall. It is suggested that the trigger factors initiating laminitis also trigger the faster growth rate of the hoof wall at the heels and that the pain of the acute stage of laminitis is due to the distortion of the sensitive laminae which occurs before any changes can be seen in the actual appearance of the hoof wall. The 'dorsal wall lifting' theory proposes that the lifting of the anterior hoof wall also pulls the sole upwards causing compression of the circumflex artery under the front of the pedal bone thus compromising the blood supply to the foot. The altered blood supply leads to reduced horn being produced at the front of the hoof whilst growth of horn at the heels is accelerated.

- **Change in sole conformation** The normally concave sole may become flat or even convex as the pedal bone rotates or sinks within the hoof capsule. The pedal bone may begin to penetrate the sole. This will show as a semicircular area of bruising before the sole is actually penetrated (see Figures 6.41a and b).

- **Increased width of the white line** In the chronic stage, there is often a widening of the white line at the ground surface due to excessive amounts of horny tissue being produced, especially at the toe. This is an area of weakness that makes the horse susceptible to abscesses and seedy toe. Foot abscesses are a common occurrence in horses with chronic laminitis.

The clinical signs and the response to treatment depend on how much damage has occurred to the laminae.

Diagnosis

The diagnosis is made on the clinical signs. Radiographic examination is essential for the following reasons.

- It is important to establish the position of the pedal bone at the outset of treatment so that subsequent progress or deterioration can be monitored.
- Radiographs will show the extent of any rotation or sinking of the pedal bone. If

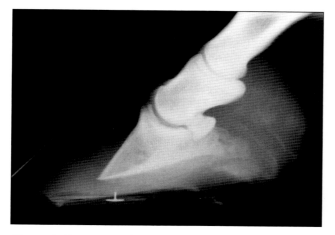

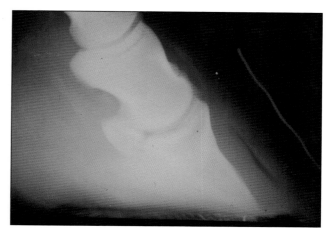

Figure 6.45 X-ray with markers showing the rotation of the pedal bone

Figure 6.46 X-ray of a 'sinker'. The pedal bone has dropped within the hoof capsule

the front of the pedal bone is no longer parallel to the front of the hoof wall, the pedal bone has rotated (Figure 6.45). If the pedal bone is not rotated but has moved downwards within the hoof capsule towards the ground, it is said to be 'sinking' (Figure 6.46). This is very important for planning the treatment and also for predicting the likely outcome. 'Sinkers' have a much more guarded prognosis.

- They will also show whether the horse has any foot changes, e.g. thickening of the dorsal hoof wall or remodelling of the toe of the pedal bone from previous episodes of the disease.

The vet will place special markers onto the hoof before taking the X-rays. A piece of wire is positioned on the front of the hoof wall extending from the coronary band towards the ground surface. This shows up on the X-ray and the vet can immediately see whether the pedal bone has dropped in relation to the coronary band or if it has rotated so that it is no longer aligned with the anterior hoof wall. If gas or fluid is trapped under the hoof wall, this will show up as a black shadow. A second marker is placed at or just behind the point of the trimmed frog.

By taking special measurements from the X-rays, your vet will be in a position to recommend the most appropriate treatment and also to gain some idea of the prognosis.

Definition of terms

Confusion sometimes arises over the terms used to describe the progression of the disease. The term 'laminitis' has traditionally been used to describe all stages of the disease but it should ideally be restricted to cases where the animal experiences foot pain but has no obvious hoof changes. Once the pedal bone has started to rotate and there is a palpable depression above the coronary band at the front of the hoof the condition becomes an

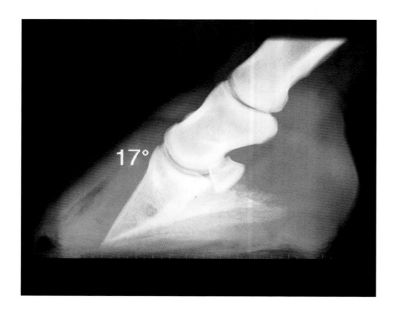

'acute founder'. If the pedal bone drops within the hoof capsule so that the coronary band depression extends all round the hoof, the affected animal is described as a 'sinker'. It is possible for the pedal bone to rotate and sink at the same time (Figure 6.47). 'Chronic founder' cases are those where there are changes to the appearance of the hoof, e.g. dropped or convex soles, concave anterior hoof wall and growth rings that are wider at the heels than the toe.

Figure 6.47   X-ray showing rotation and sinking of the pedal bone

Treatment

Laminitis should be regarded as an emergency since prompt treatment can make a significant difference to the outcome. There are 3 aims of treatment.

1   TO IDENTIFY AND TREAT ANY UNDERLYING CAUSE

Affected animals should be removed from lush or recently fertilized pastures. If the horse or pony is suffering from an infection or is toxic the treatment is likely to include:

- antibiotics
- intravenous fluids
- flunixin meglumine, a non-steroidal anti-inflammatory drug (NSAID) which has an anti-endotoxin effect, or other NSAIDs with a similar action
- uterine lavage (flushing) and removal of foetal membranes for animals with a retained placenta
- treatment to cause dilation of the blood vessels within the hoof and generally lower blood pressure, e.g. isoxuprine and acepromazine (ACP).

If the horse has gorged itself on grain:

- mineral oil may be given by stomach tube; this will have a laxative effect and by coating the intestinal wall may help to prevent the absorption of endotoxin
- probiotics may be prescribed to help restore the normal microbial population of the gut
- electrolytes.

If Cushing's disease is suspected, the animal should be tested and treated if the disease is confirmed.

2   TO PREVENT THE CIRCULATING TRIGGER FACTORS REACHING THE FEET

If the horse eats too much grain or becomes toxic for any other reason, the symptoms of laminitis may not appear for up to 48 hours. If the feet can be immediately and continuously cooled with a slurry of iced water, the blood vessels to the feet constrict and the levels of circulating trigger factors reaching the laminae are reduced. The cold may also reduce the activity of the MMPs. It has been shown that keeping the limbs cooled from the top of the cannon bone to the feet for a period of 24–48 hours can help to prevent laminitis developing in situations where it was expected. The horse tolerates the treatment well and does not find the cold water uncomfortable as we would. This needs to be performed under veterinary supervision.

3   TO RELIEVE THE PAIN AND PROVIDE EMERGENCY FIRST AID TO HELP STABILIZE THE PEDAL BONE WITHIN THE HOOF CAPSULE AND RESTORE THE BLOOD SUPPLY TO THE FOOT

The horse or pony should be managed in the following way.

- Confined to a stable with a thick, non-edible bed of wood shavings, sand or peat (45 cm [18 in] thick); these materials conform to the shape of the foot and provide some support and comfort. A comfortable bed encourages the animal to lie down more and this reduces the mechanical strain on the laminae.
- Given non-steroidal anti-inflammatory drugs such as flunixin or phenylbutazone to reduce the pain and inflammation. Flunixin and phenylbutazone may be used together in lower doses during the early stages of laminitis; phenylbutazone is considered to be the most effective analgesic while flunixin has anti-endotoxic effects. The dose should be kept to the minimum necessary to control the pain in order to avoid side effects such as gastric ulceration; this is especially important in ponies and older horses.
- Fitted with frog supports. As a temporary, emergency measure, the frog may be supported with a roll of bandage, pieces of carpet cut to the shape of the frog or a commercially available frog support pad bandaged in place. If the horse is found in the field, these should be fitted before asking the horse to walk very far; the best solution is to apply frog supports and box the horse if any distance is involved.

How to fit a frog support

- Pick out the feet and remove any residual debris with a soft brush. Examine each foot carefully. If the frog is level with the weight-bearing surface of the hoof wall or shoe, there is no need to fit a support. Keep the horse on a deep bed of shavings.
- If the frog is not level with the weight-bearing surface, use a commercially available frog support or place a roll of bandage over the frog so that it ends 1 cm ($\frac{4}{10}$ in) short of the point of the frog (Figure 6.48). When the bandage is compressed firmly,

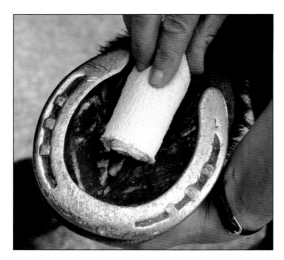

Figure 6.48 Applying a frog support

it should be level with the wall of the hoof or the ground surface of the shoe, if the horse is shod. If the frog support is too thick it will put pressure on the frog and increase the horse's discomfort.

- Wrap Elastoplast® around the foot to keep the pad/bandage in place. Take care not to cause pressure over the heels or the coronary band. The heels should be padded with a layer of cotton wool or Gamgee®.

- If the horse seems more uncomfortable with the frog supports, remove them and keep the horse on a thick shavings bed until the vet arrives.

The frog supports allow some of the horse's weight to be supported by the frog and this helps to relieve the strain on the weakened laminae. By relieving the pressure on the tip of a rotated pedal bone it reduces compression of the circumflex artery around the toe and helps to restore circulation to the foot.

An alternative first-aid support is the Styrofoam Support System. Styrofoam pads are used to provide support to the frog and also to the back half of the foot. The thick Styrofoam pad is cut so that it covers the sole of the foot and it is then taped onto the bottom of the foot and allowed to compress for 24–48 hours (Figures 6.49a and b). The pad is then removed and hoof testers are applied to determine which parts of the foot are painful. The front part of the pad is trimmed off and the back part is reapplied to the foot so that it sits 1 cm ($\frac{4}{10}$ in) behind the painful part of the foot. A second pad is applied to the whole hoof and bandaged on top of the trimmed pad. This has the effect of distributing the weight of

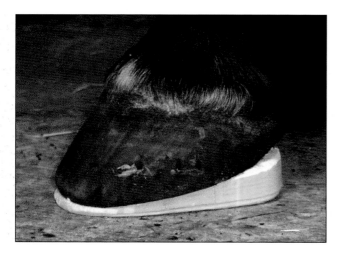 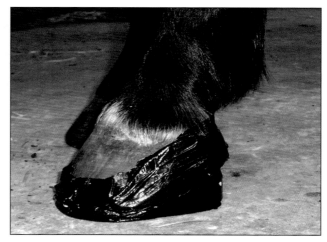

Figure 6.49a and b Styrofoam Support: a) trimmed Styrofoam pad; b) the pad is taped to the foot and allowed to compress for 24–48 hours

the horse onto the non-painful area of the foot. With this system in place, it is important to keep the horse on a firm, even surface.

OTHER MEDICAL TREATMENTS

Several drugs have been used to try and improve the blood flow to the laminae in the feet. They include:

- acepromazine
- isoxuprine
- glyceryl trinitrate patches placed over the digital vessels.

With improved methods of assessing blood flow through the laminae, the efficacy of these drugs is now being questioned. They should not be used in the developmental stage of laminitis as any increase in blood flow would increase the delivery of trigger factors to the laminae. Acepromazine is helpful for reducing the anxiety of horses and ponies in severe pain and encouraging them to lie down as well as helping to reduce blood pressure.

Management
FEEDING

Horse and ponies should be kept on a strict forage diet, supplemented with vitamins and minerals. This can be made up of hay plus an alfalfa or alfalfa/straw mix. Soaking the hay is a good way of reducing the levels of soluble carbohydrates and unmolassed sugar beet can be added. Your vet will advise you on the amount to feed. Some feeds have been approved by The Laminitis Trust for feeding to laminitis-prone horses and ponies (www.laminitisclinic.org). *Drastic starvation must be avoided or the horse will be at risk of hyperlipaemia* (see page 501)

SUPPLEMENTS

- Biotin and methionine may be added to improve the growth rate and quality of the horn.
- A proprietary mix, e.g. Farrier's Formula®, Formula Feet™, provides the essential nutrients for hoof growth.
- A liquid extract of 'chasteberry' (Hormonise) may provide symptomatic relief for animals with Cushing's disease.

EXERCISE

Exercise is *harmful at any stage until the pedal bone is stable in the foot*. Forced exercise is contraindicated, contrary to earlier beliefs. All horses and ponies experiencing laminitis should remain on box rest for at least 4 weeks after they are comfortable at walk and trot in a straight line on a hard surface without any painkillers. This is to allow the laminae time to heal and reduces the chances of subsequent rotation and sinking. Following this they can be turned out into a riding arena each day and slowly introduced to short periods of controlled walking exercise in hand.

Hoof care

The aim of hoof care is to minimize the strain on the weakened laminae to prevent rotation or sinking of the pedal bone. The forces acting on the laminae include:

- the weight of the horse
- the constant pull of the deep digital flexor tendon
- the leverage on the toe of the hoof capsule as the horse walks.

REMOVAL OF SHOES

Whether or not the shoes are removed depends on the severity of the case and the condition of the feet. If the hoof wall is strong and the sole is concave, the shoes may be removed. Where the sole has dropped, the horse will be more comfortable with the shoes left on. In cases where the foot is very overgrown or unbalanced and the shoes are contributing to the problem, they are removed carefully to minimize trauma and pain during the removal process.

CORRECTIVE TRIMMING AND SHOEING

The long-term aim of corrective trimming and shoeing is to improve the blood supply to the foot, to restore the normal alignment of the pedal bone and the hoof capsule and to correct the distortion of the hoof capsule. Distortion of the hoof capsule leads to chronic pain because it traumatises the underlying sensitive tissues. Radiographs are important for determining the best way to achieve this and the vet and farrier should work together. Using the X-rays as a guide, the farrier will:

- shorten long toes to reduce the forces on the laminae during breakover
- rasp back the front of the hoof wall until it is parallel with the pedal bone
- remove excessive heel growth in animals with chronic laminitis
- fit special shoes where required to support the frog or the whole of the back part of the foot
- if necessary, the heel will be raised to reduce the tension of the deep digital flexor tendon on the pedal bone.

The corrective trimming is done in stages over several months. Trimming is usually carried out at monthly intervals.

Shoeing

There are currently several popular methods of shoeing affected horses.

HEART BAR SHOES

There are various types of heart bar shoe. They are designed to provide support to the pedal bone by applying light, even pressure to most of the trimmed frog. This removes the pressure from the compressed blood vessels under the tip of a rotated pedal bone and helps to restore the circulation to the foot.

They require specialist fitting as an incorrectly fitted heart bar shoe can increase the horse's pain and damage the foot further. Special Imprint™ plastic heart bar shoes are now available that can be heated and moulded to fit the foot snugly and correctly. They are held in place by moulding part of the shoe into indentations drilled into the hoof wall and by a special adhesive. This avoids the pain and concussion caused by nailing shoes in place (Figures 6.50a, b and c). The shoe is seated-out to avoid any pressure on the sole (see page 147 and Figure 6.37).

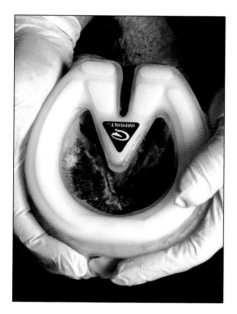

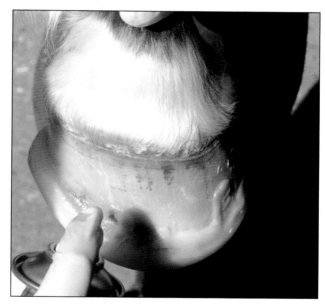

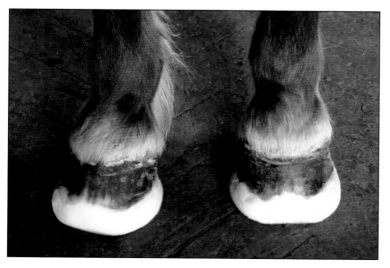

Figures 6.50a, b and c
Imprint shoes: a) and b) being fitted; c) the plastic heart-bar shoes have been moulded to the feet

THE EQUINE DIGITAL SUPPORT SYSTEM (EDSS)

This system of shoeing is used to provide support and transfer the weight bearing to the back of the foot. The weight of the horse is transferred to the frog, sole and bars. The design of the shoe brings the point of breakover back. In some circumstances it is used with special rails that are screwed in place to elevate the heels (Figure 6.51).

A VARIETY OF OTHER SHOEING SYSTEMS ARE USED

These include the use of reverse shoes (normal shoes put on back to front) and a variety of impression materials under pads to provide support. The new technique of using reverse wedge shoeing has been reported as having encouraging results. The choice of treatment depends on the stage of the disease and the circumstances of each individual case.

Surgical treatments
VERTICAL GROOVING OF THE HOOF WALL

In order to minimize distortion of the hoof capsule due to the accelerated growth rate of the horn at the heels, a vertical grooving technique has been devised. A vertical groove which extends from the coronary band to the ground surface is made through the whole thickness of the hoof wall at approximately 30 degrees on each side of the dorsal midline (Figure 6.52). This prevents the lifting of the dorsal hoof wall and the painful stretching and tearing of the sensitive tissues underneath. Styrofoam pads are applied and left on for approximately 2 weeks to protect and support the sole. The hoof wall becomes moist and softens under the tape and this helps the function of the grooves. This procedure has been used early in the acute stages of the disease and also in the chronic recurrent stages to successfully reduce the

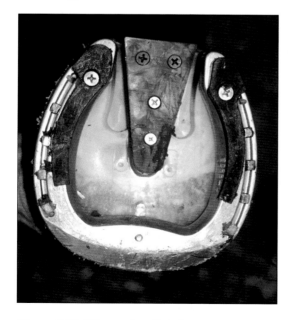

Figure 6.51 The equine digital support system (EDSS), solar view

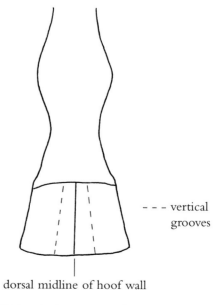

--- vertical grooves

dorsal midline of hoof wall

Figure 6.52 Vertical grooving of the hoof wall

pain experienced by affected horses and ponies. The procedure will not, however, prevent rotation or sinking in severe cases.

Dorsal wall drilling Where there is a build up of serum or blood from damaged vessels beneath the front of the hoof wall, the pressure can cause severe pain. Drilling a hole through the anterior hoof wall to release the fluid and relieve the pressure can give the horse considerable relief. This is sometimes used for acute founder and sinker cases.

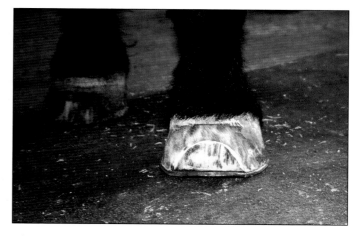

Figure 6.53 Dorsal wall resection

Dorsal wall resection Sometimes a section of the front of the hoof wall is removed when it has separated from the pedal bone (Figure 6.53). This procedure:
- allows inflammatory exudate to escape, relieving pressure and pain on the laminae
- allows removal of dead tissue and drainage of any infected pockets of tissue
- relieves the pain caused by stretching and tearing of the laminae in the dorsal part of the hoof
- allows the new horn to grow parallel to the front of the pedal bone.

Cutting the deep digital flexor tendon This procedure may be used where the position of the pedal bone is unstable and continues to rotate and penetrate the sole due to the pull of the deep digital flexor tendon. With longstanding rotation, the deep digital flexor tendon shortens and prevents the repositioning of the pedal bone. These animals tend to walk on their toes. Surgical cutting of the tendon together with corrective trimming and shoeing permits realignment of the pedal bone and the procedure usually eases the animal's pain. This operation changes the alignment of the coffin joint and causes hyperextension of the digit and so horses must be shod with extensions at the back of the shoes and raised heels for a period of approximately 3 months to reduce the strain on the joint and the superficial digital flexor tendon.

Abscesses commonly form in the feet of acutely foundered horses, causing the horse to be very lame. These should be encouraged to burst through the coronary band by tubbing several times a day or relieved by dorsal wall drilling or resection. Drainage through the sole is avoided as the sensitive tissue often swells and protrudes through the hole, taking a long time to heal. When they occur at the back of the foot it should be tubbed frequently and the coronary band should be kept soft and supple by applying udder cream.

Prognosis
The prognosis depends on a number of factors including:

- the cause of the condition
- whether the horse is laminitic, acutely foundered, a sinker or chronically foundered
- the change in position of the pedal bone within the hoof on X-ray
- the appearance of the tip of the pedal bone on X-ray; if remodelling has occurred, the animal is unlikely to become pain-free
- how promptly the correct treatment is given
- subsequent management and monitoring.

If the horse is laminitic, i.e. there is no rotation or sinking and it is managed appropriately, it should make a full recovery. Those with mild to moderate rotation have an 80% chance of recovery. If the animal is a sinker or has severe rotation the chance of recovery is reduced to 20%. Up to 80% of chronic founder cases recover if they receive the appropriate care. If there are any complications such as infection, inflammation or resorption of the pedal bone, the prognosis is very poor.

The treatment of severe cases involves many months of corrective trimming and specialist shoeing. The management of these animals is expensive and time-consuming so the commitment of the owner must be 100%. Horses and ponies vary in their ability to withstand the pain. In some cases, the suffering of the animal is so intense that euthanasia is the only reasonable course of action.

Prevention

Most cases of laminitis could be prevented by improved management. The following steps should be taken to reduce the incidence of the disease.

DIETARY CONTROL

- Obesity should be avoided. You should be able to feel your horse's ribs easily when you run your fingers over his side without being able to actually see them. There should not be any deposits of fat on the crest of the neck, over the loins or tail head or around the udder or sheath. Many show animals are at serious risk of laminitis as a result of overfeeding.
- Feed a low carbohydrate, high fibre diet. Base the diet on forage such as hay, alfalfa, and straw. Unmolassed sugar beet is another suitable food. Avoid food rich in carbohydrates such as coarse mixes and straight grains. This type of diet is adequate for most ponies, cobs and Warmblood types in light work.
- Add a broad spectrum vitamin and mineral supplement to ensure the animal's requirements are met while on a forage diet.
- Limit the grazing of susceptible animals especially in the spring and autumn. This can be achieved by:
  - restricting the time the animal is turned out
  - strip grazing with the aid of electric fencing

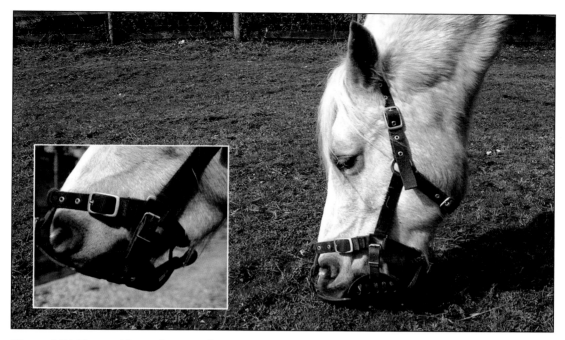

Figure 6.54 Pony with grazing muzzle

- using a grazing mask or muzzle (Figure 6.54).
- avoiding grazing of lush or fertilized grass
- restricting the animal to a small, bare paddock during the danger times and providing hay.
- If the horse has been stabled for any period of time, it should be introduced slowly to grass, gradually increasing the time in the paddock each day.
- With susceptible animals it is worth considering the fructan levels in the grass, e.g:
  - avoid turning out onto frosted paddocks where fructan levels may be high
  - avoid turning out at times of day when fructan levels are high; peak levels occur by midday, and so removing ponies from the pasture at 10 a.m. and not turning them out again until late in the evening will reduce their consumption of fructans
  - some grasses, such as timothy, contain lower levels of fructans than other species
- Ensure horses and ponies cannot have access to feed stores.

VIRGINIAMYCIN

Virginiamycin (Founderguard™) is an antimicrobial product that prevents multiplication of lactobacilli and *Streptococcus bovis*. Adding it to the feed of animals susceptible to dietary-induced laminitis reduces proliferation of these bacteria in the hind gut if carbohydrate overload is experienced. This prevents the increased acidity of the gut contents that triggers the sequence of events that leads to laminitis. This drug can help to prevent dietary-induced laminitis but *is not a substitute for good management.*

MANAGEMENT

- The feet of all ponies and horses should be regularly trimmed.
- Regular exercise is important for all animals to prevent obesity and laminitis.
- Concussion from working on hard ground should be kept to a minimum.
- Keep all feed where a loose animal cannot gain access to it.
- Ensure prompt treatment of any illness that could result in toxaemia.
- Consult your vet immediately if laminitis is suspected.

Remember that it is much easier to prevent laminitis than it is to cure it.

WHITE LINE DISEASE AND SEEDY TOE

The **white line** is the area on the ground surface of the foot where the insensitive laminae on the inner surface of the hoof wall join the horn of the sole. It is non-pigmented and in the normal, trimmed foot appears as a narrow ring of horny tissue at the perimeter of the sole (see Figures 6.2a and b). Disease occurs when this area is weakened and a cavity develops, separating the outer hoof wall from the laminae. Soil and droppings enter the cavity and bacterial or fungal invasion cause the horn of the hoof wall to break down. The cavity becomes filled with dry, crumbly, horn material. If left untreated, the lesion progresses towards the coronary band and large areas of hoof wall may become separated from the laminae. Painful abscesses sometimes form due to bacterial infection.

'White line disease' and 'seedy toe' are often used synonymously. However, 'seedy toe' is a small, focal lesion confined to the front of the toe. White line disease is more extensive and may occur at the toe, quarters or towards the heels.

Causes

Anything that weakens the white line can predispose a horse or pony to white line disease, e.g:

- living in excessively wet conditions
- long spells of dry weather or being stabled can lead to excessive drying of the hoof and cracks in the white line
- poor quality horn due to nutritional deficiencies
- chronic bacterial or fungal infection of the horn
- penetration of the white line by sharp flints
- previous white line abscesses
- the occurrence of abscesses under the sole adjacent to the white line.

Alternatively, anything that increases the mechanical strain on the white line by increasing the forces between the dorsal hoof wall and the sole can contribute to the development of seedy toe, e.g:

- long-toe, low-heel conformation
- inadequate hoof care so the toes become abnormally long
- widening of the white line in animals with chronic laminitis.

Clinical signs

These may include the following.

- Visible widening of the white line.
- Local discolouration of the white line due to bacterial infection or packing of the cavity with soil.
- Variable degrees of lameness. Many ponies and donkeys develop seedy toe which does not cause lameness but is discovered by the farrier during routine trimming. As the separation becomes more extensive, the animal may experience tender feet. Others become acutely lame a day or two before pus bursts out at the coronary band if an abscess has formed.
- Sensitivity to hoof testers in the region where an abscess is forming.
- A discharge of pus from the coronary band.
- If there is significant separation, the overlying hoof wall will sound hollow when tapped.

Diagnosis

The diagnosis is usually made on the clinical signs. If the condition is extensive, radiographs may be taken to assess the degree of separation of the hoof wall from the laminae. This also allows any changes to the pedal bone or its position within the hoof capsule from previous bouts of laminitis to be assessed.

Treatment

The key to successful treatment is prompt and adequate attention as soon as the condition is diagnosed. If the condition becomes chronic, extensive areas of hoof wall may be undermined. This means the weight of the horse will be supported by a considerably reduced number of laminae resulting in inflammation and lameness. Rotation of the pedal bone can occur.

- Any underlying conditions or predisposing factors should be treated. Long toes should be trimmed and in previously laminitic animals, the foot should be trimmed to restore a parallel relationship between the front of the hoof capsule and the pedal bone.
- As the separation is usually widest near the ground surface and narrows towards the coronet, it is often necessary to remove a portion of the hoof wall to allow access to all of the diseased tissue.
- All the dirt and any abnormal material are removed. In many cases, this is sufficient and no medical treatment is necessary.
- Any pus should be drained and all infected horn removed. When infection is present,

the exposed insensitive laminae should be treated topically with a suitable hoof disinfectant, e.g. 2.5% iodine twice a week.

- Once any infection has been dealt with, the foot should be kept clean and dry.
- A heart bar shoe may be used to provide support in cases where extensive areas of hoof wall have been resected. As many of these lesions occur at the toe, a shoe with a squared toe can be used to bring the breakover back from the toe and reduce the stress on the dorsal hoof wall.
- Once the infection has resolved and the laminae are dry, the hoof wall defect may be repaired with an acrylic material such as Equilox®. However, it is best to leave the resected area open if possible as the disease may recur under the repair. If the lesion is not too extensive, the horse can recommence work at this stage although the exercise programme may have to be modified.
- The defect will gradually grow out. A brush is used to keep the area clean.
- Hoof-wall growth may be improved in some cases by dietary supplements such as biotin and methionine.
- The feet should be kept as clean and dry as possible while the lesion grows out. Horses should not be worked or turned out in wet, muddy conditions.

Prognosis

Recurrence is common unless the underlying factors are adequately dealt with. Some horses experience repeat episodes despite good hoof care. The corrective hoof trimming can take many months. Excellent management is required while the hoof defect is growing out.

NAVICULAR SYNDROME

Navicular syndrome is a progressive, degenerative disease involving the navicular bone, its supporting ligaments, the navicular bursa and the deep digital flexor tendon (DDFT). It may affect one front foot, or more commonly both front feet, and occasionally occurs in the hind feet of horses. It rarely affects ponies. The lameness is due to pain from the heel region of the foot. The average age of onset is 7–9 years.

Anatomy

The distal interphalangeal (DIP), or coffin, joint is formed from the articular surfaces of the pedal bone, the distal end of the middle phalanx and the navicular bone. The DDFT passes over the palmar (back) surface of the navicular bone which is covered with fibrocartilage and attaches to the pedal bone. A fluid-filled sac, the navicular bursa, cushions the movement of the DDFT over the navicular bone (see Figure 6.4).

The navicular bone has several supporting ligaments, collectively known as the **navicular suspensory apparatus**. These include:

- paired **collateral suspensory ligaments** which originate on either side of the distal end of the proximal phalanx (P1) and run downwards, attaching to the outside of the middle phalanx (P2) and the upper surface of the navicular bone where they join in the midline; a branch continues from the lateral extremity of the navicular bone to insert on the lateral cartilage and the pedal bone.

- the **distal sesamoidean impar ligament** is a sheet of fibrous tissue that joins the lower surface of the navicular bone to the pedal bone, close to the attachment of the DDFT.

Causes

The disease is thought to be caused by repeated trauma to the navicular bone from its supporting ligaments and the DDFT. Certain types of conformation increase the biomechanical stress on this area. These include the following.

- Long-toe, low-heel conformation with a broken back hoof-pastern axis. During breakover, the ligaments come under excessive tension and the DDFT compresses the upper edge of the navicular bone against the other bones making up the joint; high forces are imposed on the lower part of the navicular bone from the very taut DDFT.
- Mediolateral hoof imbalance.
- Narrow, upright boxy feet.
- Small feet for the weight of the horse; concussion at the heels is increased.
- The shape of the navicular bone varies between different breeds of horse; a concave or undulating upper articular border of the bone appears to be associated with a higher incidence of navicular syndrome than a straight or convex surface; this affects the biomechanical forces that are applied to the area.

Increased concussion from working on hard surfaces may be a contributory factor. The disease is also associated with changes that can occur within the foot from prolonged periods of box rest. Without normal, regular exercise, the horse's feet tend to become contracted.

Certain breeds, e.g. the Dutch Warmblood, appear to experience a high incidence of the disease. This is likely to be the result of conformational factors.

What happens to the navicular bone?

- In each case, the forces induce changes in the fibrocartilage covering the back surface of the navicular bone. In places, the cartilage is completely eroded and the bone is exposed. This results in increased wear to the DDFT and adhesions may occur between the tendon and the bone.
- Degenerative changes occur within the bone substance.

- The supporting ligaments may tear at the site of attachment to the navicular bone.

The pain arises from within the bone and from strains and sprains to the surrounding soft tissues. Navicular bone pain may be associated with poor drainage of blood from the vessels and spaces in the bone marrow leading to raised pressure and distension of the small veins within the bone.

Clinical signs
CHANGE IN ACTION
Over a period of time there is a gradual loss of performance and shortening of the horse's stride. The toe is often placed on the ground first to reduce concussion at the heel and pressure on the navicular bone and DDFT. This gives a stiff, 'shuffling' gait and the horse may have a tendency to trip or stumble.

LAMENESS
Lameness is insidious in onset and only rarely occurs suddenly. It is usually bilateral but if the changes are more advanced in one limb, this leg will show the lameness first. In the early stages the lameness is slight and intermittent, tending to improve with exercise. It is most obvious when the horse works on a circle with the lame limb on the inside, especially when lunged at trot on a hard, flat surface. The horse often holds its neck and head rather stiffly and turned to the outside of the circle in an attempt to reduce the weight taken by the inside forelimb. Affected horses may become reluctant to jump or to increase their length of stride. The degree of lameness increases as the disease progresses and eventually the horse is continually lame.

SYMPTOMS OBSERVED AT REST
These include the following.

- Shifting the weight from one front foot to the other.
- Standing with one foot in front of the other with the heel slightly elevated; this relieves the pressure between the DDFT and the navicular bone and is known as 'pointing' the foot. When both feet are painful they are alternately pointed (Figure 6.55).
- Digging a hole in the bedding

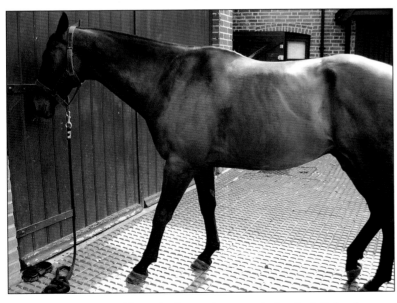

Figure 6.55 Horse with navicular syndrome pointing its left forefoot

and standing with the toes in the hole and the heels raised on the edge.

- Contraction of the heels as the disease progresses may cause the hoof to become upright and boxy, with a higher heel height. When only one foot is affected, the two front feet become dissimilar in size and shape.

RESPONSE TO FLEXION AND HOOF TESTERS

- Flexion of the lower limb is positive (i.e. results in increased lameness) in some horses with navicular syndrome.
- The response to hoof testers is not always helpful. Some horses find firm pressure applied over the centre of the frog uncomfortable. As affected horses land on the toe, there may be sensitivity in this part of the foot which can be misleading.

Diagnosis

The diagnosis is usually made on the clinical signs, the response to nerve blocks and radiography. Scintigraphy and MRI can also be helpful.

NERVE BLOCKS

- The pain is usually abolished by an injection of local anaesthetic into the navicular bursa. However, this is technically difficult and is only carried out by equine vets with experience of the technique.
- The lameness is usually significantly reduced with a palmar digital nerve block.
- In some horses, the pain from navicular syndrome is alleviated by intra-articular analgesia of the coffin joint.

The palmar digital and coffin joint blocks are not specific for navicular pain as they desensitize structures other than the navicular bone, and so the results are interpreted together with those from other tests such as X-rays.

When the pain is removed from the most obviously lame foot, the horse often shows lameness in the opposite leg. This is because the condition usually affects both front feet but is more advanced in one limb than the other. When the navicular regions of both front feet are desensitized, the horse often becomes sound and has an increased stride length.

RADIOGRAPHIC CHANGES

Changes which may be seen on the radiographs of a horse with navicular syndrome include:

- a cyst within the bone (Figure 6.56)
- bony proliferations (known as **enthesiophytes**) at the site of attachment of the supporting ligaments to the navicular bone
- enlarged vascular channels on the distal (lower) border of the navicular bone
- an increase or decrease in density of the bone

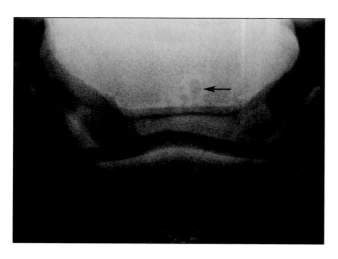

Figure 6.56 X-ray showing navicular changes: cyst-like lesions can be seen in this navicular bone

- changes to the flexor surface of the bone in contact with the DDFT, e.g. new bone deposits, loss of bone density or change in outline caused by erosions, loss of definition between the cortex (outer part) of the bone and the medulla (the central part of the bone)
- small fragments of bone on the lower border of the navicular bone.

Interpretation of the radiographs is not always straightforward as many sound horses have some changes as part of the normal ageing process. There is often poor correlation between the extent of the radiographic changes and the degree of lameness.

SCINTIGRAPHY

Scintigraphy can be useful in cases where the radiographic changes are not particularly helpful. Horses with navicular pathology show increased uptake of radioactive material due to increased bone turnover.

MAGNETIC RESONANCE IMAGING (MRI)

The use of MRI is helping to improve our knowledge of foot pain including navicular disease. Lesions within other tissues as well as bone can be seen in detail. However, this diagnostic technique is not universally available owing to the high costs and specialist knowledge and experience required to interpret the images.

ENDOSCOPIC EXAMINATION

The navicular bursa can be examined with a fine endoscope. The flexor surface of the navicular bone, the surface of the DDFT and the lining of the navicular bursa can be inspected.

Treatment – management and medication

There is no cure for navicular disease. If the horse responds satisfactorily to trimming and shoeing alone then it is unlikely to have had chronic navicular disease. Where there is navicular bone pain, the earlier treatment begins, the greater the chance of prolonging the horse's working life.

CORRECTIVE FARRIERY

This is an essential part of any treatment programme. The foot is trimmed to correct any hoof imbalance. If it is severely unbalanced, this may be done in several stages. The toe is usually shortened to ease breakover.

Egg bar and Natural Balance™ shoes are commonly fitted. Egg bar shoes are selected for horses with weak, collapsed and underrun heels or if the horse has small feet for its size. They spread the weight and transmitted forces over a wider area and this seems to help reduce the pain (Figure 6.57). The toe may be rolled to ease breakover. All shoes are fitted long and wide to give good support to the heels. The drawback to this is that in some horses there is a tendency for these long shoes to be pulled off.

Elevating the heels reduces the tension of the DDFT. This is usually done if the hoof-pastern axis remains broken back after trimming or the horse still lands on its toe. It is achieved by the use of wedge pads, a wedge heel shoe or an Equine Digital Support System (EDSS) shoe.

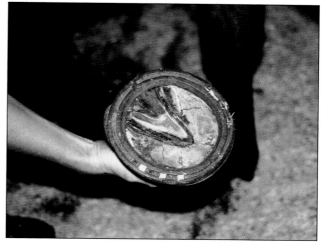

Figure 6.57 Egg bar shoe

EXERCISE

The horse should be kept in regular, daily work and turned out as much as possible. Exercise is necessary for the normal flow of blood through the foot. If the horse is lame on a circle, it should be hacked out in straight lines to start with. However, recent work with MRI has shown that many horses that were thought to have navicular disease actually have soft tissue damage involving structures such as the impar ligament within the foot. Such cases can benefit from rest.

NON-STEROIDAL ANTI-INFLAMMATORY DRUGS

Non-steroidal anti-inflammatory drugs such as phenylbutazone are sometimes necessary to allow the horse to exercise in the initial treatment period or if the disease is advanced. The lowest effective dose should be used.

ISOXUPRINE

Isoxuprine is a drug that causes dilation of blood vessels and may improve blood flow through the foot. It is administered orally. Some horses improve or become sound while on the treatment and may remain sound for up to a year after discontinuation of the medication. Other horses require continuous treatment. The treatment is most likely to have a beneficial effect in horses that are in the early stages of the disease. Those with advanced X-ray changes are unlikely to respond.

INTRA-ARTICULAR MEDICATION

Hyaluronan and/or corticosteroids injected into the coffin joint result in a temporary improvement in some cases. Injection of corticosteroids into the navicular bursa may give relief for 2–3 months.

POLYSULPHATED GLYCOSAMINOGLYCANS (PSGAG)

PSGAGs given intramuscularly every 4 days for a total of 7 treatments are reported to reduce the lameness in some patients.

NUTRACEUTICALS

Supplements containing chondroitin sulphate and glucosamine are reported to benefit some horses.

Surgical treatment

These techniques are reserved for horses that fail to respond to management changes and medication.

NAVICULAR SUSPENSORY DESMOTOMY

In this operation the collateral suspensory ligaments are cut under general anaesthesia. In one study, 76% of horses were sound after 6 months and 43% remained sound after 3 years.

PALMAR DIGITAL NEURECTOMY

If the horse becomes completely sound with a palmar digital nerve block that desensitizes the back of the foot and the sole, it may be a suitable candidate for neurectomy. With the horse under general anaesthesia, a section of the palmar digital nerve is removed. Approximately 74% of horses in one study were reported to be sound after 1 year, reducing to 63% after 2 years. This procedure must be combined with excellent ongoing foot care.

Complications of the procedure include:

- persistent lameness
- recurrence of lameness due to re-innervation of the navicular bone; the surgery can be repeated but may not be as successful the second time
- formation of a painful swelling (**neuroma**) at the cut end of the nerve
- rupture of the DDFT; the operation should not be performed on horses with obvious defects on the flexor surface of the navicular bone as the DDFT is likely to have significant lesions
- with continued use of the horse, the weakened navicular bone may fracture
- penetrating injuries to the sole and foot abscesses may go unnoticed as the sole also loses sensation with this procedure.

Prognosis

There is no cure for navicular syndrome and the disease is progressive. The outlook is always guarded, especially for performance animals.

FRACTURE OF THE PEDAL BONE

Fractures of the pedal bone (distal phalanx) are a relatively common injury. They are classified according to the location of the fracture and whether or not it extends into the coffin joint. They occur most commonly in the forelimb.

Causes

- Trauma, e.g. landing on a hard, uneven surface (forelimb) or kicking a solid object (hind limb).
- Foreign body penetration, e.g. standing on a nail or metal spike.
- A fracture may occur secondary to chronic inflammation, a bone cyst or infection of the pedal bone.
- Fractures of the extensor process of the pedal bone are associated with over-extension of the coffin joint.

Clinical signs

- In most cases there is sudden onset, moderate to severe lameness.
- Some horses show an increase in lameness over the first 24 hours due to inflammation and swelling causing a build up of pressure within the foot.
- Increased heat in the foot.
- Increased digital pulse on the affected side.
- If the fracture extends into the coffin joint there may be distension of the joint capsule just above the coronary band at the front of the limb.
- Flexion of the lower limb is painful if the joint is involved.
- The lameness is often worse when the horse turns.

Diagnosis

The diagnosis is made on the clinical signs and the results of radiography.

- In most cases the horse is sensitive to hoof testers applied close to the fracture site. However, horses with thick, hard soles may not show any reaction.
- Nerve blocks of the foot temporarily abolish the lameness.
- Many fractures are immediately obvious on X-rays (Figure 6.58). In other cases, multiple views from different angles are necessary to see the fracture line. Some fractures do not show up on the X-rays immediately after the injury occurs.

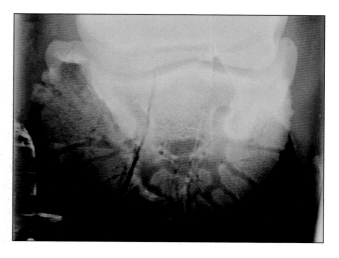

Figure 6.58 X-ray of fractured pedal bone: the fracture line is clearly visible in this pedal bone

These need to be re-examined after 10–14 days, by which time sufficient bone resorption will have taken place for the fracture to be seen.

- Nuclear scintigraphy is occasionally helpful when the fracture line is not visible on X-ray.

Treatment

Treatment is either conservative or surgical.

CONSERVATIVE TREATMENT

Fractures which do not involve the joint are treated conservatively. Some articular fractures are also treated in this way.

After balancing the foot, a bar shoe with quarter or multiple clips is used to immobilize the hoof capsule and the pedal bone. These prevent the quarters from expanding when the foot bears weight. Sometimes a shoe with a complete rim is fitted. A pad may be used to protect the sole. The Equine Digital Support System shoe can also be used to stabilize these fractures.

The foot is shod in this way every 4–6 weeks for at least 6–8 months. After this time, an ordinary bar shoe can be used. The horse is usually box rested for 3–6 months depending on the type of fracture and should not be worked for 8–12 months.

SURGICAL TREATMENT

Fractures that pass through the middle of the joint have a better prognosis if they are treated surgically. A screw is used across the fracture line to minimize movement between the two fragments and compress the fracture line. This reduces the risk of subsequent degenerative joint disease. A bar shoe with clips or a rim is then applied. Following surgery the horse is confined to a box for 2 months. Controlled walking exercise is then introduced for a further 2 months. If the horse is sound after 4 months, it can be allowed access to a small paddock for another 8 weeks.

Small fractures of the extensor process are surgically removed. Larger pieces of bone may be screwed back in place.

Aftercare

Healing progress is monitored by repeat X-rays taken every three months. This is important as pedal bones are very slow to heal and the horse often becomes sound before the fracture appears healed on the radiographs. Some fractures remain joined by fibrous tissue and will always appear abnormal on X-rays.

Possible complications

These include:

- ongoing lameness

- degenerative joint disease may be a sequel to articular fractures
- long-term use of bar shoes can cause contracted heels; this should be addressed once the fracture has healed and the horse is back in work
- the metal implant (screw) may become infected following surgery.

Prognosis

The prognosis is good for many types of non-articular fracture. If the fracture involves the joint, the prognosis is guarded. In some cases, continuing pain can be relieved by neurectomy of the palmar digital nerve.

OSSIFICATION OF THE COLLATERAL CARTILAGES OF THE PEDAL BONE (SIDEBONE)

Sidebone is a condition where bone is deposited in the paired cartilages that are attached to either side of the pedal bone. This process is known as **ossification**. It is more common in the front feet and increases with the age of the horse. Heavy breeds seem to be particularly susceptible.

The cartilages can be palpated above the coronary band towards the back of the foot (Figure 6.59 and see Figure 6.5). They extend from above the heel bulbs to halfway between the heel and toe. They are normally quite springy but become hard and unyielding when a horse has sidebone.

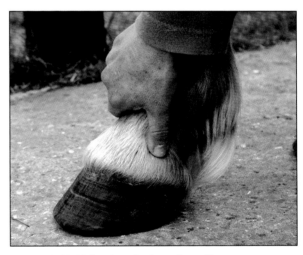

Figure 6.59 Palpating the lateral cartilages

The function of the cartilages

Together with the digital cushion they are believed to play a part in absorbing harmful concussion at the back of the foot. When the horse takes a stride and the foot contacts the ground, the frog is pushed upwards into the digital cushion and this forces the cartilages outwards. At the same time, downward movement of the pastern due to the weight of the horse has the same effect. The resultant changes of pressure within the foot are important for assisting the flow of blood through the cartilages.

Causes

This may be a normal ageing change. The process can be accelerated by increased concussion due to:

- mediolateral foot imbalance

- conformation abnormalities, e.g. toe-in horses tend to develop sidebone on the lateral side of the foot
- poor trimming and shoeing.

Ossification can also be caused by a direct injury, e.g. a wire cut to a lateral cartilage.

Clinical signs

Sidebone very rarely causes lameness. The condition develops slowly over a period of time and is usually discovered when the foot is palpated and the hardened cartilages are felt.

When it does cause lameness:
- the lameness is gradual in onset
- it is more obvious on hard surfaces
- there is occasionally heat over the affected area
- pressing the affected cartilage may cause pain
- fracture of an ossified cartilage can cause sudden-onset lameness.

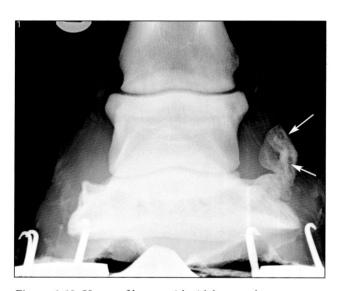

Figure 6.60 X-ray of horse with sidebone: a horse can have extensive mineralization of one or both lateral cartilages without being lame

Diagnosis

The diagnosis of sidebone is not always straightforward as there is no nerve block that selectively desensitizes that part of the foot. Many horses that are not lame have extensive mineralization of their lateral cartilages that can be seen on X-ray (Figure 6.60). Scintigraphy may be helpful in determining if there is any active remodelling of the cartilages.

Treatment

- No treatment is required in the majority of cases.
- If heat and pain are present, a combination of rest and non-steroidal anti-inflammatory drugs are recommended.
- The balance of the foot should be checked and corrected if necessary.
- The horse should be shod wide at the quarters and heels and the shoe should extend behind the heels to provide support and encourage expansion of the foot. No nails should be used any further back than the widest part of the hoof wall or they will interfere with the natural expansion of the foot when the horse bears weight.
- Fractures heal with box rest. It is sometimes necessary to remove any small bone fragments that lose their blood supply and act as a foreign body.

QUITTOR

Quittor is the name given to chronic infection of a collateral cartilage of the horse's foot.

Causes

It can be caused by:

- a penetrating injury
- a wire cut
- a blow or brushing injury to the cartilage
- the cartilage being trodden on by the opposite foot or by another horse
- a long-standing deep quarter crack or infection of the white line.

Clinical signs

These include:

- variable degrees of lameness
- one or more discharging wounds above the coronet adjacent to the infected cartilage (Figure 6.61)
- heat and swelling over the area
- pain when pressure is applied.

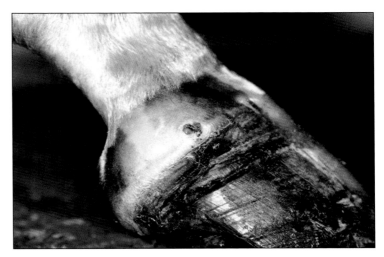

Figure 6.61 Quittor

Treatment

The only effective treatment is surgical removal of the infected area of cartilage. Broad spectrum antibiotics are given.

Prognosis

The prognosis is good if all of the damaged and infected tissue is successfully removed.

PEDAL OSTEITIS

Pedal osteitis is inflammation of the pedal bone (distal phalanx). In the past, the condition has been overdiagnosed as a cause of foot pain on the basis of foot sensitivity, the response to nerve blocks and the appearance of the pedal bone on radiographs. However, we now know that the pedal bone can be variable in appearance on X-rays and there is no nerve block that desensitizes the pedal bone without also numbing other tissues in the foot, thus it is hard to specifically diagnose the condition.

Clinical signs

Pedal osteitis usually affects both front feet.

- In the early stages the horse works normally on soft ground but shortens its stride on hard ground.
- This progresses to lameness when worked on hard ground.
- If one foot is worse than the other, the lameness may be worse on a circle.
- The lameness improves with rest, but recurs when the horse is brought back into work.

Causes

Inflammation may occur as a result of long-term concussion of the foot and chronic bruising of the sole. Horses with flat feet and thin soles that work on hard ground are particularly susceptible.

Alternatively, pedal osteitis may develop secondary to other foot problems such as:

- laminitis
- puncture wounds
- persistent corns
- foot imbalance
- fracture of the pedal bone.

Diagnosis

A diagnosis of pedal osteitis is made when:

- the pain is abolished when the foot is numbed with a nerve block
- other causes of foot pain have been ruled out
- there are marked radiographic changes on the pedal bone.

The application of hoof testers will be resented by some horses but this is an unreliable sign as many horses with thin soles react to this test by pulling their foot away.

Radiographic changes include:

- a reduction in overall density of the bone
- new bone on the front of the pedal bone giving it a rough and irregular appearance.

Treatment and prognosis

Where there is extensive deposition of new bone or considerable loss of bone density, there is no effective treatment and the prognosis is poor.

In less severe cases the horse may benefit from:

- a period of rest
- correction of any foot imbalance
- fitting of wide webbed shoes with a concave solar surface ('seated out') to protect the sole (see Figure 6.37)

- the use of egg bar shoes to maximize the weight-bearing surface
- the fitting of sole pads
- application of a topical iodine, phenol and formalin mixture to harden soft or thin soles
- modification of the exercise programme to avoid working on hard or stony ground
- administration of non-steroidal anti-inflammatory drugs such as phenylbutazone to reduce the pain and inflammation.

If the above treatments are unsuccessful, a neurectomy may be considered as a last resort. If a palmar digital nerve block completely abolishes the lameness, a section of the palmar digital nerve supplying sensation to the foot can be surgically removed.

DISEASES OF THE COFFIN JOINT

The distal interphalangeal or coffin joint has a complex structure. In addition to the joint between the middle and distal phalanges, both of these bones articulate with the navicular bone (see Figure 6.4). The joint may be affected by a number of problems which include:
- synovitis; this is inflammation of the synovial membrane of the joint
- osteoarthritis
- strain of the collateral ligaments joining the middle and distal phalanges
- fractures of the pedal bone which involve the joint
- septic arthritis (joint infection) from penetrating wounds
- subchondral bone cysts of the middle phalanx or the distal phalanx.

Signs of coffin joint pain

Lameness from coffin joint pain is relatively common in the forelimbs, but it can also be a cause of hind limb lameness. It may be sudden or gradual in onset and affect one or both limbs. It is often more obvious when the horse is worked in a circle, especially on a hard surface. If the disease is bilateral, the horse may shorten its stride or lose its enthusiasm for jumping, rather than demonstrating obvious lameness. In most cases, the disease is more advanced in one limb and lameness is apparent.

The joint capsule is often distended. A swelling may be seen just above the coronary band at the front of the foot. If the joint is flexed or rotated, the discomfort may cause the horse to snatch the foot away. The lameness may be exacerbated by a flexion test.

Predisposing causes

Horses with mediolateral foot imbalance are predisposed to strains and degenerative changes of the coffin joint. When the horse is working, most of the joint movement is flexion and extension. If the foot is unbalanced, however, the joint is tilted from side to side and this puts more strain on the supporting ligaments and joint capsule.

Long-toe, low-heel conformation or an abnormal angle of the pedal bone within the hoof capsule also increase the wear and tear of the coffin joint.

Traumatic injuries such as acute sprains can also contribute to coffin joint pain.

Diagnosis

It is not always easy to confirm that the coffin joint is the source of pain and the results of nerve blocks and radiographs have to be interpreted with care.

NERVE BLOCKS

Injection of local anaesthetic into a painful coffin joint rapidly improves the lameness. However, in some horses, the local anaesthetic can also eliminate pain arising from other areas of the foot, including the navicular bone and navicular bursa. As a general rule, if the horse responds quickly to intra-articular analgesia but does not improve with analgesia of the navicular bursa, the coffin joint is considered to be the source of pain.

RADIOGRAPHY

Several views of the foot must be taken and the images have to be interpreted with care. It is possible for there to be remodelling of the bone close to the joint, giving the appearance of degenerative joint disease (DJD), but without any pain. The horse may also experience significant joint pain in the absence of any radiographic changes.

ULTRASONOGRAPHY

This is a useful tool for detecting any damage to the collateral ligaments. It is also used to assess the degree of distension of the joint capsule.

MAGNETIC RESONANCE IMAGING (MRI)

MRI is a very useful tool for evaluating the coffin joint and the associated ligaments, but it is not universally available.

Arthroscopy and **scintigraphy** may also be helpful.

Synovitis

This is the commonest cause of coffin joint pain. The synovial membrane of the joint becomes inflamed and produces an increased amount of synovial fluid. Symptoms include:
- mild to moderate lameness
- distension of the joint capsule.

TREATMENT

This includes:

- correction of any foot imbalance with appropriate trimming and shoeing
- intra-articular medication with polysulphated glycosaminoglycans (PSGAGs), hyaluronan, or hyaluronan plus a corticosteroid
- controlled exercise following the intra-articular medication, as recommended by your vet.

PROGNOSIS

The prognosis for return to soundness is reasonable if the condition is diagnosed and treated before degenerative changes develop in the articular surface of the joint.

Osteoarthritis

Once degenerative changes that are visible on X-rays occur within the joint, the lameness is likely to become more severe and less responsive to intra-articular medication (Figure 6.62). Some horses are able to remain in work with the use of non-steroidal anti-inflammatory drugs such as phenylbutazone. The prognosis for remaining sound is guarded.

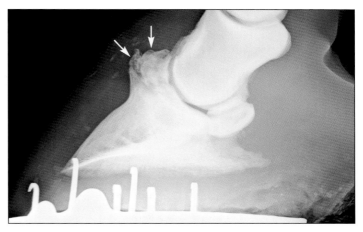

Figure 6.62 X-ray showing severe degenerative joint disease (DJD) of the coffin joint

KERATOMA

A keratoma is a benign tumour of the horn-producing cells of the foot. Abnormal amounts of horny tissue are produced on the inner surface of the hoof wall. Keratomas tend to develop at the front of the foot, between the toe and the quarters.

Causes

Keratomas usually begin at the coronary band. They are thought to form in response to direct trauma or chronic irritation from foot abscesses affecting the white line.

Clinical signs

These include the following.

- Variable degrees of lameness; this is caused by the expanding mass of horny tissue pressing on the sensitive tissues of the foot. The lameness comes on slowly and is intermittent to start with, gradually becoming more persistent and severe.
- Distortion of the hoof at the coronary band and the wall which may develop an abnormal bulge.

- If the lesion grows down to the sole, the white line is displaced towards the middle of the foot (Figure 6.63).
- Discharging tracts may form due to infection entering at the white line; the pus may escape at the coronary band or from the sole.
- The affected region is variably sensitive to hoof testers.

Diagnosis

The diagnosis is made on the clinical examination and confirmed by radiography. Pressure from the keratoma may cause resorption of bone from the pedal bone. This shows up as a semicircular defect with a smooth outline at the margin of the bone.

Treatment

Treatment involves surgical removal of all abnormal tissue. The hoof wall is resected to allow access to the abnormal horn (Figure 6.64). The exposed soft tissues are packed with iodine dressings. The hoof is stabilized by applying a bar shoe with clips on either side of the defect. If the lesion is extensive, a metal plate is screwed across the defect to aid stability. Once the exposed laminae are dry and there are no concerns about recurrence of the tumour, the defect may be filled in with an acrylic resin. At this stage the horse can start work. The defect grows out over 6–12 months.

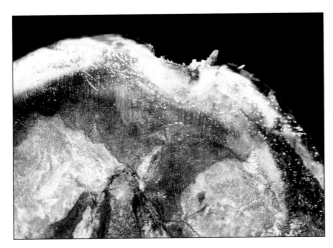

Figure 6.63 The keratoma has displaced the white line towards the centre of the foot

Figure 6.64 The hoof wall and abnormal horn have been removed

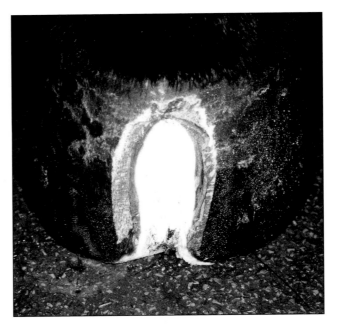

Prognosis

The prognosis is good if the entire tumour is removed and the foot can be adequately stabilized. The tumour will regrow if any abnormal tissue remains.

7

TENDON AND LIGAMENT INJURIES

STRUCTURE AND FUNCTION OF TENDONS

Tendons are bands of dense white fibrous tissue that connect muscles to bones. They are made up of parallel bundles of longitudinally aligned collagen fibrils. They have great tensile strength but are relatively inelastic.

SUPERFICIAL DIGITAL FLEXOR TENDONITIS

Anatomy

In the forelimb the superficial digital flexor muscle attaches to the medial epicondyle of the humerus, i.e. just above the elbow. The muscle tissue becomes a thick tendon before it passes through the carpal canal at the back of the knee. It then becomes a flattened band which widens at the fetlock and forms a ring through which the tendon of the deep digital flexor passes. The ring splits below the fetlock and the tendon inserts onto the back of the distal (lower) part of the proximal phalanx (P1) and the proximal (upper) part of the middle phalanx (P2). (Figures 7.1a and b.)

Strains

A strain occurs when the tendon is overstretched. The resultant haemorrhage and inflammation disrupts the normal alignment of the collagen fibrils. Strains can vary in severity from minor inflammation to severe disruption or even complete rupture of a tendon. This inflammation of the tendon is known as tendonitis. A horse with a moderate to severe tendon strain is colloquially said to have 'broken down'.

Type of horse affected

The Thoroughbred racehorse has a relatively high risk of strain to the superficial digital

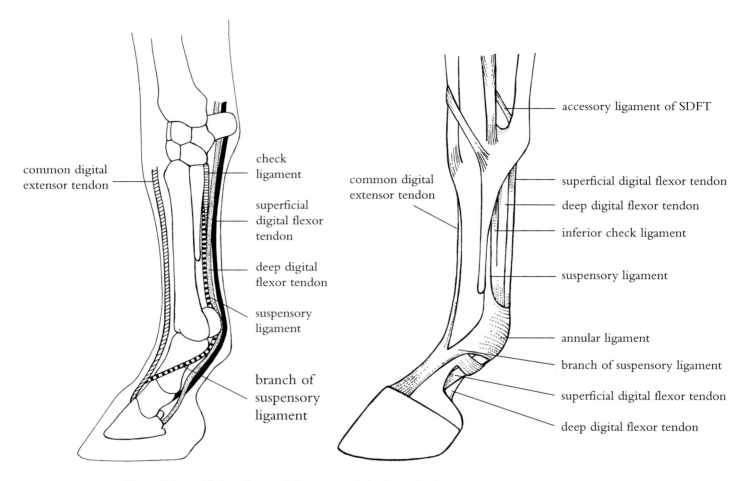

Figure 7.1a and b Tendons and ligaments of the lower limb

flexor tendon (SDFT) and the forelimb is most commonly affected. During galloping, when the forelimb contacts the ground, the fetlock is hyperextended and the SDFT is stretched to its limit. SDFT injuries also occur in other equine athletes, particularly the three-day event horse, but are less frequently found in ponies.

Causes

Predisposing factors that put extra strain on tendons include:

- poor conformation
- fatigue
- working at speed on hard, uneven ground
- inappropriate training programmes and general lack of fitness
- poor training surfaces
- weight of the rider
- age: the incidence of tendon injury increases with age due to cumulative and undetected damage as a result of training

- other illness or disease – for example, horses that continue in training with an ongoing viral infection may be more susceptible to tendon injury.

Clinical signs

These vary according to the severity of the strain. Generally the horse will show the following.

- Heat.
- Swelling.
- Lameness. The lameness may be slight to severe. In some instances the horse will bear very little weight on the affected limb, standing with the knee flexed and the heel slightly raised from the ground. Where major disruption of the tendon occurs, the fetlock sinks closer to the ground than normal. It is possible, however, for a horse to have a moderate degree of tendon damage and not show any lameness. For this reason it is *absolutely essential* that the warning signs of heat and swelling are recognized and the injury is investigated before further damage occurs. The signs may include increased warmth and very slight swelling of the tendon.
- Pain on palpation. When the affected limb is flexed, even gentle pressure applied to the tendon with the thumb and forefinger will cause the horse to withdraw the limb.
- Convex or 'bowed' profile (Figure 7.2).

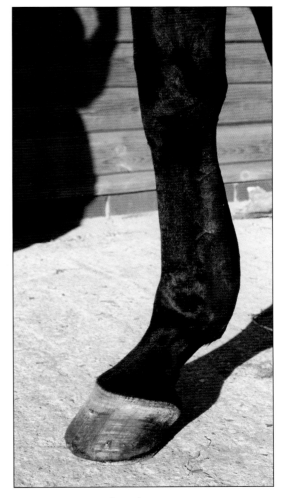

Figure 7.2 Bowed tendon

Diagnosis

The diagnosis is made on the clinical signs and the results of an ultrasongraphic examination. Scanning is essential to determine the site and the extent of the damage as it is not always possible to ascertain this by feeling the leg. It should be delayed until at least 4 days after the injury occurs for a true picture of the damage to be obtained. If examined earlier than this, the swelling makes it difficult to appreciate fibre damage. Both limbs are usually examined as degenerative changes will often be found in the other leg as well.

The procedure for scanning

The legs are clipped and scrubbed, then covered with a special gel. Modern ultrasound machines produce very good quality, detailed images which require interpretation by a vet who is used to examining them. Longitudinal and transverse images are taken at several locations between the knee and the fetlock. The signs of tendon damage include:

a

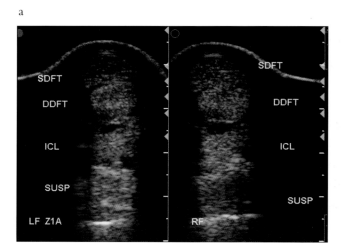

b

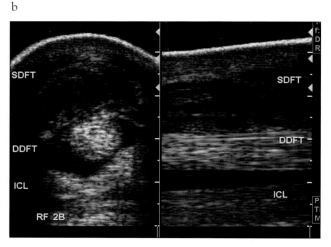

Figure 7.3a and b Ultrasound scans of the superficial digital flexor tendon showing a) normal transverse (sections across) images of the flexor tendons – SDFT = superficial digital flexor tendon, DDFT = deep digital flexor tendon, ICL = inferior check ligament, SUSP = suspensory ligament; b) transverse and longitudinal images of an injured SDFT. Note the enlarged cross-sectional area of the tendon and the dark appearance due to disruption of the tendon fibres.

- an increase in cross-sectional area of the tendon
- area(s) of decreased density of the tendon structure – these show as dark areas within the tendon (Figure 7.3b)
- change in shape of the tendon
- loss of longitudinal alignment of the fibres on the longitudinal view.

By examining all the images, the vet will know the position, the extent and the severity of the damage. Good quality images are essential so that the healing progress can be monitored at subsequent examinations. A second examination may be recommended 4 weeks later when the haemorrhage and inflammation have subsided.

Pathology and phases of healing

SDFT strains may be the result of a single catastrophic event or they may occur as a result of multiple episodes of wear and tear sustained as a result of the horse's activities. Many older horses that do not show signs of tendonitis have degenerative changes in their tendons. However, the tendon only has the capacity to cope for so long and there is a limit to the amount of damage that can be sustained before the horse goes lame.

The narrowest part of the SDFT is at mid-cannon level and this is the commonest site of injury. The lesion tends to occur in the centre of the tendon structure and is known as a 'core' lesion.

ACUTE INFLAMMATORY PHASE

This typically lasts from a few days from the time of injury up to 2 weeks later, depending on the severity of the strain. There is considerable swelling, inflammation and haemorrhage into the tendon resulting in oedema and an increased blood supply including white blood cells (neutrophils, monocytes and macrophages) which clear up the damaged tissue.

SUBACUTE REPAIR PHASE

During the healing process which starts a few days after the injury, cells called fibroblasts migrate into the areas and produce new collagen. This repair (type III) collagen is randomly arranged and it forms scar tissue which is not as strong or elastic as the original (type 1) collagen. The tendon becomes thickened and bowed and is prone to re-injury at this stage. As the inflammation subsides, so the lameness resolves.

REMODELLING PHASE

This phase of healing begins 2–3 months after the injury occurred and can last for up to 15 months. The type III collagen is gradually replaced by type I. Cross-links develop between the collagen fibrils and increase the strength of the scar tissue. Controlled exercise encourages the longitudinal alignment of the fibres. The fully healed area is thicker and stronger but less elastic than the original tendon. This puts the adjacent areas under increased strain and they are thus more prone to break down.

Treatment

The aims of treatment are to:

- relieve the pain
- reduce the swelling and inflammation
- provide support
- encourage successful healing with longitudinal alignment of the collagen fibrils.

A severe tendon injury is a medical emergency and treatment should be instigated straight away. The aim is to limit the inflammation otherwise proteolytic enzymes released to break down the damaged collagen will also digest healthy tendon tissue and increase the size of the lesion.

ACUTE PHASE TREATMENT

- Cold therapy. Immediately the injury occurs, the leg should be hosed with cold water or tubbed in a slurry of ice and water for 20–30 minutes. This should be repeated 2–3 times a day until the acute inflammation has subsided. Sophisticated cold treatment boots (Figure 7.4) and hydrotherapy spas are available.
- Between treatments, both limbs should be support bandaged.
- A cast may sometimes be applied by the vet if the tendon is severely damaged or completely ruptured.
- The horse is kept on box rest with controlled walking exercise as advised by the vet.

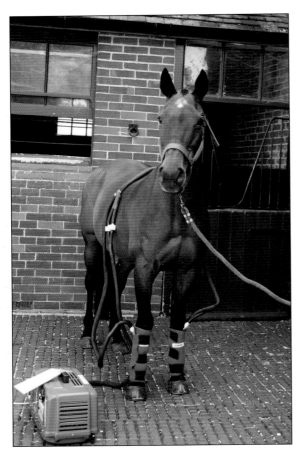

Figure 7.4 Horse having hydrotherapy: the leg wraps, with circulating cold water, are attached to a refrigeration unit

Controlled exercise introduced at the appropriate time helps to prevent adhesions forming and encourages good healing with longitudinal alignment of the collagen fibrils. Where this is not possible, passive mobilization of the region by gentle flexing of the knee and fetlock may be beneficial.

- Systemic non-steroidal anti-inflammatory drugs (NSAIDs), e.g. phenylbutazone, may be administered to reduce the pain and inflammation.

Other treatments that may be considered at this stage include the following.

- A single systemic dose of corticosteroids to reduce inflammation is sometimes prescribed.
- A course of intramuscular injections of polysulphated glycosaminoglycan (PSGAG) to reduce inflammation and encourage collagen synthesis.
- Injection of PSGAG into the lesion to inhibit proteolytic enzymes.
- Topical application of dimethyl sulphoxide (DMSO) to reduce the oedema.
- Tendon splitting may be done to increase the blood supply and speed healing of small core lesions.
- Desmotomy (cutting) of the proximal check or accessory ligament of the SDFT. This ligament attaches to the lower part of the radius on the medial side. The theory is that cutting this ligament allows the muscle belly of the SDFT to take some of the strain and so reduce that on the tendon. This treatment has been associated with a subsequent increase in injuries to the suspensory ligament which takes additional strain as a result.

SUBACUTE PHASE TREATMENT

- Controlled exercise with regular monitoring by ultrasound examination. Monitoring is essential to ensure that further damage is not occurring and should be done before any step up in the horse's exercise regime.

Additional treatments that may be considered include the following.

- Injection of hyaluronan into and around the injury to encourage healing and prevent adhesions forming.
- Injection of beta-aminoproprionitrile fumarate (BAPN) into the lesion. The drug is

no longer licensed. It prevents cross-links forming between the collagen fibrils, allowing better longitudinal alignment of the collagen fibres with controlled exercise.

- Injection of growth factors (insulin-like growth factor 1 (IGF-1) and transforming growth factor β-1 (TGF β-1) into the lesion. These are thought to play a role in stimulating the repair process and to encourage the production of type 1 collagen.

- Currently, research is being carried out on the injection of mesenchymal stem cells from bone marrow or foal umbilical cords into the lesion. Stem cells have the potential to develop into any type of tissue and the rationale is that they could help produce new tendon tissue rather than scar tissue. Bone marrow taken from the horse's sternum has been injected into damaged suspensory ligaments with some reported success. Work is now being done on culturing the stem cells, suspending them in the animal's own serum and injecting it back into the tendon. It is too early to make any conclusions about the efficacy of this treatment at this time, but the early results look promising.

- Physical therapies including low intensity laser therapy, therapeutic ultrasound, electromagnetic field therapy and extracorporeal shock wave therapy are used. These treatments will reduce the soft tissue swelling but there is little evidence that the end result is improved when compared with conservative treatment and controlled exercise.

- Hydrotherapy spas are becoming popular and seem to help healing.

- Counter-irritation including blistering and pin firing is still used on occasions if other treatments have not been successful.

REMODELLING PHASE

During this phase which can continue for 15–18 months following a severe injury, type III collagen is slowly being converted to type I. The healing process should be closely monitored by ultrasound examination. If at any stage there is an increase of more than 10% in the cross-sectional area of the tendon, the exercise is cut back. At each stage it is hoped that there will be an improvement in the tendon density and fibre pattern.

Exercise programme

This will be tailored to the individual horse. It will depend on:

- the severity of the initial injury
- the progress already made
- the temperament of the horse
- the facilities available
- the experience of the rider
- the state of the ground.

It is not possible to give guidelines to suit every horse. As a general guide, walking exercise should be initiated as soon as possible in all but the most severe cases. Consult your own vet who will recommend a programme of walking exercise to be done twice daily depending on the severity of the injury.

For the first 4–6 weeks of healing the use of a horse walker is not recommended because moving in a circle puts extra strain on the damaged tissue. Later on, the owner or trainer may find the horse is easier to manage on a walker than in hand.

At 8 weeks the tendon is usually re-examined and according to progress the walking may be increased or a short period of trotting introduced. The vet will be able to advise on each individual case. It is generally accepted that turnout in a large field puts the horse at serious risk of re-injury. Ideally the horse should be kept on a controlled exercise programme as advised by the vet for up to a year. If the horse is turned out, it should be into a small paddock where it cannot canter or build up speed.

Prognosis

This depends on the severity of the initial injury and the subsequent healing response. The appearance of the tendon on the initial ultrasound scan and at the start of canter work may be helpful in predicting whether or not the horse will stand up to fast work. Early recognition and appropriate management will influence the final outcome. No treatment has proved satisfactory or superior to others at the time of writing. In racehorses and three-day eventers, there is a high risk of recurrence.

Prevention

As treatment only has limited success, the key to this type of injury is prevention and early detection.

Attention should be paid to the following.

- Any early warning signs that might indicate tendon damage, e.g. slight heat or swelling in the metacarpal region behind the cannon bone.
- Training surfaces and exercise programmes.
- Avoiding fast work on hard, soft or uneven terrain.
- Not working fatigued horses because a stumble or uncoordinated movement can lead to severe injury due to asynchronous contraction of muscle while the tendon is taking the strain.
- Controlled exercise of growing horses less than two years old; there is evidence that this helps to develop good quality tendon tissue.
- Detection of early changes that are not clinically apparent by the use of routine ultrasonography; this applies to racehorses after a hard race and eventers after major competitions. Thermography may detect the heat associated with inflammatory changes up to 2 weeks before they are observed by the trainer or rider.
- Genetics: some horses may have a genetic predisposition to weak tendon structure; further work is being done to investigate this.

A blood test may soon become available to detect early tendon damage.

Above all else, it is important to remember that a horse may NOT be lame despite moderate tendon damage. Continued work and ignoring the warning signs may lead to permanent and irreparable damage.

STRAIN OF THE DEEP DIGITAL FLEXOR TENDON

Anatomy

The fleshy part of the deep digital flexor muscle in the forelimb lies along the back of the radius under the superficial digital flexor. It then becomes a thick tendon running through the carpal canal at the back of the knee. It continues down behind the cannon (metacarpal) bone where it is joined in the middle third by the accessory ligament which originates at the back of the knee. The tendon passes through a ring formed by the SDFT at the fetlock and then inserts on the pedal bone (third or distal phalanx). Part of the deep digital flexor tendon (DDFT) is enclosed within the digital flexor tendon sheath (DFTS) (Figure 7.5).

Causes

Injuries to the DDFT usually occur when the horse is fatigued and the going is uneven. Horses that jump are most at risk. Strains of the DDFT in the metacarpal and metatarsal region are much less common than strains of the SDFT. When they do occur it is usually in association with chronic inflammation of the accessory ligament (inferior check ligament) of the DDFT. The strains tend to occur in the fetlock and pastern regions where the tendon is enclosed within the sheath. DDF tendonitis may occur in horses with concurrent navicular disease. Recent work with magnetic resonance imaging has shown that this is much more prevalent than previously recognized.

Clinical signs

- Sudden onset of lameness, usually mild to moderate, occasionally severe. If the lameness is only slight, it may become worse if the horse is lunged on a soft surface. It is made worse with hard work and improves with rest. Flexion of the distal limb may exacerbate the lameness.
- Local heat and swelling.
- Pain on palpation.
- Distension of the DFTS if the lesion is within the sheath (Figure 7.6). With severe lesions within the hoof capsule, the horse may 'point' the limb at rest.

Diagnosis

Diagnosis of these lesions can be difficult unless the swelling is obvious. Sometimes a diagnosis can be made on the clinical signs and ultrasonography. Nerve blocks may be

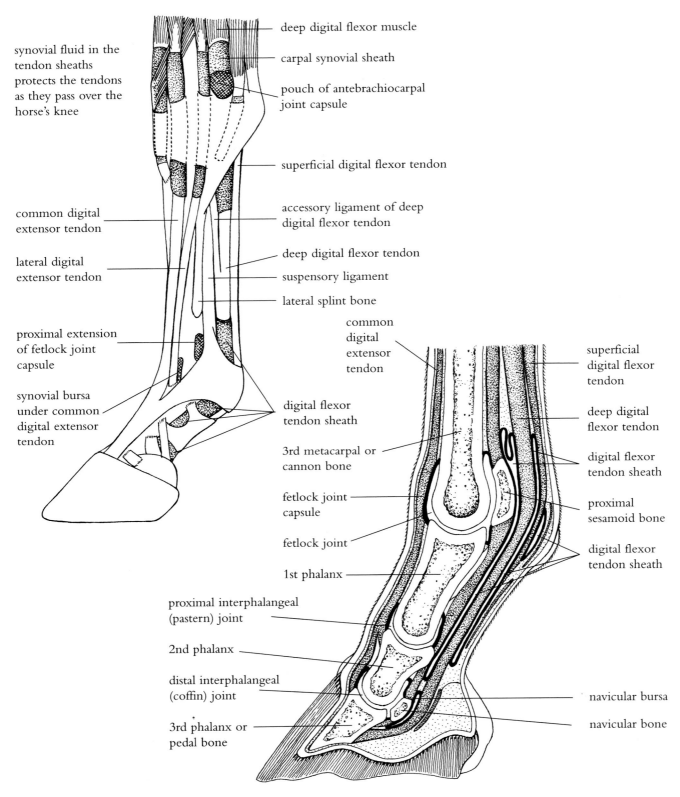

deep digital flexor muscle

carpal synovial sheath

pouch of antebrachiocarpal joint capsule

synovial fluid in the tendon sheaths protects the tendons as they pass over the horse's knee

superficial digital flexor tendon

accessory ligament of deep digital flexor tendon

common digital extensor tendon

deep digital flexor tendon

suspensory ligament

lateral digital extensor tendon

lateral splint bone

common digital extensor tendon

superficial digital flexor tendon

proximal extension of fetlock joint capsule

deep digital flexor tendon

digital flexor tendon sheath

synovial bursa under common digital extensor tendon

digital flexor tendon sheath

3rd metacarpal or cannon bone

proximal sesamoid bone

fetlock joint capsule

digital flexor tendon sheath

fetlock joint

1st phalanx

proximal interphalangeal (pastern) joint

2nd phalanx

distal interphalangeal (coffin) joint

navicular bursa

navicular bone

3rd phalanx or pedal bone

Figure 7.5 Muscles, tendons and tendon sheaths of the forelimb lateral view (top) and section through the lower limb (bottom)

helpful. Surgical exploration may be required if the lesion is within the digital sheath. However, when the damage occurs within the hoof capsule close to its insertion on the distal phalanx, this may not be picked up by ultrasonography. This may require nuclear scintigraphy, magnetic resonance imaging (MRI) or computed tomography (CT) for a definite diagnosis. Consequently, deep digital flexor tendon injuries may be under-diagnosed as a cause of foot pain and forelimb lameness in the horse.

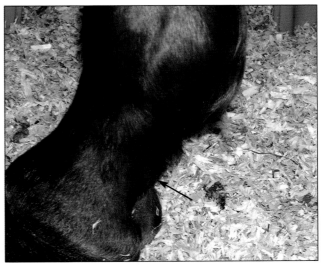

Figure 7.6 Bulge of distended digital tendon sheath

Treatment

This may include:

- box rest
- cold therapy
- support bandage
- controlled exercise
- non-steroidal anti-inflammatory drugs, e.g. phenylbutazone
- injection of hyaluronan into the tendon sheath to limit adhesions
- surgical treatment may be required if there is a tear at the edge of the tendon within the tendon sheath.

Prognosis

This depends on the site and severity of the damage, but is generally guarded.

STRAIN OF THE ACCESSORY LIGAMENT OF THE DEEP DIGITAL FLEXOR TENDON

Anatomy

The accessory (or inferior check) ligament of the deep digital flexor tendon (ALDDFT) lies between the suspensory ligament and the deep digital flexor tendon. It runs from the carpal ligament at the back of the knee to join the DDFT halfway down the cannon bone.

Desmitis or inflammation of this ligament can occur in all types of horse and pony, especially jumping animals. It usually occurs in the forelimbs and tends to be more common in the older horse. This is likely to be the result of degenerative ageing changes that occur as a result of cumulative wear and tear during the horse's working life. Desmitis of the ALDDFT may occur on its own or in association with injury to the superficial or deep digital flexor tendons. Adhesions frequently develop between these structures.

Clinical signs

- Sudden-onset lameness.
- Local swelling in the upper third of the metacarpal region.
- Heat.
- Pain on palpation.
- In severe cases, the horse may stand with the knee slightly flexed and the heel slightly raised from the ground.

Diagnosis

Diagnosis is made on the clinical signs and ultrasonography. Diagnostic scanning is essential for assessment of the severity of the injury.

Treatment

This may include the following.

- Box rest.
- Cold therapy.
- Controlled exercise.
- Non-steroidal anti-inflammatory drugs (NSAIDs) may be given.
- Desmotomy (surgical cutting) of the ALDDFT, which may be done if the healing does not progress after six months; the procedure removes the strain on the scar tissue and relieves the pain and lameness. Following surgery, the ligament still heals by forming scar tissue but it is longer in length and less subject to strain.

Healing

Healing should be monitored by repeat ultrasound examinations. The horse should not be turned out or do any more than controlled exercise until the ligament has healed, which is likely to take a minimum of 6 months and up to 1 year. The ligament will remain permanently thickened.

Prognosis

For acute injuries that are recognized and treated appropriately, the prognosis is reasonably good. Chronic injuries have a much less favourable outcome. With very severe strains, adhesions may develop between the ALDDFT and the superficial digital flexor tendon. In these cases the prognosis is poor.

BRUISED TENDONS

The flexor tendons at the back of the cannon bone are covered only by skin so they are very vulnerable to bruising from kicks or overreaches.

Clinical signs and diagnosis

The clinical signs are similar to those for a tendon strain. There may be visible signs of external trauma or the history may be known, but frequently the only clues will be soft tissue swelling and tenderness. Diagnostic ultrasound is often required to differentiate oedema and swelling around the tendon and bleeding within the tendon due to bruising, from a more serious tendon strain.

Treatment

The treatment is similar to that described for tendon strains. Where the overlying skin is damaged and infection is a complicating factor, the wound will need to be thoroughly cleaned and antibiotics are administered.

Prognosis

In general, the prognosis is more favourable and the recovery period is shorter than for strained tendons.

Prevention

Boots and bandages may provide protection, especially when lungeing or jumping. However, overtight bandages and badly fitting boots that rub especially in wet, muddy conditions can cause problems of their own.

SEVERED TENDONS

A severed tendon is a medical emergency. With prompt diagnosis, good wound management and adequate support, the prognosis is good for extensor tendons and variable for flexor tendons. Veterinary attention should be sought immediately.

Extensor tendons

The common and lateral digital extensor tendons in the forelimb and the long and lateral digital extensor tendons in the hind limb are vulnerable to injury as they lie just below the skin. Injury usually occurs between the knee or hock and the fetlock. The function of the extensor tendons is to extend the toe.

CLINICAL SIGNS

If an extensor tendon is severed, the horse will often bring the affected limb forward with a characteristic flip of the lower limb at walk. There is a tendency for the fetlock to knuckle when walking but the horse will bear weight normally at rest.

DIAGNOSIS

Diagnosis is made on the clinical signs, exploration of the wound and possibly ultrasonography.

TREATMENT

The wound is clipped and carefully cleaned. Any dead or damaged tissue is removed. Antibiotics are administered together with tetanus antitoxin if the horse is not vaccinated. The horse is kept on box rest and the limb is usually immobilized with a heavy bandage, a splint or a cast for 3–6 weeks. During the following 6 weeks the horse is started on a programme of controlled walking exercise. If there are no complications and no tendency for knuckling at the fetlock joint, the exercise may then be gradually increased. Healing and full return to normal function can take up to 6 months. Healing can be monitored by serial ultrasound examinations.

Flexor tendons

Laceration of a flexor tendon is a serious injury. The deep and superficial digital flexor tendons, together with the suspensory ligament support the fetlock joint.

CLINICAL SIGNS

These depend on the degree of tissue damage. The horse will generally be very lame. However, these injuries are sometimes overlooked if the injury has occurred at speed. This is because there is a gliding action between the skin and the tendon as the horse moves, so the skin wound may not lie directly over the tendon laceration when the horse is at rest.

If the superficial digital flexor tendon (SDFT) has been severed, the horse may stand normally. If the injury is very painful, it may bear weight on the toe to prevent movement of the tendon. If the opposite limb is lifted, the fetlock joint will have a 'dropped' appearance and be slightly closer to the ground (Figure 7.7). If both the SDFT and the deep digital flexor tendon (DDFT) are cut, the toe will lift off the ground when the limb bears weight (Figure 7.8).

DIAGNOSIS

Diagnosis is made on the clinical signs and ultrasonography.

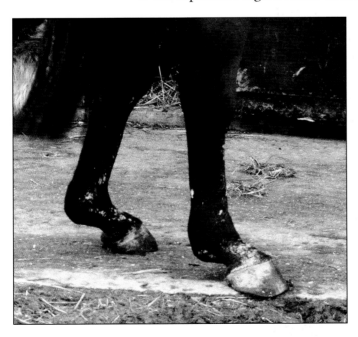

Figure 7.7 Both fetlocks of this horse have dropped following severe tendon injury

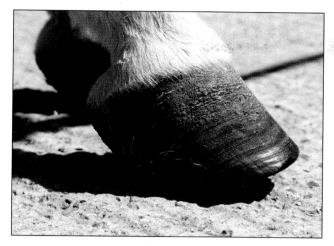

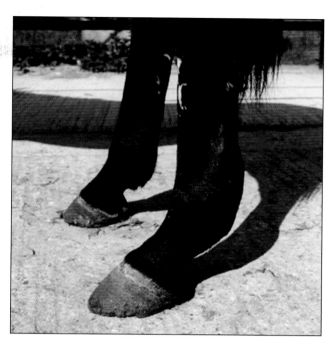

Figure 7.8 With a severe tendon injury the toe lifts off the ground when the limb bears weight

Figure 7.9 A severed superficial digital flexor tendon left this horse with a permanently thickened limb

TREATMENT

General anaesthesia may be required for the wound to be thoroughly inspected and cleaned, then dead or contaminated tissue is removed surgically. If the digital flexor tendon sheath is involved, this must be flushed and medicated with antibiotics. Wherever possible, the tendon is sutured and then immobilized in a cast for several weeks. A heel support is sometimes incorporated in the cast to reduce the pull on the tendon and allow healing to occur. Following removal of the cast, the horse may be shod with raised heels which are gradually lowered over the next few weeks. If both flexor tendons were ruptured, heel extensions are used to provide further support. Controlled walking exercise is introduced after the initial 3-month period of box rest. Healing is monitored by ultrasound examinations. The horse should not be turned out until it is sound at walk and trot and the appearance is good on clinical and ultrasound examination. Healing takes up to 12 months.

PROGNOSIS

The prognosis for straightforward extensor tendon lacerations with no complications is good. If treated immediately and appropriately, approximately 50% of horses with a single flexor tendon laceration are able to return to work after a year. Those with rupture of both the SDFT and the DDFT have a guarded prognosis. The most common cause of residual pain and lameness is adhesions between the tendon and the surrounding tissues or within the tendon sheath. Depending on the site of the injury, annular ligament constriction may be a cause of subsequent lameness.

THE STRUCTURE AND FUNCTION OF LIGAMENTS

Ligaments are bands of tough, fibrous tissue that support the joints and hold the bones in place. Injuries to these structures should be treated promptly to minimize the risk of permanent damage.

SUSPENSORY LIGAMENT INJURY

Anatomy

The origin of the suspensory ligament in the forelimb is the palmar carpal ligament at the back of the knee and the top of the cannon bone. It runs down the back of the cannon bone as a broad flat band between the two splint bones. Above the fetlock it divides into medial and lateral branches. Each branch attaches to one of the proximal sesamoid bones before running obliquely across the pastern to join the common digital extensor tendon. The function of the suspensory ligament is to prevent overextension of the fetlock joint (Figures 7.10a and b).

Injuries to the suspensory ligament

Inflamation of a ligament is known as desmitis. Injuries to the suspensory ligament usually occur during fast work or with athletic manoeuvres such as those performed in

a) Position of the suspensory ligament

b) Back view of cannon region

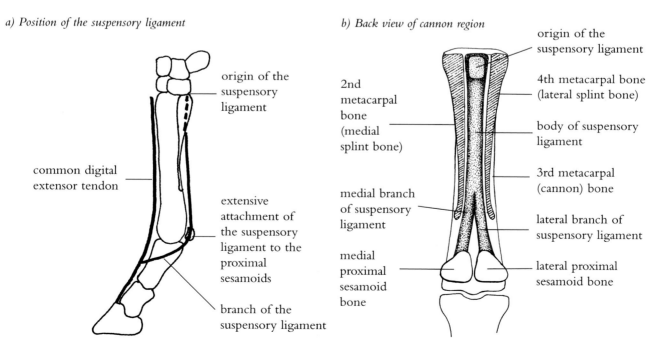

Figures 7.10a and b Position of the suspensory ligament

dressage. There is an increased incidence with age, and age-related degenerative changes occur. Suspensory ligament injuries occur in three separate regions:

- proximal suspensory desmitis
- desmitis of the body of the suspensory ligament
- desmitis of the branches of the suspensory ligament.

Proximal suspensory desmitis of the forelimb

This is a relatively common injury in athletic horses. The injury affects the proximal part of the ligament, close to its origin. It may affect one or both limbs.

CLINICAL SIGNS

- Lameness:
    - mild to moderate lameness which is sudden in onset
    - the lameness may be more obvious when the horse works on a soft surface
    - it may be exacerbated when the affected limb is on the outside of a circle
    - it often resolves rapidly with rest but recurs with hard work
    - if the condition is bilateral, the horse may appear to move badly rather than look lame
    - with chronic lesions the horse may remain lame
    - flexion of the distal limb accentuates the lameness in some but not all cases.
- Heat and slight swelling may be present in acute cases but neither are a consistent sign.
- Pain may be elicited on deep palpation of the origin of the ligament.

If the injury is severe, a fragment of cannon bone may become detached at the origin of the ligament. This is known as an avulsion fracture. The lameness is usually unilateral, sudden in onset and moderate to severe.

DIAGNOSIS

Because of the intermittent nature of the lameness and the lack of obvious heat and swelling, the diagnosis is often confirmed using one or more of the following techniques.

Diagnostic analgesia

Nerve blocks are often used in order to confirm a diagnosis of proximal suspensory desmitis. However, these have to be interpreted with care as they can eliminate other sources of pain which may also be contributing to the lameness.

Ultrasonography

Good quality images are essential for diagnosis of this condition and monitoring of the healing process. Both forelimbs are examined as the changes may be bilateral. Some injuries show only very subtle ultrasongraphic changes and in unilateral cases comparison with the other limb may be helpful.

Radiography

There are not usually any radiographic changes with acute proximal suspensory desmitis. With a chronic injury, there may be increased bone density or new bone deposition at the top of the cannon bone. When the lameness is sudden in onset and severe, radiography is used to rule out an avulsion fracture of the cannon bone at the site of origin of the suspensory ligament.

Scintigraphy

Scintigraphy does not reliably detect proximal suspensory desmitis. However, it can be helpful in the diagnosis of proximal suspensory desmitis when it is accompanied by an avulsion fracture or if other diagnostic techniques have been inconclusive.

TREATMENT

Treatment consists of the following.

- Box rest.
- Controlled exercise for 3–6 months.
- Correction of any foot imbalance.
- Regular monitoring of healing by ultrasound examinations until the ligament has healed. In some horses the affected area never returns to a normal appearance. Rest and controlled exercise in these cases is continued until the ligament appears the same in sequential examinations.
- Non-steroidal anti-inflammatory drugs, e.g. phenylbutazone, as necessary.
- Shock wave therapy. This is normally reserved for horses with chronic lesions not responding to conservative therapy. Three treatments are usually given at 2-week intervals.

Other treatments that may be used include:

- local or systemic injections of polysulphated glycosaminoglycan (PSGAG)
- local injection of corticosteroid or hyaluronan
- topical dimethyl sulphoxide (DMSO)
- injection of counter-irritants has anecdotally been reported to be successful in some cases.

PROGNOSIS

This depends on the severity of the injury and how quickly it is diagnosed and treated appropriately. More damage can be done if the horse is kept in work. On the whole the prognosis is good: 85–90% of horses with acute injuries respond well to conservative management.

Proximal suspensory desmitis of the hind limb

This injury can occur in any type of horse but is commonly seen in dressage horses. Poor conformation may be a contributory factor. Horses with straight hocks, abnormally sloping pasterns and long-toe, low-heel conformation are at risk.

CLINICAL SIGNS

- Lameness, which can be mild to severe. Onset of lameness may be gradual or sudden. It is usually more persistent following rest than the same condition in the forelimb. This may be due to compression of the plantar metatarsal nerves when the ligament swells within the confined space between the cannon bone and the two splint bones, leading to persistent pain and lameness. Flexion of the limb may accentuate the lameness as may working on a circle. The lameness may be more obvious when the horse is ridden.
- Heat and swelling may be present but this is not a consistent sign.
- Deep palpation of the origin of the ligament may be painful.

DIAGNOSIS

Diagnostic techniques are as for the forelimb, i.e:

- nerve blocks
- ultrasonography
- radiography; as these lesions are often chronic by the time the cause of lameness is diagnosed, radiographic changes of the proximal cannon bone are more commonly seen than in the forelimb
- scintigraphy.

Very often a combination of the above techniques is required for diagnosis of this condition.

TREATMENT

Whatever the treatment, the prognosis for return to soundness is poorer than with similar forelimb injuries especially if the horse has radiographic changes or has been lame for more than 3 months. The possible treatments include:

- box rest
- correction of any foot imbalance and use of egg bar shoes to limit extension of the fetlock
- controlled walking exercise in hand building up to 30–60 minutes daily over a 12-week period
- non-steroidal anti-inflammatory drugs, e.g. phenylbutazone
- local infiltration of corticosteroid, hyaluronan, PSGAG or homeopathic remedy.

If the horse is sound after 12 weeks, the work is gradually increased. In horses that are still lame after 3 months:

- extracorporeal shock wave therapy is successful at abolishing the lameness in some cases.

If lameness persists and the diagnosis is re-confirmed by nerve blocks, the following options exist:

- fasciotomy (surgical release) of the deep fascia in the region allows the damaged ligament to swell and releases the pressure on the ligament and the local nerves
- neurectomy of the lateral plantar metatarsal nerve is combined with the above
- injection of bone marrow aspirated from the horse's sternum into the damaged ligament appears to improve the speed and quality of healing in some horses; the bone marrow contains stem cells and growth factors which together can stimulate the production of high-quality collagen.

The results of these procedures are encouraging with many more horses returning to their former activities. However, the prognosis is far worse in horses that are affected by proximal suspensory desmitis of the hind limbs when compared with the forelimbs.

Desmitis of the body of the suspensory ligament

The body of the suspensory ligament is the middle part that lies from 10–12 cm (4–5 in) below the knee or hock to approximately halfway down the cannon bone where it divides into medial and lateral branches. Injuries of this type are common in horses that jump fences at speed.

Inflammation of the suspensory ligament in this region may be associated with splint bone injuries. The new bone formed can impinge on the suspensory ligament.

CLINICAL SIGNS

These include:

- lameness
- heat
- swelling
- pain on gently squeezing the ligament
- thickening of the ligament.

DIAGNOSIS

Diagnosis is made on the clinical signs and ultrasonography.

TREATMENT

The aim of treatment is to relieve pain, reduce inflammation and swelling, provide support and encourage healing. It includes:

- cold therapy
- support bandages
- box rest
- controlled exercise
- non-steroidal anti-inflammatory drugs, e.g. phenylbutazone.

It may also include:
- topical DMSO
- local injection of hyaluronan or PSGAG
- pin firing has been used in chronic cases
- if the injury is associated with a splint bone fracture, surgical removal of the fractured part of bone may be necessary.

Progress is not easily monitored by serial ultrasound examinations as the ligament contains some muscle tissue which looks the same as an injured area of ligament. Also, some lesions persist, despite disappearance of the lameness, making it difficult to advise when the horse should resume work. Comparison with the opposite limb is often helpful. As the ligament heals, the scar tissue causes the ligament to become enlarged.

PROGNOSIS
Recurrence of suspensory strains is relatively common, therefore the prognosis is guarded.

Injury to the branches of the suspensory ligament
This is a common injury in all types of horse. Usually a single branch is injured.
Foot imbalance may be a predisposing factor.

CLINICAL SIGNS
- Lameness which may range from mild to severe depending on the severity of the injury.
- Localized heat.
- Swelling which may be severe. This injury may be accompanied by swelling of the fetlock joint and/or the digital flexor tendon sheath making palpation difficult.
- Pain on palpation of the affected branch.

DIAGNOSIS
Diagnosis is made on the clinical signs and ultrasonography. Radiography is usually carried out to eliminate involvement of the distal part of the splint bones or the proximal sesamoid bones. Possible lesions include:
- fractures of the splint and proximal sesamoid bones
- new bone deposition on the sesamoid bones or within the suspensory ligament.

TREATMENT

Treatment depends on the severity of the lesion. It may include:

- cold therapy
- box rest
- a controlled exercise programme
- topical DMSO
- NSAIDs, e.g. phenylbutazone, as necessary
- balancing the feet by appropriate trimming and shoeing
- low intensity laser therapy
- ultrasound therapy
- shock wave therapy
- ligament splitting may be performed if there is a core lesion.

Healing is monitored by regular ultrasound examinations. As with suspensory body injuries, the lesions may not return to a normal appearance on ultrasound scans so they are not always helpful in deciding when to resume full work.

PROGNOSIS

The prognosis depends on the severity of the injury and whether it is associated with a fracture or inflammation of the sesamoid bones. Horses suffering from severe ligament damage are prone to re-injury of the suspensory ligament.

ANNULAR LIGAMENT SYNDROME

Anatomy

The annular ligament of the fetlock joint lies at the back of the fetlock between the two sesamoid bones. It forms part of a canal through which the superficial and deep digital flexor tendons pass on the way to their attachments on the middle phalanx and the distal phalanx (pedal bone). This canal is lined by the synovial membrane of the digital flexor tendon sheath. Inflammation or desmitis of the annular ligament has several causes and is referred to as 'annular ligament syndrome'. (See Figures 7.1b and 7.5.)

Causes

- Direct trauma, e.g. an overreach or cut.
- Indirect trauma, e.g. repeated overextension of the fetlock whilst exercising.
- Swelling of the superficial or deep digital flexor tendons close to the fetlock as a result of injury can exert pressure and cause inflammation of the annular ligament.
- Inflammation or infection of the digital flexor tendon sheath (DFTS) can cause pressure on the ligament.

Whatever the cause, the inflamed ligament becomes thickened which reduces the space within the fetlock canal. Pressure is then exerted on the ligament by the flexor tendons, leading to persistent inflammation and pain.

Clinical signs

Acute injury is characterized by heat, swelling and pain on palpation of the region. The degree of lameness is variable.

Chronic injury is more common. In these cases:

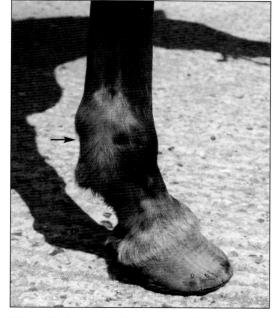

Figure 7.11 Annular ligament syndrome

- the lameness is usually slight to moderate
- it improves slightly with rest but becomes worse with exercise
- it is often worse after a flexion test
- the lower limb has a characteristic appearance with an obvious constriction in the swollen digital sheath (tendinous windgall) at the back of the fetlock (Figure 7.11)
- the horse may stand with the heel slightly raised from the ground to avoid pressure on the inflamed ligament.

Diagnosis

Diagnosis is made on the following.

- The clinical signs.
- The results of diagnostic analgesia. The horse may improve with analgesia of the digital sheath or with a low four- or six-point nerve block.
- Ultrasonography. The palmar annular ligament cannot normally be seen on an ultrasound examination as it is only 1–2 mm ($\frac{1}{10}$ in) thick. However, subcutaneous thickening, a thickened ligament and digital sheath effusions are all readily visible.
- Radiography may be used to rule out the presence of an avulsion fracture or new bone at the site of insertion of the ligament on the proximal sesamoid bones.
- Sampling the fluid within the tendon sheath (synoviocentesis) to check for infection and allow analysis of the tendon sheath fluid.

Treatment

Acute injuries normally respond to:

- box rest
- systemic NSAIDs, e.g. phenylbutazone, if necessary
- injections of hyaluronic acid and corticosteroids into the DFTS to reduce inflammation.

Chronic injuries often fail to respond to the above treatment. In these cases, surgical release of the inflamed and thickened ligament may be required. A minimally invasive approach is possible with a small incision or using a tenoscope (arthroscope). Following surgery, the horse is kept on box rest with controlled exercise to reduce adhesions.

Prognosis

If the palmar annular ligament is inflamed with no other complications, then the prognosis following either box rest or surgery is reasonably good. However, if there is an associated tendon injury or adhesions within the digital sheath, the outlook is less favourable.

CURB

Traditionally, a curb is the name given to a swelling that develops at the back of the leg below the point of the hock when the plantar ligament is strained. The origin of the plantar ligament is the upper part of the calcaneus. It attaches distally to the fourth tarsal bone and the head of the lateral splint bone (Figure 7.12). However, now that there are sophisticated ultrasound machines capable of producing excellent images, it is recognized that there are several possible causes of swelling in this area. These include:

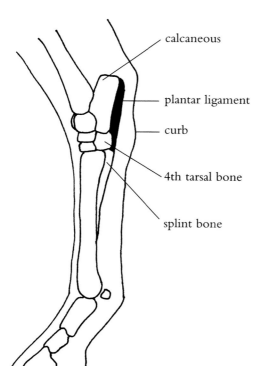

calcaneous

plantar ligament

curb

4th tarsal bone

splint bone

- strain of the plantar ligament with swelling of the surrounding tissues
- injury to the superficial digital flexor tendon (SDFT) with associated soft tissue swelling
- injury to the deep digital flexor tendon (DDFT) with associated soft tissue swelling; this is not common and affected horses experience severe swelling and lameness
- swelling of the soft tissues of the region with no apparent injury of the plantar ligament, the SDFT or the DDFT
- infection of the soft tissues around the above ligament and tendons
- some horses have a prominent head of the fourth metatarsal (lateral splint) bone; this is known as a 'false curb' and can be differentiated from a true curb by careful palpation or radiography.

Figure 7.12 Position of the plantar ligament of the hock

Causes and predisposing factors

The injury occurs most commonly in Thoroughbreds and animals with sickle- or cow-hock conformation. The causes include:

- direct trauma
- excessive tension placed on the ligament by poor conformation
- violent extension of the hock, e.g. bucking and kicking out.

Clinical signs

- Variable degrees of lameness from mild to severe depending on which structures are affected. Not all horses are lame.
- Swelling on the back of the limb below the hock which may be hot and inflamed. Alternatively there may be an area of thickening due to fibrous tissue without any obvious heat (Figure 7.13).
- The horse may experience pain on firm palpation of the area with an acute injury.

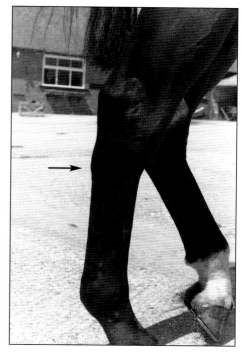

Figure 7.13 A curb

Diagnosis

Diagnosis is made on the clinical signs and ultrasonography. Any lameness should be investigated as curbs do not always produce lameness.

Treatment

Treatment is not always necessary. If the horse is not lame, and the swelling is not sore, it may just be regarded as a blemish. Other cases are managed by:

- box rest with introduction of in-hand walking exercise after 2 weeks
- cold therapy
- NSAIDs, e.g. phenylbutazone, as necessary.

Other possible treatments include:

- Shock wave therapy
- local injection of corticosteroids to reduce the swelling.

Prognosis

The prognosis depends on which structures are damaged and ultrasonography is essential to establish this. Horses with plantar ligament desmitis generally respond well to conservative therapy if given adequate rest. The affected area frequently remains permanently thickened once healing is complete.

8

JOINT INJURY AND DISEASE

DISEASES OF JOINTS

Horses experience a wide range of joint problems. Joint disease is a common cause of lameness and ultimately loss of use of the horse, thus early diagnosis and treatment are essential if these are to be avoided. Examples of joint disease include sprains, degenerative joint disease and infection.

The structure of a synovial joint

A synovial joint is made up of bones covered with articular cartilage and the soft tissues which surround it. These include the synovial membrane, joint capsule, ligaments, tendons and muscle (Figure 8.1).

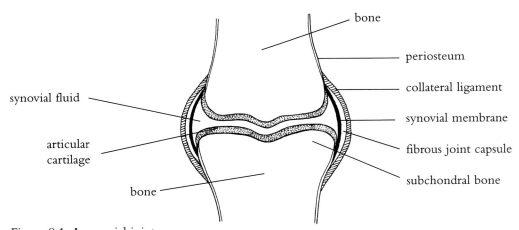

Figure 8.1 A synovial joint

HYALINE CARTILAGE

The articular surfaces are covered with hyaline cartilage which allows them to glide over one another with minimal friction when the horse moves. It is made up of collagen fibrils within a proteoglycan matrix and water. The collagen fibrils give tensile strength and structural support to the articular cartilage. The proteoglycan matrix compresses a little to allow distribution of the load during weight bearing. When the cartilage is compressed, a thin film of water is squeezed from the matrix onto the surface of the cartilage and this keeps the cartilage surfaces apart and is important for lubrication of the joint. When the joint is no longer under pressure and the cartilage expands, the water is pulled back into the matrix. The cells responsible for producing cartilage are called chondrocytes; these make up only 2% of the tissue volume.

Articular cartilage has no blood vessels or nerves. It relies on synovial fluid for nutrition. Nerve endings in the joint capsule, ligaments, muscles and subchondral bone give rise to pain when a joint is injured, but a lesion confined only to articular cartilage is not painful. While an animal is growing there is some remodelling of articular cartilage, but in adults, the turnover and capacity for repair is limited.

SUBCHONDRAL BONE
Articular cartilage provides little shock absorption; this is provided by the underlying bone and the soft tissues surrounding the joint. The subchondral bone immediately under the articular cartilage is deformable when under pressure and so is able to support and protect the articular cartilage.

THE JOINT CAPSULE
The joint capsule is composed of two layers.
- An outer fibrous layer which is attached to the periosteum of the bone. The collateral ligaments are often incorporated into the joint capsule and together they provide stability to the joint.
- An inner synovial membrane which lines the joint where there is no articular cartilage. It secretes synovial fluid.

SYNOVIAL FLUID
Synovial fluid nourishes the articular cartilage and has a lubricating role within the joint. One of the major components of synovial fluid is hyaluronan which gives the fluid its characteristic viscosity.

OTHER PERIARTICULAR SOFT TISSUES
These include ligaments, tendons and muscles.
- Ligaments join together and stabilize the bones making up a joint.
- Tendons are responsible for movement of a joint as they transfer force from a muscle to the opposite side of a joint.
- Both tendons and muscles absorb some of the forces that are generated during movement and so protect the articular surfaces from potentially damaging forces.

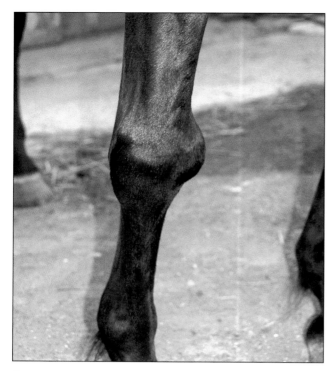

Figure 8.2 An arthritic knee

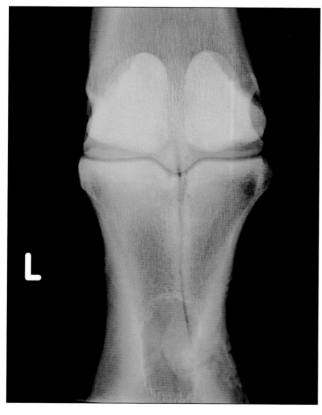

Figure 8.3 X-ray of a split pastern; the fracture line is clearly visible

THE DIAGNOSIS OF JOINT DISEASE

Diagnosis of joint disease is usually by clinical examination (see Examination of the Lame Horse on page 86), followed up by further investigations.

Clinical examination

Signs of joint disease may include:

- swelling of the joint, known as a synovial effusion; the joint becomes distended due to increased production of synovial fluid
- swelling of the soft tissues around the joint
- bony enlargement (Figure 8.2)
- heat around the joint
- tenderness on palpation of the soft tissues; although articular cartilage has no nerve supply, there are many free nerve endings in the tissues around a joint and these become more sensitive if the joint is inflamed
- pain on flexion or extension of the joint
- decreased range of motion of the joint
- abnormal posture
- lameness which may be sudden or gradual in onset
- muscle wasting.

It is often helpful to compare the injured joint with the same area on the opposite limb.

Radiography

Radiographic signs of joint disease include:

- narrowing or disappearance of the joint space due to cartilage degeneration and loss
- increase of bone density directly below the joint; this is known as sclerosis
- decrease of bone density directly below the joint; this is known as lysis
- spurs of new bone at the joint margins

- intra-articular fractures (Figure 8.3)
- osteochondrosis lesions
- bone cysts below the cartilage
- thickening of the soft tissues around the joint
- calcification of soft tissue attachments, e.g. ligaments, tendons, joint capsule.

The radiographs must be interpreted with care as early lesions will not show up on the X-rays. A 40% change in bone density must occur for the lesion to be visible. As cartilage does not show up on radiographs, erosions confined to the articular surface will not be seen. There is often poor correlation between the severity of radiographic changes and the degree of lameness. The presence of bony changes around a joint may reflect previous trauma and is not necessarily the cause of the current lameness. Nerve blocks are important in determining whether the changes seen are significant.

Intra-articular and regional analgesia – nerve blocks

Nerve blocks are often used to localize the cause of the lameness or to confirm that a particular joint is the source of the pain. If local anaesthetic injected into a joint abolishes the lameness, then the cause is usually within the joint. The result is not always straight-forward because analgesia of a particular joint may only reduce rather than eliminate the lameness, showing that other factors are playing a part (see Nerve Blocks, page 99). It is important to be aware that there is a risk of infection when a joint is injected with local anaesthetic or medication

Ultrasonography

Ultrasonography is increasingly used in the diagnosis of joint disease as the modern, sophisticated ultrasound machines provide excellent images of the soft tissues of a joint and the bony surfaces.

Magnetic resonance imaging (MRI)

Magnetic resonance images provide good detail of the joint structure and can detect pathological changes in the tissues before they are visible on X-ray or with ultrasound. The limitation is the cost of the procedure and the fact that with some machines it has to be done under general anaesthesia. The joints that can be imaged in this way include the hock, knee, fetlock, pastern and coffin joints. The technique has improved our ability to diagnose the various causes of palmar foot pain.

Scintigraphy

Scintigraphy will highlight any regions of increased blood flow and active remodelling of bone. It may be helpful in localizing joint problems that do not yet show up on radiographs. The technique is also useful for imaging joints such as hips that cannot be X-

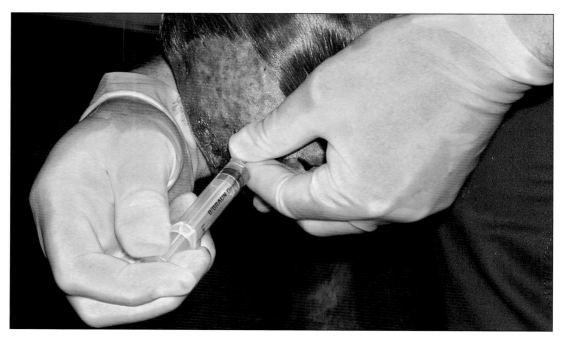

Figure 8.4 Synovial fluid is being withdrawn from this horse's knee to see if the injury penetrated the joint capsule

rayed in the standing horse. It can provide valuable information when multiple joint problems are contributing to the lameness.

Synovial fluid examination

Valuable information can be obtained by examination of the synovial fluid. The joint to be examined is prepared by clipping and thorough cleaning with a surgical scrub. The fluid is withdrawn with a sterile needle and syringe (Figure 8.4) and examined for the following.

- Appearance. Normal synovial fluid is clear and straw-coloured. Cloudiness is indicative of acute inflammation or infection. Streaks of blood are likely to be due to bleeding caused by the needle, but uniformly red synovial fluid is due to haemorrhage into the joint caused by injury or infection.
- Viscosity. The synovial fluid from an inflamed joint is less viscous than normal synovial fluid due to a reduction of hyaluronan.
- Cytology and protein concentration. The numbers of white blood cells and the protein levels are elevated in an infected joint.

Arthroscopy

The synovial membrane and the articular surfaces of some joints can be inspected with an arthroscope (see page 115). This allows detection of lesions not yet visible on radiographs, as well as examination of intra-articular ligaments and menisci.

JOINT SPRAINS

A sprain occurs when the fibres of the joint capsule or the supporting ligaments are stretched and torn. It may be mild with just a few disrupted collagen fibrils and limited haemorrhage into the ligament. Moderate sprains have variable degrees of ligament tearing and some loss of function, but the ligament remains intact. Severe sprains result in considerable haemorrhage and possible rupture of a ligament with major disruption to the joint.

Causes

It is usually the result of a twist or wrench when the horse slips or works on uneven ground.

Clinical signs

The symptoms are similar, regardless of which joint is affected. There is:

- heat
- lameness
- distension of the joint capsule due to increased production of synovial fluid
- soft tissue swelling around the joint (Figure 8.5)
- pain and increased lameness when the joint is flexed

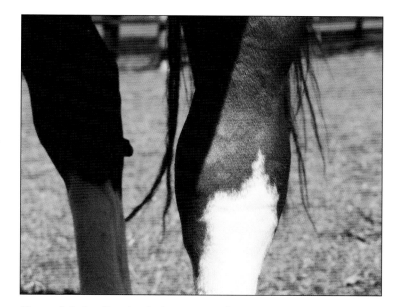

Figure 8.5 Swollen hock due to a sprain

- partial or complete dislocation may occur if the ligaments of a joint rupture.

Treatment

The aim of treatment is to:

- alleviate pain
- stabilize the joint
- reduce the inflammation of the synovial membrane and the joint capsule; if damaged, the cells in the synovial membrane release enzymes which can damage the articular cartilage
- prevent permanent fibrous thickening of the joint capsule which would limit its range of motion
- prevent the development of osteoarthritis.

Treatment is likely to include the following.

- Box rest.

- Cold therapy for at least the first 48 hours.
- Support bandaging where practical.
- Non-steroidal anti-inflammatory drugs, e.g. phenylbutazone.
- Application of a cast for moderate and severe sprains where there is joint instability to minimize movement and allow healing.
- Controlled exercise is introduced as soon as possible as prolonged immobility of joints leads to muscle wasting and weakening of the tendons, ligaments, the joint capsule and articular cartilage.
- Passive flexion of the affected joint if in-hand walking is not possible to help prevent adhesions.
- Sodium hyaluronate may be injected into the joint space to decrease inflammation within the joint.
- Low intensity laser or magnetic therapy may be beneficial.
- Swimming exercise can be useful in maintaining the horse's condition without straining the joint.
- Surgery may be necessary following ligament rupture; arthroscopy may be performed to evaluate and repair the damage.

If the lameness persists for more than 2 weeks, X-rays should be taken to see if there are any bony changes at the sites of attachment of the joint capsule or collateral ligaments to the bone.

Prognosis

If the horse is appropriately managed and there is no major damage to the collateral ligaments, the prognosis is good for mild sprains. As the severity of sprain increases, so does the risk of subsequent development of degenerative joint disease.

DEGENERATIVE JOINT DISEASE (OSTEOARTHRITIS)

Osteoarthritis is a disease of the articular cartilage within a joint. Cartilage degeneration and loss is followed by development of new bone on the joint surfaces and margins, hence the name degenerative joint disease (DJD)

Causes

It may develop following:

- sprains
- repeated low-grade trauma due to poor conformation and normal work
- unsuitable training programmes

- a fracture
- infection
- osteochondritis dissecans (see page 235)

The incidence of DJD increases with the age of the horse and is a reflection of wear and tear.

The course of the disease

The thickness of articular cartilage is limited as it has no blood supply and relies on diffusion of nutrients from the synovial fluid. Thus it can only withstand a certain amount of shock absorption during athletic exercise. Consequently, forces are absorbed by the soft tissues surrounding the joint and the underlying subchondral bone. This can cause microfractures in the bone immediately under the articular cartilage. Initially the repair of these improves the strength of the bone and its ability to absorb the shock. However, continued stress results in increased density of the bone with subsequent loss of deformability and the risk of mechanical damage to the articular cartilage is increased.

The chondrocytes are responsible for the maintenance of the cartilage matrix. Under normal circumstances they maintain a balance between breakdown and repair. Once the cartilage has been damaged by mechanical trauma, they release destructive enzymes which further break down the cartilage. Cells within the synovial membrane also release degradative enzymes; these include prostaglandins, cytokines and matrix metalloproteinases. Together these contribute to destruction of the articular cartilage as the rate of destruction exceeds the rate of repair. As a result the cartilage becomes thinner and less able to withstand normal forces. Small fissures develop and the surface of the cartilage becomes fibrillated. Eventually fissures develop through the full thickness of the articular cartilage and pieces of cartilage and the exposed subchondral bone are released into the joint space. As the cartilage is lost, secondary changes occur in the surrounding bone and soft tissues. This is seen on radiographs (Figures 8.6a and b) as:

- loss of joint space
- increased density of the bone immediately below the area of damaged cartilage
- development of bony spurs or osteophytes around the joint margin; these are covered with hyaline or fibrocartilage and are thought to develop as an attempt to stabilize a joint by increasing the surface contact area.

If the course of the disease is unchecked, eventually the underlying bone may become less dense due to resorption or lysis, and weakened leading to fragmentation. The end result is ankylosis where the joint space is totally destroyed and the bones become permanently fused together.

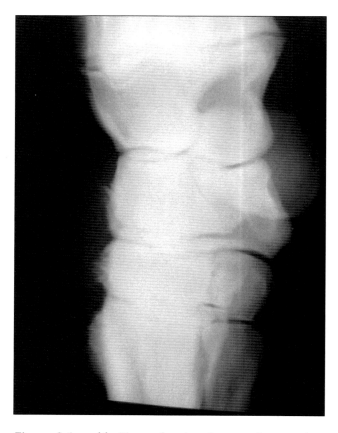

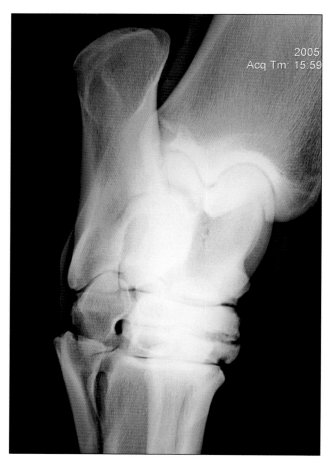

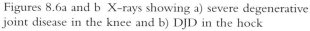
Figures 8.6a and b X-rays showing a) severe degenerative joint disease in the knee and b) DJD in the hock

Clinical signs

These are variable, depending on the cause of the problem and the joint(s) affected. There may be:

- heat
- distension of the joint capsule due to increased production of synovial fluid
- soft tissue swelling around the joint
- lameness which may be sudden or gradual in onset
- pain on passive motion of the joint
- pain on flexion of the joint.

In advanced cases there may be:

- joint enlargement due to thickening of the synovial membrane and joint capsule due to deposition of fibrous tissue and new bone in response to the inflammation
- a reduced range of joint movement.

Diagnosis

Diagnosis of osteoarthritis is made from:

- the history
- clinical signs
- radiography
- nerve blocks
- ultrasonography
- scintigraphy
- arthroscopy
- magnetic resonance imaging (MRI).

THE TREATMENT OF DEGENERATIVE JOINT DISEASE (DJD)

Once articular cartilage has been damaged, it is rarely completely repaired. The aim of treatment is therefore to:

- remove the cause if possible (e.g. modify training programmes, treat infection, correct foot balance)
- relieve pain
- reduce joint capsule and soft tissue inflammation
- limit inflammation of the synovial membrane
- restore normal synovial fluid quality and volume
- improve joint mobility
- stop the cartilage destruction
- encourage cartilage healing.

The response to treatment will depend on:

- the stage of the disease
- the age of the horse
- the location of the injury
- whether the lesions are superficial or extend right through the cartilage
- the size of the defect.

Medication
NON-STEROIDAL ANTI-INFLAMMATORY DRUGS (NSAIDs)

This group of medicines, which includes phenylbutazone, inhibits the production of substances such as prostaglandins which are part of the inflammatory process and cause damage to articular cartilage. They have analgesic properties and also help to bring down the horse's temperature if it is raised.

Examples of this type of medication include phenylbutazone, flunixin meglumine, meclofenamic acid, acetyl salicylic acid, ketoprofen, carprofen and naproxen. Unfortunately these drugs inhibit some beneficial actions of prostaglandins as well as the harmful ones and this occasionally can lead to problems with long-term administration.

Toxic effects of this group of drugs include:

- gastric ulceration
- kidney damage
- liver damage
- urticaria and other skin rashes
- bone marrow depression causing anaemia.

Symptoms include anorexia, weight loss, diarrhoea and anaemia. However, side effects are uncommon if the drugs are used at recommended levels. They are more likely to be seen in ponies, foals and older or debilitated animals.

There is also concern that with long-term use, some NSAIDs have a detrimental effect on cartilage metabolism. Others may have a protective effect. There is much research going on in this area at present and it is hoped that, as a result, new drugs will be developed to overcome these problems.

The use of NSAIDs should be combined with a programme of regular, light work. If the work is strenuous and intermittent, the joint changes may be accelerated.

INTRA-ARTICULAR MEDICATIONS

These treatments are injected directly into the joint following careful preparation and cleaning of the site. They include the following 3 treatments.

1 Corticosteroids

Intra-articular corticosteroids are used in arthritic joints because of their potent anti-inflammatory effects. Their use is often accompanied by a rapid and marked reduction in pain. Deleterious effects on articular cartilage have been associated with repeated high doses and insufficient rest periods following injection. These can largely be avoided by lower doses and judicious use of these preparations.

As corticosteroids have such potent anti-inflammatory effects, there is a risk that early signs of joint infection following an injection could be delayed with potentially serious consequences. There is also a small risk of laminitis following intra-articular injection of a corticosteroid.

Corticosteroids are often used in conjunction with hyaluronan.

2 Hyaluronan

Hyaluronan is a component of articular cartilage and synovial fluid. It is responsible for lubricating the joint and gives synovial fluid its viscosity. When a joint is inflamed, there is an increase in synovial fluid production and the hyaluronan is diluted and broken down. There are several preparations of hyaluronan available for intra-articular injection in the horse. They have anti-inflammatory effects and some analgesic activity. They may stimulate synthesis of hyaluronan by the synovial membrane. There are many theories as to how they work, but their mode of action is still incompletely understood. They are most effective if used early in the course of disease. There is an intravenous preparation of hyaluronan which may be of some benefit in reducing lameness and synovial effusion associated with inflamed joints. Again, its mechanism of action is unclear.

3 Polysulphated glycosaminoglycan (PSGAG)

This product is composed mainly of chondroitin sulphate. As well as being a constituent of articular cartilage, it has anti-inflammatory effects owing to its ability to inhibit prostaglandin synthesis and cytokine release. It also inhibits the activity of enzymes which break down the articular cartilage in horses with DJD. The product is injected into the joint or administered by intramuscular injection. When given by intramuscular injection, 7 doses are given at 4-day intervals.

Risks associated with intra-articular injections

- Joint infection.
- There may be a short-term increase in joint effusion and lameness shortly after injection due to inflammation of the synovial membrane. This is known as 'post-injection flare'. It usually resolves in 1–3 days.
- Further damage may occur within the joint as a result of overuse while the horse is under medication, particularly with corticosteroids.

ORAL NUTRACEUTICALS, E.G. GLUCOSAMINE AND CHONDROITIN SULPHATE

There are numerous preparations commercially available containing one or both of these substances. They are used in the formation of the proteoglycan matrix of articular cartilage. Both substances are reported to increase proteoglycan synthesis by chondrocytes and to protect articular cartilage by inhibiting the synthesis of degradative enzymes that are released in inflamed joints. Although the scientific evidence to date is limited, these products are reported to be of some benefit in providing relief for the painful symptoms of arthritis. Some horses seem to experience less pain and increased range of motion of affected joints as a result of their anti-inflammatory effects. Recent studies of gait analysis in mature riding horses with multiple areas of stiffness, demonstrated that supplementation with glucosamine and chondroitin sulphate improved the symmetry of gait, especially for the hock joint.

These preparations are given to the horse in its feed. Glucosamine is absorbed well from the small intestine and trials have shown it to be as effective as ibuprofen in relieving the symptoms of osteoarthritis of the knee in human patients. In contrast with NSAIDs, there are no known problems of toxicity with long-term administration. The supplement needs to be fed for 2–3 weeks before the results are seen. Chondroitin sulphate, on the other hand, is broken down before being absorbed in the small intestine. The reported beneficial effects may be due to the biological activity of the breakdown products but this is the subject of continuing research and debate.

Management

Where soft tissue inflammation is a contributory factor, treatment may include:

- rest
- cold therapy for the first 48 hours to reduce the pain, inflammation and swelling
- support bandaging
- immobilization if the joint is unstable
- passive flexion to reduce oedema and maintain joint mobility and circulation
- heat may be applied following the initial period of cold therapy in order to increase the circulation, decrease the stiffness and discomfort and improve the range of motion of the joint
- walking in hand
- swimming if facilities are available (Figure 8.7).

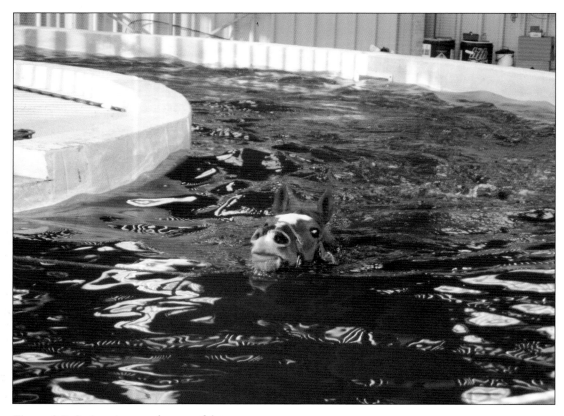

Figure 8.7 Swimming can be a useful treatment

Physiotherapy

The following treatment modalities may help.

- Massage to alleviate muscular stiffness.
- Low intensity laser therapy.
- Magnetic therapy.
- Therapeutic ultrasound.

Acupuncture

Acupuncture is helpful in relieving the muscle tension and pain that can develop in association with degenerative joint disease. If unresolved, the muscle tension can cause increased pressure on the cartilage of the joint surfaces and further degenerative changes.

Corrective farriery

Where foot imbalance is considered to be a contributory factor in the development of joint disease, this should be addressed. With painful lower-limb joints, shortening or squaring-off the toe brings the breakover point of the stride further back and can reduce the discomfort.

Topical applications

Dimethyl sulphoxide (DMSO) may be used on its own or with corticosteroids as a topical application to reduce inflammation and oedema following joint injury. However, this treatment is now less readily available in the UK. It is also reported to reduce pain and fibrosis.

Topical NSAIDs in the form of gels are used in man. These preparations, rubbed into painful joints are coming onto the market in the USA for equine use.

Surgical management of joint disease

With increased use of arthroscopy, joint problems are being diagnosed earlier in the course of the disease. Damage to the articular cartilage can be seen and treated before it shows up on radiographs. Surgical treatments include the following.

- Joint lavage. This technique involves flushing the joint out to remove debris from cartilage breakdown and the harmful inflammatory mediators that lead to ongoing cartilage destruction.
- Removal of cartilage fragments attached to the joint surface that have developed as a result of injury or developmental problems (Figure 8.8)
- Arthrodesis. This is a procedure that can be used in some cases when the pain from degenerative joint changes cannot be relieved by management or medication. It is sometimes recommended for certain joints that have relatively little movement including the proximal interphalangeal (pastern) or distal tarsal (hock) joints. The

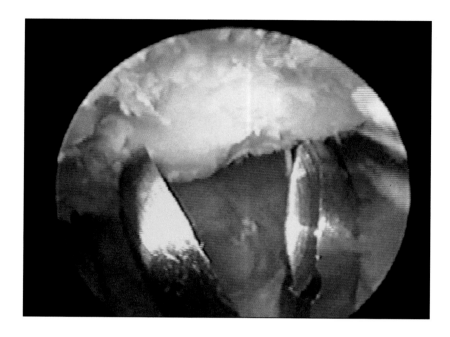

cartilage surface of the joints is surgically removed and the opposing bones are held together with plates and screws in the same way as a fracture. If the operation is successful, the bones fuse and the horse may become pain free. Fusion of the bones is known as **ankylosis**. Whether or not the horse can return to work depends on which joint is involved and the level of work expected from it.

Figure 8.8 Damaged cartilage fragments can be removed during arthroscopy

Techniques for the future

The big problem with degenerative joint disease is that once articular cartilage has been damaged, it has very little capacity for repair. As a result, a number of new techniques are currently under investigation.

MICROPICKING

The aim of this technique is to allow cells from the bone marrow to enter the damaged cartilage and assist healing. With the horse under general anaesthetic, tiny cracks are made in the subchondral bone beneath the damaged cartilage to allow access of these cells.

CARTILAGE TRANSPLANTS

A piece of healthy cartilage is removed from one site in the body and transplanted into the damaged cartilage in the hope that it will encourage healing. However, one of the problems is that in order to heal one area, damage is created elsewhere. If cartilage is used from another horse, there may be problems of tissue rejection as well as ethical issues to be considered.

CELL TRANSPLANTS

Recent work has involved transplanting special cartilage cells into diseased joints. These cells may be obtained by taking a small piece of the horse's cartilage and extracting the cells so that they can be cultured in the laboratory. Once they have multiplied sufficiently, they are placed back into the joint.

Another technique is to take **stem cells** from the bone marrow of the sternum and induce them to become cartilage cells in the laboratory. These can then be replaced back into the joint to help heal the cartilage.

Gene therapy

With this type of therapy, the horse's genetic code is manipulated so less of the destructive chemicals that cause cartilage breakdown are produced, together with more of the components of healthy cartilage. There are two ways of introducing the new genes:

- a virus containing the therapeutic genes can be injected directly into the joint
- a biopsy of the synovial membrane is taken and the cells are infected with a virus containing the new genes; these are grown in the laboratory and then re-introduced into the joint.

This research is still very new and long-term studies need to be carried out to see if this genetic modification has any harmful effects on the horse in the long term.

COMMON EXAMPLES OF DEGENERATIVE JOINT DISEASE IN THE HORSE

Bone spavin

Bone spavin is DJD (osteoarthritis) of the distal joints of the hock. The anatomy of the hock is complex as it is made up of several joints (Figures 8.9a and b). Most movement occurs at the tarsocrural joint and only a small amount of gliding movement is possible in the proximal intertarsal, the distal intertarsal and the tarsometatarsal joints which are low-motion joints. DJD of the distal hock joints is a common cause of hind limb lameness in the horse. It most commonly affects the distal intertarsal and the tarsometatarsal joints. The

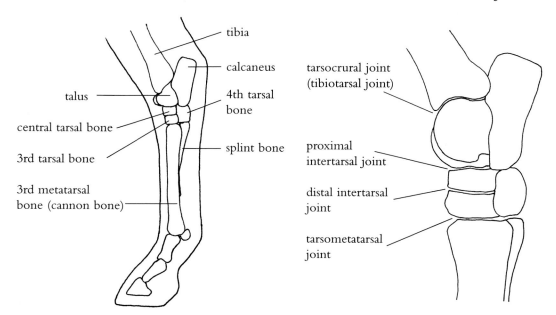

Figures 8.9a and b Lateral view of a) the bones of the hock and b) the joints of the hock

proximal intertarsal joint is only occasionally involved. When it occurs it is usually a more serious problem.

CAUSES

- Poor conformation. Horses with cow hocks, sickle hocks or excessively straight conformation are susceptible (Figures 8.10a–e). With cow hocks and sickle hocks, the medial aspect of the joint experiences greater stresses than the lateral aspect.
- Constant wear and tear due to compression and rotational forces generated when the horse jumps or stops quickly.
- The tendency to develop the condition may be inherited in some horses.
- The type and level of difficulty of work may be a factor.
- Bone spavin may be a sequel to a specific injury.

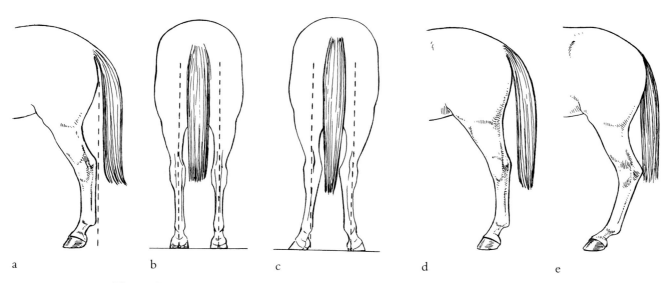

Figures 8.10a–e Hock conformation: a) normal conformation side view: a line dropped from the point of the buttock (tuber ischii) is parallel to the cannon bone; b) normal conformation rear view: a line dropped from the point of buttock bisects the limb; c) cow hocks: the hocks are close together and the feet are wide apart and turned outwards; d) straight behind: this horse has an abnormally straight hind limb, there is too little angulation of the hock and stifle joints; e) sickle hocks: there is an excessive angle of the hock joints

CLINICAL SIGNS

Change in hind limb action

The horse is uncomfortable flexing the hock, so the height of the hind foot flight arc is reduced. The hind limbs take shorter strides and the horse tends to land on its toe. Some affected horses swing the limb towards the midline as it is brought forward and then move it laterally and land on the outside edge of the foot. The toe may be dragged causing abnormal wear of the shoe. Irregular rhythm or dragging of the toe may be noticed or heard when riding.

Lameness

- Lameness which is usually gradual in onset.
- As the condition is often bilateral, the horse may show hind limb stiffness rather than a unilateral lameness.
- The stiffness is most apparent at the start of exercise and wears off as the horse warms up.
- Where only one limb is affected or the changes in one limb are more advanced than in the other, the horse appears unlevel or lame.
- Lameness may be more obvious with the horse lunged on a circle or when it is ridden.
- If the horse has a few days of hard work the lameness may become more pronounced.
- If the horse is rested and turned out for a few days the lameness often becomes less pronounced.

Flexion

Affected horses are often uncomfortable when the hind limb is held in the flexed position for shoeing. In advanced cases, flexion of the hock may be markedly reduced.

Most affected horses show a positive reaction to a spavin or hock flexion test. If the hock is flexed for a minute and the horse is trotted off on a hard flat surface, the lameness is usually accentuated for a variable number of strides. It must be remembered that this test is not specific for hock pain as other joints are flexed at the same time. A negative spavin test does not rule out a diagnosis of bone spavin.

Swelling

Horses can have distal hock pain with no change in the appearance of the limb. However, as the osteoarthritis progresses, a soft tissue or bony enlargement may develop on the medial or dorsomedial aspect of the hock at the level of the distal intertarsal or tarsometatarsal joints (Figures 8.11a and b). If the disease is bilateral or the horse has naturally boxy hocks this can be difficult to appreciate.

Poor performance

With bilateral hock pain the horse may show poor performance rather than lameness. Signs include:

- reluctance to turn, or perform either an upward or downward transition with proper engagement of the hind limbs
- reluctance to canter on a particular lead or becoming disunited at canter
- jumping badly or refusing jumps as a result of the pain.

Muscle pain and wasting

Many horses with distal hock joint disease experience muscle pain. The lumbar and hindquarter muscles may be sore. Chronic disease may lead to wasting of the muscles of the hindquarters.

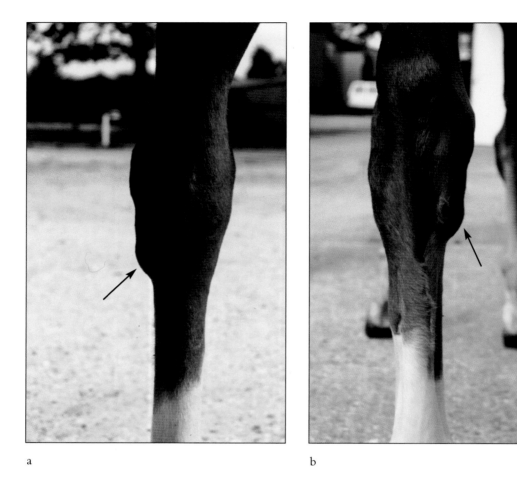

a   b

Figures 8.11a and b Two views of bone spavin: a) from the front; b) from behind

DIAGNOSIS

Diagnosis is made on:

- the history
- the clinical signs
- nerve blocks
- radiography
- scintigraphy.

Nerve blocks

Intra–articular anaesthesia (i.e. nerve blocks of the hock joint) is important for early diagnosis of DJD of the distal hock joints in some horses because radiographic changes may not be visible at this stage of the disease. In other cases, however, the horse may not become lame until the radiographic changes are advanced.

Radiographic changes

These include:

- spurs of new bone at the joint margins
- increased or decreased density of the subchondral bone directly under the articular cartilage
- widening of the joint space
- narrowing or loss of the joint spaces (see Figure 8.6b).

There is poor correlation between the extent of the radiographic changes and the degree of lameness. Horses may have extensive changes at the time the lameness is first recognized. Others may be severely lame with no changes visible on radiographs.

The use of scintigraphy

Scintigraphy is not usually necessary but is helpful in cases where:

- the horse is uncooperative and cannot be safely nerve blocked
- multiple joint problems are contributing to the lameness.

Horses can have positive scintigraphy results despite having no changes on X-ray and so the technique is useful in these cases.

TREATMENT

Once degenerative changes are present, the aim of treatment is to slow down progression of the disease and provide pain relief so that the horse can stay in work. The options include the following.

Corrective trimming and shoeing

This is an important part of any treatment programme for horses with hock pain. The mediolateral balance of the feet should be checked and the toe shortened to facilitate breakover. Rolling the toe and slight raising of the heel can be helpful. Natural Balance® shoes which are set back from the toe may improve the horse's comfort and action.

Non-steroidal anti-inflammatory drugs (NSAIDs), e.g. phenylbutazone

The minimum dose is used as necessary to keep the horse in work. Problems from long-term administration are rarely encountered.

Intra-articular medication

Intra-articular medication with corticosteroids is often very effective at reducing distal hock joint pain by reducing inflammation of the synovial membrane. These preparations may be used in combination with hyaluronan. Polysulphated glycosaminoglycan (PSGAG) is also used. The horse is walked in hand or only lightly exercised for a few days following treatment.

Systemic hyaluronan and PSGAG

A course of intravenous hyaluronan or intramuscular PSGAG may be beneficial in addition to the intra-articular use of these drugs.

Sodium tiludronate

This is a new treatment which may inhibit bone resorption and reduce the associated pain. It is given as a single intravenous injection. This is repeated after 60 days if no improvement is seen. It is too early to say whether this treatment is successful enough for routine use.

Oral administration of glucosamine and chondroitin sulphate (see pages 223–4)

Surgical arthrodesis

This technique involves drilling out some of the articular cartilage so that bridges of bone form across the joint space and immobilize the joint. The technique has a better success rate for riding horses than for competition animals, particularly dressage horses where hock action is crucial. In one study, 59% of horses were able to return to their former level of performance. Most horses recover within 6 months but some do not become sound for up to 1 year.

Chemical fusion of the distal hock joints

Injection of sodium monoiodoacetate into the distal hock joint spaces causes degeneration and collapse of the articular cartilage, allowing the adjacent bones to fuse. Suitable cases have to be selected carefully to ensure that the distal hock joints are not in communication with the proximal intertarsal or tarsocrural joints. (Communication between the synovial cavities of the hock joints of horses is variable.) This technique destroys the pain receptors in the synovial membrane of treated joints, thus allowing the horse to exercise which speeds up ankylosis of the joint. The drug is not licensed in the UK and treatment can be painful.

Cunean tenectomy

The cunean tendon runs obliquely across the medial aspect of the hock. Removing a section of this tendon results in an improvement in some horses. This was considered to be due to a reduction of pressure on the medial side of the distal hock joints. The technique has currently become less popular.

Extracorporeal shock wave therapy

Some horses which fail to improve with medical therapy do improve following shock wave therapy. This is considered to be due to an analgesic effect rather than any affect on ankylosis of the joints. The long-term results have not yet been evaluated.

Neurectomy of the tibial and deep peroneal (fibular) nerves
A partial tibial and deep peroneal neurectomy can be performed to relieve the pain from DJD of the distal hock joints. A success rate of 60% has been reported.

PROGNOSIS

If caught in the early stages, a combination of light work, corrective trimming and shoeing, intra-articular medication and/or NSAIDs may return the horse to soundness. However, the prognosis is guarded for any horse with bone spavin. The condition is often bilateral, even if the lameness is more obvious in one limb. Some horses will respond well to a long and gentle warm up before doing any serious work, as this allows the initial stiffness to wear off.

It is difficult to predict which horses will become sound enough to continue their former level of work. Previously, it was thought that if the horse could be kept in work to encourage ankylosis of the affected joints, they were more likely to be pain free in the long term. However, some horses with completely fused distal tarsal joints remain lame and others with incomplete fusion may be sound. Each horse must be individually assessed.

DJD of the proximal interphalangeal joint (high ringbone)

The proximal interphalangeal (PIP) joint has relatively little movement but has to bear the weight of the horse on a small surface area. Thus it is known as a high-load, low-motion joint. DJD or osteoarthritis of the PIP joint is known as **high ringbone**. The degenerative changes affect the distal end of the proximal phalanx and the proximal end of the middle phalanx. The condition is usually seen in older horses and is more common in the forelimbs (Figure 8.12).

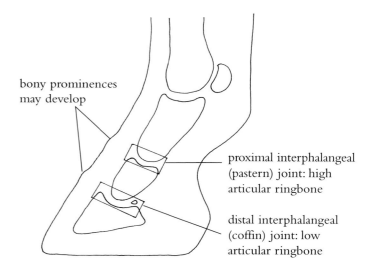

bony prominences may develop

proximal interphalangeal (pastern) joint: high articular ringbone

distal interphalangeal (coffin) joint: low articular ringbone

Figure 8.12 Sites of articular ringbone

CAUSES

Trauma leading to inflammation of the soft tissues surrounding this low-motion joint is considered to be the initiating factor. These tissues repair by fibrosis and this reduces the range of movement further and subjects the articular cartilage to abnormal stresses. Small areas of the joint surface bear an increased load and damage to the cartilage occurs.

Injuries leading to osteoarthritis of the PIP joint include:
• direct blows to the bone

- a sprain causing tearing of the periosteal attachments of:
    - the collateral ligaments
    - the distal sesamoiden ligaments
    - the extensor tendon
    - the joint capsule
- puncture wounds and wire cuts that damage the periosteum or collateral ligaments
- fractures of the proximal or middle phalanx
- joint infection.

Osteoarthritis of the PIP joint can also develop secondary to:
- poor conformation
- osteochondrosis
- certain types of work, e.g. it is relatively common in polo ponies which make sharp turns and quick stops.

CLINICAL SIGNS

These depend on whether the injury is acute or chronic. There may be:
- swelling in the pastern region which can be localized or diffuse (Figure 8.13)
- heat over the joint
- pain when the joint is flexed or rotated
- variable degrees of lameness.

The lameness is usually more obvious at trot and may be exacerbated on a hard surface. It tends to show up more when the horse is worked on uneven ground or on a circle with the affected limb on the inside. Affected horses show a positive response to a flexion test of the lower limb and are often uncomfortable when turned in a short circle.

DIAGNOSIS

Diagnosis is made on the clinical signs and is confirmed by nerve blocks and radiography.

Radiographic changes include:
- osteophytes at the joint margins
- new bone around the joint
- narrowing or disappearance of the joint space
- subchondral bone sclerosis.

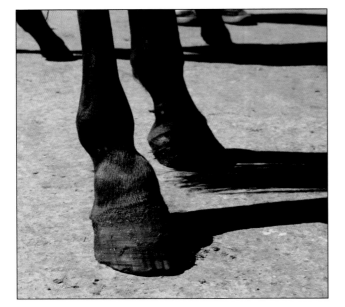

Figure 8.13 High ringbone

In some cases where radiographic changes are not visible, the diagnosis may be confirmed by scintigraphy.

TREATMENT

Once osteoarthritis has developed, the treatment options are limited. They include:

- rest in the early stages of disease
- trimming the foot to correct any foot imbalance and shortening the toe
- shoeing with Natural Balance® shoes to ease breakover
- non-steroidal anti-inflammatory drugs, e.g. phenylbutazone, which may allow the horse to continue in work
- intra-articular injections of corticosteroid and hyaluronan
- oral administration of glucosamine and chondroitin sulphate
- intravenous hyaluronan or intramuscular glycosaminoglycan
- surgical arthrodesis (where the joints are fused surgically) is an option for consideration in some horses; the operation is not commonly performed and is more of a salvage procedure for high-value animals that are being retained for breeding purposes.

PROGNOSIS

The prognosis for horses with osteoarthritis of the PIP joint is guarded. It is more favourable in cases involving a hind limb.

OSTEOCHONDROSIS (OCD)

Osteochondrosis is disease that causes localized abnormalities in the cartilage and bone of young growing animals. As the skeleton grows, cartilage is converted to bone by a process known as **endochondral ossification**. In affected animals, this process is interrupted leaving thickened areas of cartilage on the joint surface which extend into weakened underlying (subchondral) bone. These areas are very prone to injury and fissures develop in the cartilage and lead to inflammation of the joint. Small pieces of cartilage may become detached and move around within the joint. When a flap of articular cartilage lifts away from the joint surface but remains attached, the condition is known as **osteochondritis dissecans**.

Causes

Exactly how the disease develops is still poorly understood. It probably occurs as a result of a combination of some of the following factors.

GROWTH RATE AND BODY SIZE

Studies suggest that in particular breeds such as Warmbloods, larger foals that grow rapidly are more likely to develop OCD of their stifle and hock joints.

NUTRITION

- Overfeeding of high-energy diets to foals is associated with an increased occurrence of OCD. It is thought that the high level of insulin produced to reduce the blood sugar level has an adverse affect on the development of cartilage, possibly by suppressing the output of thyroid hormones that influence normal cartilage development.
- Feeding excessively high levels of phosphorus or calcium is associated with an increased incidence of OCD.
- Copper deficiency can result in a high incidence of OCD lesions in growing foals. Attention should be paid to the copper levels in the diet of the pregnant mare as well as that of the foal.
- Excessively high levels of zinc in the diet can interfere with copper uptake and lead to OCD.

TRAUMA AND BIOMECHANICAL STRESS

Because OCD lesions occur in particular locations, it is likely that biomechanical factors play a part in their development. They tend to develop in sites with high biomechanical loading where the cartilage layer is relatively thick. Factors such as poor conformation, high body-weight and inappropriate levels of exercise would have a direct influence on the forces experienced in these areas.

However, this is not the whole story as the common sites for OCD in the equine hock are not the areas with the thickest cartilage. Factors such as shearing forces and trauma may damage the blood supply and contribute to the development of lesions.

GENETIC PREDISPOSITION

Studies have revealed that the progeny of some stallions have a significantly higher incidence of OCD, despite being reared under a wide range of environmental conditions.

GENDER

There is no evidence that either male or female foals are more prone to the development of OCD lesions.

Sites affected

The most commonly affected sites are the:

a   stifle

b   hock

c   fetlock

d   shoulder.

The lesions are usually bilateral, even if the horse shows unilateral lameness.

Clinical signs

These include:

- mild to severe lameness
- joint swelling
- very young foals may lie down more than expected
- the disease may be asymptomatic.

It is thought that most OCD lesions develop by the time the foal is 5 months of age. However, affected animals may not show any clinical signs until they are backed and begin work. OCD may occur together with other developmental disorders such as:

- physitis (painful enlarged growth plates)
- angular limb deformities
- subchondral bone cysts
- contracted tendons
- cervical vertebral malformation.

Diagnosis

Diagnosis is usually made on the clinical signs (which can be very subtle) and confirmed by radiography (Figure 8.14) Ultrasonography and scintigraphy can be helpful. Arthroscopy allows direct inspection of the joint surfaces and detection of lesions not yet visible on radiographs. Intra-articular analgesia may be used to confirm that a lesion seen on radiographs is the cause of the lameness.

Treatment and management

This depends on the:

- age of the animal
- the degree of the lameness
- the location of the lesion
- the severity of the lesion
- the intended use of the horse.

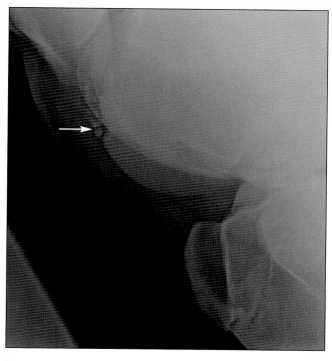

Figure 8.14 X-ray of ostoechondrosis of the stifle joint

In some cases, conservative management with restricted exercise and a balanced diet is effective and the lesions will heal. In other cases, arthroscopic removal of bone fragments and debridement of damaged articular cartilage and bone are necessary. Intra-articular injections of hyaluronan or corticosteroids may be considered.

Prognosis

The prognosis ranges from excellent to guarded, depending on the site and extent of the lesion.

Prevention

Correct management and feeding of the pregnant mare and foal can reduce the incidence of developmental diseases such as OCD. However, our understanding of all of the factors contributing to the disease process is not sufficient to completely eliminate the risk of it occurring.

JOINT INFECTION (SEPTIC ARTHRITIS) IN ADULT HORSES

Bacterial infection of a joint is a medical emergency. It can lead to rapid, irreversible destruction of the articular cartilage of the joint, leading to permanent lameness, loss of use and subsequent destruction of the horse.

Causes

Bacteria may enter a joint:

- from a penetrating wound into or close to a joint (Figure 8.15)
- from direct trauma, e.g. the lateral aspect (outside) of the elbow joint has little soft tissue covering and can easily be entered by a kick from another horse
- with an intra-articular injection
- during surgery
- in the bloodstream from a site of infection elsewhere in the body; this is most commonly seen in young foals (see page 241).

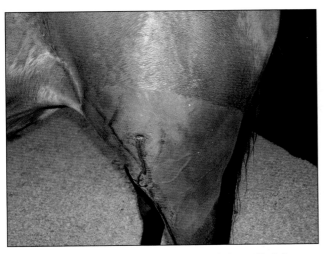

Figure 8.15 This wound has penetrated the stifle joint and a trickle of leaking synovial fluid can be seen

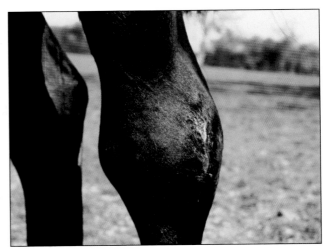

Figure 8.16 Infected hock joint

What happens when bacteria invade a joint?

Bacteria colonize the synovial membrane and cause an acute inflammatory response. This leads to the release of enzymes that can damage the articular cartilage. Ultimately, the cartilage may be completely eroded so the infection invades the subchondral bone resulting in a septic osteomyelitis (bone infection).

Clinical signs

- Sudden onset of severe and sometimes non-weight-bearing lameness.
- Distension of the joint capsule (Figure 8.16)
- Heat over the joint.
- Swelling around the joint.
- Decreased range of movement of the joint.
- Pain on passive flexion and palpation of the joint.
- There may be a wound near the joint. If the wound is large and draining freely, there is unlikely to be a build up of pressure within the joint and hence less lameness.

Diagnosis

Diagnosis is made on the clinical signs and the history. Lameness may occur almost immediately when a wound penetrates a joint and thus can be confused with a fracture. If a horse is lamer than expected with a tiny wound, the possibility of a joint infection should be considered.

Infections resulting from joint injection are usually apparent within 2 days, but signs may be delayed if the joint has been injected with corticosteroids or the horse is on non-steroidal anti-inflammatory drugs such as phenylbutazone.

The diagnosis may be confirmed by the following.

SYNOVIAL FLUID EXAMINATION

- Normal synovial fluid is clear and a pale straw colour. If the joint is infected, it can be cloudy, flocculent (contain debris) due to fibrin clots, darker yellow or orange in colour and sometimes contains blood.
- Synovial fluid from an infected joint has a reduced viscosity.
- The white blood cell count is usually raised to above 30×10^9/L with more than 90–95% neutrophils.
- The protein level is raised to above 40g/L.
- Bacteria may be seen under the microscope.
- The fluid should be cultured to try and grow and identify the species of bacteria involved and determine its sensitivity to different antibiotics.

RADIOGRAPHY

Radiographs are taken to determine the following.

- To rule out traumatic damage to bone.
- To assess whether there is any infection in the bones making up the joint; infection in the bone is known as **osteomyelitis** or **septic osteitis**. If bone is infected it may show up as areas of reduced bone density (lysis) or there may be an irregular pattern of new bone production. The joint space may be widened or narrowed depending on the stage of the disease.

SCINTIGRAPHY

Scintigraphy may be helpful in the early detection of bone infection but is rarely necessary.

ULTRASONOGRAPHY

Ultrasonography can be helpful for evaluating whether swelling is due to enlargement of the joint or to thickening of the periarticular tissues. It may detect fibrin material within the joint and thickening of the synovial membrane.

ARTHROSCOPY

Arthroscopy under general anaesthesia allows direct inspection of the articular cartilage, the synovial membrane and the joint fluid. It allows confirmation of the diagnosis and may be part of the treatment protocol.

BLOOD TESTS

Blood may be taken for haematology. The horse's total white cell count may be raised with an increased percentage of neutrophils. The plasma fibrinogen may also be raised. However, these changes may not occur until several days after the joint infection has become established.

INJECTION INTO THE JOINT TO CHECK FOR LEAKAGE

It is not always easy to tell whether a wound directly over a joint has breached the joint capsule. In these cases, it can be helpful for the vet to inject sterile fluid into the joint at a site well away from the contaminated area, to see if the fluid then leaks from the wound.

Treatment

Early diagnosis and prompt treatment have a big influence on the outcome of joint infections. The aim of treatment is to remove the bacteria and the harmful inflammatory products along with any foreign material.

Treatment may include the following.

- Immediate intravenous injection of broad spectrum antibiotics while awaiting the results of bacterial culture and antibiotic sensitivity.
- Joint lavage (flushing out) and drainage, usually best performed under general anaesthesia. This removes the inflammatory mediators and also fibrin clots and other

debris which may have bacteria trapped inside and therefore protected from the antibiotics.

- Debridement (surgical removal) of any infected or damaged articular cartilage and bone. This may be done arthroscopically or via an arthrotomy (open joint surgery) incision. Any infected or severely damaged synovial membrane can be removed at the same time. The advantage of looking inside the joint with the arthroscope is that the damage can be seen and dirt and debris removed.
- Injection of antibiotic directly into the joint cavity.
- Injection of antibiotic into infected bone.
- Implantation of antibiotic impregnated beads into joints with chronic or resistant infections.
- Analgesic and anti-inflammatory drugs such as phenylbutazone to reduce the pain and inflammation. This is important in the early stages to reduce the likelihood of laminitis developing in the uninjured limb while the infected limb is non-weight bearing. These should be stopped as soon as possible as they may mask the early signs of recurrence of infection.
- Application of bandages to reduce joint swelling and limb oedema. This helps to reduce the discomfort and improve the blood supply to the region.
- Box rest is essential in the early stages.
- As the patient responds to treatment and the pain is less intense, passive joint movement and physiotherapy are important to reduce stiffness and fibrosis of the joint capsule, so improving the joint function.
- Once the lameness has resolved, walking in hand is gradually introduced.

Monitoring of progress

It is essential that the affected joint is closely monitored as it begins to improve. Any recurrence or increase of heat, swelling or lameness should be investigated immediately with follow-up synovial fluid samples.

Prognosis

Prompt diagnosis and aggressive treatment of adult horses with no cartilage damage or foreign material within the joint cavity carries a reasonably good prognosis. If the diagnosis is delayed or the joint has pre-existing osteoarthritic changes, the outlook becomes more guarded.

JOINT ILL IN FOALS (SEPTIC ARTHRITIS)

Causes

Infection of a foal's joints is most likely to occur if the foal has received inadequate or poor quality colostrum resulting in insufficient immunity to protect it against infection. This is known as failure of passive transfer of immunity (FPT). Foals born prematurely are particularly at risk as are those born to mares with placental problems.

The infection may originate at the umbilicus (navel) or it may be the result of spread of the infection in the blood from elsewhere, e.g. if the foal has pneumonia, enteritis (gut inflammation) or any other cause of septicaemia (blood poisoning). There are many different bacteria that can cause joint ill in foals. Dirty environmental conditions increase the risk of umbilical infection. Any physical trauma to a joint increases its susceptibility to infection.

Clinical signs

- Sudden-onset severe lameness in one or more limbs.
- Reluctance to stand (Figure 8.17).
- Warm, distended and painful joint or joints (Figure 8.18).
- Increased temperature.
- Raised pulse and respiratory rates.
- The foal's lack of desire to suck and an enlarged udder in the mare.

Diagnosis

Diagnosis is as described for adult horses with the addition of:

- blood culture to try and identify the bacteria involved
- measurement of IgG levels (see pages 604 and 679)
- full haematology and plasma fibrinogen.

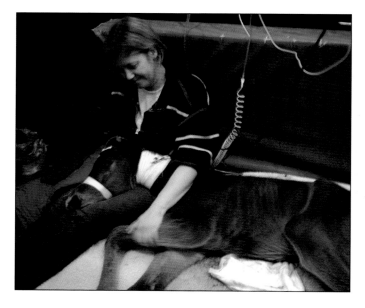

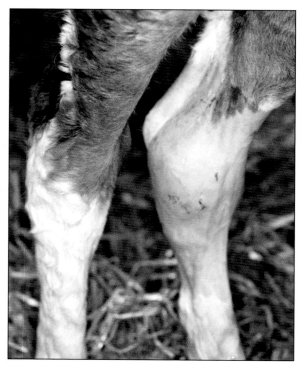

Figure 8.17 Foals with joint ill can be very poorly and need intensive care

Figure 8.18 Swollen infected hock joint in a foal

Radiography is more frequently carried out in foals as they are much more likely to develop osteomyelitis than adult horses.

Treatment

As with adult horses, joint infection should be regarded as an emergency. The source of infection should be identified and addressed, e.g. chest infection, umbilicus. The treatment is likely to include:

- systemic broad spectrum antibiotics
- intra-articular antibiotics
- joint lavage
- surgical removal of infected bone and administration of antibiotics directly into the bone where necessary
- box rest
- bandaging and physiotherapy
- non-steroidal anti-inflammatory drugs are used with care as they cause gastric ulceration in foals; they may be given together with omeprazole or ranitidine to try to prevent this.

Prognosis

The prognosis is guarded to poor. The treatment can be expensive and there is no guarantee of success. Even if the infection is eliminated, the damage to the joint may prevent the foal from developing into a successful athlete. Many foals are euthanased owing to persistent lameness.

LYME DISEASE

Lyme disease is caused by the spirochaete *Borrelia burgdorferi*. It is transmitted to humans and horses by ticks which acquire the infection from feeding on infected rodents and deer, which act as reservoirs of the disease. In the UK and Europe, the tick *Ixodes ricinus* is the vector. Clinical infection of the horse in the UK is uncommon and the incubation period is unknown. Once the horse is infected, the spirochaete multiplies and spreads in the blood to other sites in the body, especially the joints. This can happen months or even years after the acute phase of the disease. Many other organs may be affected.

Clinical signs

The clinical signs may include the following.

- Swollen joints.
- Stiffness or lameness in one or more limbs.
- A temperature.

- Depression.
- Lethargy.
- Limb swelling.
- Enlarged lymph nodes.
- Inflammation of the eye; the spirochaete may cause recurrent uveitis.
- Neurological signs. Encephalitis (brain inflammation) may develop. Reported symptoms include a head tilt, paralysis of the tail, difficulty eating, glazed eyes, profuse sweating and aimless wandering.
- Young foals have been known to die of the disease, but this is rare.

Diagnosis

A presumptive diagnosis of Lyme disease is often made from the clinical signs and a positive antibody titre.

However, the diagnosis is not always straightforward as the organism is difficult to culture. Sometimes the spirochaetes can be seen in samples of blood, cerebrospinal fluid, urine or joint fluid when they are examined under the microscope, using special techniques.

The presence of antibodies in a blood sample proves only that the animal has been exposed to the infection at some stage of its life, not that it is the cause of the current illness. Significant antibody levels may not be detectable in the blood early in the course of the disease, so false negative results do occur. More than one blood sample may be required to check the significance of any blood test results.

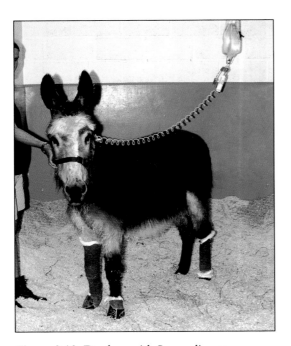

Figure 8.19 Donkey with Lyme disease receiving intravenous fluids and medication; despite multiple joint involvement it did recover

Treatment

This includes:
- antibiotics; a number of antibiotics may be effective: intravenous tetracycline and/or oral doxycycline are most commonly used (Figure 8.19)
- non-steroidal anti-inflammatory drugs can be used to reduce the inflammation and pain; they are not always given straight away as the vet may wish to monitor the response to the antibiotics, to help confirm the diagnosis
- general supportive nursing care should be given
- specific treatment will be given to horses with anterior uveitis.

Prevention

- If possible, avoid grazing horses in tick-infested areas.
- Remove ticks on a daily basis as the ticks must feed for quite a long time before the disease is transmitted.

Prognosis

The prognosis is guarded unless the condition is diagnosed and appropriately treated straight away. Antibiotic treatment is not always effective and the organism can be difficult to eliminate from the body. Long-term infection can result in permanent joint damage, lameness and debility.

THE HORSE'S KNEE (CARPUS)

Anatomy

The veterinary term for the horse's knee is the **carpus**. It is a complex structure made up of three joints and two rows of small bones (see diagrams). Most of the movement takes place at the **antebrachiocarpal** and **middle carpal** joints (Figures 8.20a and b).

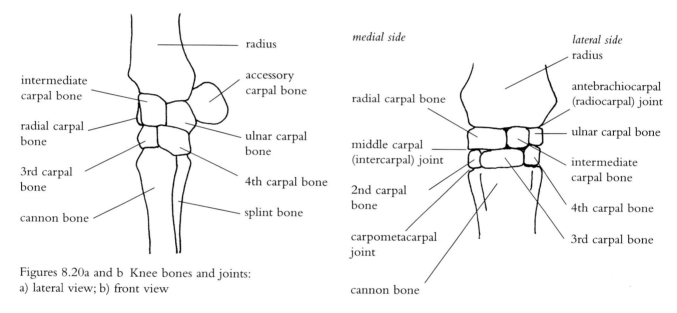

Figures 8.20a and b Knee bones and joints:
a) lateral view; b) front view

Carpal joint inflammation
CAUSES

The carpus is susceptible to injury from falls, kicks and hitting fences as well as general wear and tear. Young racehorses in particular are prone to joint inflammation and degenerative changes due to the stresses of training and racing. Faulty conformation, e.g. back at the knee and offset knees, predisposes the Thoroughbred racehorse to carpal disease (Figures 8.21b and e).

CLINICAL SIGNS
These include:
- lameness
- shortening of the stride

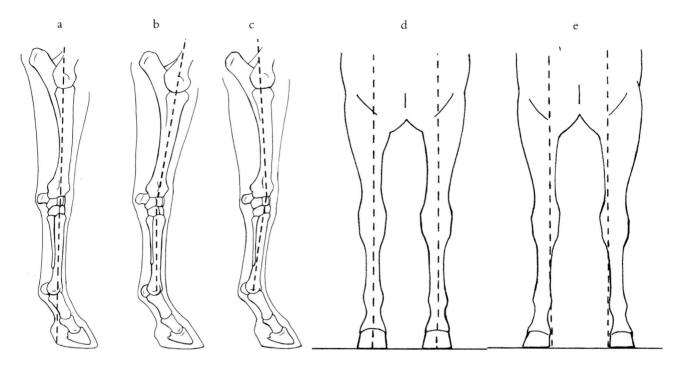

Figures 8.21a–e Knee conformation: side view – in the normal horse a vertical line from the tuber of the scapular spine passes through the elbow joint, knee (carpus) and fetlock to meet the ground behind the heels – a) normal; b) back at the knee; c) over at the knee; front view – in the normal forelimb, a line dropped from the point of the shoulder bisects the limb – d) normal; e) offset (bench) knees, the cannon bone is offset to the lateral side

- a base-wide gait when the condition affects both knees
- distension of the joint capsule
- increased heat over the front of the knee
- pain when firm pressure is applied
- pain on flexion; this can be severe and the horse may rear to avoid flexion
- a reduced degree of flexion
- a tendency to stand with the knee slightly flexed.

DIAGNOSIS

Diagnosis is made on:
- the clinical signs
- intra-articular nerve blocks
- radiography
- synovial fluid analysis to rule out infection if the joint is acutely inflamed
- scintigraphy may help to localize the problem in some cases.
- arthroscopy is sometimes used to examine the tissues and help establish the prognosis.

TREATMENT

Treatment may include:

- box rest with short periods of in-hand walking exercise
- cold treatment in the early stages
- non-steroidal anti-inflammatory drugs, e.g. phenylbutazone, to reduce the pain and inflammation
- ultrasound, low intensity laser or magnetic field therapy
- passive flexing of the knee several times a day to keep the joint mobile
- intra-articular administration of hyaluronan, polysulphated glycosaminoglycan (PSGAG) or corticosteroid.

A thick bed should be provided to minimize the risk of further trauma when lying down.

PROGNOSIS

This depends on the degree of damage that has occurred before treatment begins. If faulty conformation is the cause, the prognosis is poor. Affected racehorses should have their training and racing programmes reassessed. Ongoing joint inflammation ultimately leads to osteoarthritis.

Carpal chip and slab fractures

Carpal chip and slab fractures are predominantly a racehorse injury. Chip fractures are small fragments of bone that break off the top or bottom of individual carpal bones in response to the stresses of training and racing. The radial, intermediate or third carpal bones and the distal aspect of the radius are most commonly involved. The pieces can remain attached or float around the joint space. Slab fractures are larger and extend throughout the whole length of the bone. These most often occur in the third carpal bone.

CAUSES

- The fragments of bone break off in response to repeated concussion and overloading of the front of the carpal bones.
- Back-at-the knee conformation may predispose to this type of injury.
- Tired horses are most likely to sustain injury.
- Poor racing and training surfaces.
- Working at very fast speed.
- Foot imbalance causes uneven distribution of forces within the limb.

CLINICAL SIGNS

These depend on the type of fracture. They include:

- variable degrees of lameness: small, undisplaced fractures may cause slight lameness, whereas large chip or slab fractures can be very painful and cause severe lameness

- heat and swelling over the front of the knee
- a tendency to stand with the knee slightly flexed
- reduced flexion and severe pain on flexion in horses with large chip or slab fractures
- pain on palpation of the front of the joint.

DIAGNOSIS

The diagnosis is made on the results of clinical examination, intra-articular analgesia and radiography. Multiple X-ray views of the carpus, including some with the knee flexed, are required to show up the different bone surfaces. Repeat views may be necessary 10–14 days later as some fractures do not show up initially. Arthroscopy is helpful as the joint surfaces and ligaments within the joint can be seen and the damage is often more extensive than that seen on the X-rays. Scintigraphy is useful for detecting early stress fractures.

TREATMENT

Treatment may be surgical or conservative. Small or incomplete chip fractures that are not displaced may be treated conservatively with an extended period of box rest and gradual introduction of controlled exercise. Larger chips or thin slabs should be surgically removed as soon as possible after the injury has occurred to minimize the risk of subsequent degenerative joint disease (DJD). Larger slab fractures are treated by screwing them back in place.

One of the problems associated with carpal fractures is damage to the articular cartilage. At the moment this can only be accurately assessed by arthroscopy. It is hoped that in the future, examination of the blood or joint fluid for specific substances released when cartilage is injured, will help to determine the presence and degree of damage. Treatments that help to limit this damage include:

- non-steroidal anti-inflammatory dugs, e.g. phenylbutazone, to reduce the pain and inflammation
- intra-articular injections of hyaluronan or polysulphated glycosaminoglycan (PSGAG)
- intramuscular injections of PSGAG.

New techniques have been developed and are being used experimentally. These include:

- cartilage resurfacing using cartilage taken from another site
- transplantation of cartilage cells or stem cells from the horse that have been grown in the laboratory; these are then injected back into the diseased joint and help it to repair.

PROGNOSIS

The prognosis is reasonable if the horse is promptly and appropriately treated. Many horses are able to continue racing. Multiple fractures carry a poorer prognosis.

Broken knees

'Broken knees' is the name used to describe an injury where the horse loses the skin from the front of its knees, usually as a result of a fall. It occurs when a horse slips on a hard surface such as a road.

CLINICAL SIGNS

The injury may just involve the superficial layers of skin or the whole skin thickness may be lost (Figure 8.22). Because the knees tend to scrape along the road surface they are usually badly grazed and often have dirt ground into the tissue. There is a moderate amount of bleeding. The tendon sheaths that run across the knee may be opened and on occasions the joint capsule may be damaged, allowing synovial fluid to escape and joint contamination to occur.

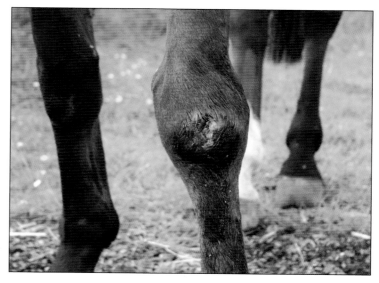

Figure 8.22 Broken knees: this wound has gone right through the skin; scarring from an earlier similar injury can be seen on the opposite knee

TREATMENT

- The wounds should be thoroughly cleaned and inspected so the damage can be assessed. If clear synovial fluid leaks from the wound or the horse is obviously lame, the vet should be called straight away.
- The first step in the treatment is to hose the wound and then clean it with an appropriately diluted antiseptic scrub and sterile saline.
- Where necessary, the vet will cut away any severely damaged tissue and remove as much of the dirt as possible.
- Antibiotics are likely to be given unless the wound is very superficial.
- Non-steroidal anti-inflammatory drugs, e.g. phenylbutazone, will help to reduce any swelling or discomfort.
- As with any wound, the tetanus vaccination status of the horse should be checked. If it is not covered, tetanus antitoxin and the first vaccine will be given.

WOUND MANAGEMENT

These wounds cannot be sutured as:

- there is skin loss
- they are usually contaminated
- the injury is on the front of the knee which flexes with every stride the horse takes; any sutures would simply pull through the tissue and the wound would break down.

The wound must heal by granulation. Damaged tendon sheaths usually heal and stop leaking within a few days. The wound should be covered with a non-stick dressing (e.g.

Melolin® or Rondopad®) and a layer of Gamgee®. The easiest way to keep the dressing in place is to use either a wide crepe bandage (15 cm [6 in] for a horse) or a tubular bandage and fix this in place with Elastoplast®. Alternatively, the dressing may be held in position with a Pressage® bandage. A support bandage is applied to the lower limb.

While the wound is healing, the horse should be kept on box rest. When healing is progressing satisfactorily, in-hand walking exercise can begin. Under no circumstances should the horse be turned out and allowed to get down onto unprotected knees and roll. If proud flesh forms, the vet will remove it and make recommendations on how to manage any further growth. Regular low intensity laser therapy can stimulate and speed up healing which may take 4–6 weeks.

PROGNOSIS

Despite variable amounts of unsightly scar tissue, the prognosis is good for uncomplicated cases.

PREVENTION

If the horse is known to slip or stumble, knee boots worn for road work will afford considerable protection. Road nails can be very helpful in areas where the road surface is abnormally slippery. Keeping the toes short and rolling the toes may also reduce the likelihood of the horse stumbling.

THE STIFLE JOINT

Anatomy

The stifle joint of the horse is the equivalent of the human knee. It is made up of three bones – the femur, the tibia and the patella (kneecap). The patella is attached to the tibia by the medial, middle and lateral patellar ligaments. The quadriceps femoris muscle which lies along the front and both sides of the femur attaches to the patella.

As the stifle joint extends and flexes, the patella glides up and down in a groove at the lower end of the femur. This groove is called the trochlea. The trochlea has a prominent medial ridge with a knob-like extension on the upper edge. The medial side of the patella has a cartilage extension which overlies the medial ridge of the trochlea.

This arrangement allows the stifle joint to be locked in an extended position. The joint is extended by contraction of the powerful quadriceps femoris muscle. As the joint is fully extended, the patella glides to the upper limit of the trochlea groove. If the patella is then moved medially, the knob of the medial ridge of the trochlea projects between the medial and middle patella ligaments (Figures 8.23a and b).

This locking mechanism allows the horse to stand for long periods without experiencing muscle fatigue. The opposite hind limb is rested. To unlock the stifle, the horse's

a) *Medial view*

b) *Cranial view*

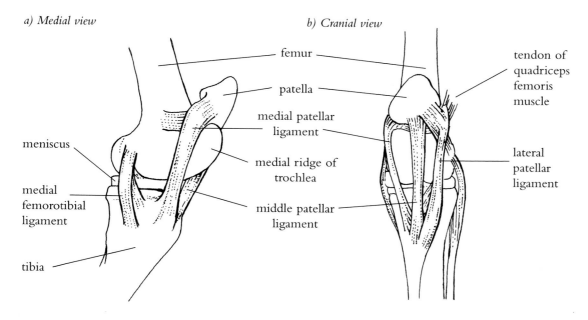

Figures 8.23a and b Ligaments of the stifle joint

weight is shifted to the opposite hind limb. The quadriceps muscle pulls the patella in an upward direction. The patella is then moved laterally and returned to the trochlear groove.

The stifle joint may be affected by:

- traumatic injuries
- osteochondrosis
- bone cysts
- infection
- degenerative joint disease.

The equine stifle joint also has the unique problem of upward fixation of the patella.

Upward fixation of the patella

This is a condition where the horse or pony is temporarily unable to unlock the stifle from the extended position. The medial patellar ligament stays hooked over the medial trochlear ridge. The problem may occur in one or both hind limbs.

CAUSES

Horses with very straight hind limbs are prone to upward fixation of the patella. Young, unfit or poorly muscled animals are also particularly susceptible. The condition is common in Shetland ponies and may be hereditary. Any condition causing debility or sudden loss of quadriceps muscle tone can lead to the condition in susceptible animals, hence it is seen in horses that have lost weight as well as muscle tone.

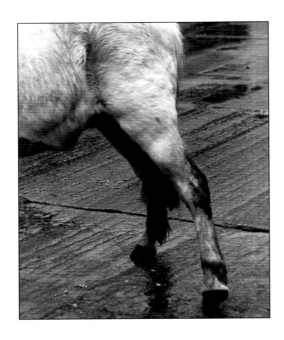

CLINICAL SIGNS

- The stifle and hock are locked in extension and unable to flex and so if the horse is made to move it hops forwards with the leg extended behind it (Figure 8.24).
- The fetlock is flexed and the toe is dragged on the ground.
- The condition tends to occur after the animal has been standing still.
- It can lock for a few strides or for a prolonged period of time.
- When the stifle unlocks a 'snapping' sound may be heard and the limb may jerk up quickly in a fashion resembling stringhalt.

Figure 8.24 Upward fixation of the patella

In some horses and ponies, the limb does not lock but tends to 'catch' with every stride. This is known as 'delayed patella release'. It is most noticeable if the horse is observed walking downhill or turned in a short circle with the affected limb on the inside. It may be seen when the horse turns round in the stable or walks forwards after standing still. It may also be observed on the downward transition from trot to walk or seen if the horse is standing square and rocked from side to side.

The condition does not usually cause lameness, but the femoropatellar joint may become distended due to inflammation of the synovial membrane in longstanding cases. These horses may find walking downhill very uncomfortable and be unhappy working in deep going.

DIAGNOSIS

Diagnosis is made on the history and the clinical signs but can be difficult in horses where the condition occurs only intermittently. Radiographs of the stifle may be taken to eliminate joint pathology such as osteochondrosis.

TREATMENT

- The first line of treatment is to increase the fitness of the affected animal and improve its quadriceps muscle tone. The exercise programme will depend on the age and type of horse. Very young animals can be walked in hand. The recommended exercise for older animals is walking and trotting in straight lines. They may be led or ridden as appropriate.
- If the horse is sore, non-steroidal anti-inflammatory drugs such as phenylbutazone may be administered.

- The animal should be turned out rather than stabled.
- If the horse is debilitated for any reason, this should be addressed. The diet should be checked and routine worming and dentistry carried out.
- If the limb remains locked, it may release if the horse is walked backwards. If not, then the vet will try to dislodge the locked patella manually.

A youngster should be allowed to mature if possible before any further action is taken. When the above measures do not provide relief, then the following options may be considered.

- Injection of the medial patellar ligament(s) with irritants to tighten the ligament.
- Surgical cutting of the medial patellar ligament. This procedure is called a medial patellar desmotomy. It is usually performed under local anaesthetic in the standing horse, under sedation. The technique is rarely the first option because of complications that have been reported following surgery, e.g. persistent low-grade postoperative lameness and fragmentation of the patella.
- Recently, a new procedure has been developed for treatment of upward fixation of the patella. The upper third of each medial patellar ligament is split while the horse is under general anaesthetic. Horses begin in-hand walking exercise the day after surgery. Immediate resolution of the condition is reported in some cases, in others it takes up to 2 weeks. The healing process causes the ligament to become 2–3 times its original thickness and this stabilizes the joint and prevents the upper part of the ligament from catching or hooking easily over the medial ridge of the femoral trochlea. No long-term complications have been reported.

PROGNOSIS

The prognosis is good when the condition resolves as the horse becomes fitter. Occasionally the condition will recur if the horse loses fitness and condition or needs box rest for any other reason.

The prognosis is reasonable for horses undergoing medial patella desmotomy if care is taken with their rehabilitation. Some animals have a slightly restricted gait following surgery and long-term complications have been reported.

A recent study indicates that the prognosis is good for horses treated by splitting of the medial patellar ligament.

9

SYNOVIAL EFFUSIONS

Synovial membranes sometimes produce an abnormal amount of synovial fluid in response to low-grade trauma. This can cause swelling without any heat or lameness. The examples considered here include:

- joints – e.g. articular windgalls, bog spavin
- tendon sheaths – e.g. tendinous windgalls
- bursae – e.g. hygroma of the knee, capped hock, capped elbow.

JOINTS

Articular windgalls
Cold, painless distensions of the fetlock joint capsule are known as articular windgalls (Figure 9.1).

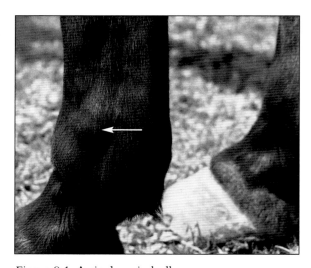

Figure 9.1 Articular windgall

CAUSES
The cause is low-grade trauma of the fetlock joint. This may be related to conformation. For example, they are common in stocky animals with upright conformation, probably as a result of concussion. In young or athletic horses, the appearance of articular windgalls is an indication that that the horse's work is traumatizing the joint.

CLINICAL SIGNS
These swellings can be seen on either side of the limb, between the back of the cannon bone and the suspensory ligament. Applying pressure to the swelling on one side of the joint causes the swelling on the opposite side to enlarge. They often fluctuate in size according to the horse's exercise regime. In some horses they are only present after a spell of heavy work, whereas in others they are a permanent feature.

TREATMENT

As the condition is not associated with lameness, no treatment may be necessary apart from modification of the exercise programme. Application of stable bandages may help to reduce the swelling.

If distension of the fetlock joint capsule is associated with any heat or pain, the treatment is as described in the section on joint sprains.

Bog spavin

Bog spavin is the name given to a synovial effusion of the tarsocrural joint of the hock. The joint capsule can become markedly distended. One or both hocks may be affected.

CAUSES

- Poor conformation which puts abnormal strain on the joint. The condition tends to occur in horses with cow hocks, sickle hocks and straight hocks. The persistent low-grade trauma causes inflammation of the synovial membrane resulting in effusion. If no other pathology is found, the condition is known as **idiopathic synovitis**.

However, the following conditions can also be accompanied by swelling of the tarsocrural joint:
- osteochondrosis (OCD)
- osteoarthritis
- acute trauma such as a sprain
- infection
- fracture of the hock.

CLINICAL SIGNS

- Swelling of the joint capsule. There are usually two obviously fluid-filled swellings that develop below the point of the hock. The largest is on the front of the hock towards the inside and the second swelling is further back on the outside of the limb (Figures 9.2a and b). Applying pressure to one of the swellings will cause the other to enlarge and the tension in the joint to increase.
- The horse may or may not be lame. Severe swelling can cause a mechanical lameness by restricting flexion of the hock resulting in a shortened stride.
- Lameness may be caused or increased by flexion of the joint.
- Heat may be present.

DIAGNOSIS

Diagnosis is made on the clinical signs. If an underlying lesion is suspected, any of the following diagnostic procedures may also be used:

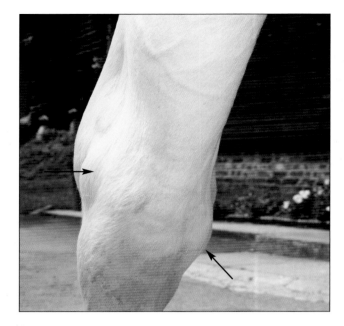

a

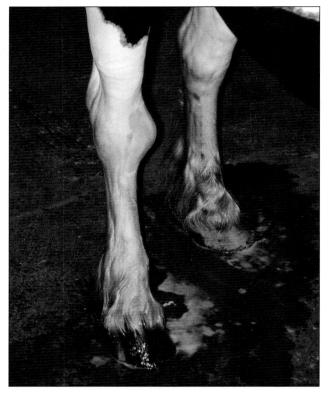

b

Figures 9.2a and b Bog spavin: effusion of the tarsocrural joint, a) bog spavin; b) very large bog spavin

- radiography, which is necessary to detect OCD lesions, any osteoarthritic changes or a fracture
- examination of the joint fluid
- intra–articular nerve blocks may be helpful if the horse is lame
- scintigraphy.

TREATMENT

Any underlying pathology within the joint must be appropriately treated and those conditions listed above are discussed elsewhere. Where the condition is idiopathic (i.e. of no known cause) the following options may be considered:

- no treatment
- drainage of the excess fluid and injection of corticosteroid with or without hyaluronan; the hock is then bandaged and the horse's activity is restricted for 2 weeks.

PROGNOSIS

The prognosis is guarded as treatment is effective in only 50% of cases. The hock is not the easiest area to bandage comfortably and the swelling often recurs. However, provided the condition is not accompanied by any lameness, most horses are able to perform satisfactorily.

TENDON SHEATHS

Tendon sheaths are long thin sacs of synovial fluid that surround and protect tendons as they pass over bony prominences. They are lined by a synovial membrane, similar to joints.

Tenosynovitis

Tenosynovitis is inflammation of the synovial membrane within the tendon sheath. It can be caused by wear and tear, an acute injury or infection.

Idiopathic tenosynovitis

It is possible for a tendon sheath to become distended by increased production of synovial fluid without any obvious inflammation. Examples include tendinous windgalls and thoroughpin and these do not cause pain or lameness.

TENDINOUS WINDGALLS

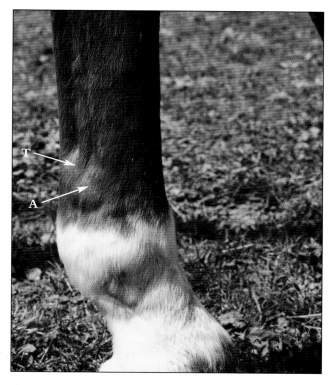

Figure 9.3 Articular (A) and tendinous (T) windgalls

These are enlargements of the digital flexor tendon sheath (DFTS). The swellings are located just above the fetlock, between the suspensory ligament and the flexor tendons. They are often larger on the hind limb. The cause is considered to be low-grade trauma. They may swell when the horse is in the stable and reduce with exercise. Tendinous windgalls are considered to be a cosmetic blemish and are rarely of clinical significance. In a young horse they can be an indication that too much is being asked of it. The application of stable bandages will sometimes reduce the swelling. No specific treatment is necessary. (Figure 9.3.)

THOROUGHPIN

A thoroughpin is a swelling of the tarsal sheath which encloses the deep digital flexor tendon as it passes over the hock. The swelling occurs in front of the Achilles tendon just above the point of the hock (Figures 9.4a and b). The condition tends to be more common in horses with straight hocks. It is rarely associated with lameness and the swelling may be spontaneously resorbed over a period of time. Treatment is rarely necessary. If the swelling is large, drainage followed by a local injection of corticosteroid may reduce the blemish.

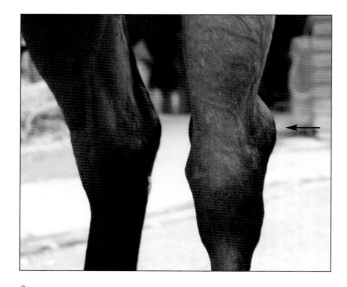

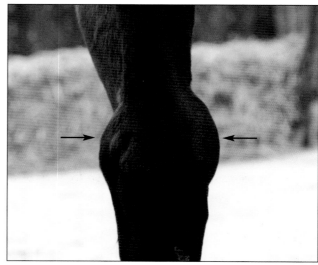

a   b

Figures 9.4a and b Thoroughpin: a) front view; b) rear view

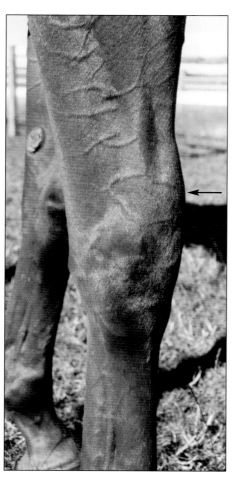

Figure 9.5 Tenosynovitis of the common digital extensor tendon sheath

Acute tenosynovitis

Common examples include:

- tenosynovitis of the common digital extensor tendon sheath as it passes over the knee (Figure 9.5)
- inflammation of the digital flexor tendon sheath (DFTS) at the back of the fetlock and pastern
- inflammation of the tarsal sheath.

CAUSES

The acute inflammation can be the result of:

- a direct blow, e.g. hitting a jump (extensor tendon sheaths) or an overreach (DFTS)
- strains during exercise, e.g. tarsal sheath and DFTS
- injury to the tendon, e.g. the deep digital flexor tendon within the DFTS.

CLINICAL SIGNS

The distension of the tendon sheath in these cases is accompanied by:

- heat
- pain
- pain on palpation of the swelling
- lameness
- the horse may stand with the heel slightly raised from the ground with an acute injury to the DFTS.

DIAGNOSIS

Diagnosis is made on:

- the clinical signs
- ultrasonography – this is essential to identify any accompanying damage to the tendon or adhesions within the sheath
- examination of a sample of synovial fluid which may be taken to check for any infection if the swelling and lameness are severe
- tenoscopy, e.g. endoscopic examination of the digital sheath and the tendon within it; the procedure is generally reserved for serious or chronic injuries as it has to be carried out under general anaesthesia.

TREATMENT

Treatment in the early stages includes:

- box rest
- cold therapy
- bandaging
- non-steroidal anti-inflammatory drugs, e.g. phenylbutazone.

As the inflammation subsides, controlled walking exercise is introduced prior to a gradual return to ridden work. If the condition does not resolve and there is no injury to the tendon or infection present, the tendon sheath may be injected with a combination of hyaluronan and corticosteroid to reduce the inflammation.

PROGNOSIS

The prognosis is good provided there is no tendon damage and the condition is recognized early and treated promptly and appropriately. Failure to manage this condition correctly may lead to chronic tenosynovitis.

Chronic tenosynovitis

If an acute tenosynovitis fails to respond to treatment, the tendon sheath remains distended by a persistent synovial effusion and may become permanently thickened by fibrous tissue. Adhesions may develop within the sheath and between the sheath and the tendon. By this stage, the swelling may be cold and painless.

CAUSES

The causes can include:

- a single acute trauma
- repeated minor injuries, i.e. wear and tear
- injury to the tendon within the sheath.

DIAGNOSIS

Diagnosis is as described for acute tenosynovitis.

TREATMENT

Treatment is necessary when the condition affects the horse's performance. It is likely to include:

- drainage of excess synovial fluid and injection of hyaluronan and corticosteroid followed by bandaging
- surgical exploration of the tendon sheath and removal of the thickened synovial membrane with resection of adhesions if the condition fails to respond to the above treatment
- treatment of annular ligament thickening if it is either causing, or the result of, chronic tenosynovitis of the DFTS
- physiotherapy following surgery is beneficial.

PROGNOSIS

The prognosis is variable, depending on which tendon sheath is affected, the severity of the condition and the use of the horse. It is less favourable if adhesions are present.

Septic or infectious tenosynovitis

Infection of a tendon sheath is a serious medical emergency. The digital flexor tendon sheath (DFTS) is the most susceptible to injury and the condition is described here.

CAUSES

- The commonest route of infection is through a puncture wound or laceration at the back of the pastern. This may be caused by a thorn or other sharp object.
- It may occur following an injection into the DFTS.
- Occasionally infection my spread in the bloodstream to the tendon sheath from an abscess or infection elsewhere in the body.

CLINICAL SIGNS

These include:

- sudden onset severe lameness
- the horse may stand with its heel raised from the ground
- on occasions these wounds cause such extreme pain that the horse will not bear weight on the limb
- swelling of the tendon sheath; this may be masked due to a generalized and severe cellulitis of the fetlock and pastern regions
- the wound may be open and leak synovial fluid; small puncture wounds, however, can easily be overlooked if they seal up quickly

- the horse may have a temperature, increased respiratory rate and tremble.

DIAGNOSIS

Prompt diagnosis is essential otherwise inflammatory enzymes can damage the tendon within the sheath and the fibrin produced causes adhesions to develop. Diagnosis is made on:

- the clinical signs
- analysis of synovial fluid taken from the tendon sheath (Figures 9.6a and b); infected synovial fluid has a higher protein and white cell count than normal
- ultrasonography
- radiographs may be taken to rule out damage to underlying bone.

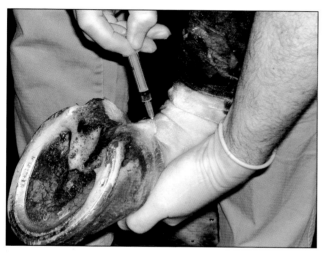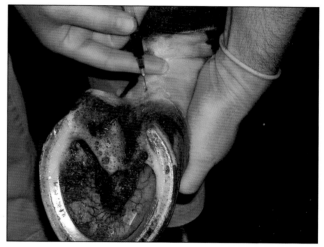

Figures 9.6a and b Sampling fluid from the digital flexor tendon sheath: a) a sample of synovial fluid is taken from the DFTS to determine whether it has been contaminated by the wound at the back of the fetlock; b) normal synovial fluid is clear and straw-coloured but the dark colour of the synovial fluid being withdrawn here indicates that the DFTS has been breached

TREATMENT

Treatment includes:

- administration of broad spectrum antibiotics
- surgical drainage and flushing of the infected sheath to remove bacteria and other debris (Figure 9.7)
- surgical removal of any adhesions or grossly infected and thickened synovial membrane
- infusion of antibiotics into the tendon sheath
- a drain may be implanted so the sheath can be regularly flushed and infused with antibiotics

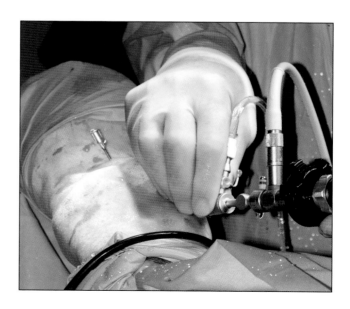

Figure 9.7 Flushing an infected tendon sheath

- the annular ligament may be surgically cut to release the pressure on the tendon sheath
- administration of non-steroidal anti-inflammatory drugs, e.g. phenylbutazone
- box rest and bandaging
- early introduction of walking in hand or passive flexing of the distal limb to reduce adhesions forming
- elevating the heel in the early stages may make the horse more comfortable
- when the tendon sheath has healed and the infection resolved, the sheath may be injected with hyaluronan as this is reported to reduce adhesions forming
- if there is extensive soft tissue injury, a cast may be applied once the tendon sheath has healed to minimize movement of the soft tissues.

PROGNOSIS

The prognosis is guarded once infection has become established within a tendon sheath.

BURSAE

A bursa is a small sac of synovial fluid, lined with synovial membrane which acts as a natural cushion or padding over a bony prominence. They may be congenital or acquired.

Congenital bursae are present in all horses at birth and they occur in areas where a tendon glides over a bony prominence. The fluid-filled sac cushions the tendon and protects it from friction as the tendon moves. Examples include:
- the navicular bursa, which lies between the navicular bone and the deep digital flexor tendon
- the bicipital bursa, which protects the tendon of the biceps brachii muscle as it passes through the groove at the front of the humerus close to the shoulder
- the supraspinous bursa, which lies between the ligamentum nuchae and the dorsal processes of the third and fourth thoracic vertebrae.

Acquired bursae are not present in every animal. They develop under the skin as a reaction to repeated trauma. Examples include:
- capped hock
- capped elbow
- hygroma of the knee.

Bursitis

Bursitis is inflammation of a bursa and is usually due to trauma or infection. Traumatic bursitis may be acute or chronic. Acute bursitis can occur as the result of a direct blow and bicipital bursitis is an example of this. Chronic bursitis is usually the result of repeated trauma, for example, capped hocks. A few of the more common examples will now be described.

ACUTE BURSITIS

Bicipital bursitis is usually accompanied by lameness and pain on deep palpation. It can be caused by a kick or a blow to the point of the shoulder and there may be heat and some local swelling. Diagnosis is made on the clinical signs and confirmed if necessary by local analgesia, ultrasound examination or scintigraphy. Treatment includes box rest and controlled exercise. Cold therapy may be beneficial. Local injections of corticosteroid into the bursa may be given and non-steroidal anti-inflammatory drugs such as phenylbutazone can be administered orally.

CHRONIC BURSITIS (CAPPED HOCKS, CAPPED ELBOWS, HYGROMA OF THE KNEE)

Capped hocks are cold, painless swellings which develop on the point of the hock (Figures 9.8a and b).

Causes
- Inadequate bedding.
- Leaning against the stable wall or trailer ramp.
- A blow to the point of the hock.

Prevention
- Provide a thick, banked bed.
- Protect the hocks when travelling.

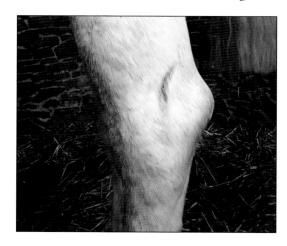

a

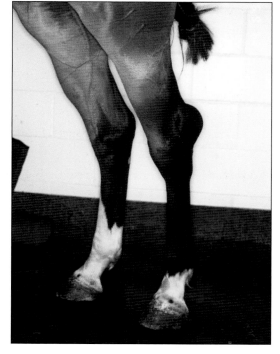

b

Figures 9.8a and b Capped hocks: a) capped hock; b) a more extreme example of a capped hock

Capped elbows are subcutaneous bursae which develop on the point of the elbow. The fluid-filled swelling is usually cold and painless.

Causes

They are caused by repeated knocks from the heel of the front shoe when the horse lies down, or during fast work.

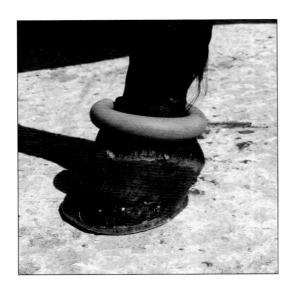

Prevention

Using a sausage boot around the pastern may provide some protection by limiting flexion of the lower limb (Figure 9.9).

Hygroma of the knee; this presents as a swelling on the front of the knee (Figure 9.10).

Causes

- Inadequate bedding.
- Knocking a fence.
- Repeatedly banging the stable door.

Figure 9.9 Sausage boot

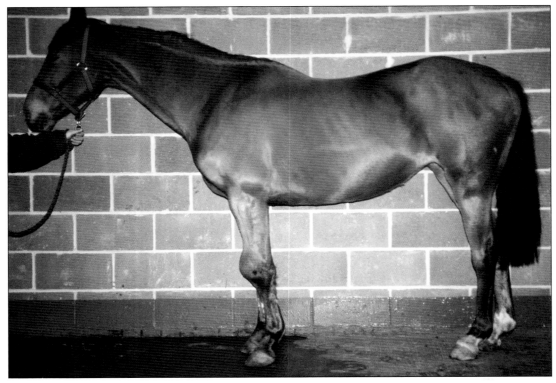

Figure 9.10 Horse with a large carpal hygroma

Prevention

- Provide a thick, comfortable bed.
- Pad the door with thick foam rubber or replace it with a wooden bar or chain during the day.
- Protect the knees when travelling.

Treatment

- Removal of the cause of the problem is essential. If the problem is identified promptly, no further treatment may be necessary.
- If the swelling is large and unsightly, the fluid may be drained by the vet and the area bandaged. However, the improvement may only be slight or temporary as the swelling often reforms and effective bandaging of these sites is not easy. Following drainage of the bursa, corticosteroids may be injected to reduce inflammation.
- Very large swellings that do not respond to medical treatment can be removed surgically under general anaesthesia. This would be considered when the swelling was sufficient to affect the horse's gait as can occur with a large hygroma of the knee.

SEPTIC BURSITIS

A bursa can become infected if it is penetrated by a sharp object. Examples include the following.

- Infection of the navicular bursa following penetration by a nail or other sharp object.
- Fistulous withers which presents as a painful swelling over the withers that may or may not discharge (Figure 9.11). The condition can be caused by blunt trauma or a penetrating wound, but in many cases there is no obvious cause (idiopathic). The bacterium *Brucella abortus* may be involved and as this infection can cause serious problems in people, any discharges are cultured to identify the bacteria present.

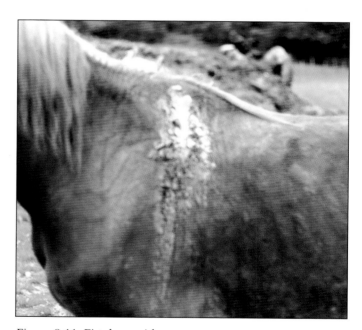

Figure 9.11 Fistulous withers

Treatment

In both cases the infection is serious. Drainage is established together with surgical removal of all dead and infected tissue. Even with intensive antibiotic therapy, the prognosis is guarded as the recurrence rate is high.

10
CONDITIONS AFFECTING BONE

PERIOSTITIS

Periostitis is inflammation of the periosteum which is the thin membrane that covers bone. It may be thought of as a protective 'clingfilm' wrapper around the bone. The periosteum is composed of two layers:
- an outer fibrous layer
- an inner cellular layer containing blood vessels and cells that can differentiate into **osteoblasts**. These cells are able to produce new bone.

The periosteum is important for:
- attachment of tendons and ligaments to bone
- nutrition of bone
- growth of young bone
- repair of bone fractures.

Causes
The periosteum can become inflamed following:
- repeated stress
- a direct blow
- tearing of the attached ligaments.

The resultant haemorrhage lifts the periosteum away from the bone and this stimulates the osteoblasts to produce new bone.

Clinical Signs
A tender, bony swelling develops. This is often accompanied by heat and inflammation of the surrounding soft tissue. If the affected area is pressed, the horse will often react by moving away. As the inflammation subsides, the bony lump remodels, becoming smaller and painless.

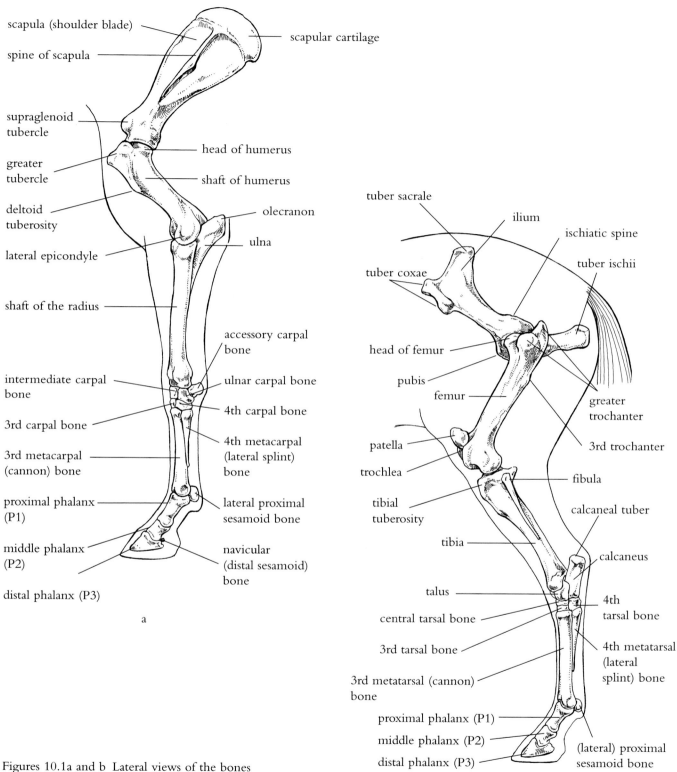

scapula (shoulder blade)
spine of scapula
scapular cartilage
supraglenoid tubercle
greater tubercle
head of humerus
shaft of humerus
deltoid tuberosity
olecranon
lateral epicondyle
ulna
shaft of the radius
accessory carpal bone
intermediate carpal bone
ulnar carpal bone
4th carpal bone
3rd carpal bone
4th metacarpal (lateral splint) bone
3rd metacarpal (cannon) bone
proximal phalanx (P1)
lateral proximal sesamoid bone
middle phalanx (P2)
navicular (distal sesamoid) bone
distal phalanx (P3)

a

tuber sacrale
ilium
ischiatic spine
tuber coxae
tuber ischii
head of femur
pubis
femur
greater trochanter
3rd trochanter
patella
fibula
trochlea
calcaneal tuber
tibial tuberosity
calcaneus
tibia
4th tarsal bone
talus
central tarsal bone
4th metatarsal (lateral splint) bone
3rd tarsal bone
3rd metatarsal (cannon) bone
proximal phalanx (P1)
middle phalanx (P2)
(lateral) proximal sesamoid bone
distal phalanx (P3)

b

Figures 10.1a and b Lateral views of the bones of the fore and hind limbs: a) left forelimb; b) left hind limb

Radiographic changes

The new bone is visible from approximately two weeks after the injury occurs. While the inflammation is still active, the new bone appears less dense than the normal bone and has a fuzzy and irregular outline. As the inflammation subsides, the bony lump remodels. It acquires a smooth contour and remains as a bony lump or **exostosis**.

Examples of periostitis include sore shins and splints.

Sore (bucked) shins

The veterinary term for sore shins is dorsal metacarpal (metatarsal) disease. The condition usually affects the forelimbs; the hind limbs are only occasionally involved. In this condition, the dorsal aspect (front) of the third metacarpal (cannon) bone becomes inflamed and sore. It is very common in 2-year-old Thoroughbred horses in training.

CAUSES

The disease occurs when the immature bones of young, growing Thoroughbreds are subjected to the stresses of racing and training. Fast exercise causes compression of the front of the cannon bone. In response to this, the bone remodels and becomes thicker as an adaptation to the demands placed on it. If the speed and distance in the training programme are increased too quickly, however, the bone cannot adapt fast enough and the resultant stress on the bone causes inflammation and pain.

CLINICAL SIGNS

These may include:

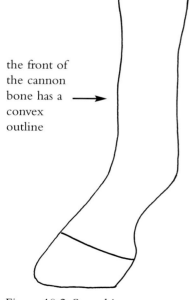

the front of the cannon bone has a convex outline →

- heat
- pain when the shins are palpated
- an alteration of gait ranging from a slight shortening of stride or stiffness, to severe lameness
- reduced performance level
- the front of the cannon bone may become convex in outline (Figure 10.2)
- improvement with rest but the soreness recurs with further exercise.

There are 3 stages of the disease.

Stage 1

Periostitis of the dorsal and dorsomedial (at the front and towards the inside of the leg) surface of the cannon bone causes the horse to appear stiff or bilaterally lame. These horses are sore on

Figure 10.2 Sore shin

palpation but there is no change in the contour of the cannon bone. No changes are visible on radiographs. This is a common occurrence in 2-year-old Thoroughbreds in training.

Stage 2

New bone is deposited on the dorsomedial aspect of the cannon bone as a result of continued stress from training and racing. The shins develop a convex profile and are sore on palpation. Affected horses are characteristically sore after exercise and between 2–4 years of age. New bone is visible on radiographs.

Stage 3

If the horse is not adequately rested and continues in training, stress fractures can develop on the weaker, dorsolateral (front, outside) aspect of the cannon bone, approximately two thirds of the way down. This results in acute, localized pain on palpation and severe lameness. The fractures are usually visible on radiographs and tend to occur in 3–4-year-olds.

DIAGNOSIS

The diagnosis is usually made on the clinical signs and confirmed with radiography. Scintigraphy is sometimes helpful in detecting areas of increased bone activity. Areas of increased heat may be detectable on thermographic images.

TREATMENT

Stage 1

- Box rest for 5–10 days with short periods of in-hand walking on soft ground
- Cold hosing.
- Application of topical anti-inflammatory preparations.
- Non-steroidal anti-inflammatory drugs (NSAIDs), e.g. phenylbutazone, to reduce the inflammation and pain.
- When re-introduced to training, the demands made on the horse should be reduced to significantly less than when the problem occurred.

Stage 2

- Rest for up to 6 weeks, although some cases take as long as 4 months to settle.
- NSAIDs.
- Topical anti-inflammatory preparations.
- If the condition is chronic, the healing may be accelerated by a procedure known as **osteostixis** or **dorsal cortical drilling**. Several holes are drilled at intervals through the affected area of the cannon bone. This improves the blood supply to the area. It is usually performed under a general anaesthetic but may be possible under sedation with

local anaesthesia. The horse then has 1 month of box rest, with in-hand walking introduced after 2 weeks. Light training may be resumed as early as 3–4 months depending on the clinical signs and healing which is monitored by taking X-rays.

- Swimming allows a horse to keep fit without putting strain on the limbs.

Stage 3

There are two approaches to treatment of a stress fracture. Some can be screwed back in place. This operation requires a general anaesthetic and may be combined with osteostixis around the fracture site. The screw may be removed after 8 weeks or left in place. Return to training may be possible from approximately 4 months after the surgery.

The alternative is conservative treatment which entails a period of rest with NSAIDs as necessary. Horses with severe or multiple fractures are generally treated conservatively because of the risk of a catastrophic break of the bone while recovering from general anaesthesia.

Extracorporeal shock wave therapy has recently been used for the treatment of metacarpal stress fractures. The early results are promising but more studies need to be carried out.

PREVENTION

Training

With careful planning of the training programme, sore shins should be preventable. Research has shown that working at high speed subjects the dorsal surface of the third metacarpal bone to compressive forces, whereas trotting puts it under tension. The bone remodels differently for each of these gaits. In order for the bone to adapt to the stresses of racing, trotting should be restricted to the warm-up period and not be used to increase fitness. By early introduction of short, high-speed workouts into the training programme twice a week, the bone will adapt to the stresses of racing. Galloping should be restricted to one mile. If training is interrupted for any reason, it should recommence at slower speeds and shorter distances than those used prior to the break in routine. Training on hard surfaces increases the likelihood of the disease.

Monitoring

The dorsal surface of the metacarpus should be palpated regularly and especially after racing or hard training. If there is any soreness, the horse should not be raced and the training programme should be modified.

PROGNOSIS

If appropriately managed, the prognosis for stage 1 is good. The prognosis for stages 2 and 3 is fair provided the training programme is modified. Once a horse is 4 years old, sore shins are unlikely to be a problem as the cannon bone is mature and better able to withstand the forces of fast exercise.

Splints

Each limb of the horse has a long, thin splint bone attached to either side of the cannon bone by a strong (interosseous) ligament composed of dense fibrous tissue. If the periosteum of the splint bone or the ligament becomes inflamed, a bony swelling known as a 'splint' develops. The most common site for a splint is on the medial side (inside) of the forelimb, 6–8 cm (2–3 in) below the knee. They tend to occur in horses between 2 and 4 years of age.

ANATOMY

The cannon and splint bones of the forelimb are all metacarpal bones (in the hind limb they are metatarsals). The medial splint bone is the second metacarpal, the cannon bone is the third metacarpal and the lateral (outside) splint bone is the fourth metacarpal. The splint bones are positioned on either side and towards the back of the cannon bone (Figure 10.3). The suspensory ligament lies as a flat band between the two splint bones.

Both the medial and lateral splint bones articulate with the lower row of bones of the horse's knee and hock. When the limb bears weight, they are displaced downwards in the young horse, so there is slight movement between the splint and cannon bones. Splints are more common on the medial side of the forelimb because the medial splint bone bears more weight and provides more support to the cannon bone than the lateral one. If the interosseous ligament tears, it can lift the periosteum of the splint bone to which it is attached, resulting in bleeding, inflammation and soft tissue swelling. As the inflammation subsides, the swelling becomes smaller as the fibrous tissue reaction is replaced by bone forming the splint (Figure 10.4).

As the horse ages, the ligament becomes strengthened by deposition of bone within its substance. By the time a horse is 6 years old, the ligament is more stable and less likely to be strained.

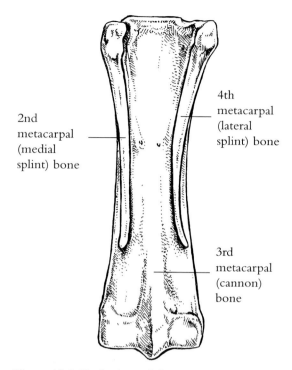

2nd metacarpal (medial splint) bone

4th metacarpal (lateral splint) bone

3rd metacarpal (cannon) bone

Figure 10.3 Back view of the cannon and splint bones

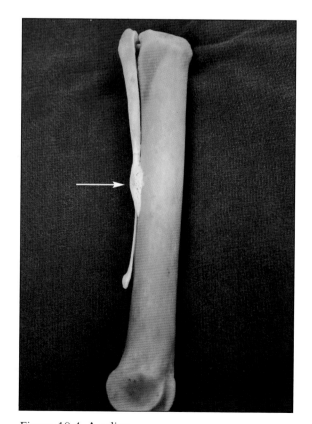

Figure 10.4 A splint

CAUSES

Any of the following factors can contribute to the development of splints.

- Poor conformation. Horses with bench knees where the cannon bone is positioned more laterally than normal, take yet more weight on the medial splint bone and have a high incidence of splints.
- Interference from the opposite limb. Horses with base-narrow, toe-out conformation tend to swing their limbs inwards as they move and strike the inside of the opposite limb. The direct blow causes bleeding under the periosteum and soft tissue inflammation.
- External trauma, e.g. a kick from another horse. This is a common cause of splints on the outside of a limb.
- Poor trimming and shoeing can lead to interference with the opposite limb.
- Working a young horse on hard ground.
- Overworking a young horse.
- Carrying too much weight can predispose a young horse to developing splints.

CLINICAL SIGNS

- Heat, pain and soft tissue swelling develop over the affected splint bone, usually in the upper third of the cannon bone.
- There may be a single swelling, or several, along the length of the splint bone (Figure 10.5).
- Applying pressure to the area is painful and the horse will usually draw the limb away.
- Variable degrees of lameness. The horse may be:
  - sound
  - sound at walk, lame at trot
  - lame at walk and trot; lameness from developing splints tends to increase with work, especially on hard or rough ground; it may be gradual or sudden in onset.
- As the inflammation settles, the swelling becomes smaller and the lameness resolves.

COMPLICATIONS

New bone formed high up on the splint bone may cause arthritis of the knee joint. Extensive deposits of new bone can interfere with the suspensory ligament causing chronic lameness.

DIAGNOSIS

Diagnosis is often made on the clinical signs. Palpation of the splint bone with the leg flexed is usually painful.

Radiographs are useful as they:

- show whether the splint is active or settled; initially the new bone is less dense than the original splint bone and it has an irregular outline; as the splint settles down it appears more dense and smooth

- determine the extent of the new bone and its position in relation to the knee joint and the suspensory ligament
- reduce the chance of a fracture of the splint bone being overlooked.

Ultrasonography is used to determine if the splint impinges on the suspensory ligament.

    Local infiltration of anaesthetic can be helpful in confirming whether a splint is causing lameness.

    Scintigraphy is occasionally helpful to identify 'blind splints' where the swelling of the interosseous ligament is confined to the medial surface of the splint bone. It cannot be palpated, but is an area of inflammation that may impinge on the suspensory ligament and cause lameness.

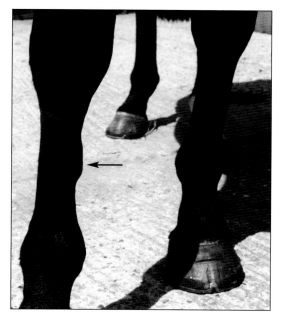

Figure 10.5 A large splint

TREATMENT

The aim of treatment is to reduce the inflammation and pain. It is likely to include some of the following.

- Box rest or confinement to a small area until firm palpation of the splint does not cause any pain. The length of time required is extremely variable and each case should be individually assessed. It usually takes between 2 and 6 weeks, but some horses need a longer period of rest. The sooner a developing splint is recognized and treated, the better chance it has of healing quickly. If the horse is put back into work too early, signs are likely to recur.
- Cold treatment, e.g. hosing or application of ice packs, for 20–30 minutes, 2–3 times daily for the first 2–3 days.
- Support bandaging to prevent further injury from knocks.
- Non-steroidal anti-inflammatory drugs such as phenylbutazone help to settle the inflammation and relieve the pain
- Topical applications of dimethyl sulphoxide (DMSO) may help.
- Injection of corticosteroids into the lesion is believed to reduce the soft tissue swelling by some practitioners.
- If pain persists for longer than 6 weeks, pin firing may be considered.
- Any foot trimming or shoeing problems should be addressed.

Surgery

Surgery may be necessary if:

- the splint impinges on the suspensory ligament causing lameness
- it is so large that it is repeatedly knocked by the other limb.

Splints are sometimes removed for cosmetic reasons. However, the trauma of the surgery may cause more new bone to form in their place.

RETURN TO WORK

Once the condition has resolved, the horse can slowly be brought back into work. The use of protective boots or exercise bandages is recommended and working on hard ground should be avoided.

PREVENTION

- Avoid working young horses on hard ground.
- Avoid breeding from horses with poor conformation. Make all possible efforts to monitor and help a foal's limb conformation, e.g. by appropriate foot trimming in the early weeks to avoid preventable limb deformities.
- Use brushing boots or bandages for exercise, particularly if the horse moves close in front or behind.
- Make sure the feet are correctly trimmed and shod on a regular basis.

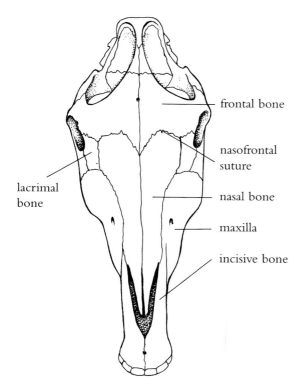

lacrimal bone

frontal bone

nasofrontal suture

nasal bone

maxilla

incisive bone

Figure 10.6 The bones of the horse's skull

PROGNOSIS

The prognosis is good unless the splint is exceptionally large or encroaches on the suspensory ligament or knee joint.

Suture periostitis
ANATOMY

The skull is made up of a number of bones which join together at very close-knit junctions called **sutures** (Figure 10.6). Inflammation at these sites is called suture periostitis. One example is nasofrontal suture periostitis which occurs when the suture line between the nasal bones and the frontal bones becomes inflamed.

CAUSE

The most likely cause is trauma and it may develop following a blow to the face. However, on occasions it occurs with no known history of trauma.

CLINICAL SIGNS

These include:

- localized swelling (Figure 10.7)

- heat and pain are sometimes present but it may also occur as a cold and apparently painless swelling
- in severe cases, the swelling obstructs the nasolacrimal duct so tears spill onto the horse's face instead of draining to the nostrils.

DIAGNOSIS

The diagnosis is made on the clinical signs. Occasionally an X-ray is needed to rule out the possibility of an underlying fracture or other cause of facial swelling.

TREATMENT

- Non-steroidal anti-inflammatory medication may help to settle the condition.
- If the affected area is painful, the horse should not be ridden.
- Flushing the blocked nasolacrimal ducts with sterile saline and a dilute antibiotic solution may be helpful.

PROGNOSIS

The condition usually resolves spontaneously over a period of 2–4 months. The bony swelling reduces in size and may disappear altogether. Some horses are left with a permanent blemish.

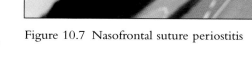

Figure 10.7 Nasofrontal suture periostitis

Sesamoiditis

Sesamoiditis can be defined as inflammation of the proximal sesamoid bones.

ANATOMY

There are two small proximal sesamoid bones at the back of the fetlock, one on either side of the limb. The suspensory ligament divides into medial and lateral branches in the lower third of the metacarpal and metatarsal regions. The medial branch attaches to the top and outside of the medial sesamoid bone and the lateral branch attaches to the top and outside of the lateral sesamoid bone before they run obliquely across the first phalanx (P1) to join the common digital extensor tendon. The lower edges of the sesamoid bones are attached to the first and second phalanges (P1 and P2) by three ligaments. The two sesamoid bones are directly joined by the intersesamoidean ligament. (See figures 7.10a and b.)

In this condition, a periostitis occurs at the sites of ligament attachment and new bone deposits (called enthesiophytes) may be formed. Degenerative bony changes may also occur as a result of the inflammation or altered blood supply. The condition is seen most commonly in animals that do fast work; racehorses are particularly susceptible and it is commonly reported in Standardbreds. Sesamoiditis may be associated with suspensory ligament injuries.

CAUSES

- Tearing of the suspensory or distal ligament attachments when the fetlock joint is over-extended. This tends to occur when tired horses work or jump at speed.
- An acute sprain.
- Direct trauma, e.g. an overreach.
- Long-toe conformation increases susceptibility to this injury.

CLINICAL SIGNS

These include some of the following.

- There may be a loss of performance before the lameness is apparent. The horse may shorten its stride and move in a more upright fashion as extension of the fetlock pulls the ligaments and is painful.
- Variable degrees of lameness. It can occur as an acute injury with severe lameness or as a chronic progressive condition with low-grade lameness.
- The lameness may be most evident at the start of exercise and on hard surfaces.
- Heat over the outside edge of the sesamoid bones.
- Pain on palpation of the sesamoid bones and attached ligaments.
- Soft-tissue swelling or thickening at the back of the fetlock.
- Flexion of the fetlock may be painful and increase the degree of lameness.
- The condition improves after a period of rest.

DIAGNOSIS

This is made on:

- the clinical signs
- nerve blocks; the lameness should be abolished by a low four-point nerve block; however, this is not specific for this condition and does not rule out pain coming from other areas such as the fetlock joint
- radiography; possible radiographic changes include:
  - new bone (enthesiophytes) laid down at the site of ligament attachments
  - calcium deposits within the suspensory ligament
  - decrease in bone density
  - an increase in the size and number of vascular channels within the bone.

With the exception of a fracture, the X-ray changes are unlikely to be seen until approximately 3 weeks after the injury has occurred. Early changes can be detected using scintigraphy. Ultrasound examination of the surrounding soft tissues is routine as they may also be very painful and it is important to try to confirm the primary site of pain as treatment may vary, depending on the structures involved.

TREATMENT
- In the acute stages, cold treatment and support bandaging are beneficial.
- Non-steroidal anti-inflammatory drugs, e.g. phenylbutazone, help to reduce the inflammation and pain.
- Box rest to start with and introduction of controlled exercise as advised by the vet.
- Physiotherapy.
- Corrective foot trimming if necessary.
- Topical anti-inflammatory medications can be applied.

The period of rest depends on the severity of the injury. When the horse is brought back into work, the exercise programme should be modified. Swimming is helpful in some cases if the facilities are available.

Chronic cases are difficult to treat successfully. Treatments such as pin firing and blistering have been used with limited success. Shock wave therapy is used with variable results.

PROGNOSIS
The prognosis depends on the severity of the injury. It is generally guarded as the condition tends to recur.

PHYSITIS

Physitis is the name given to the condition where there is inflammation and abnormal bone activity in the growth plates of foals and young horses. The growth plates most commonly affected are:
- the distal (lower) end of the radius just above the knee
- the distal end of the cannon bone in the fore and hind limbs
- the distal tibia.

As with osteochondrosis, there is a disturbance of endochondral ossification of the growing bones. The condition usually occurs in the fetlock region of foals aged between 3 and 6 months and at the distal radius in animals between 8 months and 2 years.

Causes
Physitis is a developmental orthopaedic disease thought to be a consequence of overloading and compression of the affected growth plates. This may occur owing to:

- overfeeding of foals and yearlings
- mineral imbalance, e.g. incorrect calcium/phosphorus ratios or low copper levels
- high body-weight
- too much exercise of young animals
- severe lameness in one limb can lead to the development of physitis in the other limb as a result of increased weight bearing
- angular limb deformity leads to uneven pressure on the growth plate and may cause physitis.

Clinical signs

These include:

- warm, painful enlargement of the growth plate, usually on the medial side
- pain on palpation of the region
- shortening of the stride or mild lameness that may be exacerbated by flexion
- change in contour of the limb
- the condition may affect just one limb or occur bilaterally.

Diagnosis

Diagnosis is usually made on the clinical signs and may be confirmed by radiography.

Treatment

Treatment includes:

- box rest or restricted exercise; this may be necessary for between 2–8 weeks
- assessment of the diet; it may be necessary to reduce the energy intake while ensuring adequate intake of minerals such as calcium, phosphorus, copper and zinc
- reduction of body-weight if the foal or yearling is too heavy
- non-steroidal anti-inflammatory drugs, e.g. phenylbutazone, if the animal is very lame
- corrective hoof trimming if necessary
- correction of any angular limb deformity.

Prognosis

The prognosis is good provided the condition is recognized and appropriately managed.

ANGULAR LIMB DEFORMITIES IN FOALS

A foal may be born with an angular limb deformity (congenital) or the condition may develop in the first few weeks or months of life (acquired). In each case there is a medial (inward) or lateral (outward) deviation of the limb distal to the carpus (knee), tarsus (hock) or fetlock. A medial deviation is known as **varus** and a lateral one as **valgus**. The commonest deformity is **carpal valgus** where the lower part of the cannon bone deviates outwards giving the foal a knock-kneed appearance (Figure 10.8). The next most common deformity is **fetlock varus** where the pastern is deviated medially from the fetlock. One or several joints may be affected.

Causes

The condition is caused by asymmetric growth of the physis or growth plate of the lower part of the radius, tibia and cannon bones. For example, if the distal growth plate of the radius grows more on its medial side, this results in carpal valgus. Faster growth on the lateral side of the lower part of the cannon bone results in fetlock varus. The imbalance of the growth rate on either side of the growth plate is usually due to one side being subjected to abnormal pressure which retards or stops longitudinal growth of the bone at that site. This can be caused by:

- laxity of the ligaments and soft tissues around the joint allowing excessive movement
- delayed or defective ossification of the small cuboidal bones of the knee and hock – this is often associated with prematurity; the affected bones may not be able to withstand the weight of the foal and become compressed or misshapen
- malpositioning of the growing foal in the mare's uterus before birth
- overfeeding of young foals so they become 'top heavy'
- Over-exertion of young foals
- any injury leading to reduced weight bearing on one limb can lead to an angular deformity in the sound limb as the foal adjusts its stance and action to compensate
- trauma to the growth plate.

Clinical signs

- The signs may be slight or immediately obvious as a valgus or varus conformational deformity. Sometimes a combination of varus and valgus is seen (Figure 10.9). The condition may occur with a toe-in or toe-out conformation.
- Localized heat and swelling may be present.
- The foal may show a degree of lameness.

Heat and lameness are associated with trauma or collapse of the carpal or tarsal bones.

Diagnosis

A prompt assessment and diagnosis is essential as most of the growth of the distal cannon bones occurs within the first 2–3 months of a foal's life. That of the distal radius and tibia occurs in the first 6 months and treatment is most effective within this period of rapid growth. However, many foals born with an angular limb deformity improve dramatically within the first few days of life. A proper assessment should be delayed until this time, when the foal has found its feet.

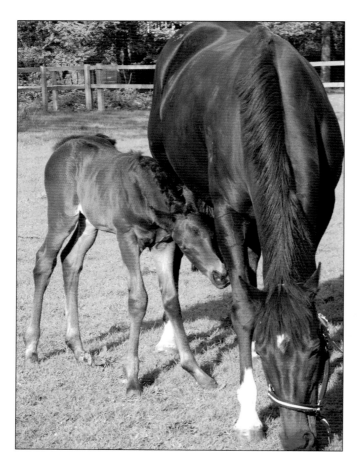

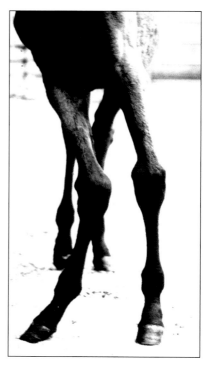

Figure 10.8 Foal with carpal valgus (left)

Figure 10.9 A 'windswept' foal with multiple angular limb deformities (above)

The foal should be assessed standing squarely and also at walk. The breakover of each foot is noted. Radiography is helpful in assessing the degree of deformity and essential for identifying any bony abnormality. A video recording of the foal is useful for monitoring progress.

Treatment

Treatment is either conservative, i.e. with management changes, or surgical, depending on the severity of the condition and the age of the foal. Many foals are born with a minor degree of carpal valgus that improves spontaneously and requires nothing more than a few days of restricted exercise.

CONSERVATIVE TREATMENT

This may include:

- confinement to a large stable or small barn for newborn foals with ligament laxity
- restricted exercise in a small paddock
- appropriate trimming of the foot to balance it
- use of glue-on shoes with extensions to encourage normal alignment of the limb and breakover

- correct nutrition
- foals with incomplete ossification of the carpus or tarsus need restricted exercise and support from bandages and possibly splints or casts to prevent collapse or fracture of the affected bones.

All foals managed conservatively should be closely monitored. Many mild or moderate angular limb deformities will resolve spontaneously, but those which fail to improve or worsen should be treated surgically.

SURGICAL TREATMENT

The aim of surgical treatment is either to accelerate or slow down growth on one side of the growth plate in order to straighten the limb. Growth can be slowed down on the faster-growing side by placing staples or screws and wire across the growth plate. This allows the other side of the limb to catch up and the implants are removed once the limb is straight. The slower-growing side can be encouraged to lengthen by a technique which involves cutting and elevating the periosteum which relieves the tension across the growth plate and encourages the bone to grow. A combination of these techniques may be used.

Other treatments such as shock wave treatment have been used recently.

Prognosis

The prognosis is good for foals with mild or moderate deformities that are recognized and treated promptly. Recent research has shown that mild carpal valgus may serve as a protective mechanism against the chance of a carpal (knee) fracture or joint strain in racing Thoroughbreds. Traditionally, knock-knees and turned out toes have been treated with foot trimming or even surgical intervention to achieve a straighter leg. This may actually be counter-productive in changing a desirable conformation for the worse.

The prognosis is more guarded for those with severe deformities and abnormalities of the carpal or tarsal bones.

FRACTURES

A fracture can be defined as a break in the continuity of a bone. Recent advances in surgical techniques, repair materials and anaesthesia mean that a wide range of equine fractures can now be successfully treated. The prognosis depends on which bone is involved and the nature of the fracture. Fractures of the upper limb have a poor prognosis but many fractures of the lower limb can be repaired.

Types of fracture

Fractures can be divided into several main categories.

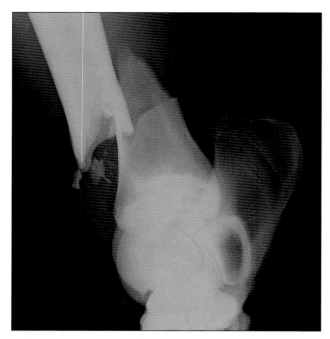

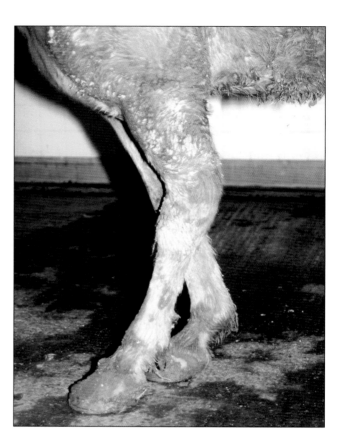

Figure 10.10 X-ray of a severe irreparable fracture of the tibia

Figure 10.11 Broken leg in abnormal position; the pony has a fractured radius

- **Simple fractures** have a single fracture line and the bone is in 2 pieces.
- **Comminuted fractures** have 2 or more fracture lines and a minimum of 3 fragments (Figure 10.10).
- **Closed fractures**: the skin over the fracture has not been broken.
- **Open or compound fractures**: the skin over the fracture site has been broken. These fractures are nearly always contaminated and have a more guarded prognosis.
- **Articular fractures** involve the articular surface of a joint.
- **Avulsion fractures**: a fragment of bone is torn away at the site of attachment of a ligament or tendon.
- **Complete fractures** divide the bone into 2 or more pieces.
- **Incomplete or fissure fractures** affect only part of a bone and do not completely divide it into 2 pieces.
- **Chip fractures**: a small fragment of bone is loosened or detached.

Many fractures are obvious as soon as they have occurred. The horse may be unable to bear weight on the limb and be in considerable pain. The leg may be in an abnormal position (Figure 10.11) and crepitus (grating sensation of broken bones rubbing together) may be heard or felt. With open fractures, the bone may even protrude from the wound.

However, other fractures are more difficult to diagnose in the field as there may be no immediate signs apart from variable degrees of lameness. In these cases, it is essential that appropriate first aid is given prior to moving the horse. If you suspect that a horse may have a fracture, leave him where he is and keep him as still as possible until the vet arrives. The vet will examine the horse and advise you on the right course of action. If treatment is considered, the vet will apply a suitable splint to:

- stabilize the limb
- prevent further injury to the bone or surrounding soft tissues
- stop further contamination and infection of open wounds
- allow the horse to travel safely to a hospital for further assessment.

The management of the horse at this stage can have a big influence on the eventual outcome. Any uncontrolled movement could turn a potentially repairable fracture into a complete disaster necessitating euthanasia.

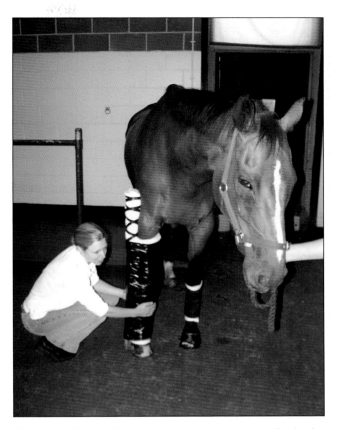

Figure 10.12 A splint being applied to a horse's forelimb

There are several different bandaging and splinting techniques and the choice is determined by the type and location of the fracture. Your vet will decide which is the most appropriate, following examination of the horse. If possible, the joints above and below the fracture site will be immobilized. Once the splint has been applied, the horse is usually more comfortable.

On arrival at an equine hospital the horse will have X-rays to help make a diagnosis and to determine how serious the injury is. On the whole, open, comminuted and articular fractures have the worst prognosis.

Fracture of the splint bone

Fracture of a splint bone is a relatively common injury.

CAUSES

These include the following.

External trauma

- Being struck by the foot of the opposite limb.

- A penetrating wound.
- A kick from another horse. This is a common cause of fracture of the fourth metatarsal (outside splint) bone in the hind limb.

Internal trauma

During fast exercise, the splint bone is subject to biomechanical stress. The medial splint bone of the forelimb articulates with bones of the knee joint and experiences compressive forces. The lower part of the splint bone is attached to the suspensory ligament and also by fibrous tissue to the proximal sesamoid bones. It can be fractured in the following ways.

- Too much force on the medial splint bone during high-speed exercise can cause it to fracture.
- If the fetlock is overextended, the tension on the splint bone can be enough to cause a fracture between the distal (lower) and middle third of its length.
- Inflammation and thickening of the suspensory ligament can put pressure on the splint bone and push the lower third away from the cannon bone. This makes it more susceptible to fracture from biomechanical stresses.

This type of injury is common in 5–7-year-old racehorses.

CLINICAL SIGNS

These may include:

- heat, pain and swelling over the splint bone
- pain when the fracture site is pressed
- a variable degree of lameness
- an open wound over the fracture site when the fracture is caused by an external injury such as a kick
- a discharging sinus over the splint bone; this is a small wound in the cannon area which does not heal.

DIAGNOSIS

The diagnosis is usually confirmed by radiographic examination (Figure 10.13). If the wound is infected, radiography is repeated after a few days to check for infection of the splint bone. Ultrasonography is used to determine whether the suspensory ligament is involved and the extent of any damage.

TREATMENT

The treatment depends on:

- the location of the fracture
- whether the fracture is simple or in many pieces

- if there is a wound overlying the fracture site
- if infection has entered the wound and become established in the bone.

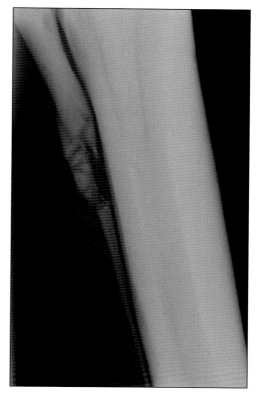

Uncomplicated fractures with little displacement of the distal third of the splint bone usually heal well with support bandaging and 6 weeks of box rest. The bony callus that develops as the bone heals often remodels leaving only a small bony lump. If there is a superficial wound, this is thoroughly cleaned and the horse is given antibiotics. Healing progress can be monitored by radiographic examination.

Significantly displaced fractures of the distal third of the splint bone are sometimes removed surgically. This is because they can form large amounts of fibrous tissue and bony callus in their attempts to heal and this can impinge on the suspensory ligament, causing lameness.

High fractures involving the upper third of the splint bone may need to be stabilized with a bone plate or screws following removal of the lower piece of bone. This is especially important for high fractures of the medial splint bone of the forelimb as it

Figure 10.13 X-ray of a fractured splint bone

is important for stability of the knee joint. If the knee is stable, some fractures in this location will heal with conservative management (box rest) providing there is no infection present.

Wounds overlying fractures need to be thoroughly cleaned and any contaminated or severely damaged tissue must be surgically removed. Antibiotics are prescribed and the bone should be monitored by radiographic examination for any secondary infection.

With all fracture types, non-steroidal anti-inflammatory drugs such as phenylbutazone are given as necessary to reduce the pain and inflammation.

COMPLICATIONS

- Infection may enter a wound and become established in the splint bone. This is especially common with severe kick injuries where earth and other foreign materials are left deep within the wound. In this case surgery is necessary to remove the infected bone and all the damaged tissue. Antibiotics are given and the horse will need at least 6 weeks of box rest.
- If a piece of infected bone is left in the wound, pus will discharge onto the skin surface

through a sinus. This will not heal until the piece of bone is removed.

- Sometimes a small piece of bone separates from the splint bone, loses its blood supply and dies. This is known as a **sequestrum**. A tract develops between the sequestrum and the skin surface, discharging pus. This can occur some time after the original injury. The fragment and any infected tissue must be removed surgically in order for the wound to heal.

PROGNOSIS

The prognosis is good for most splint bone fractures if there is no damage to the suspensory ligament and they are recognized and appropriately treated. Fractures of the upper third of the medial (inside) splint bone of the forelimb have a more guarded prognosis, especially if the bone is in many pieces and infection is present.

INFECTION OF BONE

Septic or infectious osteitis

Septic or infectious osteitis is inflammation of bone due to infection. There is no involvement of the marrow cavity.

CAUSES

Such injuries occur on the cannon and splint bones as the result of a kick from another horse. As there is only skin covering the bone at these sites, the periosteum may be exposed and damaged. Another common site is the pedal bone which may become infected when a horse stands on a sharp, penetrating object.

PATHOPHYSIOLOGY

Bacteria colonize the superficial layers of bone and these may die. The dead piece of bone is called a **sequestrum** and this causes a chronic discharge through a non-healing skin wound.

CLINICAL SIGNS

- Variable degrees of lameness. A horse with an infected pedal bone may be very lame, while an animal with an area of infected cannon bone may be only slightly lame.
- A non-healing, discharging wound.

DIAGNOSIS

Diagnosis is made on the history, the clinical signs and radiography.

Radiographic changes include:
- soft tissue swelling

- resorption of bone may be seen a few days after the injury occurs
- periosteal reaction and new bone may be visible 7–14 days post injury
- it usually takes 2–3 weeks before a sequestrum is clearly visible on the radiograph.

TREATMENT

Treatment involves removal of all unhealthy bone, granulation and scar tissue. This may require general anaesthesia. The wound is then bandaged and the horse rested until healing is complete. Antibiotics and tetanus antitoxin will be administered.

PROGNOSIS

The prognosis is generally good.

Osteomyelitis

Osteomyelitis is an infection of bone that involves the marrow or medullary cavity (i.e. the inside of the bone).

CAUSES

- It can occur as a result of a penetrating wound.
- Open fractures where the skin is broken and the bone is exposed are likely to be contaminated with bacteria and foreign material.
- It can develop following fracture repair despite the administration of antibiotics at the time of surgery.
- It may develop as an extension of a joint infection.
- Bone may become infected in foals that have abscesses elsewhere in the body or are septicaemic. Bacteria that get into the bloodstream are able to colonize bone because the blood flow through it is quite slow.

CLINICAL SIGNS

These include:

- severe lameness
- soft tissue swelling
- pain on palpation and manipulation of the affected area
- heat
- poor wound healing
- development of a discharging sinus
- sudden worsening of lameness following fracture repair; this can occur any time between 1 and 4 weeks after surgery.

DIAGNOSIS

Diagnosis is made on the clinical signs and imaging techniques.

Radiographic changes include:

- loss of bone density
- new bone formation
- the presence of a sequestrum (see page 286)

Unfortunately the very early signs of osteomyelitis cannot be seen on radiographs. The changes caused by infection are not visible until 50–70% of the bone has been demineralized and this may take up to 21 days.

Scintigraphy using labelled white blood cells which collect at sites of infection is very useful, but not widely available.

Ultrasound can be useful in detecting small pockets of pus building up around surgical implants such as bone plates and screws. With ultrasound guidance these can be aspirated and cultured to determine which bacteria are present and their antibiotic sensitivity.

TREATMENT

The treatment depends on the cause of the infection and how well established it is. It is likely to include the following.

- Surgery to remove any dead or grossly infected soft tissue or bone.
- Removal of any infected implants such as bone plates and screws.
- Bone grafts may be useful to promote healing of infected fractures.
- Administration of broad spectrum antibiotics for a minimum of 3 weeks. These are usually injected for 7–10 days and followed up with oral antibiotics.
- Antibiotic-impregnated beads may be placed at the wound site. This technique gives high antibiotic concentrations at the site of infection.
- Antibiotics may be infused directly into the medullary cavity.
- Antibiotics can be delivered to the wound site by regional intravenous infusion. A tourniquet is applied to the limb above the area of infection. The diluted antibiotic is then injected into a superficial vein under pressure. Antibiotics delivered in this way or by intramedullary infusion reach higher tissue concentrations than can be achieved by systemic dosing.
- Non-steroidal anti-inflammatory drugs to reduce the associated pain and inflammation may be helpful in adult horses, but are used with caution in foals due to the risk of gastric ulceration.

PROGNOSIS

The prognosis is generally guarded. It depends on the severity and location of the infection and how well established it is.

CYSTIC LESIONS WITHIN BONE (BONE CYSTS)

Bone cysts (known as osseous cyst-like lesions [OCLLs] or subchondral bone cysts [SBCs] are round or oval-shaped cystic lesions that usually occur in the subchondral bone, directly beneath the articular cartilage of a joint. Cysts that develop in young animals that are still growing often migrate away from the joint surface as the skeleton matures.

They can occur in horses of any age but are often found in young animals less than 4 years old. The most common sites are the stifle, fetlock, pastern, coffin and elbow joints.

Causes

The exact cause of these lesions is unclear. They can develop wherever there is a defect in the articular cartilage or subchondral bone. This may be the result of trauma or a developmental defect such as osteochondrosis. In some cases, a number of factors may contribute to their development.

Pathophysiology

Synovial fluid is thought to flow through cracks in the damaged articular cartilage into the subchondral bone. Mechanical factors, including weight bearing, then lead to resorption of bone and the formation of a cyst-like structure.

Clinical signs

- Mild to moderate lameness that may be sudden in onset.
- The lameness may be intermittent and improve with rest.
- Flexion may be resented.
- The affected joint may be distended.
- Lameness is not always apparent, particularly with lesions deep in the bone such as those seen in areas of the carpus (knee). Cyst-like lesions that are close to a joint surface are more likely to be associated with lameness.

Diagnosis

Diagnosis usually requires intra-articular analgesia in addition to radiography as not all bone cysts cause lameness. Lesions are sometimes seen as incidental findings on radiographs of sound horses. Since the local anaesthetic takes some time to diffuse from the joint into the subchondral bone cyst, it may be necessary to wait for up to one hour before the full effect of the analgesia is seen. The lameness may be reduced rather than abolished.

Treatment

Conservative treatment consisting of management changes and medication is normally tried in the first instance, as surgery is not always successful. However, your vet will decide on the best course of action depending on the location and severity of the lesion and the use and age of the horse.

CONSERVATIVE TREATMENT

- Box or pasture rest to allow the bone the opportunity to remodel and heal.
- Non-steroidal anti-inflammatory drugs (NSAIDs) such as phenylbutazone.
- Intra-articular injection of corticosteroids, hyaluronic acid or polysulphated glycosaminoglycan to reduce inflammation and encourage healing.

SURGICAL TREATMENT

When the cyst-like lesion does not respond to conservative treatment or occupies a large area of the joint surface, surgery may be indicated. This involves removing the lining of the cyst cavity and all the debris from within the joint capsule. Following surgery the horse is usually given:

- antibiotics
- NSAIDs
- a period of box rest followed by the introduction of controlled walking exercise
- field rest for a further 3–12 months.

PROGNOSIS

Horses under 3 years of age with small lesions have the best chance of becoming and staying sound. Success rates following surgery in young horses can be up to 75%. The prognosis is poor if degenerative changes have occurred in the joint.

11
MUSCLE DISEASE AND NEUROLOGICAL CONDITIONS

SKELETAL MUSCLE INJURY AND DISEASE

Introduction

The skeletal muscles attach via tendons to bones and work in a co-ordinated fashion to control the voluntary movements of the horse's body. They also act to support the body while the horse is at rest. In order to do this they require:

- a good blood supply to provide oxygen and nutrients
- an intact nervous system.

Muscles are susceptible to a number of problems. These include:

- strains, tears and ruptures
- pain induced by pressure from poorly fitted saddles or bad riding
- muscle shortening and myofascial pain (see page 374)
- muscle atrophy
- metabolic disorders
- functional abnormalities due to neurological problems.

The diagnosis of muscle problems is usually made from:

- the history
- gentle movement of the horse's neck, limbs and thoracolumbar spine to test the range of movement and detect any pain or restriction
- observation of the horse at rest and in motion
- palpation for heat, swelling, pain, atrophy, fibrosis
- blood tests to check muscle enzyme levels (CK, AST, LDH, see pages 680–81) and myoglobin
- muscle biopsy.

Ultrasonography, scintigraphy, thermography and electromyography are also useful in some cases. Electromyography is a procedure that measures the electrical activity in skeletal muscles. Normal skeletal muscle has little electrical activity unless the horse moves or a muscle is stimulated to contract. In some conditions, the diseased muscle has abnormal, spontaneous bursts of electrical activity.

Muscle strains and tears

Any muscle that is subjected to unaccustomed activity is likely to have some soreness, 24–48 hours later. This usually resolves quite quickly, provided the horse is allowed to recover and does not overexert himself again.

Muscle strains and tears may be the result of:

- a traumatic event such as a fall
- a sudden uncoordinated muscle contraction due to slipping or working on uneven ground
- continuing to work a tired horse
- failure to warm the horse up properly prior to strenuous exercise
- an inadequate cooling-down period following fast work; the horse should be walked on a loose rein for at least 10 minutes.

CLINICAL SIGNS

These include:

- an abnormal posture
- stiffness or lameness
- muscle swelling
- heat and/or pain on palpation
- increased muscle tension or spasm
- decreased range of motion.

TREATMENT

The aim of treatment is to relieve the pain and spasm, and to restore the normal circulation and function of the muscle with minimal scarring. This may be achieved by:

- rest
- controlled exercise
- massage
- gentle stretching
- heat treatment
- acupuncture or acupressure
- low intensity laser therapy
- therapeutic ultrasound
- electromagnetic therapy

- transcutaneous electrical stimulation (TENS)
- H-wave (muscle stimulation)
- chiropractic or osteopathic treatment.

The recommended treatment will depend on the type of injury and the stage of healing. Your vet may recommend physiotherapy to assist the horse's recovery. This should be followed by a rehabilitation programme to build up the muscle strength and reduce the potential for re-injury.

Muscle atrophy

When skeletal muscles lose their normal bulk, they are said to **atrophy** or waste away. There are a number of circumstances under which this happens.

- If a horse is undernourished, the muscles may be broken down into amino acids and used as a source of energy. The muscle atrophy will be generalized and symmetrical throughout the horse's body (Figure 11.1)
- When a muscle is not used for a period of time, it decreases in size. This is known as **disuse atrophy**. It commonly occurs when a limb is immobilized in a cast or if it cannot function in its normal manner due to a fracture. An example is atrophy of the gluteal muscles following a pelvic fracture (Figure 11.2). In some cases, this type of atrophy is reversible when normal function is restored. However, if the atrophy is severe, the horse will take longer to recover and some of the muscle may be replaced by fibrous tissue.
- If the nerve supply to a muscle is damaged, the muscle will undergo **neurogenic atrophy**. An example is neurogenic atrophy of the supraspinatus and infraspinatus muscles of the shoulder following damage to the suprascapular nerve. Due to the loss

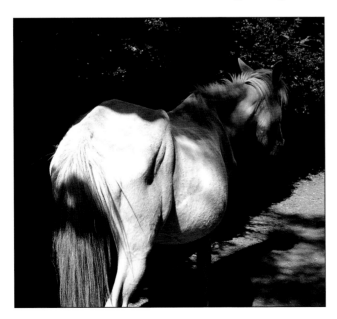

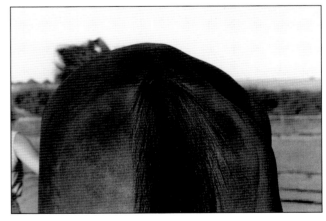

Figure 11.1 This malnourished pony has generalized muscle wasting (left)

Figure 11.2 Gluteal muscle atrophy in a horse with a pelvic fracture (above)

of muscle, the scapular spine becomes abnormally prominent and the condition is known as **sweeny.** If the nerve recovers, the muscle volume and function may be restored. However, if the nerve injury is severe, the affected muscles never recover and are replaced by fibrous and fatty tissue.

EXERTIONAL RHABDOMYOLYSIS SYNDROME (ERS)

This is a syndrome where the skeletal muscle fibres of the horse become damaged and die in response to exercise. The lumbar muscles and the gluteal muscles in the hindquarters are most commonly affected. It can occur as an acute single event or as a mild recurrent form. The condition is also known as azoturia, tying-up, set fast, exertional myopathy, Monday morning disease and paralytic myoglobinuria.

Clinical Signs

The symptoms characteristically start within 10–30 minutes of the onset of exercise.

- The horse experiences painful cramp-like symptoms which vary in severity from slight stiffness of gait to being unable to move at all, hence the name 'tying-up'. In extreme cases, collapse and death can occur.
- Initially, the horse may feel as though he is rolling from side to side and the hindquarters gradually sink.
- The horse becomes anxious and is increasingly reluctant to move forwards.

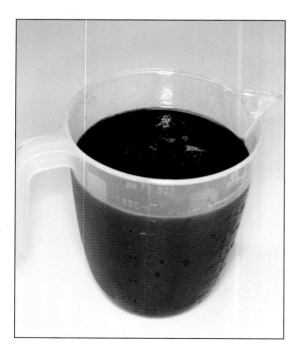

Other symptoms include:
- excessive sweating
- muscle fasciculation (small spontaneous tremors)
- an increase in heart and respiratory rates
- pawing the ground and mild colicky signs
- repeated attempts to urinate as adopting the normal stance for this is uncomfortable
- passing urine which varies in colour from normal, through reddish brown to dark chocolate; the discolouration is due to a pigment called myoglobin which is released from the damaged muscle fibres (Figure 11.3)

Figure 11.3 Discoloured urine from a horse with exertional rhabdomyolysis syndrome

- resentment of pressure on the affected muscle groups which may include the gluteals, the lumbar muscles and those that make up the hamstrings, i.e. the biceps femoris, semitendinosus and semimembranosus
- dehydration
- raised temperature
- the horse becomes recumbent (unable to stand) in very severe cases.
- kidney failure and death may occur as a result of circulatory failure and damage to the kidney tubules by myoglobin.

Immediate action

- Call the vet as soon as the condition is suspected
- Stop the horse as soon as the gait begins to alter; forcing it to move will increase the amount of damage that occurs.
- If conditions are wet or cold, put rugs or coats over the horse's back to keep it warm.
- Arrange transport home or find temporary stabling nearby. A trailer is preferable to the steeper ramp of a lorry.

Diagnosis

The diagnosis is made on the history, the clinical signs and the results of blood tests. When the muscle cells are damaged, creatine kinase (CK) and aspartate aminotransferase (AST) leak from the cells into the bloodstream. The timing of the blood sampling is important as the CK reaches its maximum level approximately 4–6 hours after the episode and usually returns to normal within 2 days. AST peaks at 24 hours and takes about 2 weeks to return to normal. The enzyme levels do not always correlate with the clinical signs. Horses with severe symptoms, for example, can show a relatively small increase in enzymes.

In horses with the chronic form of the disease where the symptoms are not so acute, the condition may be diagnosed with the aid of:

- a muscle biopsy which can show characteristic degenerative changes in the muscle fibres
- an exercise test: blood samples are taken before exercise and between 4 and 6 hours afterwards
- scintigraphy, as some horses will show increased uptake of the radiopharmaceutical by affected muscle (this is rarely necessary).

Causes

Exertional rhabdomyolysis is a complex syndrome and why it occurs is not fully understood. Some or any of the following factors may play a role.

- Inappropriate exercise for the horse's level of fitness. Pushing the horse too fast or for too long can trigger an attack.
- Feeding full rations high in starch (cereals) with only irregular exercise increases the

likelihood of ERS. It commonly follows a day off work with no reduction in rations.

- Electrolyte imbalance is suspected as a cause. Sodium, potassium, magnesium and calcium are important for the normal function of nerves and muscles. A combination of regular hard work causing sweating and an inadequate diet may cause depletion of any of these and lead to poor performance and possibly ERS.

- The composition of the diet can affect the horse's ability to regulate the electrolytes in the body. Electrolytes such as sodium (Na^+), potassium (K^+), magnesium (Mg^{2+}) and calcium (Ca^{2+}) have a positive charge and are known as cations. Electrolytes such as chloride (Cl^-) and phosphate (PO_4^{3-}) have a negative charge and are called anions. The balance of the cations and anions in the diet, known as the dietary cation/anion balance (DCAB) has an effect on the horse's metabolism. A diet consisting mainly of forage has a high DCAB and this enables the horse to absorb and use the electrolytes efficiently. Diets containing a lot of cereals and restricted forage tend to be acidic and have a low DCAB. Electrolytes such as calcium may be lost from the body in processing the acid diet even though the horse needs them for other metabolic processes. Diets with a low DCAB can predispose to ERS.

- Viruses such as the equine influenza virus and equine herpesvirus 1 appear to increase some horses' susceptibility.

- Temperament can be a factor as nervous excitable animals seem to be more at risk.

- Hormonal factors may play a part as the incidence is higher in females, particularly when they are in season.

- Horses experiencing ERS are rarely deficient in vitamin E or selenium so a deficiency of either is unlikely to be a cause. However, both of these antioxidant micronutrients scavenge the damaging free radicals that are generated by exercise. It may be that horses with ERS generate more free radicals than normal horses, thus accounting for why supplementation anecdotally appears to help in some cases.

- Genetic factors may be important. Work in the United States has identified an inherited form of recurrent equine rhabdomyolysis (RER).

- Horses with polysaccharide storage myopathy (PSSM) are prone to experiencing RER.

- Stress and climatic factors can trigger ERS.

- Endurance horses may develop ERS due to a combination of overheating, dehydration, electrolyte imbalance and exhaustion.

- Anything that reduces the blood flow to skeletal muscle can predispose a horse to ERS. Examples include lameness and muscle tension.

- Abnormal calcium transport at cellular level is another area currently being investigated.

Treatment

The aim of treatment is to:
- minimize the pain and anxiety

- prevent further muscle damage
- restore fluid and electrolyte balance
- maintain adequate kidney blood flow to minimize the accumulation of myoglobin in the tubules as it is toxic and may cause permanent kidney damage.

The management and medication of affected animals varies with the severity of the condition. The following may be included in the treatment.

- Analgesic and anti-inflammatory drugs to relieve the pain and inflammation.
- A tranquilliser to relax the horse. Acepromazine (ACP) will decrease the horse's anxiety and may increase the blood flow through the muscles. If the horse is in severe pain, a combination of detomidine and butorphenol may be used.
- Intravenous fluid therapy to combat dehydration and shock and maintain the circulating blood volume.
- Electrolytes and fluids which can be given by stomach tube. If electrolytes are put in the drinking water, a separate supply of fresh water should also be offered.

Analgesics are usually only necessary for the first couple of days. Both analgesics and tranquillisers have to be given with care as their use in a severely dehydrated horse can contribute to kidney damage.

Management in the recovery stage
STABLE MANAGEMENT

In the acute stage of the disease, the horse should be stabled to stop further damage occurring to the muscles. It should be kept warm and dry in a well-ventilated stable that is free from draughts. A thick, dry bed should be provided.

DIET

The diet should be restricted to good quality hay with a broad spectrum mineral supplement. Fresh drinking water should be available.

TURNOUT

As soon as the horse appears to be comfortable and is not showing any signs of lameness or stiffness, it may be led out in hand for a few minutes at a time or turned out for short periods into a small paddock. The temperament of the horse must be taken into consideration as persistent excitement and galloping around will exacerbate the condition and delay recovery.

RETURN TO WORK

Work should not recommence until the muscle enzymes have returned to normal which can take up to 2 weeks or more. The reintroduction to work should be gradual and exercise should be regular.

Prevention

Some horses are susceptible to recurrent attacks of ERS. The following measures may reduce the likelihood of recurrence.

DIET

- A high-forage diet with good quality hay and a broad spectrum mineral and vitamin supplement is recommended. The composition of the diet influences the horse's ability to absorb electrolytes. A horse on a diet which is composed mainly of good quality forage is able to absorb and use electrolytes more efficiently than a horse on a high-cereal, low-forage diet.

- Concentrates high in starch (i.e. mainly cereals) should be avoided and replaced wherever possible with feeds high in oil and digestible fibre as an energy source. Several small feeds a day are preferable to two large ones. Hard feed should be reduced if the horse has any time off work and sudden changes of diet should be avoided. The recommendation to increase the work of a horse ahead of its feed should be followed, i.e. the level of work should be increased before more food is given.

- The diet should have a DCAB above 300milliequivalents/kg. Discuss this with an equine nutritionist.

- A bio-available calcium source such as calcium gluconate may be beneficial in replacing the calcium lost in processing an acid diet.

- Recent research suggests that chromium and certain B-complex vitamins may help some horses, probably owing to their role in carbohydrate metabolism.

- Electrolytes given following periods of heavy sweating such as strenuous exercise or travelling can help to replace depleted electrolytes and prevent ERS. By analysing blood and urine samples taken at the same time, the vet may be able to identify a specific electrolyte imbalance which could be helped by dietary supplementation.

EXERCISE ROUTINE

- Training programmes should be carefully planned and adhered to so that the demands on the horse are increased gradually.
- The horse should always be warmed up gently before commencing fast work.
- Sudden increases in the speed or duration of exercise should be avoided.
- Days off should be avoided in susceptible horses. It has been shown that CK levels are higher after exercise when the horse has just had a day off.
- An exercise sheet should be used to keep the horse warm in cold or wet weather.
- Regular turnout, especially on a day off, may reduce the occurrence of the condition.

MINIMIZING STRESS

Reducing stress of any kind will benefit susceptible horses.

MEDICATION

- A low dose of ACP prior to exercise may help prevent ERS in excitable horses.
- Suppressing the oestrous cycles of affected mares and fillies with progesterone is sometimes helpful.
- Drugs such as dantrolene and phenytoin which influence nerve and muscle cell function appear to help prevent the disease in some horses. However, these drugs are expensive and cannot be given to competing horses as they would be considered an illegal substance.

Prognosis

This is variable depending on the individual horse, its management and intended use. Some horses have a single attack and make a full recovery. Others have repeated episodes despite careful management. With recurrent cases, muscle wasting and scarring can eventually occur and this limits the ability of the horse to work.

EQUINE POLYSACCHARIDE STORAGE MYOPATHY (EPSSM)

Equine polysaccharide storage myopathy (EPSSM) is a metabolic disorder. Affected horses are thought to have an abnormally rapid uptake of glucose from the bloodstream and to store glycogen and an abnormal polysaccharide within their skeletal muscle fibres. These horses experience painful muscle contraction while exercising but the physiology is not fully understood. It is most prevalent in draught horses, Quarter Horses and Warmbloods, but is now recognized in many other breeds. The condition is considered to be hereditary.

Clinical signs

- Muscle pain, spasm or swelling.
- Stiffness.
- Reluctance to work.
- Exercise intolerance.
- Recurrent exertional rhabdomyolysis (RER).
- Abnormal hind limb gait.
- Increased incidence of 'shivers' or 'shivering'.
- Intolerance of trimming and shoeing the back feet.
- Muscle wasting.
- Progressive weakness.
- Inability to stand up in severe cases.
- An increased likelihood of myopathy following a general anaesthetic.
- Behavioural problems, probably as a result of pain.

The muscles of the back, rump and hamstrings are most severely affected, i.e. the longissimus dorsi, gluteals, semimembranosus and semitendinosus.

Diagnosis

A biopsy of skeletal muscle taken from the semitendinosus or semimembranosus muscles is the only was to confirm a diagnosis of EPSSM. It should be sent to a specialist pathology laboratory where muscle samples are regularly examined. When viewed under the microscope, abnormal polysaccharide inclusions can be seen in the muscle.

Laboratory findings may be helpful. Many affected horses have raised creatine kinase (CK) and aspartate aminotransferase (AST) levels in their blood 4–6 hours post exercise due to release of these enzymes from damaged muscle cells.

Treatment

Treatment is likely to include:

- non-steroidal anti-inflammatory drugs such as flunixin meglumine or phenylbutazone to relieve the pain and reduce inflammation
- tranquillizers such as acepromazine or detomidine to reduce anxiety
- intravenous fluids if the horse has severe RER to prevent damage to kidney tubules from myoglobin
- turnout into a small paddock as soon as the horse is comfortable enough.

Dietary changes

Most horses improve when fed a diet that is high in fat and fibre, and low in starch and sugar. A forage-based diet supplemented with vegetable oil, minerals and vitamins is usually recommended. Whether this leads to reduced muscle glycogen concentrations is uncertain. Horses usually respond to the dietary changes within four months.

Exercise

Affected horses should be turned out daily and kept in regular work. Sudden changes in the intensity of the exercise should be avoided.

Prognosis

The prognosis for horses that respond well to dietary changes is reasonable. Many are able to continue to perform adequately with careful management.

HYPERKALAEMIC PERIODIC PARESIS (HYPP)

This is a muscle disorder affecting Quarter Horses and their crosses, American Paint horses and Appaloosas. It is an inherited trait and the gene responsible has been identified in descendents of the Quarter Horse sire *Impressive*. In most horses, intermittent clinical signs begin by 2 to 3 years of age with no apparent abnormalities between episodes.

Causes

- The genetic defect results in a functional abnormality of skeletal muscle cell membranes leading to periods with high serum potassium levels and muscle weakness.
- Diets high in potassium (such as alfalfa and molasses) may induce signs along with sudden dietary changes.
- Episodes may be triggered by stress including transport, sedation, fasting and anaesthesia.

Clinical signs

- Affected horses experience episodes of muscle tremors and weakness, which may produce collapse.
- Facial muscle spasm and prolapse of the third eyelid may occur.
- The episodes typically persist for 15–60 minutes.
- Respiratory distress may occur in some cases.

Diagnosis

A definitive diagnosis can be made by a DNA test from tail hairs or a blood sample.

Treatment

- Low-grade exercise may stop the muscle trembling if an episode is detected early.
- Feeding grain to reduce potassium levels can help.
- Severe cases may require medical treatment including intravenous fluids.
- However, most cases are manageable, particularly when the owners are aware of the condition.

Prevention

- Steps should be taken to decrease the potassium levels in the diet.
- Regular exercise and turnout is beneficial.
- Stress levels should be kept to a minimum.

Prognosis

The majority of affected animals survive although the disease is occasionally fatal if an animal experiences recurrent and severe episodes. These horses should not be used for breeding and special care should be taken if or when such animals require a general anaesthetic.

FIBROTIC OR OSSIFYING MYOPATHY

This is a condition where some of the muscle fibres at the distal (lower) end of the semitendinosus muscle are replaced with fibrous tissue or occasionally by bone.

Clinical signs

The horse has an abnormal hind limb gait which can appear short and choppy. This is due to the mechanical restriction rather than pain.

Due to the loss of elasticity of the muscle, the extension of the stifle joint is limited. This causes a shortening of the cranial (forward) phase of the stride. The limb is often advanced, then jerked back slightly before being slapped onto the ground. It is most obvious at walk.

The condition can affect one or both hind limbs. Sometimes it is possible to palpate a firm, non-painful thickening in the semitendinosus muscle at the lower end of the hamstrings, behind the stifle. Abnormal tension, sensitivity and 'jumpiness' on palpation are often present in the affected muscle. In some horses, muscle wasting may be visible.

Causes

The usual cause is repeated tearing or straining of the semitendinosus muscle. The muscle fibres are gradually replaced with fibrous tissue and adhesions may develop between the semitendinosus and the other hamstring muscles, i.e. the biceps femoris and the semimembranosus. The condition is most commonly seen in horses that make quick turns at speed and sliding stops, e.g. polo ponies.

The condition can also occur following a series of irritant intramuscular injections.

Diagnosis

The diagnosis is made on the clinical signs and the findings of the clinical examination. Occasionally, ultrasonography or radiography may be used to confirm the presence of fibrotic or calcified tissues.

Treatment
ACUTE INJURY

Prompt treatment of an acute hamstring injury may reduce the amount of scar tissue and the likelihood of the condition occurring. This is likely to include:

- non-steroidal anti-inflammatory drugs, e.g. phenylbutazone

- controlled exercise
- physical therapy including massage, stretching, laser, ultrasound.

CHRONIC INJURY

Once the condition is established, there are several options.

- If the symptoms are only mild and the use of the horse or pony is not affected, no treatment is necessary apart from taking care to avoid activities that may aggravate the condition.
- Regular physiotherapy or acupuncture helps to release tension in the semitendinosus muscle.
- If the gait is severely restricted, surgery may be considered to try and restore a more normal action. The tendon of the muscle may be cut just above its attachment onto the top of the tibia or the muscle itself may be severed at the site of the scar tissue. Alternatively the affected part of the muscle and the tendon can be surgically removed. Physiotherapy is important after all of these procedures to minimize adhesions and further scar tissue.

Prognosis

The prognosis is variable following surgery as the condition will recur in some horses.

SHIVERING

Shivers or shivering is a condition where the horse intermittently flexes a hind limb, lifting it abnormally high and holding it away from the body. This is an involuntary action, accompanied by quivering of the hind limb muscles and the tail. The first signs are usually seen when the horse is between 2 and 4 years of age.

Cause

The cause is unknown. The following have been suggested:

- mild spinal cord lesions
- arthritic degeneration of the lumbar spine
- pain
- equine polysaccharide storage myopathy (EPSSM)
- It has been suggested that shivering may be inherited; the condition is seen in draught breeds and Warmbloods more than other breeds.

Clinical signs

- It characteristically occurs when the leg is lifted or the horse is pushed backwards. It is also likely to be seen when the horse moves off after standing still or is turned in a small circle (hence these procedures are included in a prepurchase examination).

- The first sign may be an intermittent reluctance to lift the hind limb for shoeing or to walk backwards.
- When the limb is lifted, the leg is flexed in an exaggerated fashion and often held away from the body for several seconds.
- The tail head is usually raised and may quiver.
- The thigh muscles often tremble spontaneously.
- The signs are not seen at trot or canter.
- The signs may be worse if the horse is exercised infrequently, the weather is cold or the horse is anxious.
- The condition can vary from day to day and may not be apparent some of the time.
- The condition is progressive and may eventually affect the forelimbs.
- Severely affected animals may experience generalized muscle wasting.

Diagnosis

Diagnosis is usually made on the history and the clinical signs.

Treatment

There is no effective treatment. If the horse has an underlying EPSSM then a high fat and low sugar and starch diet may help. Regular exercise helps in some cases.

Prognosis

The condition is progressive and some horses are euthanased as they are unfit for work. A frequent problem is that it becomes impossible for the farrier to fit their shoes safely. However, on occasions the horse will continue to perform adequately in spite of the shivering and the progression of the disease is unpredictable.

STRINGHALT

Stringhalt is a condition where the hocks of one or both hind limbs flex in an exaggerated fashion when the horse is walking (Figure 11.4).

Clinical Signs

- One or both hind limbs may be affected.
- The affected limb jerks upwards from the ground in an involuntary fashion.
- The condition may be mild with just slight hyperflexion of the limb or very obvious with the fetlock striking the abdominal wall with every stride.
- It is most obvious when the horse is walking, turning or backing.
- The symptoms may occur with every stride or intermittently.

- In some horses the problem is less obvious at trot and canter.
- The condition is often worse in cold weather or after the horse has rested.
- Anxiety is reported to exacerbate the condition in affected horses, but the condition does not appear to concern the horse.

Diagnosis

Diagnosis is made on the clinical signs.

Causes

Degenerative changes in particular nerves are associated with stringhalt but

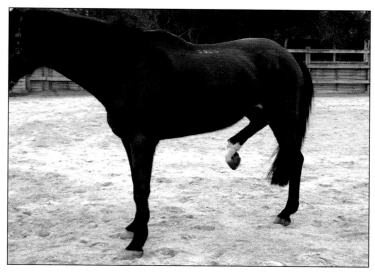

Figure 11.4 Stringhalt

the cause of these changes is unknown. There are two forms of the disease. 'True' or 'classic' stringhalt occurs worldwide as isolated cases and a suggested cause is trauma to the lateral digital extensor tendon as it crosses the front of the hock or the cannon bone.

The second form of the disease occurs mainly in Australia and New Zealand. Groups of horses grazing together may be affected. It tends to occur on poor pasture in summer or autumn in fields with toxic weeds following a long, dry spell of weather. The weed *Hypocheris radicata* has been implicated. This plant has green leaves in a rosette form, with small dandelion-like flowers on a long stem. It is likely that other, as yet unknown, factors are also involved.

The Australian form of the disease is more severe. It is often bilateral and may affect the forelimbs and the muscles of the larynx as well.

In either form, the cause of the jerky hyperflexion of the hock joint is not understood. Altered sensation or muscle reflexes as a result of the nerve degeneration may be responsible.

Treatment

- Horses mildly affected by classic stringhalt may be able to perform their work with no treatment.
- Severely affected horses may improve after an operation to remove part of the lateral digital extensor muscle and its tendon.
- With the Australian stringhalt, the first step is to remove the horse from the pasture. Some horses will recover spontaneously over 6–12 months, although others may take up to 3 years. A drug called phenytoin which is normally used as an anticonvulsant may help these horses owing to its action on nerves and muscles.

Prevention

Prevention of classic stringhalt is not possible as the cause is not known. With the Australian type, poor quality pastures with toxic weeds should be avoided, especially in the summer and autumn of dry years.

Prognosis

With classic stringhalt, this depends on the severity of the condition, the use of the horse and the response to surgery. The outcome of Australian stringhalt is very variable. Some horses make a full recovery when removed from the pasture. Others are so severely affected that euthanasia is the humane option.

WOBBLER SYNDROME

The horse has 7 cervical vertebrae (C1–7) – see page 320. Wobbler syndrome occurs when developmental abnormalities of the cervical vertebrae cause narrowing (known as stenosis) of the vertebral canal. This results in compression of the spinal cord, leading to gait abnormalities and incoordination. The condition is also known as cervical stenotic myelopathy and cervical vertebral malformation. There are two recognized forms of the disease.

1   **Static stenosis** With static stenosis, there is constant narrowing of the vertebral canal which is not influenced by movements of the neck. It typically affects the vertebrae of the lower neck, C5–7, and the condition is usually diagnosed when the horse is between 1–4 years of age.

2   **Dynamic stenosis** With dynamic stenosis, the compression tends to affect the vertebrae in the middle of the neck, between C3 and C6, and it only occurs when the neck is flexed. The symptoms are usually noticed earlier and the condition tends to be diagnosed before the horse reaches 2 years of age.

Wobbler syndrome is seen particularly in well-nourished, fast-growing foals and young animals, especially male Thoroughbreds.

Causes

A number of factors may contribute to the development of wobbler syndrome.

- There may be a hereditary predisposition.
- A large body size and periods of rapid growth.
- Dietary factors, e.g. overfeeding of high energy diets or copper deficiency can lead to osteochondrosis (OCD) lesions of the vertebral joints.
- Trauma.

Clinical signs

The signs may develop suddenly following a traumatic incident or they may occur very slowly over an extended period of time. They are usually progressive.

- When the condition is gradual in onset, the first sign may be occasional clumsiness. A fall may be blamed, whilst the reality is that the wobbliness/clumsiness caused the fall.

- The hind limbs are affected first. Signs include slight, intermittent stiffness or lameness with a tendency to stumble or drag the toes. This is a result of reduced joint flexion during movement. The toes may become worn or squared.

- The horse may not be aware of the position of its hind limbs and so develop an incoordinated, rather wobbly gait. This loss of co-ordinated movement is known as **ataxia**. It is most obvious when the horse is walking or turning in small circles. On turning, the horse may throw one leg outwards in an abnormally wide position in order to maintain balance.

- If asked to walk backwards, the horse may stand with its legs wider apart than normal, lean back and be slow to move the hind limbs. The forelimbs may be dragged backwards and then tread on the hind limbs.

- The muscles of the hind limbs are abnormally weak. If the tail of a normal horse is pulled to one side as it is led forwards, the horse will resist the pull and continue in a straight line. A weak horse is easily pulled to one side and a severely affected animal may stagger or fall over. This is known as the 'sway test' (Figure 11.5).

- At canter and gallop, the horse may 'bunny hop'.

- The forelimbs are less commonly affected unless C5–7 have severe lesions. These horses may cross their forelimbs when walking or move with an abnormally wide or stilted forelimb gait.

- Moderate to severely affected horses may have cuts on the inside of the forelimbs and the bulbs of their heels from overreach and brushing injuries.

- Neck pain is occasionally, but not consistently, present.

If the symptoms appear to develop suddenly after a fall, it may be that they were subtly present before and the fall has exacerbated the spinal cord compression.

Diagnosis

The diagnosis is made on the following.

- The clinical signs.

- Neurological examination. Any neurological deficits

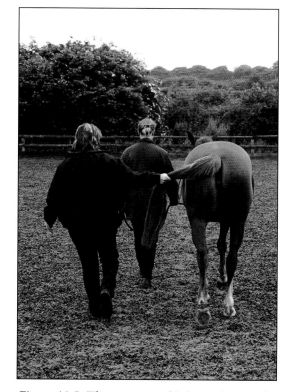

Figure 11.5 The sway test: this horse is normal

may become more obvious if the horse is asked to walk over obstacles or examined on a slope. Elevating the horse's head can accentuate any abnormality.

- The appearance of the neck vertebrae on radiographs. Measurements of the width of the vertebral canal may show it to be narrower than normal. The radiographs must be of excellent quality and examined by a vet who has considerable experience in this field.

- Narrowing of the vertebral canal can exist without being obvious on plain radiographs. **Myelography** is sometimes necessary to demonstrate compression of the spinal cord. With the horse under general anaesthesia, a water-soluble contrast medium is injected into the subarachnoid space which surrounds the spinal cord and contains cerebrospinal fluid (CSF). In a normal horse, this contrast media shows up as a white column on either side of the spinal cord. At sites of compression, the columns on both sides of the cord are reduced in diameter by more than 50% or obliterated altogether. Radiographs are taken in the neutral and flexed positions. Myelography is relatively safe, but complications including seizures do occasionally occur.

Treatment
MANAGEMENT

The condition is often progressive, but this is not always the case. Sometimes the clinical signs remain stable for long periods. Some horses learn to cope with the condition and live happily as companions. Riding these horses is not recommended as there are reports of sudden worsening of signs following an apparently minor incident. A horse with spinal cord compression is potentially dangerous as it may suddenly fall as the result of a sudden stop or turn. Breeding from these animals is not recommended as there is a hereditary predisposition for development of the disease in some cases.

Conservative management

In foals under 1 year of age that have symptoms of wobbler syndrome due to dynamic stenosis of the vertebral canal, conservative management can help to relieve the compression of the spinal cord. This involves the following.

- Restricting the protein and energy levels of the diet to 65–75% of the recommended intake for the size and weight of the foal. A balanced vitamin and mineral supplement is given with increased levels of vitamins A and E and a specific level of selenium. Low quality (6–9% protein) timothy hay is provided as roughage. The aim of this is to slow the growth rate of bone and improve bone metabolism in the hope that the vertebral canal will enlarge and relieve the compression of the spinal cord.

- Confining the foal to the stable for up to 6 months reduces the repeated compression of the spinal cord caused by neck flexion and movement.

- The feed and water should be provided at a height that is easily reached. Hay should be loose so the animal does not have to repeatedly flex his neck, pulling it from a net.

- Corticosteroids or non-steroidal anti-inflammatory drugs such as phenylbutazone may be given to reduce inflammation at the site of compression. These can produce a temporary reduction of neurological signs.

SURGICAL TREATMENT

Fusion of adjacent cervical vertebrae has been used for the treatment of both dynamic and static stenosis. With the horse under general anaesthesia, the intervertebral disc is drilled out and screws are used to fix adjacent vertebrae in an extended position. The vertebrae fuse together as healing progresses. If the operation is successful, this eliminates dynamic compression of the spinal cord immediately. Remodelling of the lower cervical vertebrae after fusion can result in gradual decompression of the spinal cord of horses with static compression over a period of weeks to months.

There is an alternative surgical procedure (called a subtotal dorsal laminectomy) for horses with static compression. This provides immediate decompression of the spinal cord, but has a higher incidence of postoperative complications.

Following surgery, recovery and rehabilitation take up to 1 year. There is unlikely to be any further improvement after this time.

Prognosis

The prognosis depends on the severity of the spinal cord damage and the duration of clinical signs before the surgery is performed. Horses that are operated on within 1 month of the signs developing have a better chance of returning to athletic function than those that have experienced symptoms for longer than 3 months.

The prognosis is more guarded for horses with static stenosis of the vertebral canal. In these cases, both surgical procedures can have fatal postoperative complications including vertebral fracture, spinal cord oedema and screw failure.

Surgical fusion of the vertebral bodies is reported to improve the horse's neurological signs in 44–90% of cases. Between 12–60% return to some type of athletic function and of these approximately 60% are able to be used for their intended purpose. Horses with static compression that undergo a subtotal laminectomy show some improvement in 40–75% of cases.

Insurance

Insurance for these cases can be complicated since the affected horse is unlikely to die from this disability. A policy that covers death only will not pay out for a horse affected by wobbler syndrome. If you have taken out more extensive insurance cover for loss of use, it is likely that a proven wobbler would be a justifiable claim. Each case needs to be individually assessed. Special diagnostic X-rays may help, but the most important consideration is whether the horse can cope safely for all concerned. If it cannot do so, then euthanasia may have to be considered.

Prevention

Dietary management to reduce the growth rate of susceptible, fast-growing foals may help to prevent the condition. Dietary and exercise restriction may prevent neurological signs developing in foals when neck radiographs suggest that spinal cord compression may occur.

EQUINE MOTOR NEURON DISEASE (EMND)

Equine motor neuron disease (EMND) is a debilitating condition that affects adult horses. It causes a generalized muscle wasting and weakness due to degeneration of the lower motor neurons that carry nerve impulses from the brainstem or spinal cord to the skeletal muscles. The clinical signs are not obvious until 30% of the motor neurons have died or become dysfunctional.

Causes

The condition is not fully understood, but it is thought that the affected lower motor neurons are damaged by free radicals produced by metabolism of the skeletal muscles. These harmful substances are normally neutralized by antioxidants such as vitamin E, supplied in the diet. Horses suffering from motor neuron disease have abnormally low vitamin E levels in their plasma and body tissues. Predisposing factors include the following.

- Little or no access to pasture for several months of the year. Horses rely on green forage for their supply of vitamin E. Experimentally, the disease has been induced in horses that were deprived of access to pasture for more than 18 months.
- A diet high in cereal with only poor quality hay.
- Recent work has shown that EMND can occur in grazing horses as a result of reduced absorption of vitamin E by the gut or excessive utilization of vitamin E due to exposure to enviromental oxidants.

Exposure to unknown neurotoxins may also trigger the disease. The death of the motor neurons leads to neurogenic atrophy of the muscles they innervate.

Clinical signs
These include:
- trembling
- weakness
- atrophy (wasting) of the postural muscles especially the triceps, quadriceps, neck, shoulder, back and sacral muscles
- muscle fasciculations (fine involuntary tremor-like movements)

- frequent shifting of the weight between the hind limbs and inability to stand still for any length of time
- the limbs may be positioned close together under the body in an abnormal posture, with most of the weight on the hind limbs (Figure 11.6)
- some horses develop a stringhalt-like gait or stand with slight buckling of the forelimbs
- lying down more than usual
- the head of the tail may be raised
- poor performance and exercise intolerance
- an abnormally low head carriage
- sweating
- abnormal brown pigment deposits on the retina of the eye.

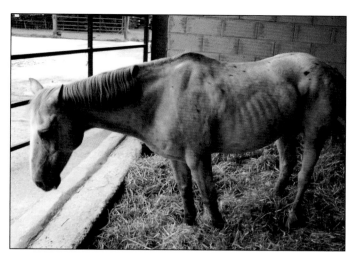

Figure 11.6 Horse with equine motor neuron disease

Affected horses lose muscle and weight, despite having a normal appetite. There are two recognized stages of the disease. In the **subacute** form, the symptoms develop quickly and are very obvious. Some horses deteriorate rapidly and have to be euthanased. In 70% of cases, however, after a period of 2–8 weeks, the condition stabilizes and the horses enter a **chronic** stage where the trembling and muscle fasciculations subside and the horse may not lie down as much. These horses still tire easily and fail to gain weight despite having a good appetite. They may remain this way for months or years, or the symptoms may be slowly progressive. A second, acute episode sometimes occurs 1–6 years later, necessitating euthanasia of the horse. Some horses appear to develop the chronic form of the disease without experiencing a subacute episode.

Diagnosis

The diagnosis is made on:
- the clinical signs
- abnormally low vitamin E levels in the blood
- mild to moderate elevation of the muscle enzymes creatine kinase (CK) and aspartate aminotransferase (AST)
- abnormal deposits of brown pigment on the retina of the eye
- electromyography which may reveal abnormal electrical activity in the affected muscles.

The condition is confirmed by taking a biopsy of a particular muscle at the top of the tail (the sacrocaudalis dorsalis medialis muscle). Characteristic changes are seen in the appearance of the muscle fibres and there is an increase in fibrous tissue. It is the resultant contracture of this muscle that causes the tail head to be raised.

Treatment

There is no treatment that can repair the damage to the nervous system. Supplementing the diet with around 5000–7000 international units of vitamin E per day and turnout onto green pasture improves some horses. Sometimes the muscles increase in size, but in general they remain wasted.

Prognosis

The prognosis is poor.

- Approximately 30% of cases continue to deteriorate and do not stabilize. These are usually euthanased within a year of the onset of clinical signs.
- Around 70% stabilize for a period of 1–6 years. Of these, about 40% improve with vitamin E supplementation. However, they are not safe to ride. There are reports of horses suddenly deteriorating when put back into work. Affected horses may fall and injure themselves or their rider.

Prevention

If vitamin E deficiency is the only cause of the disease, it should be preventable by providing horses with adequate levels in their diets. Experimental work has shown that the diet must be very deficient in vitamin E for at least 14 months before horses develop equine motor neuron disease.

Horses with no access to grass or green hay, or at pasture for less than 3 months a year (e.g. some competition horses or laminitic ponies) are the most susceptible and their diets should be supplemented. Ask your vet to recommend a product as some of the combined vitamin E and selenium preparations do not contain enough vitamin E for deficient horses. Increasing the amount of a combined supplement may raise the selenium content of the diet to toxic levels.

If one horse in a yard develops EMND, all similarly managed horses should be assessed and supplemented in case they are affected but not yet showing clinical signs.

TETANUS (LOCKJAW)

Tetanus is a life-threatening disease caused by toxins released by the bacterium *Clostridium tetani*. Spores of this bacterium are widespread in the environment and are found in dust, faeces and soil. They are commonly present in the intestinal contents of horses. If the spores enter a wound where there is damaged tissue and an anaerobic environment (with no oxygen), they germinate into bacteria which produce the potent toxins. These toxins migrate along the peripheral nerves to the central nervous system and interfere with normal nerve function. The disease is characterized by extreme sensitivity to stimuli, increasing stiffness and muscle spasms. It is usually fatal.

High-risk situations

Situations which are most likely to lead to infection include:

- puncture wounds contaminated with soil, e.g. hoof punctures
- stake wounds
- umbilical infections in the foal
- castration wounds
- contamination of the uterus during assisted foaling.

Clinical signs

The incubation period is usually between 7 and 21 days, but it can be longer. The signs include:

- abnormal sensitivity to sound or touch
- a stiff gait (Figure 11.7a)
- prolapse of the third eyelid which may cover half of the eye
- very erect and rigid ears
- a raised tail head
- a worried expression with retraction of the eyelids and flared nostrils due to muscle spasm
- inability to open the mouth due to spasm of the masseter (powerful chewing) muscles, hence the name lockjaw
- regurgitation of food and water from the nostrils and drooling of saliva from the mouth as swallowing becomes more difficult; partially chewed hay may be held in the mouth
- colic.

As the disease progresses there is:

- progression of the muscle spasms
- rigid extension of the limbs causing difficulty in moving and turning; affected animals may adopt a 'saw-horse' stance
- progressive stiffness and extension of the neck making it difficult to eat from the floor
- rapid, shallow respirations and flared nostrils (Figure 11.7b)
- muscle spasm or convulsions when stimulated by light, noise or touch
- constipation and urine retention
- the horse or pony may fall over and lie with all limbs extended, unable to rise (Figure 11.8)
- in the final stages the horse may develop a temperature and sweat profusely
- death inevitably follows from dehydration, malnutrition and respiratory failure over a period of 5–10 days in severe cases.

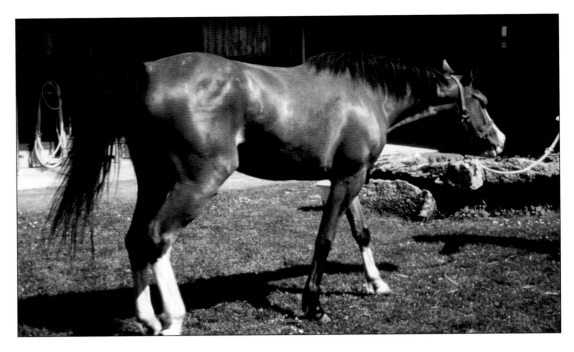

Figures 11.7a and b Tetanus: a) note the stiff limbs, extended neck and raised tail head of this horse with tetanus; b) this pony with tetanus has flared nostrils

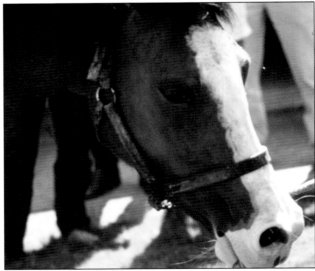

Diagnosis

The diagnosis is made on the history and the clinical signs. A puncture wound may be found and an affected animal is unlikely to be up-to-date with its vaccinations.

Treatment

This is only undertaken if the disease is diagnosed early in its course. Where the horse is already unable to rise, the prognosis is very poor and euthanasia is the kindest course of action. Even if the disease is diagnosed in the very early stages, the horse may require weeks or months of nursing. The treatment is expensive and labour intensive.

MEDICAL TREATMENT

This includes the following.

- Large doses of tetanus antitoxin to neutralize toxin that is still circulating and has not yet affected the nervous system. However, this does not penetrate the nervous tissue, so antitoxin is sometimes injected into the cerebrospinal fluid around the brainstem and spinal cord to try and neutralize toxin here before it causes more damage. The antitoxin does not reverse the clinical signs that have already developed.
- High doses of penicillin are given for at least a week to kill the bacteria.
- Sedatives and tranquillizers, e.g. acepromazine or barbiturates are used to control the anxiety, muscle spasms and convulsions.
- All dead or damaged tissue should be removed from any wound. It should be thoroughly cleaned and flushed with an oxidizing agent such as hydrogen peroxide, then left open to the air. The exposed tissues may be injected with penicillin and tetanus antitoxin.

NURSING

- The patient should be nursed in a quiet, dark stable with a deep bed of wood shavings. Long straw or paper tends to wind or clump around the horse's legs.
- The nursing routine should be quiet and efficient so the horse is disturbed as little as possible. External noises and stimuli should be minimized. Plugging the horse's ears with cotton wool is helpful.
- If the horse cannot swallow, a gruel mixture or soaked, complete cubes and fluids may be given by stomach tube. This is often sutured in place. Intravenous fluids may be necessary.
- When the horse can swallow, soft, palatable food and water should be placed in easy reach.
- If the horse has difficulty urinating or passing droppings, it may be catheterised and have the rectum evacuated manually.
- If the horse is in danger of falling over, it may be supported by a sling.

Prognosis

Most horses with tetanus will die. Once they have become recumbent, the prognosis is very poor. Some mild cases recover over a period of weeks or months if they are diagnosed early and treated aggressively. An improvement should be seen within two weeks. Tetanus is more common in foals as most adult horses are vaccinated against the disease. In severe cases, foals may die within 3 days.

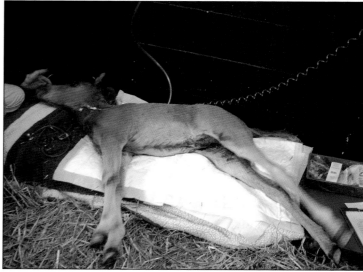

Figure 11.8 A foal with tetanus

However, they have a better chance of survival than adult horses because their smaller size makes them easier to nurse and manage.

Prevention

The loss of a horse from tetanus is a double tragedy because of the suffering involved and the fact that the disease is effectively prevented by vaccination with a very safe and effective vaccine.

- The primary vaccination course of tetanus toxoid includes 2 doses given 4–6 weeks apart. Regular boosters are given thereafter. The exact schedule may vary slightly according to the recommendations of different vaccine manufacturers and whether it is combined with vaccination against equine influenza. Your vet will advise you on this.
- Vaccinated pregnant mares should have a tetanus toxoid booster 4–6 weeks prior to foaling. This ensures the foal receives maximum protection from the antibodies in the colostrum.
- Foals usually begin their vaccination programme between 4–5 months of age.
- Foals of unvaccinated mares or those that do not receive adequate colostrum for any reason should be given tetanus antitoxin at birth.
- Horses that are unvaccinated or are of doubtful vaccination status should be given tetanus antitoxin if they have a wound or require surgery. A vaccination programme should be started straight away in addition to the administration of the antitoxin which provides immediate temporary protection for approximately 10–14 days.
- A horse or foal that has recovered from tetanus is not immune to the disease; regular vaccination is essential.

BOTULISM

Botulism is a disease characterized by neuromuscular paralysis caused by the toxins of *Clostridium botulinum*. This bacterium grows in neutral to alkaline soils, decaying vegetable matter and rotting animal carcases. It reproduces by producing spores. It is anaerobic, which means that it can only live in an environment that has no oxygen.

Causes

In an anaerobic environment, these bacteria produce 8 different neurotoxins; types B and C are the commonest causes of botulism. The disease usually occurs when feedstuffs are contaminated with decaying plant matter or dead animals, e.g. rodents. Stagnant water sources contaminated by carcases are another source of the toxin.

There are 3 recognized routes of infection.

1   Ingestion of the toxin. This is often referred to as **forage poisoning** as the source is

often dead animals accidentally included in big bales of silage or hay.

2 Ingestion of spores from the environment which develop into toxin-producing bacteria in areas of tissue damage, e.g. gastric ulcers in foals.

3 Contamination of wounds such as umbilical stumps and castration wounds with *Clostridium botulinum* which then produces toxin that circulates around the body.

The toxin interferes with the release of the neurotransmitter acetylcholine at various nerve endings including neuromuscular junctions. The muscles cannot function properly without stimulation from the nerves and paralysis is the result. The sensory nerves are not affected and nor is the central nervous system, so affected animals often remain bright and alert, despite their weakness or paralysis.

Clinical signs
The severity of the clinical signs varies with the dose of toxin.

FOALS
The disease is seen in foals as young as 1–2 weeks of age. In severe cases, the foal may be found paralysed and unable to stand, or even dead. If the intoxication is less severe, the first signs may be a stiff-legged gait and muscle weakness, with more time spent lying down than usual. Due to loss of muscle tone of the tongue and difficulties with swallowing, milk may dribble from the mouth or return down the nostrils. The muscle tone of the eyelids and tail also becomes weak. These foals are still bright and alert. As the disease progresses, they have difficulty standing and develop muscle tremors. At this stage they are known as 'shaker foals'. Eventually they are no longer able to stand and have difficulty breathing. They ultimately die as the result of paralysis of the respiratory muscles.

ADULTS
Botulism can affect any age of horse and the symptoms vary from mild weakness to rapid collapse and death, depending on the dose of toxin. The following signs may be seen.

- Loss of tongue tone and weakness or paralysis of the pharyngeal muscles often leads to difficulties picking up and swallowing food. The horse may have a normal appetite but only be able to chew very slowly. Saliva or food may drop from the lips or appear at the nostrils. Affected horses often play with

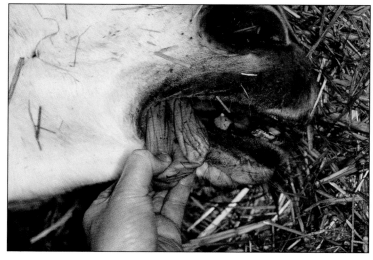

Figure 11.9 This pony suffering from botulism has no tongue tone and is unable to stand. The mucous membranes are a poor colour

water but are unable to drink. If the tongue is gently pulled forwards, there is less resistance than normal and the horse may be slow to pull it back into the mouth.

- Bad breath from accumulated food retained in the mouth.
- Weak eyelid and tail muscles.
- Dilated pupils.
- A weak, short-striding and shuffling gait.
- Muscle tremors of the shoulder and flank muscles.
- Increasing weakness and fatigue.
- Lying down for long periods with increasing difficulty getting up (Figure 11.9)

In the advanced stages, there may be paralysis of the bladder, little gut motility and constipation. Respiration becomes increasingly difficult and the horse dies of respiratory failure.

Diagnosis

The diagnosis is made on the history and the clinical signs. In the UK the disease is usually associated with feeding big bale silage and it can affect a number of horses within a group simultaneously.

Treatment

- Botulism antitoxin given early in the course of the disease greatly increases the horse's chance of survival. This is given as a slow, intravenous infusion. It binds with toxin in the circulation and prevents the disease progressing. However, it does not affect the toxin already bound to the neuromuscular junctions or change the existing clinical signs. The antitoxin is very expensive and not readily available. Administration is essential for any horse with severe signs, but it does not guarantee its survival. Mildly affected animals that have only been exposed to a small dose of toxin may survive without it.
- Good nursing is vital for these patients. If they are unable to stand, they must be provided with thick, comfortable beds and turned regularly to prevent pressure sores. Bandaging the legs with thick padding will afford some protection.
- Regular turning also helps to reduce congestion of the lungs of recumbent horses. Wherever possible, they should be propped up onto their sternums.
- A nasogastric tube can be sutured in place or passed several times a day to ensure the horse has enough food and water. An appropriate gruel or soaked complete diet and fluid/electrolyte mixture will be recommended by the vet.
- Horses that are dysphagic (have difficulty swallowing) may be at risk from inhalation pneumonia. Those horses that cough while attempting to eat should be muzzled to reduce this risk and fed by stomach tube.
- Antibiotics are used if wound infection is thought to be the source of the problem, if the horse is unable to get up or if the horse is considered to be at risk of developing aspiration pneumonia.

Prevention

In certain parts of the United States, a vaccine is successful in preventing the disease in areas where it commonly occurs. This is not available or necessary in the UK where the outbreaks are infrequent, but the following precautions apply.

- Every attempt should be made to minimize the inclusion of soil and dead animals when silage is made.
- Bags of silage should be stored in such a way that they are unlikely to be spoiled or damaged. If they are accidentally split open or spoiled by rodents, they should be discarded.
- Wounds should be effectively treated to avoid bacterial infection.
- Stress levels should be minimized to prevent gastric ulcers. If present, they should be treated.

Prognosis

- This depends on:
- the dose of toxin absorbed
- the speed of progression of the clinical signs
- the timing of the administration of antitoxin.

Horses that are exposed to a large dose of toxin and are already recumbent when they are found may die despite the administration of antitoxin. However, if antitoxin is given early in the course of the disease and the toxin dose was low, 70–90% recover. Mildly affected animals that have been exposed to a low dose of toxin may recover without treatment. Complete recovery may take weeks or months.

12
THE HORSE'S SPINE AND PELVIS

THE HORSE'S SPINE

Anatomy

The horse has 7 cervical vertebrae (C1–7), 18 thoracic vertebrae (T1–18), 6 lumbar vertebrae (L1–6), 5 fused sacral vertebrae which make up the sacrum and 15–21 coccygeal vertebrae (Figure 12.1). The spinal cord runs through the spinal canal in each vertebra from the top of the neck to the sacral region. A pair of spinal nerves (one on each side of the horse) leaves the spinal cord and emerges from the vertebral column at the intervertebral foramen between adjacent vertebrae (Figures 12.2 and 12.3).

The thoracic and lumbar vertebrae have dorsal spinous processes (DSPs) which can be palpated in most horses. The longest one is normally T6 which is usually the highest point of the withers (variable between T4 and T6). The DSPs of most of the thoracic vertebrae point slightly backwards. The caudal thoracic spinous processes and those of the lumbar vertebrae point slightly forwards. T15 or T16 has a vertical spinous process and is known as the **anticlinal** vertebra. The supraspinous ligament runs along the top of the DSPs.

The bones of the spine are connected by a complex array of ligaments and muscles. The shape and angle of the articular surfaces plus the arrangement of attached ligaments and muscles determine the amount of movement in each part of the spine. There is more flexibility in the cranial (front) part of the thoracic spine which allows more lateral flexion than in the caudal (back) part or the lumbar spine. The lumbosacral joint is the most mobile part of the horse's back. It allows flexion and extension but limited lateral flexion. The sacrum is attached to the pelvis by the sacroiliac joint.

NECK INJURIES

Anatomy

The body of each of the 7 cervical vertebrae articulates with that of the adjacent vertebrae. In addition, there are paired facet joints between adjacent vertebrae on each side of the spine.

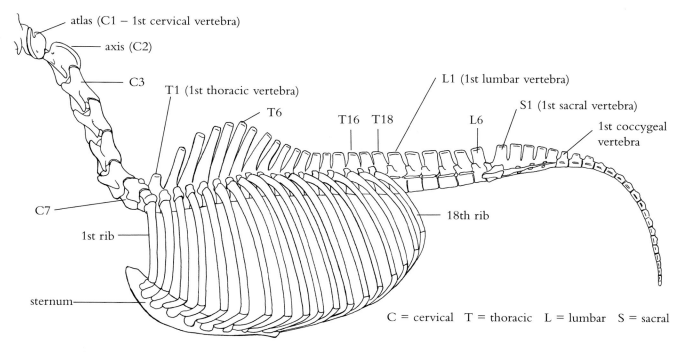

Figure 12.1 The spine

atlas (C1 – 1st cervical vertebra)

axis (C2)

C3

C7

1st rib

sternum

T1 (1st thoracic vertebra)

T6

T16 T18

L1 (1st lumbar vertebra)

L6

S1 (1st sacral vertebra)

1st coccygeal vertebra

18th rib

C = cervical   T = thoracic   L = lumbar   S = sacral

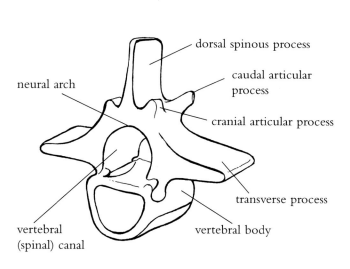

Figure 12.2 A typical equine vertebra – craniocaudal view

dorsal spinous process

caudal articular process

cranial articular process

neural arch

transverse process

vertebral (spinal) canal

vertebral body

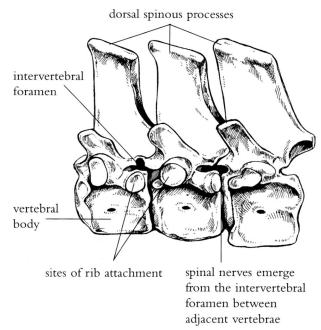

Figure 12.3 Last 3 thoracic vertebrae, lateral view

dorsal spinous processes

intervertebral foramen

vertebral body

sites of rib attachment

spinal nerves emerge from the intervertebral foramen between adjacent vertebrae

The first cervical vertebra is called the atlas. It articulates with the skull at the atlanto-occipital joint. The movement is mainly flexion and extension with a little oblique lateral movement. The second cervical vertebra is the axis. The atlanto-axial joint between C1 and C2 allows rotation of the head from side to side. The remainder of the articulations between C2 and C7 permit both flexion and extension, and lateral flexion. The base of the neck allows the most movement.

The vertebrae are joined by a number of ligaments. The powerful, elastic nuchal ligament runs in the midline from the skull to the fourth thoracic vertebra. The atlantal bursa lies between the atlas and the nuchal ligament (Figure 12.4).

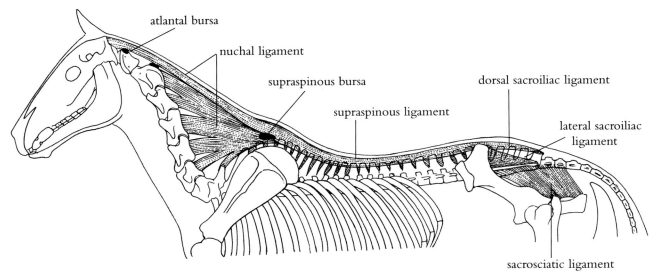

Figure 12.4 Ligaments of the neck, back and pelvis

Causes

The horse's neck is very susceptible to injuries from:

- falls (Figure 12.5)
- pulling back when tied up
- getting the head stuck through a gate or a fence
- catching the headcollar on a gate catch or other object
- hitting the poll on a low beam or door frame
- rearing up and falling over backwards
- colliding with solid objects, e.g. fences or another horse
- intramuscular injections given into the neck; these occasionally cause temporary bruising and soreness or an abscess to form.

Types of injury

The following injuries occur:

- muscle strains

- injury to the nuchal ligament where it inserts onto the occiput or the atlantal bursa (from pulling back or rearing up and sustaining a blow to the region)
- fractures
- bruises and abscesses.

Clinical signs

These may include:

- obvious signs of external trauma, e.g. skin and muscle damage
- muscle swelling or wasting
- holding the neck in an unusual position

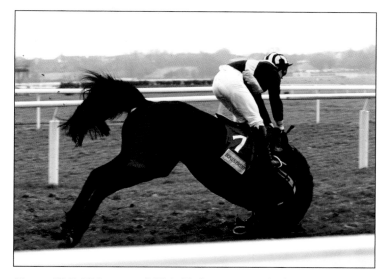

Figure 12.5 This type of fall is likely to injure the horse's neck

- an abnormal head carriage or head tilt
- difficulty lowering the head to the ground; the forelimbs may be widely separated when the horse grazes
- reduced range of motion; horses with reduced lateral flexion of the neck often tilt their heads markedly when attempting to reach a titbit held beside their shoulder
- pain on palpation
- patchy sweating
- dislike of bridling or being brushed or handled around the head.

Signs which show up at exercise include:

- mild forelimb stiffness or lameness
- reluctance to go onto or stay on the bit
- difficulty bending.

Serious injuries such as fractures that compress the spinal cord may present as incoordination of the limbs or an inability to stand.

Diagnosis

Diagnosis is made using some of the following.

- The clinical examination. This includes an assessment of the horse at rest and while exercised. The neck is palpated to locate sore areas and any muscle swelling or atrophy. The range of motion is tested by tempting the horse with a titbit such as a carrot.
- Radiography may be helpful in identifying fractures or other bony changes such as osteoarthritis.
- Scintigraphy may help to detect fractures that are difficult to see on radiographs.
- Ultrasonography can be used to evaluate the neck tissues.

The upper part of the neck can be examined with magnetic resonance imaging (MRI), but this is not widely available and requires general anaesthesia.

Treatment
This depends on the type of injury.

MUSCLE STRAINS
Following a thorough assessment, these may be treated by a combination of rest, non-steroidal anti-inflammatory drugs (e.g. phenylbutazone), physiotherapy, acupuncture and chiropractic or osteopathic treatment.

INJURY TO THE INSERTION OF THE NUCHAL LIGAMENT
The area may be injected with corticosteroids and sometimes a homeopathic substance, Traumeel®. Acupuncture, physiotherapy and shock wave therapy may help.

FRACTURES
Some neck fractures heal successfully without surgery if the horse is kept on box rest. The hay and water should be positioned at head height and the hay must be thoroughly shaken and fed loose to minimize neck movements. Pain relief from non-steroidal anti-inflammatory drugs (NSAIDs) may be necessary in the early stages, but this is kept to a minimum to discourage the horse from moving its neck too much. The horse is not tied up until the bone has healed. This is monitored by taking repeat X-rays.

The prognosis depends on the site of the fracture and whether there is any compression of the spinal cord causing ataxia (unsteadiness). In the early stages there may be spinal cord compression from soft tissue swelling, but this may disappear in a few days. Prolonged ataxia is a poor prognostic sign.

Certain fractures can be surgically treated. Others result in catastrophic damage to the spinal cord and necessitate immediate euthanasia.

BRUISES AND ABSCESSES
These should be treated as described on page 72.

Osteoarthritis
Degenerative ageing changes may be seen on X-rays between the facet joints of the lower neck vertebrae (C5–7). In many cases these are of no clinical significance. Severe bony changes, however, may ultimately cause compression of the spinal cord resulting in hind limb weakness and ataxia. Alternatively, compression of the cervical nerves as they leave the vertebral canal through the intervertebral foramen can result in local or referred pain. This can cause neck pain and stiffness, muscle wasting and forelimb lameness.

TREATMENT

Affected horses usually show a disappointing response to rest and NSAIDs. Injection of corticosteroids into or around the joint may provide temporary relief.

Chronic neck stiffness

A number of horses experience chronic neck stiffness but have no changes on radiographs. Many of these horses improve with treatments such as rest, acupuncture and chiropratic or osteopathic treatment, but remain restricted. In selected cases, manipulation under general anaesthesia significantly improves the horse's range of motion and level of comfort. Techniques such as this should only be performed by properly trained and experienced operators following a veterinary assessment.

Wobbler syndrome (see page 306)

BACK PAIN IN THE HORSE

Back pain may originate from the:
* skin
* associated muscles
* ligaments
* vertebrae (bone)
* nerves – due to trauma or compression.

Predisposing factors

* Certain types of conformation seem to predispose a horse to particular types of back pain. Animals with long backs may be predisposed to muscle and ligament strains. Horses with particularly short backs are more likely to develop vertebral lesions.
* The type of work may be a contributory factor. For example, dressage horses are often sore in the area beneath the back of the saddle owing to the rider sitting deep and asking for collection and impulsion.

Causes of back pain

These include:
* falls, jumping awkwardly, slipping
* inadequate warming up prior to strenuous exercise
* over-use, i.e. repetitive strain injury
* over-exertion of fatigued muscles
* being asked to perform at a level that is beyond the horse's capability or level of training and fitness

- failure to give the horse a 10 minute cooling-down period at walk following fast work
- incorrectly fitted or poorly maintained saddles (see Saddle Fitting on pages 335, 551–4)
- bad riding
- pain elsewhere in the body, e.g. hind limb lameness, causing the horse to alter its gait and put abnormal stresses on the back muscles, producing secondary back pain
- dental problems can lead to secondary back pain
- chronic stress, which leads to increased body tone and tight, shortened muscles
- metabolic problems, e.g. equine rhabdomyolysis syndrome
- certain viral infections.

Clinical signs

The first signs are often behavioural and the observant owner will notice a change in temperament. The horse may become uncharacteristically grumpy, less outgoing and lose its enthusiasm for work. It may resent being groomed. Some horses will start to fidget and move away or look worried when approached with a saddle (Figure 12.6). This can progress to dipping of the back, grunting, trying to bite and even collapsing when the girths are done up. When the rider mounts, the horse may dip or arch its back and jump forwards when asked to move off.

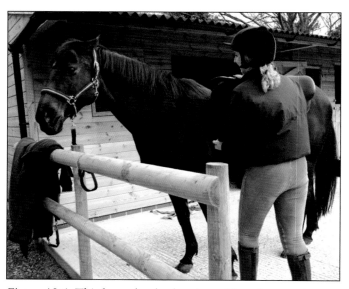

Figure 12.6 This horse has back pain and is unhappy when approached with the saddle

Other possible symptoms of back pain include:
- loss of performance
- reluctance to stay on the bit
- shortness of stride in front
- 'hopping' on the transition from walk to trot
- poor hind limb impulsion and failure to track up
- working with a high head carriage and hollow back with little engagement of the hindquarters
- moving uncharacteristically wide or close behind
- intermittent unilateral or bilateral hind limb lameness
- dragging the toes of the hind limbs and abnormal wear on the shoes
- increased stiffness especially when turning or working on a circle
- changing legs at canter or going disunited
- refusing to jump or altered jumping technique

- bucking
- swishing of the tail or holding the tail to one side
- looking cross, putting the ears back and shaking the head from side to side when asked to perform certain movements
- reluctance to rein back
- discomfort going downhill
- localized heat and swelling
- abnormal sensitivity to palpation
- abnormal curvature of the spine due to localized muscle spasm
- muscle wasting
- reluctance to lift the hind limbs for shoeing
- difficulty adopting the stance to urinate
- lying down or rolling less than usual
- standing in an unusual posture in an attempt to alleviate the pain.

Diagnosis

Diagnosing back pain in a horse is usually straightforward, but pinpointing the cause can be extremely difficult. Many horses are very stoical and will put up with considerable discomfort before exhibiting any signs. Ultimately there may be several contributory factors.

Difficulties arise because:
- there are so many possible causes
- the back pain may be a primary condition or it may be secondary to another, as yet undiagnosed, problem, e.g. hock pain
- it is not possible to directly palpate the vertebrae with the exception of the dorsal spinous processes
- obtaining images of the back is expensive and can only be done on premises that have the specialized equipment.

The techniques that may be used in the investigation of back pain include:
- a full clinical examination
- radiography (X-rays)
- local analgesia
- scintigraphy
- ultrasonography
- thermography
- blood tests.

THE HISTORY

A detailed history will be taken first. The vet will want to know when the problem started, what the symptoms are, the current level of fitness and the intended use of the horse. Any previous traumatic incidents should be noted as back pain may gradually develop following a traumatic incident some time ago.

The clinical examination

The clinical examination should include a thorough check of the whole horse to make sure there is no underlying illness or other physical problem. This includes:

- a dental inspection
- an assessment of foot balance
- visual inspection for obvious problems and to check the horse's symmetry
- palpation
- manipulation
- observation of the horse in hand, on the lunge and under saddle.

In addition the following should be checked:

- the suitability and fit of the bit
- the fit of the bridle
- the fit and condition of the saddle
- the type and condition of the girth
- the weight and ability of the rider
- the exercise programme of the horse
- the horse's suitability for the expected level of performance
- the horse's diet and amount of turnout.

Examination of the horse's back
INSPECTION AT REST

The horse is observed at rest in his stable for any postural abnormalities that could be caused by back pain. It is then led out of the stable for further inspection.

With the horse standing square, the vet will:

- check its general conformation
- note the condition and degree of muscling
- note the conformation of the back: an abnormal dipping of the thoracic part of the spine is known as **lordosis** (sway or dipped back) (Figure 12.7); increased arching of the lumbar spine is known as **kyphosis** (roach back); lateral deviation of the spine is known as **scoliosis**, which is observed most easily by standing on a mounting block and viewing the horse from above (Figure 12.8)
- inspect the foot balance
- look for any localized swelling or muscle wasting
- check for areas of hair loss in the saddle or girth region
- note any scars, lumps or white hair in the saddle region

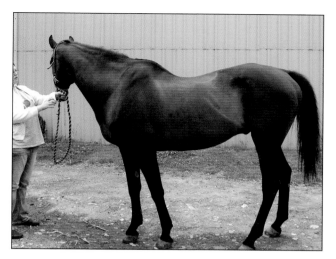

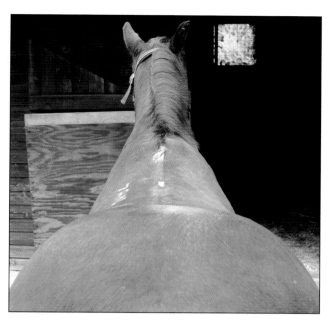

Figure 12.7 Lordosis of the spine, i.e. sway backed

Figure 12.8 Checking the alignment of the horse's spine from above

- check the symmetry or otherwise of the bony prominences of the pelvis, i.e. the tubera sacrale and the tubera coxae.

PALPATION

- The horse is gently stroked along the muscles of the back and the vet will feel for any areas of heat, pain or swelling. Any lumps or scars will be noted. The pressure is very light, using flat fingers to begin with to relax the horse and familiarize it with the procedure. This is repeated several times and the pressure is gradually increased. A normal horse will dip its back (ventroflex) when firm pressure is applied to the thoracolumbar region and arch its back (dorsiflex) in response to firm pressure applied from either side of the sacrum backwards towards the tail. This should be a fluid movement that is repeatable without causing any muscle spasm or resentment. Horses with back pain will often grunt and swish their tails while dipping in a jerky, exaggerated fashion. Some will try to bite or lash out. The muscles may go into spasm and feel much harder than the adjacent muscle or fasciculate (show tiny, repeated contractions). Other horses will tense their backs and go rigid rather than dip or arch their backs. In each case, the results must be interpreted taking factors such as the temperament of the horse into consideration. A sensitive or nervous horse without back pain may give an exaggerated response while many cobs and thick-set ponies show very little response.
- The dorsal spinous processes are individually palpated to feel for any misalignment or localized tenderness and swelling of the supraspinous ligament.

MANIPULATION

These tests are performed to check the range of movement and the suppleness of the spine. A blunt instrument is run smoothly along the muscles on either side of the spine from the withers to level with the tail. The spine extends (seen as dipping or ventroflexion) as the instrument passes along the thoracic and lumbar regions, and flexes (seen as arching or dorsiflexion) from the tuber sacrale backwards.

Extension and flexion of the thoracic and lumbar vertebrae can also be tested by gently pinching the muscles on either side of the spine over the lumbar and croup regions respectively. Lateral flexion can be tested by stroking the horse across its back muscles from the spine outwards. The range of movement of the neck is also checked.

EXAMINATION IN HAND

The horse is observed moving in hand on a loose rein at walk and trot on a firm surface. The vet is looking for any:

- lameness that may be contributing to the back pain
- gait abnormalities: horses with mild back pain may move close behind with a plaiting action; horses with moderate to severe back pain often adopt a wide, straddling hind limb gait; any restriction of hind limb action or dragging of the toes will be noted.

Flexion tests

These should be negative. A positive test can be indicative of a limb problem developing.

Observation of the horse turning

The horse is assessed when turning around at the end of each trot up and when turned in a tight circle on each rein. A horse with back pain often has reduced lateral flexibility of the spine and shows resistance to turning or signs of discomfort. He may pivot round his hind limbs rather than crossing them over on the turn. Localized spasm of the muscles may be observed or behavioural signs such as the ears going flat back and swishing of the tail.

Walking backwards

Finally, the horse is asked to walk backwards for several steps by gently pushing on its chest. The horse may lift its head and be reluctant to do this. Spasm or fasciculation of the back muscles may be seen or the horse may move in a circle rather than a straight line. Swishing of the tail is common in horses with sore backs (see Figure 4.7).

EXAMINATION ON THE LUNGE

This may be done with and without the tack. The horse is observed on the lunge at walk, trot and canter. The vet is looking for any stiffness of the back and reluctance to bend. Any behavioural signs of discomfort are most likely to be observed during transitions. If the facilities and the temperament of the horse permit, this should be repeated at walk and trot on a hard surface.

If the result is different when the horse is tacked up, a problem with the saddle (or less commonly the bridle or teeth) should be suspected.

TACKING UP

The horse should be observed for any signs of anxiety or discomfort when approached with the saddle or being girthed up. The fit of the saddle for both the horse and the rider is assessed, together with the condition of the saddle, numnah etc (see Saddle Fitting page 335, and Girth Sensitivity page 552–6).

RIDDEN EXERCISE

The horse is observed as the rider mounts and as it moves off. The horse is then assessed performing its usual work unless the degree of pain prohibits this. The history is very important as a good rider may feel a change in performance before it is visible to an observer. The pain may only be apparent with certain movements. Each horse is normally seen at walk, trot and canter on both reins. In certain cases, the horse will be observed jumping or performing lateral work.

This part of the examination also gives the vet the opportunity to assess the ability of the rider to see if they are contributing to the horse's problem. Sometimes the rider's expectations of the horse are unrealistic. Finally, some horses are capable of carrying more weight than others. A rider that is too heavy for the horse is sure to cause problems. The back is palpated again following the exercise.

Investigation of back pain

By now, the cause of the pain may be obvious or further investigations may be necessary. They may include the following.

BLOOD TESTS

When there is severe muscle spasm and soreness, the vet may take a blood sample to check for muscle damage. The level of the muscle enzymes creatine kinase (CK) and aspartate aminotransferase (AST) in the blood increases if muscle damage has occurred.

RADIOGRAPHY

Very powerful X-ray machines are needed to take X-rays of the horse's back. Even then, only limited parts of the spine can be seen. Radiographs are useful to identify conditions such as impingement or overriding of the dorsal spinous processes (DSPs).

LOCAL ANALGESIA

Once a potential problem has been identified, e.g. impingement of DSPs, local anaesthetic can be infiltrated around and between the suspect processes, sometimes using ultrasound guidance. If the horse is much more comfortable when ridden after a period of approximately 20 minutes, the impingement is confirmed as the source of the pain.

SCINTIGRAPHY (BONE SCAN)

Scintigraphy is useful for locating lesions such as vertebral fractures which are too deep in the body to be seen on X-rays. It shows up any areas of bone remodelling and can be useful to confirm the presence of inflammation of the dorsal spinous processes. However, many horses with no signs of back pain have abnormal patterns of uptake of the radioactive drug. The results therefore have to be interpreted with great care even by vets experienced in this technique.

ULTRASONOGRAPHY

Ultrasound is useful for examining the spinous processes and attached ligaments. The articular and transverse processes can also be seen with this technique.

THERMOGRAPHY

Thermography is increasingly being used as part of the examination of a horse with back pain. Horses with chronic back pain often have cold areas with decreased blood flow rather than inflamed 'hot spots'.

SUMMARY

Diagnosing the cause of back pain can be very difficult and is not always possible. There may be a number of contributory factors. Because the investigative techniques can be expensive and are not universally available, some form of treatment may be tried first, providing there are no special concerns following a thorough clinical examination.

Treatment of back pain
MANAGEMENT CHANGES AND PHYSICAL THERAPIES

The first step is to identify and remove any obvious causes.

Management changes may include:

* alterations to the existing saddle or purchase of a new one
* modification of the horse's training programme
* schooling for the horse and lessons for the rider
* turning the horse out
* feeding from the floor to encourage the horse to stretch its spine and separate the spinous processes.

The treatment depends on the cause of the pain and its severity. The aim in every case is to remove the pain so that the horse can continue to be exercised in a way that will restore muscle function and strength and prevent muscle wasting.

In many cases, a horse will require a period of rest for acute injuries. This should be combined with some form of physical and/or medical therapy so that normal function is restored to the muscle as soon as possible

Possible treatments include the following.

- Physiotherapy, including the use of massage, heat, stretching, low intensity laser therapy, ultrasound, magnetic field therapy, muscle stimulation etc.
- Acupuncture.
- Manipulation (osteopathy and chiropractic).
- A rehabilitation programme, which is an essential part of the treatment. The re-introduction to exercise should be gradual and include a gentle warm-up. For some horses, exercise may begin on the lunge without a saddle, then progress to lungeing with a saddle before ridden exercise commences.

MEDICAL TREATMENT

Treatment may include the following.

- Non-steroidal anti-inflammatory drugs, e.g. phenylbutazone, to reduce the inflammation and pain. However, many horses with chronic back pain show a poor response to these drugs.
- Local injection of corticosteroids for overriding DSPs or osteoarthritis of the small facet joints between adjacent vertebrae.
- Local injection of muscle relaxants or Sarapin® (see page 359) for overriding DSPs.
- Mesotherapy. This is a treatment that works in a similar way to acupuncture. Small amounts of a selected medication are injected into the dermis of the skin on either side of the spine. The selected sites are chosen because they are innervated by the same segmental nerve as the painful area. Stimulation of these sites can block the pain signals from the lesion travelling from the spinal cord to the brain. This is known as the gate mechanism of pain, where the treatment 'closes the gate' to pain.

SURGERY

Resection of impinging or overriding DSPs is sometimes carried out if conservative treatment is unsuccessful.

Prognosis

The prognosis depends on the cause of the pain and the severity of the problem. Some of the common conditions are discussed in more detail later.

BACK PAIN – WHO IS QUALIFIED TO TREAT YOUR HORSE?

Under the 1911 Protection of Animals Act, it is illegal for anyone apart from the owner to treat a horse without prior permission from the vet. This law exists to protect animals from potential injury in the hands of unqualified operators. The Veterinary Surgery (Exemptions) Order 1962 was introduced to allow therapies such as physiotherapy, chiropractic and osteopathy to be used under supervision of a vet. The vet is consulted first, to establish a veterinary diagnosis and rule out any underlying conditions that may be aggravated by the above treatments. These therapies may be used in conjunction with conventional veterinary treatment.

Most equine vets work closely with qualified therapists. It is important to establish good communication channels so that everyone involved is treating the horse as part of the same team. In the past, some vets have been reluctant to acknowledge the benefits of complementary therapies. Fortunately this situation is changing, resulting in effective treatment for many horses.

Qualifications
PHYSIOTHERAPY

A 'chartered physiotherapist' has a high level of academic and practical training in all aspects of physiotherapy. They have the letters MCSP (Member of the Chartered Society of Physiotherapy) after their names. The Association of Chartered Physiotherapists in Animal Therapy (ACPAT) has introduced a Post Graduate Diploma/Master of Science degree in Veterinary Physiotherapy. This is run in collaboration with the Royal Veterinary College. Only people with this degree can call themselves 'Veterinary Physiotherapists'.

CHIROPRACTIC

Qualified chiropractors are members of the General Chiropractic Council. Again they have extensive training in human chiropractic techniques. The McTimoney College of Chiropractic runs an MSc course in animal manipulation.

OSTEOPATHY

All qualified osteopaths have taken a 4–5 year BSc course in human osteopathic medicine at an accredited college. A Society of Osteopaths in Animal Practice (SOAP) has now been formed in association with the General Osteopathic Council. Members must have a letter from a vet with whom they work regularly. Post graduate courses in animal osteopathy are now available.

ACUPUNCTURE

Acupuncture using needles can only be done by a veterinary surgeon with special training in this field.

Treatment from unqualified persons

The important thing to remember is that obtaining treatment from an unqualified person is against the law and may cause harm to the horse. In the past such treatments were sought after as the number of qualified therapists was insufficient to cope with the demand. While good results were obtained in some cases, the operators will not have undergone the formal training necessary to recognize situations in which manipulation is inappropriate. The pain or stiffness may be secondary to a slight lameness that has been overlooked or systemic illness. It is obviously important to address the cause of the problem as well as to treat the symptoms.

A professional therapist will always work with your vet. The law is changing with regard to the granting of protected titles to make it clear who is properly trained. In the past, it has sometimes been difficult to establish just who is a legitimate therapist. Be cautious as it is not uncommon to encounter horses with serious problems that could have been avoided if veterinary help had been sought at an earlier stage.

PROBLEMS CAUSED BY THE SADDLE

A large number of horses experience back pain as a direct result of an ill-fitting saddle. Most horses change shape as they mature or at different times of the year according to their work routines and management. Saddle-induced pain is discussed in some depth on page 551 (Saddle Sores).

Regular checks by a qualified and recommended saddler will help to avoid these problems. They should be carried out annually or as soon as a problem is suspected. Buying a new saddle is not always easy as both saddles and horses come in many shapes and sizes. Some basic guidelines are given below.

SADDLE FITTING

Examining and fitting a saddle

Saddles come in many different styles, e.g. dressage, jumping, general purpose etc. They are available in different widths and lengths. It is important that the selected saddle is comfortable for both the horse and the rider. Traditionally, the shape and size of the saddle is based on its tree which is usually made of wood. Fitting should always be performed by a qualified saddler. It is a good idea to send the saddler a wither pattern before their visit in order to give them an idea of the shape of your horse. They can then bring along the saddles most likely to fit the horse as well as suit the rider's requirements.

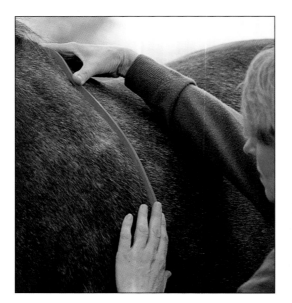

Figure 12.9 Use of a flexi-curve to take a wither pattern

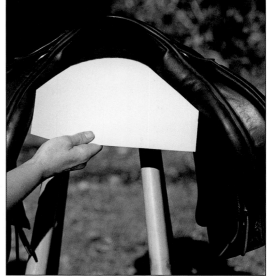

Figure 12.10 How to use the wither pattern

HOW TO TAKE A WITHER PATTERN

The wither pattern is taken using a flexible bar called a flexi-curve. With the horse standing square, the middle of the flexi-curve is positioned over the top of the withers and shaped so that it follows the contour of the wither and lies behind the scapula on each side of the horse (Figure 12.9). It is then lifted off and laid onto a large piece of paper or card. A line is drawn under the curve and the template is cut out. This should fit snugly under the front of any saddle purchased for the horse with 5–6 cm (approximately 2 in or 3 fingers) clearance under the centre of the pommel (Figure 12.10).

CHECKS ON THE SADDLE (Figure 12.11)

Once suitably sized saddles have been selected, the following checks should be made before placing them on the horse.

- The stitching and quality of the leather should be checked. There should be no creases or cracks in the leather panels or the flaps of the saddle. The leather should be smooth and supple.
- The flocking under the panels should be smooth and even with no hard lumps or soft patches. The panels should not be overstuffed and hard as this can lead to bruising of the horse's back. They should have a little 'give' to allow the muscles of the back to work properly. Insufficient flocking, however, can lead to severe discomfort as the horse may be able to feel the points or the stirrup bars.
- The saddle should be checked for symmetry of the tree, the panels, stirrup bars and the girth straps. The best way to do this is to stand the saddle on its pommel on the floor and view it from above. A twisted tree or asymmetrically positioned stirrup bars

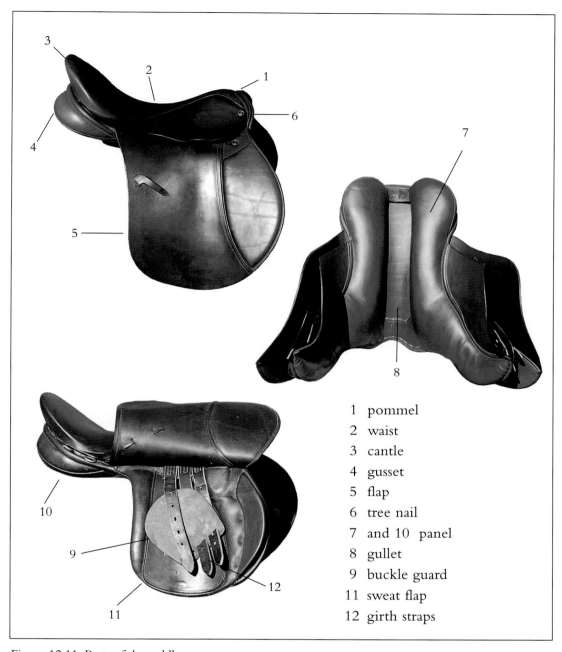

1 pommel
2 waist
3 cantle
4 gusset
5 flap
6 tree nail
7 and 10 panel
8 gullet
9 buckle guard
11 sweat flap
12 girth straps

Figure 12.11 Parts of the saddle

or girth straps will cause the saddle to twist round on the horse and cause discomfort.

• If a saddle is dropped or purchased second-hand, it should be checked for a broken tree. Hold the pommel of the tree against your stomach and pull the cantle towards you with both hands. Then put the saddle down and see if there is any movement when the pommel is pushed down and pulled up on both sides. Any abnormal movement or noise could indicate a damaged tree.

STEPS IN FITTING THE SADDLE

- Stand the horse squarely on a level surface.
- Position the saddle. It is surprising how many people still place the saddle too far forward on the horse's back. The saddle should be gently placed over the withers and slid backwards until it is *behind* the scapula (shoulder blade). It should not cover the scapula as this will restrict the horse's action. It will also cause the saddle to swing from side to side across the midline each time the horse takes a stride. This can cause friction and soreness. Positioning the saddle too far forward may also cause the rider's weight to be tipped towards the back of the saddle.
- Now check the length of the saddle. It should not extend beyond the last (18th) thoracic vertebra. This can be determined by following the line of the last rib up to the spine.
- The width is checked at the front of the saddle by straightening one's fingers and sliding them between the saddle and the horse from the withers downwards. The contact should be even all the way down with no areas of increased pressure. There should be a 3-finger clearance of the pommel over the withers. If the gap is more than this, the tree may be too narrow. If it is less, the tree may be too wide or the saddle may have insufficient flocking (Figures 12.12a and b).
- If the width seems correct, do up the girths loosely on the first and third straps and check again. The girths should be placed over the seat of girth which is located as a depression in the horse's ventral midline approximately 10 cm (4 in) behind the elbow.
- Now place your hand so that your fingers are underneath the seat of the saddle as far forward as possible. Run your palm backwards along the horse's back under the panels to check that the pressure is even. Any blockages, or absence of contact will lead to pressure points for the horse.
- With the girths done up, the back of the saddle should not be lifted easily from the horse's back.
- Next stand back and check the balance and symmetry of the saddle sitting on the horse. The seat should be horizontal and not tip uphill or downhill (Figure 12.13). Saddles that tip backwards concentrate the weight of the rider at the back of the saddle and may cause bruising and pressure sores; saddles that tip forwards may be too wide.
- The rider should now mount from a mounting block and the fitting and balance of the saddle are checked again. The rider should sit centrally and not be tipped forwards or backwards. Any reaction from the horse should be noted.
- With the rider in place, the clearance of the gullet should be checked. This should be sufficiently wide (approximately 6 cm [$2\frac{1}{2}$ in]) and deep so that there is good clearance of the dorsal spinous processes of the horse's vertebrae. However, if the gullet is too wide there may be insufficient clearance and the weight will not be spread evenly over the strongest back muscles on either side of the midline.
- The gap between the pommel and the withers should still accommodate 3 fingers.

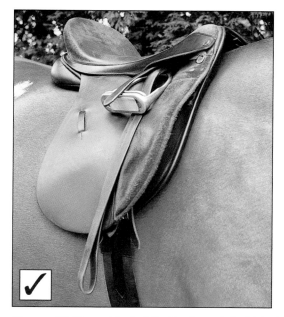 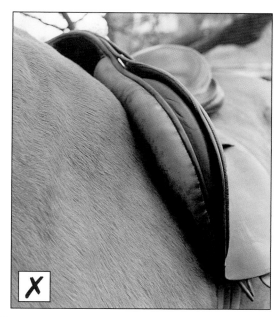

Figures 12.12a and b Saddle fit: a) good fit; b) bad fit

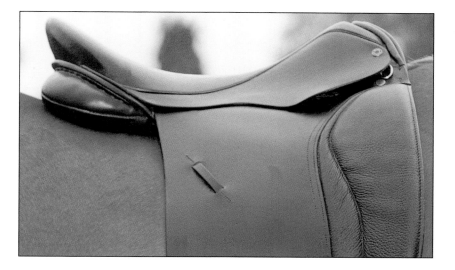

Figure 12.13 A well–fitting saddle (left)

- If all is well, the horse should be observed working at walk, trot and canter. If a jumping saddle is being purchased, the horse should be seen going over a couple of fences. A well-fitted saddle will stay in balance and not rock from side to side. It must not interfere with movement of the shoulders.
- When the saddle is removed, the sweat or dust pattern should be symmetrical on either side of the horse's back.
- There are sophisticated tools such as pressure-measuring pads which record the pressure exerted on the horse's back from the saddle. These are used for research purposes in the development of new saddles and also for assessing the saddle comfort with individual problem horses.

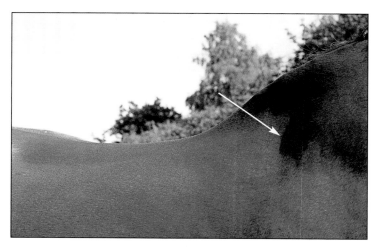

Figure 12.14 A horse with deep hollows either side of the withers due to muscle wasting

Individual horse problems

Not all horses are symmetrical. If a horse has a specific injury there may be unilateral loss of muscle. In this case, the saddle can be adjusted as required. Equally, if a horse loses or gains weight dramatically, its saddle will need to be altered.

Horses that have worn saddles that are too narrow for them develop hollows just below the withers on both sides, behind the top of the shoulder blades (Figure 12.14). Fitting a saddle to this shape will not allow correct development of these wasted muscles. In these cases, temporary padding using a wither pad under a wider saddle may provide the solution. This should be fitted by a qualified saddler. A common mistake is to place a pad under a saddle that is too narrow to lift it away from the withers. This actually compounds the problem and increases the pressure.

Common problems with traditional saddles

- The problem areas with traditional saddles tend to be the 'points' and the stirrup bars (Figure 12.15). The arched part of the tree that forms the pommel continues down on either side of the withers and has squared off ends that are called the **points**. These sit over the thoracic part of the trapezius muscle behind the shoulder blades. If there is any error with the fitting or flocking of this region, the points press into the muscles causing nerve damage and muscle wastage. The horse experiences chronic pain which may be exacerbated on turning.

- The weight of the rider is transmitted from the stirrup bars onto the arch at the front of the saddle and thence to the tree points. This occurs particularly when the rider adopts the forward position for cross-country riding. It is important that the stirrup bars are in the correct position for the rider. If they are too far forward, for instance, it is impossible for the rider to remain in balance.

- If the saddle is fitted too far forwards, the back of the scapula will push against the tree point as the limb is extended.

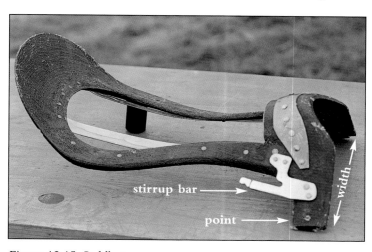

stirrup bar

width

point

Figure 12.15 Saddle tree

This causes the back of the saddle to swing across to the opposite side of the horse's back. The withers become pinched and bruised resulting in a shortened, choppy gait. The back may also become sore.

New innovations

Saddles are responsible for a great deal of pain and misery if they are not correctly fitted and maintained. As a result, new ideas are being developed all the time.

AIR FLOCKING

In recent years, a combination of air and foam has been used to flock the saddle panels instead of the traditional wool, felt or foam. The claim for this method is that it allows the panels to be softer and continually mould to the horse's shape, thus avoiding pressure points and also allowing impact absorption. These saddles also need regular, professional fitting and maintenance.

TREELESS SADDLES

Recently, a number of treeless saddles have been introduced onto the market. They are fitted to the size, weight and needs of the rider, rather than the horse. The manufacturer's claim that as it is flexible and has no rigid parts, the saddle will mould to the shape of the horse and not cause injury. Once the rider has a saddle that is suitable and comfortable, it should fit any horse whatever their conformation. The reports so far are encouraging, but long-term use is still being monitored.

HEAT-SENSITIVE PANELS

New materials that mould to the shape of the horse as they warm up are now being used for some saddle panels. When removed from the horse, they revert back to the original shape. Such materials are being used with traditional saddles as well as treeless models and the results are encouraging.

Numnahs and pads

Numnahs and pads can be helpful fitted under a saddle whilst a horse is building up muscle. If the saddle fits well, they are not necessary. A discussion of the huge range available is beyond the scope of this book but there are some general rules when using a numnah.

- The numnah should be shaped across the top in such a way that it follows the contour of the horse's spine rather than being cut straight (Figure 12.16).
- It should be large enough to extend beyond the saddle all the way round. If it is too short at any point, the saddle will sit on the edge of the numnah and this will cause a pressure point.
- The numnah should be pulled up into the gullet along the whole length of the saddle. It should not press on the withers and spine. (Figures 12.17a and b.)

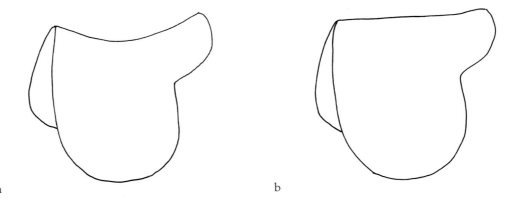

a   b

Figures 12.16a and b Correctly and incorrectly shaped numnahs: a) correctly shaped to follow the curve of the spine; b) too straight across the top

- There should be no ridges or wrinkles.
- Numnahs and pads should be washed regularly in a non-biological detergent.
- A variety of numnahs and pads are available for horses with wasting of the muscles on either side of the withers or under the saddle. Your saddler is the best person to advise on the most appropriate choice. These numnahs and pads are made of many different materials. There is also a numnah on the market with four air bags which can be adjusted individually. This can be helpful for asymmetric horses and riders, and those horses that are changing shape quickly.

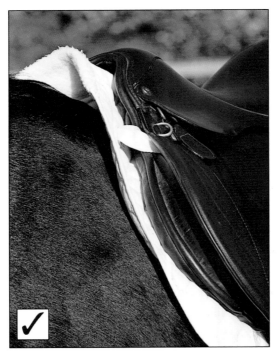 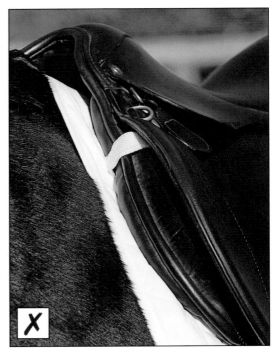

Figures 12.17a and b Correctly and incorrectly fitted numnahs: a) correctly pulled up into the saddle's gullet; b) incorrectly pressing on the horse's back

COLD BACKS AND PAIN IN THE GIRTH REGION

The term 'cold-backed' is used to describe horses that persistently dip their backs and hindquarters when mounted. They are often short striding for the first 10 minutes of exercise. In some cases the reaction is extreme and the horse collapses as the girth is tightened.

Causes

In the past these symptoms have been attributed to 'bad behaviour' or habit, possibly following an episode of back pain. A number of causes of back pain can trigger this type of behaviour. However, it is increasingly being recognized that some of these horses are suffering from hypersensitivity or pain in the girth and wither regions.

Why does this happen?

The causes of pain in the girth region are still not fully understood. One theory is that, during the birth process, the thoracic vertebrae that form the withers and the associated ribs are traumatized. Recent research indicates that up to 20% of newborn foals have a degree of ribcage trauma and as many as 5% sustain rib fractures. This may lead to irritation of the 2nd–6th thoracic nerves that innervate the girth area and heightened sensitivity of the local muscles behind the elbow.

Many horses tolerate a low grade of discomfort. However, this may be exacerbated by a fall or the horse going over backwards and landing on its withers. This is often when the real problems begin. Alternatively, a saddle that is too narrow and pinches the withers may trigger the problem.

Once this has started, anxiety and fear on the horse's part may increase the pain and lead to the extreme reactions sometimes encountered.

Clinical signs

- Many horses are sensitive in their girth regions. In some, however, running a finger down the girth region behind the elbow causes the muscles to jump so markedly that it causes discomfort and anxiety.
- These horses have no visible lesions but they are often uncomfortable when brushed.
- Tightening the girth causes the horse to swish its tail, toss its head, grunt in discomfort or move away. Less obvious signs include a change in facial expression or breathing pattern. Some horses will momentarily stop chewing hay.
- The horse may turn round and try to bite the handler or kick out at the girth.
- Some affected animals will breathe in to expand the chest as the girth is done up in an attempt to stop it being tightened.
- Many of these horses have pain in the trapezius muscle (which is supplied by the same

thoracic nerves) that is directly under the front of the saddle. Firm stroking of this muscle often causes the horse to give a violent shudder of the muscles over the girth area and to move away.

- Severely affected horses jump or even collapse when the girth is tightened or immediately afterwards.
- Once the horse is girthed up it may move in a short-striding and restricted fashion for the first few minutes of exercise. Some horses will leap forwards when asked to walk on.
- Others hump their backs and buck, especially on the transition to canter.

Diagnosis

Diagnosis of girth-region pain is made on the clinical signs. The horse should have a full examination to rule out any other contributory factors such as lameness, poor saddle fit or unsuitable girths (see Girth Galls on page 555).

Treatment

Suitable treatments include:
- sensitive handling, as rough grooming or girthing up may cause the problem or be a contributory factor
- chiropractic
- osteopathy
- acupuncture or acupressure
- physiotherapy, including massage
- removal or treatment of any underlying problems.

A combination of these treatments may be used.

Management

These horses need thoughtful handling to overcome the association between saddling up and discomfort. The following action should be taken.
- Regular saddle-fit checks.
- Use of a wide, comfortable girth; well-maintained leather ones are the most comfortable. Some dressage girths, for example, can dig into the soft skin behind the horse's elbow when the horse moves (Figures 12.18).
- Girths with elastic at one end can inadvertently be over-tightened. This can pull the saddle to one side and interfere with the horse's breathing. To avoid this, the elastic should be on the horse's right side (offside) and once the rider is mounted, the girth should only be tightened from the left side (nearside).
- Always use a mounting block. Take care to avoid poking the horse's ribcage with your toe when mounting.

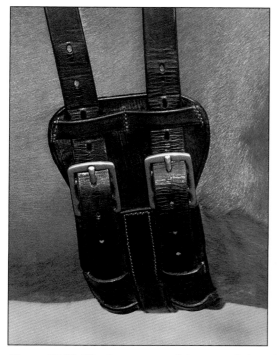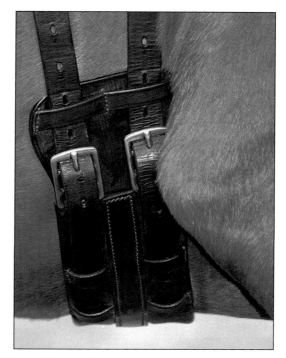

Figure 12.18 The long straps of dressage girths, which buckle low down on the horse's side, can cause discomfort to the horse because the buckles can come into contact with the horse's elbow

The following steps may help.

- Tack the horse up at least 10 minutes before mounting.
- Take care that the girth is sitting in the correct position. Many people position the saddle and girth too far forwards. The girth should sit a short distance back from the elbow. Do the girth up loosely to start with.
- Pulling the forelimbs forwards one at a time will help the girth to sit in the correct position. It also checks that the soft skin in this region is not being pinched underneath the girth.
- Walk the horse around and tighten the girth progressively during this period.
- Avoid over-tightening the girth as this will increase the discomfort and may affect the horse's breathing.
- Make sure the horse stays warm whilst waiting to be ridden.
- Lead the horse around or lunge it with the tack on for a few minutes prior to mounting.
- Once mounted, the rider should lower their weight gently into the saddle. Some horses are more comfortable if the rider stands up in the stirrups for a short period before sitting down.
- If possible, going downhill should be avoided at the start of the ride.

Prognosis

With appropriate care, the prognosis is reasonable as many horses respond well to treatment.

STRAINED MUSCLES

Causes

A back muscle strain usually results from:

- falls
- awkward movements
- over-exertion
- inadequate warming up prior to strenuous exercise.

Clinical signs

These include:

- areas of muscle spasm or swelling
- heat and pain on palpation
- stiffness
- dipping the back when mounted
- reduced hind limb impulsion.

Diagnosis

Diagnosis is made on the clinical examination and blood tests may be taken to check the muscle enzyme levels. Creatine kinase (CK) and aspartate aminotransferase (AST) are elevated if there is significant muscle damage.

Treatment

Treatments include:

- a period of rest
- non-steroidal anti-inflammatory drugs, e.g. phenylbutazone
- physiotherapy
- acupuncture
- manipulation (osteopathy or chiropractic)
- controlled exercise as part of a rehabilitation programme.

IMPINGEMENT AND OVERRIDING OF THE DORSAL SPINOUS PROCESSES (KISSING SPINES)

Each of the thoracic and lumbar vertebrae has a dorsal spinous process (DSP). As discussed earlier in this chapter, the DSPs of the majority of the thoracic vertebrae point in a slightly backwards direction. The caudal thoracic and lumbar vertebrae point slightly forwards. The 15th or 16th thoracic vertebra, known as the anticlinal vertebra, points directly upwards. A gap of at least 4 mm ($\frac{2}{10}$ in) between each spinous process is desirable.

In some horses, the spinous processes are too close to each other and may impinge (touch) or override (Figures 12.19 and 12.20). The region most commonly affected is between T12 and L2. Impingement occurs particularly in the caudal thoracic region where the weight of the rider is concentrated and the spaces between the processes are narrowest. As a result, the bone remodels and areas of increased and/or decreased bone density can be seen on radiographs.

Causes

- The condition may be congenital. Horses with short backs are most likely to be affected.

- Many horses with impinging DSPs are asymptomatic. The onset of pain may be triggered by a fall.

- Horses that jump tend to experience the most problems as the DSPs of the middle and caudal thoracic regions may impinge when the horse lands after a fence.

- Impingement may occur as the horse ages and its back becomes more hollow.

Clinical signs

There are many horses with impingement and remodelling of their DSPs that do not appear to have back pain. When the DSPs are a source of pain, the symptoms are very variable. They tend to develop gradually as the horse's work becomes more advanced and physically demanding. Possible

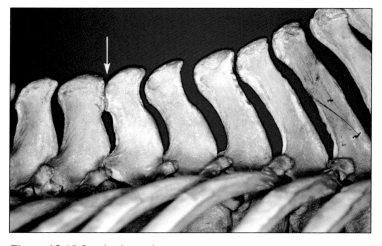

Figure 12.19 Impinging spines

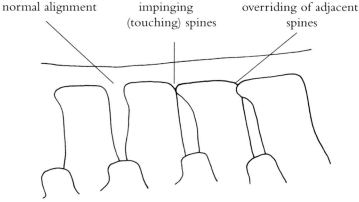

Figure 12.20 Impingement and overriding of the dorsal spinous processes

symptoms include:

- resentment of being brushed, rugged up, saddled, mounted or ridden
- change of temperament and loss of enthusiasm for work
- groaning or sinking as, or after, the girth is tightened
- dipping or humping the back when mounted
- leaping forwards suddenly after mounting
- loss of performance
- poor hind limb impulsion
- discomfort going downhill
- bucking when the aids are applied
- reluctance to jump
- muscle guarding or spasm
- tail swishing and obvious discomfort when ridden.

Diagnosis

Horses with impinging DSPs dislike dipping their backs when a blunt instrument is run along each side of the spine. They often hold themselves rigidly with the muscles in spasm.

Radiography and scintigraphy can be valuable aids to diagnosis.

Radiographic changes include:

- less space than normal between adjacent spinous processes
- Impingement or overriding of adjacent spinous processes
- bone remodelling of the affected processes.

Scintigraphy is useful for identifying areas of active bone remodelling. However, the results of both of these imaging techniques have to be interpreted with care as many apparently normal horses have visible bony changes on radiographs and active remodelling occurs in horses without back pain.

A positive diagnosis is made if local analgesia of an area which looks suspicious on the X-rays or scans abolishes the pain.

Treatment

The first line of treatment is likely to include some of the following.

- A period of rest. Many horses initially respond to rest, but the symptoms recur when they resume work.
- Non-steroidal anti-inflammatory drugs such as phenylbutazone may relieve the discomfort sufficiently for mild cases to continue light work.
- Local injection of corticosteroids between, or close to, the affected DSPs.
- Physiotherapy.
- Acupuncture.

- Controlled exercise to strengthen the back.
- Avoidance of activities such as jumping which are painful for the horse.

If there is no improvement after 6 months, then surgery may be considered. The top part of one or more spinous processes may be removed with the horse under general anaesthesia. Following the surgery, the horse has a short period of box rest and then starts a rehabilitation programme which includes long reining, lungeing and physio-therapy.

Prognosis

The prognosis is guarded. Many horses are kept in work with regular exercise and treatment as necessary. In one study, over 70% of horses undergoing surgery were able to resume their normal work.

FRACTURES OF THE PELVIS

Anatomy

Each half of the pelvis is made up of three fused bones, the ilium, the ischium and the pubis (Figures 12.21a, b and c). The two halves join in the midline at the pubic symphysis. The large wing of the ilium extends from the tuber sacrale to the tuber coxae, both of which are easily palpated as bony prominences. The tubera sacrale form the highest part of the hindquarters and are sometimes referred to as 'jumper's bumps'. The body or shaft of the ilium extends backwards from the ilial wing and fuses with the ischium and pubis to form the acetabulum which is part of the hip joint. The ischium and pubis make up the bony floor of the pelvis. The most caudal part of the ischium, the tuber ischii, can be felt as a bony prominence below the tail head on either side of the horse. The upper limit of the pelvic cavity is formed by the sacrum. This is attached to the ventral (lower) surface of the wing of the ilium at the sacroiliac joint.

Several powerful muscles used in locomotion attach to the bones of the pelvis. The propulsive forces of the hind limbs are transmitted to the horse's body through the pelvis.

Causes

These include the following.
- Falls, e.g. slipping and falling sideways on a hard surface or during a competition.
- Rearing up and falling over backwards.
- Knocking the tuber coxae on a gate post or stable door frame.
- Uncoordinated attempts to get up whilst being cast.
- 'Stress' fractures: in young racehorses, the bones of the pelvis constantly remodel as an adaptation to the powerful forces experienced during training. Stress fractures occur if

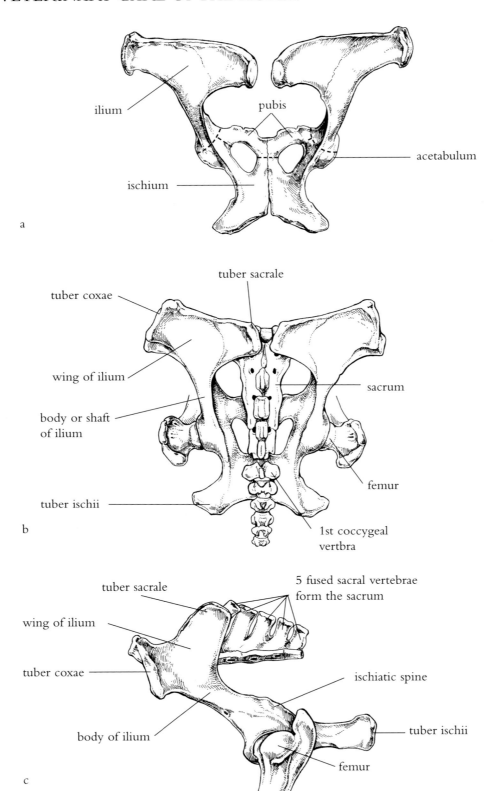

Figure 12.21a, b and c Bones of the pelvis: a) pelvic bones (without the sacrum), viewed from above showing the ilium, ischium and pubis; b) viewed from above including the sacrum; c) lateral view

these forces exceed the capacity of the bone to withstand them and are common in young racehorses.

Clinical signs

These depend on the site of the fracture. The commonest sites are the wing and shaft of the ilium. All fractures are associated with a sudden onset of moderate to severe lameness. In the case of stress fractures in young horses, this may be preceded by periods of intermittent, slight hind limb lameness, poor performance or altered hind limb gait. The fracture usually affects only one side of the pelvis giving a unilateral lameness. Occasionally, catastrophic bilateral stress fractures occur and the horse is unable to walk or support itself comfortably.

FRACTURES OF THE ILIAL WING

The wing of the ilium is the commonest site for a stress fracture.

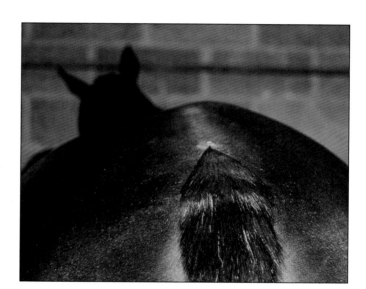

Figure 12.22 This horse had a fracture of the left side of the pelvis

- Incomplete fractures (consisting of tiny microfractures that do not go all the way through the bone) are associated with a shortened stride, poor propulsion and loss of performance.
- Complete fractures cause variable degrees of lameness. A moderate to severe lameness may be present for the first 48 hours followed by a marked improvement.
- The horse will sometimes change its gait and plait behind at trot.
- The tuber sacrale on the affected side may be lower than the opposite tuber sacrale due to displacement of the fractured part of the bone (Figure 12.22).
- Pressing firmly on the skin over the displaced tuber sacrale is usually very painful and causes muscle spasm.
- There may be gradual wastage of the gluteal muscles with an incomplete stress fracture. Marked wasting of the muscles occurs within two weeks of a complete fracture occurring (Figure 12.23).
- Bilateral complete fractures are very serious and often necessitate destruction of the horse.
- Ilial wing fractures close to the sacroiliac joint may cause instability and pain in this region, leading to chronic problems.

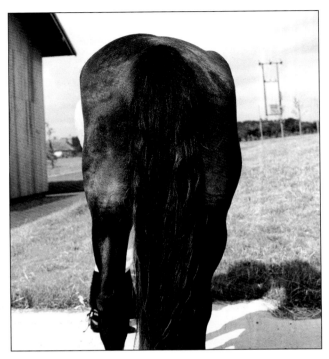

Figure 12.23 Marked muscle wastage following a pelvic fracture

FRACTURES OF THE ILIAL SHAFT

Fractures of the ilial shaft occur following falls or in response to the stresses of fast exercise. The signs are:

- very severe lameness; the horse is often unable to bear any weight on the limb, especially if the fracture passes through the hip joint
- the iliac arteries may be severed by the sharp edges of bone and cause the horse to go into shock and die from blood loss
- the height of the two tubera coxae and tubera sacrale are no longer the same resulting in pelvic asymmetry
- the overlying muscles are often in spasm.

FRACTURES OF THE TUBER COXAE

The tuber coxae may fracture as the result of a blow, a kick or in response to training stresses. The condition is sometimes referred to as a 'knocked down hip'. The clinical signs are:

- moderate to severe lameness for the first couple of days followed by a rapid improvement
- severe muscle spasm
- a haematoma may form at the fracture site
- soft tissue swelling
- asymmetry of the paired tubera coxae when viewed from behind
- the fractured piece of bone often migrates forwards and downwards to under the skin in the flank region
- sometimes a discharging sinus develops over the fractured piece of bone
- if the skin is broken at the fracture site, the sharp bone may prevent the skin healing over and closing the wound.

FRACTURES OF THE PUBIS AND ISCHIUM

These fractures are much less common than fractures of the ileal wing and shaft. If the tuber ischii is fractured by the horse falling over backwards, there is often:

- obvious soft tissue swelling
- pain and crepitus (grating of bone) on palpation
- patchy sweating on the back of the thigh from nerve damage
- the tail may be held to the affected side as a result of muscle spasm.
- wasting of the attached muscles

Diagnosis

Diagnosis of pelvic fractures is made on the following.

- The clinical signs.
- Rectal examination. The fracture or an associated haematoma may be felt on the inside of the pelvis. If the horse is asked to walk forwards slowly, or gently rocked from side to side, crepitus may be felt or heard.
- Crepitus may also be heard by placing a stethoscope over the gluteal muscles and rocking the horse gently from side to side.
- Palpation and manipulation of the bony landmarks and muscles of the pelvis which is painful.
- Ultrasonography is very useful for diagnosing fractures of the ileal wing and shaft.
- Scintigraphy (a bone scan) is often used to diagnose a pelvic fracture. The increased bone turnover at the fracture site causes increased uptake of the radioactive material. However, this may not be evident for several days after the fracture has occurred.
- Radiography is not routinely used because the large amount of overlying muscle means that poor images are obtained. The very powerful X-rays needed are hazardous to the people helping with the procedure. Occasionally they are taken with the horse lying on its back under general anaesthetic. This has the additional risk of further injury being caused during the horse's recovery from the anaesthetic.

Treatment

This involves the following.

- A minimum of 2–3 months box rest. If the shaft of the ilium is fractured, the horse is tied up for the first month to reduce the risk of the iliac arteries being severed as the horse lies down and gets up. Daily walking exercise is introduced as advised by the vet.
- Non-steroidal anti-inflammatory drugs, e.g. phenylbutazone, are administered to control inflammation and pain.
- If the horse is non-weight-bearing on one hind limb, the supporting limb is at risk of laminitis. If possible, a frog support should be fitted. If the horse is unable to stand on the affected limb to allow this, the horse should be kept on a very deep, supportive bed. A support bandage should be applied to the other limbs.
- If the horse is in distress and experiencing severe pain, a small dose of acepromazine helps to relieve the anxiety.
- Following the period of box rest, the horse should be turned out into a tiny paddock for at least a further 2 months.

The healing may be monitored by repeat ultrasound examinations. Complete healing takes up to 1 year in some cases.

Prognosis

The prognosis is very poor if the fracture involves the acetabulum (hip joint). Those fractures that affect the shaft of the ilium have a guarded prognosis. Horses with incomplete, minimally displaced fractures of the ileal wing have a reasonably good prognosis with appropriate care and rest. Fractures of the tuber coxae and tuber ischii also have a reasonable prognosis.

Displacement of the bone or large amounts of bony callus formed during healing may restrict the diameter of the pelvic cavity sufficiently to make breeding of affected mares inadvisable. Pregnancy increases the strain on the pelvis and should not be considered without conferring with your vet or until healing is complete.

SACROILIAC DISEASE

Anatomy

The sacroiliac joint connects the pelvis to the vertebral column (Figures 12.24a and b, and see Figure 12.4). The upper surface of the wing of the sacrum articulates with the ventral surface of the wing of the ilium. The joint capsule is attached closely to the edge of the joint. The strong ventral sacroiliac ligament surrounds the joint and provides a strong attachment between the sacrum and the ilium. All the power from the hind limbs is transmitted to the vertebral column through this joint. It is therefore designed for stability rather than movement. A small amount of flexion and extension occurs.

Additional strong ligaments join the sacrum and the pelvis, helping to support and stabilize the joint. Pain arises when these ligaments are strained and subsequent joint instability may lead to degenerative, osteoarthritic changes. However, our understanding of sacroiliac disease is incomplete because the joint lies under a large muscle mass and is not accessible to many of our diagnostic techniques and imaging methods.

Causes

Acute sacroiliac disease may be caused by:
- an acute traumatic injury, e.g. slipping or falling during work or flipping over backwards
- any injury that causes pelvic rotation can strain the sacroiliac ligaments and joint
- complete fractures of the ilial wing (see page 351) can cause instability of the sacroiliac joint.

Chronic sacroiliac disease:
- may be the result of long-term overuse of the horse leading to sacroiliac joint osteoarthritis rather than a single traumatic incident.
- can develop if an acute injury is not rested sufficiently
- may develop secondary to a lower hind limb lameness that changes the horse's gait and puts strain on the sacroiliac ligaments.

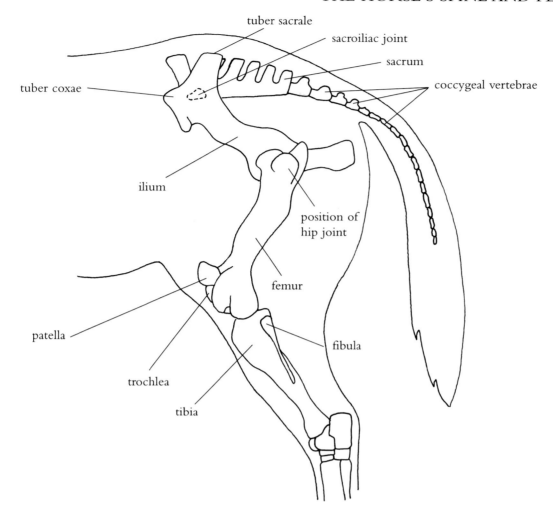

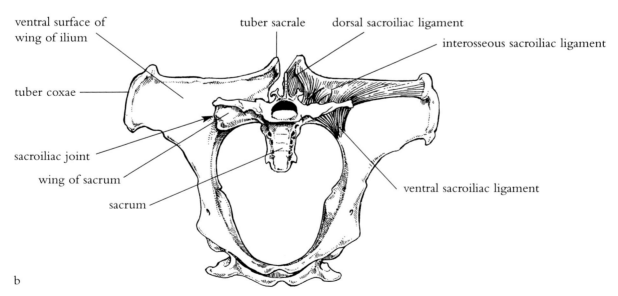

Figure 12.24a and b a) Lateral view of the stifle, hip and sacroiliac joints of the horse; b) cranial view of the pelvic anatomy showing position of sacroiliac joint

Clinical signs

These are variable and depend on whether the horse has an acute injury or chronic disease. If the injury is acute, the horse is likely to show the following.

- Significant hind limb lameness on the affected side.
- Painful spasm of the overlying gluteal muscles.
- Pain when firm pressure is applied to the tubera sacrale and surrounding soft tissues.
- If the sacroiliac ligaments rupture and the joint surfaces are partially or completely torn apart (known as subluxation and luxation respectively), there may be an upward displacement of the tuber sacrale on the side of the injury which was not present before the injury occurred. Bilateral disruption and displacement can occur. These injuries are uncommon.
- With a complete ileal wing fracture, the tuber sacrale is often displaced downwards on the affected side (see Figure 12.22)

Horses with chronic injuries are likely to experience a deep, aching pain and may show the following.

- Loss of performance.
- Lack of hind limb engagement and propulsion resulting in a shortened stride.
- Mild, intermittent, unilateral or bilateral hind limb lameness.
- The lameness occurs on the affected side. It is not usually exacerbated by flexion of the limb. However, if the horse is forced to stand on the affected limb during a flexion test or routine shoeing of the opposite limb, it may show resentment and discomfort. The farrier may be the first to notice this.
- Gait abnormalities, e.g. rolling excessively from side to side, dragging the toes of the hind feet, an outward swing (circumduction) of the lower limb when the hind limb is brought forwards.
- Stiffness of the horse's back.
- Loss of enthusiasm for work and resistance to certain movements, e.g. bucking on transition from trot to canter.
- Repeatedly changing legs at canter or becoming disunited.
- Reluctance to jump.
- The significance of slight asymmetry of the tubera sacrale is the subject of much debate as it can be an incidental finding in clinically normal horses. In the past it was considered to be the result of joint subluxation but this is now disputed. It may result from differences in the thickness of overlying soft tissues as a result of asymmetric muscle or ligament forces acting on the pelvis from previous injuries (Figure 12.25). Horses with level tubera sacrale can experience sacroiliac pain. The horse must be standing square on a firm, level surface when the symmetry of the pelvis is assessed.
- Muscle wasting may occur on the affected side.

Diagnosis

Diagnosis of sacroiliac disease can be very difficult because of the inaccessibility of the joint. Other causes of hind limb lameness must be ruled out, e.g. back pain and distal hock joint pain. Nerve blocks may be used to check that the lameness is not coming from the limbs.

A number of tests may be used to establish a diagnosis. They include the following.

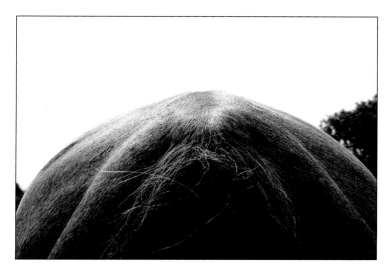

Figure 12.25 Slight asymmetry of the tubera sacrale is not always significant

PALPATION AND MANIPULATIVE TESTS

- Firm palpation of the tuber sacrale and surrounding soft tissues may be painful and cause the horse to sink down. Painful spasm of the gluteal and hamstring muscles may be elicited. Pressing on the dorsal spinous processes of the caudal lumbar and the sacral vertebrae may cause the same response.

- A number of manipulative tests can be used to detect discomfort in the sacroiliac region, e.g. squeezing the opposing tubera sacrale together or applying rhythmic downward pressure to each of the tuber coxae. These are just two of several tests your vet may use.

- The tubera sacrale normally move together when the horse moves. If there is a luxation or ilial wing fracture, they can be seen or felt to move independently at walk.

- Apart from identification of fractures and severe instability of the joint, rectal examination is not usually helpful.

- Flexion of the affected limb does not exacerbate the lameness.

INJECTION OF LOCAL ANAESTHETIC

Because the joint is so small and deep (it only contains about 1ml of synovial fluid), accurate injection of local anaesthetic is not possible. However, injecting local anaesthetic close to the joint and allowing it to diffuse locally may alleviate the pain. This test is not completely reliable.

SCINTIGRAPHY (BONE SCAN)

This is one of the most commonly used imaging techniques. In some cases it is very informative and helps to confirm the diagnosis. However, the results are not always conclusive, even with expert interpretation.

ULTRASONOGRAPHY

Ultrasound examination is useful for imaging of the more superficial associated structures, e.g. the wing of the ileum and the dorsal sacroiliac ligament. The ventral ligaments and joint margins are examined using a rectal probe.

RADIOGRAPHY

Radiographs are not generally helpful owing to the depth of the joint and the thickness of overlying muscle and bone.

POST MORTEM EXAMINATION

The significance of degenerative changes of the sacroiliac joint is uncertain as they are found in many sound horses examined at post mortem.

Treatment

The pain from sacroiliac injuries may arise from 2 sources:

1   inflammation of the ligaments (known as desmitis)
2   joint pain which occurs when there is instability and arthritis of the joint.

The treatment for these conditions is as follows.

ACUTE AND CHRONIC SACROILIAC LIGAMENT INJURIES (INCLUDING SACROILIAC SUBLUXATION)

Horses with sacroiliac ligament injuries need an extended period of strict rest and controlled exercise in order to allow the ligaments to heal. A premature return to work will impair healing and may lead to chronic disease.

- A 6-week period of strict box rest is recommended for horses with acute injuries.
- The sacroiliac region may be iced or hosed with cold water for the first 48 hours. This may be followed up by heat treatment (see page 363) for 1–2 weeks.
- After 4–6 weeks, short sessions of walking out in hand may be introduced and gradually increased over the next 8 weeks.
- After 3–4 months of box rest, the horse may be allowed access to a small outside run (no larger than a stable) and in-hand walking is continued for a further 3 months.
- Back stretches and strengthening exercises can be started approximately 1 month after the injury has occurred and continued throughout the 6-month period of extended rest.
- The healing of the ligament should be monitored by ultrasound examination every 8 weeks and the exercise programme adjusted accordingly. Walking over poles and low obstacles may be included.
- Once healing of the ligament has been confirmed by ultrasound, the horse may then be turned out into a small paddock. This often takes 4–6 months but some horses require up to 1 year of confinement.

- Once the horse is sound and the ligament has healed, the horse may gradually be re-introduced to ridden exercise. Regular light exercise on a horse walker or lungeing with side reins or a chambon for several weeks helps to build up the horse's strength before light, ridden exercise is commenced. A lightweight rider is recommended if possible. It often takes 6–12 months of rest and controlled exercise before the horse is ready to attempt more athletic work.

- Non-steroidal anti-inflammatory drugs, e.g. phenylbutazone, may be prescribed for the first couple of weeks to reduce the associated inflammation and pain.

- Acupuncture, osteopathic or chiropractic techniques and physiotherapy are helpful for pain relief and relieving muscle spasm.

- Local injections of corticosteroids or Sarapin® are sometimes helpful in settling the inflammation and pain. Sarapin® is a substance that alters transmission of nerve impulses in the nerve fibres that transmit chronic pain signals. Its use is reported to alleviate the pain in some horses.

- Injection of sclerosing agents to cause thickening of the sacroiliac ligaments may increase the joint stability and can alleviate the lameness. However, there is potential for nerve damage with disastrous consequences.

Following a period of rest, horses with chronic disease should be kept in regular, light work to strengthen the supporting muscles. The exercise programme or use of the horse may have to be modified as trotting, galloping and jumping all put stress on the sacroiliac ligaments.

CHRONIC SACROILIAC ARTHRITIS
Horses with degenerative changes of the sacroiliac joint are treated in the following way.

- The joint may be injected with corticosteroid and following 48 hours of box rest and controlled exercise the horse is turned out for 7 days.

- An in-hand exercise programme is given to build up the strength of the back and croup musculature for 4–8 weeks before ridden exercise commences.

- Back stretches and strengthening exercises are helpful.

- Regular ridden exercise is introduced over 2–3 months.

- The horse should be kept as fit as possible to prevent recurrence of the disease. This usually requires daily work.

- Acupuncture, chiropractic adjustments and physiotherapy can be helpful.

- Non-steroidal anti-inflammatory drugs may be necessary for the first 2–3 weeks.

Prognosis
The prognosis is guarded. Many horses with sacroiliac problems are not able to return to their previous level of performance. Many exhibit intermittent, low-grade lameness which reduces with rest and recurs with work.

13
THERAPIES

PHYSIOTHERAPY

The purpose of physiotherapy is to assist the natural healing of the tissues following an injury. It helps to restore normal function to the injured part of the body and provides relief from pain. Physiotherapy also has an important role in rehabilitation. Specific exercises and techniques are used to optimize tissue repair and build up strength and mobility.

Who performs physiotherapy?

Physiotherapy should only be undertaken by a **chartered physiotherapist**, or **veterinary physiotherapist** who is a member of the Association of Chartered Physiotherapists in Animal Therapy (ACPAT). A chartered physiotherapist has extensive training in human physiotherapy and the letters MCSP after their name. A veterinary physiotherapist has an additional Post Graduate Diploma/Master of Science degree in Veterinary Physiotherapy.

Physiotherapy may be carried out with permission from the treating vet, once a diagnosis has been made. In order to select the most appropriate treatment, the physiotherapist will take a detailed history and examine the horse thoroughly. This involves a comprehensive assessment of the whole horse, not just the injured part.

What conditions are likely to respond to physiotherapy?

- Soft tissue injuries, e.g. muscles, tendons, ligaments, joints.
- Back pain.
- Neck problems.
- Muscle tension.
- Muscle wasting.
- Nerve injury.
- Wounds that are slow to heal.
- Poor performance.

Physiotherapy can also play an important role in the restoration of function following surgery. Many competition horses enjoy and benefit from physiotherapy as part of the preparation before a competition as well as to assist recovery afterwards.

Physiotherapy treatments

These usually involve a combination of the following.

APPLICATION OF COLD AND HEAT (see below)

MANUAL TECHNIQUES

- Soft tissue and joint mobilization and manipulation (Figure 13.1).
- Stretching (Figure 13.2).
- Massage.

THE USE OF THERAPEUTIC MACHINES

These include:

- magnetic field therapy
- low intensity laser therapy
- muscle stimulators
- TENS
- therapeutic ultrasound.

EXERCISE THERAPY

Controlled exercise is a very important part of the rehabilitation programme following an injury. It is essential that the demands on the horse are increased very slowly to build up strength and muscle tone before normal exercise is resumed. The programme will depend on the nature of the injury and how long the horse has been off work. It should be designed to develop suppleness and balance while gradually building up muscular strength. In the early stages the horse is likely to benefit from exercise without the

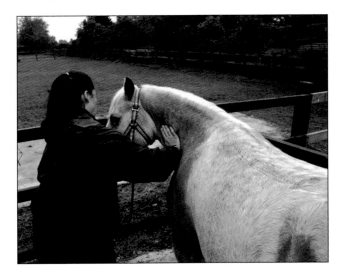

Figure 13.1 Physiotherapist performing manual therapy on a pony's neck

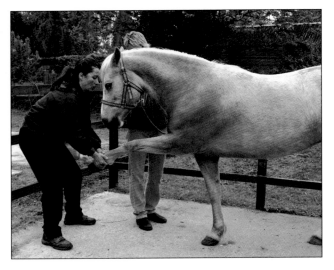

Figure 13.2 Soft tissue mobilization through stretching

weight of a rider. He may have become accustomed to moving in a certain way to alleviate pain and need help to restore the normal movement pattern.

The following may be used for rehabilitation:

- horse walker
- treadmill
- swimming pool (see Figure 8.7)
- cold water hydrotherapy unit
- training aids such as the Chambon or Pessoa
- application of weights to a limb
- application of materials such as sticky tape in a way that heightens sensation in particular muscle groups and causes the horse to alter its gait, helping to re-establish a normal movement pattern.

The use of all of these aids requires experience and an in-depth understanding of the goals of treatment. Incorrect use has the potential to aggravate the existing injury or even create a new problem. The rehabilitation programme should be drawn up following consultation between the vet and the physiotherapist.

Some of these treatments are now discussed in more detail.

Cold treatment

Cold treatment is used for bruises and strains of tendons, muscles, joints and ligaments. It is of maximum benefit immediately after the injury occurs and in the following 24–48 hours. The low temperature causes constriction of the blood vessels which decreases the amount of haemorrhage in the damaged tissue; it also helps to relieve pain. In order to minimize further swelling when the cold treatment has finished, injuries to the lower limb should be appropriately bandaged.

Cold can be applied in several ways.

COLD HOSING

This is done for 20 minutes, 3 times a day.

ICED WATER

The affected limb is immersed in a bucket of cold water with added ice. This is usually done for 15 minutes, 3 times a day. Standing a horse is a stream is an effective way of providing cold treatment if there is a suitable one nearby. Special boots are available for cold water treatment of lower limb injuries. Some can be attached to refrigeration units to control the temperature of the circulating water (see Figure 7.4).

CRUSHED ICE, FROZEN PEAS

These can be applied to the injured area over a thin layer of material such as a tea towel. Frozen substances must not be placed in direct contact with the skin or ice scald may occur. These are left on for up to 30 minutes.

COMMERCIALLY AVAILABLE COLD PACKS AND BANDAGES

These can be stored ready for use in the freezer. They stay cold for approximately 15 minutes.

Heat treatment

Heat treatment is often used in conjunction with massage and controlled exercise. It should not be used within the first 24–48 hours after an injury occurs as it may provoke further haemorrhage.

Heat increases the blood supply to the damaged tissue. This provides increased oxygen and more white blood cells to clear up the debris. The improved blood and lymph flow promote resorption of blood and fluid from the injured area. The warmth helps to relieve muscle spasm and reduce the pain, making the horse more comfortable and relaxed. It also improves the horse's range of motion.

Superficial heat does not penetrate far beneath the skin. It can be applied by:

* infra-red lamps (Figure 13.3)
* heated pads or blankets
* hot poultices
* hot tubbing.

Deep heat is provided by ultrasound.

Massage

Massage is used to improve the circulation through the tissues. It can be used to reduce oedema and relieve muscle spasm. Skilled massage can help to prevent adhesions forming and help break down existing ones. Many horses enjoy massage; in addition to pain relief, it helps them to relax.

Magnetic field therapy

There are two types of magnetic therapy available.

Static magnets are incorporated into boots,

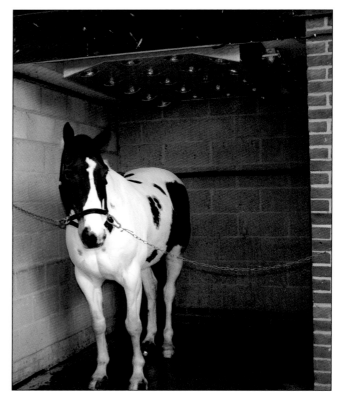

Figure 13.3 Infrared heat lamps

tendon wraps and blankets for the horse or can be bandaged directly in place. These magnets vary in strength. They can be left on the horse without constant supervision for up to 12 hours at a time.

Electromagnetic field therapy units produce low frequency pulsed magnetic fields. These may be operated by batteries or require an electricity supply. The settings of the instrument can be varied according to the condition being treated. The treatment times are shorter but the horse must be supervised throughout the duration of the treatment.

The effects of magnetic fields on body tissues are not fully understood. Living tissues generate electromagnetic fields around them. When tissues are injured, the normal electrical charge across the cell membrane is disturbed and this disrupts cell metabolism. Applied magnetic fields of the appropriate strength are able to influence the passage of chemical ions through cell membranes and help to restore the normal electrical charge. Electromagnetic field therapy has proved useful for:

- improving the circulation
- pain relief
- fracture healing
- treatment of sore shins.

It is contraindicated in the presence of infection.

Low intensity laser therapy (LILT)

Low intensity lasers are used in equine practice to stimulate wound healing, tissue repair and also for pain relief. The machine emits a narrow, focused beam of red or infra-red (invisible) light which penetrates a variable depth into the tissues. The wavelength of the light governs the depth of penetration and the power and wavelength can be altered by selecting different probes.

The laser assists healing by stimulating the production of collagen and blood vessels as well as activating various cells such as mast cells and macrophages involved in tissue repair and immune response. This can result in:

- faster healing
- increase in tensile strength of the repaired tissue
- reduction of scarring
- stimulation of the immune system
- control of infection
- reduction of inflammation
- pain relief
- acupuncture point stimulation.

Pain relief may be due to stimulation of acupuncture points causing release of endorphins and serotonin which influence pain pathways and suppression of pain-detecting nerve endings. When acute injuries are treated, the horse's exercise should be controlled so further damage is not caused by over-use of the injured limb while the pain is reduced.

Laser treatment can speed up the healing of wounds in equine practice and reduce the speed of bacterial multiplication in infected sites. The more powerful lasers are effective for treatment of superficial ligament and tendon injuries as they can penetrate up to 3 cm (1 in) below the skin surface. Chronic injuries require more stimulation than acute conditions and a mild inflammatory response may be seen at the start of treatment. Although this can cause the patient to experience increased discomfort for a short period of time, it will start off the healing process.

FREQUENCY OF TREATMENT

This depends on the type of injury. Initial treatment may be daily for 2–3 days, then 2 or 3 times a week. It should be used as soon as possible after the injury occurs. A response should be seen after 2–3 treatments.

PRECAUTIONS AND CONTRAINDICATIONS

- The laser beam can cause permanent damage to the retina of the eye so protective glasses should be worn by the owner and the therapist. The beam should never be pointed at or into the eye.
- The beam should not be applied over the uterus of a pregnant mare.
- If steroid has been injected, the laser should not be used over the injection site for 48 hours.

Muscle stimulators

Muscle stimulators produce an electrical signal that stimulates muscles to contract. They are used to:

- identify muscle pain or weakness (Figure 13.4)
- restore muscle strength and function following an injury
- maintain muscle tone and blood supply following nerve damage and reduce muscle atrophy
- keep the muscles functioning when the horse is on strict rest for injuries such as fractures or joint and tendon problems

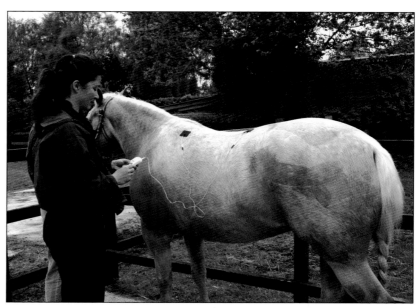

Figure 13.4 Physiotherapist using neuromuscular electrical stimulation to identify muscle pain or weakness

- increase the circulation
- provide pain relief.

The frequency (measured in Hertz) can be adjusted for different therapeutic effects. Low frequency treatment creates visible muscle contractions which aid lymphatic drainage and venous return of blood. High-frequency treatments provide pain relief. More than one frequency can be used at one time.

Transcutaneous electrical nerve stimulation (TENS)

These instruments can be used for pain relief. The pads are placed so that the current passes through the painful area. It works by preventing pain signals from the area reaching the brain. It also stimulates the release of natural opioids.

Therapeutic ultrasound

An ultrasound machine converts electrical energy into high-frequency sound waves. These penetrate the tissues and produce minute vibrations and heat. Ultrasound has the following effects on injured tissue:

- assists natural healing
- encourages resolution of inflammation
- encourages the growth of new capillaries in the damaged tissue
- stimulates collagen synthesis
- improves the alignment of collagen fibrils.

It is used for:

- muscle, ligament and tendon injuries
- to relieve muscle spasm
- treatment of stiff or arthritic joints
- encouraging resorption of haematomas after the first 48 hours
- improving blood flow through damaged tissue
- to increase the elasticity of scar tissue.

The ultrasound machine should only be used by an experienced operator. If used incorrectly, it can cause serious overheating and damage to bone. Ultrasound should not be used over tumours, open wounds, infected tissues, the brain, the eyes or the reproductive tract. Nor should it be used to treat epiphyseal plates or fractures.

Summary

The appropriate use of physiotherapy assists the natural healing of the tissues. The quality of the repaired tissue is optimized and in some cases this will improve the likelihood of the horse returning to its previous type of work and level of performance.

EXTRACORPOREAL SHOCK WAVE THERAPY (ESWT)

What is shock wave therapy?

Shock waves were used in human medicine over 20 years ago to break down kidney stones (lithotripsy). More recently it has been shown to stimulate bone formation and ligament healing. Thus it has proved a useful tool in the treatment of conditions such as tennis elbow, plantar fasciitis and stress fractures.

Shock waves are high-energy acoustic (sound) waves that build up to high amplitude in a very short period of time. These shock waves travel through the tissues until they encounter an interface between different types of tissue, e.g. soft tissue/bone. At the boundary between different tissues the resistance to the flow of the shock waves is altered and the result is that mechanical energy is released.

How does it work?

How this release of energy affects healing is not fully understood. It is thought to stimulate the body's own healing. The proposed mechanisms include:

- increased activity of osteoblasts (bone forming cells)
- stimulation of new blood vessel growth
- stimulation of nerve endings (nociceptors) which release neurotransmitters and block pain signals from reaching the brain (gate theory)
- induction of cytokines, e.g. TGF-β1 which play a role in healing.

Radial and focused shock waves

There are two different types of shock wave therapy. Radial shock waves do not penetrate so far into the tissues and expose the site being treated and the surrounding tissues to similar pressures. Focused shock waves can be accurately delivered to the site of injury with less pressure exerted on the neighbouring tissues. Both types have a number of probes so the depth of penetration can be altered.

With both systems the energy is transferred between the shock wave probe and the body with the aid of a coupling gel.

What conditions is it used for?

Shock wave therapy has only recently been used in equine veterinary medicine. It has been used for the following conditions with some success.

- Tendonitis.
- Ligament injuries.
- Fractures, e.g:
    - stress fractures, e.g. of the tibia
    - splint bone fractures

- proximal sesamoid fractures
- non-union fractures (i.e. fractures that are not healing properly).
- Periostitis (inflammation of the periosteum of a bone), e.g. 'bucked shins'.
- Navicular syndrome.
- 'Kissing spines'.
- Sacroiliac conditions.
- Back pain.
- Osteoarthritis of the distal tarsal joints (bone spavin).
- Osteoarthritis of the interphalangeal joints (ringbone).

The procedure

The treatment can be painful and noisy, so is usually carried out with the horse sedated. The coat is clipped and then cleaned to remove any scale or dirt. Alcohol and a coupling gel are applied. With fine-coated horses it may be possible to treat without clipping.

The appropriate head of the unit will be selected according to the type of injury and the depth of the injury from the skin surface. The energy settings and number of shocks also depends on the condition being treated and the type of tissue.

The probe is placed on the skin over the area to be treated. It is gently rocked during treatment to reduce the possibility of bruising.

Number of treatments

This is still a subject of ongoing discussion and depends on the type of injury. Bones generally require 1 or possibly 2 treatments. Acute suspensory ligament and tendon injuries are given 2 or 3 treatments at 2-week intervals. Chronic injuries usually require 2 or 3 treatments at 3-week intervals. As a general rule, chronic soft tissue and bone lesions usually need higher energy and shock wave numbers than acute injuries.

Management following treatment

Following shock wave therapy, the horse usually has up to a week of box rest with walking exercise in hand. This is to ensure that the horse does not over-exert itself and cause further injury during the initial period of pain relief following the treatment. It is then given a rehabilitation programme appropriate to the condition being treated.

Adverse reactions

Few adverse reactions have been reported. Occasionally the horse will experience increased pain following treatment. Hair loss or regions of white hair growth are a rare occurrence. Haematomas and cell damage can occur if the pressure generated is too high.

Advantages of shock wave therapy

- The treatment is minimally invasive.

- It has few known side effects.
- It takes a short time to perform (10–20 minutes)

Disadvantages of shock wave therapy

- Tissue damage can be caused if the energy or number of shocks is too high.
- There is a risk that the pain relief following treatment will allow the horse to do too much with potentially catastrophic results. Thus it is essential that an accurate diagnosis has been made prior to therapy.
- The cost of the equipment is high.

Contraindications

The following areas should not be treated with shock waves:

- the head
- the heart or lungs as cardiac arrhythmias and tears in the lung tissue can occur
- large nerves and blood vessels
- infected sites
- tumours, e.g. sarcoids
- growth plates of young animals; an exception is its use to specifically affect the growth plate of some foals with angular limb deformities.

Summary

Shock wave therapy is proving to be a useful tool in the treatment of an increasing number of conditions. However, much of the reported success is anecdotal and further research needs to be carried out in order to determine the best treatment protocol for each condition.

14
COMPLEMENTARY THERAPIES

EQUINE ACUPUNCTURE

The history of acupuncture

Acupuncture has been used for more than 3000 years in China. In the UK it has been widely practised in human medicine since the 1970s and most pain clinics now have an acupuncturist as part of their team.

In the veterinary world, acupuncture is increasingly being acknowledged as a useful treatment for a wide range of conditions. This is particularly exciting as it offers another option for patients not responding to conventional veterinary treatment. Insurance companies recognize this and include acupuncture in their cover for veterinary fees.

Who can do acupuncture?

Only a qualified veterinary surgeon is allowed to perform acupuncture on animals. In-depth training and certification is provided by the Association of British Veterinary Acupuncturists (ABVA) and the International Veterinary Acupuncture Society (IVAS). Mastery of acupuncture takes years of study and practice.

What is acupuncture?

Acupuncture involves inserting fine, stainless-steel needles through the skin at specific points called acupuncture points. This is known as **dry needling** (Figure 14.1). The needles commonly used for horses vary in length from a few millimetres ($\frac{1}{4}$ in) to 8 cm (3 in). Once inserted, the needles may be withdrawn immediately or left in place for 20–30 minutes. While in situ, they may be manipulated by hand for stronger stimulation of the point.

There are other types of acupuncture which include the following.

- Electroacupuncture. This is most commonly used for treatment of chronic pain. Electrodes from a battery-operated unit are attached to the inserted needles and the points are stimulated electrically causing muscle contraction. It is particularly effective for treating chronic neck, back or lumbosacral pain (Figure 14.2).

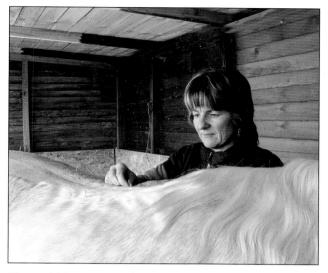

Figure 14.1 Inserting the acupuncture needles; this is known as 'dry needling'

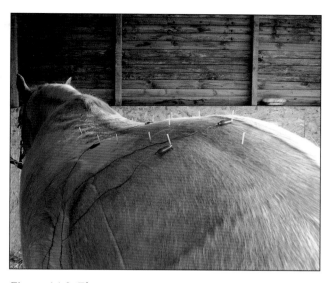

Figure 14.2 Electroacupuncture

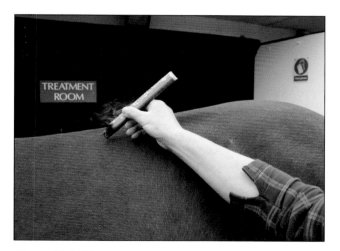

Figure 14.3 Moxa

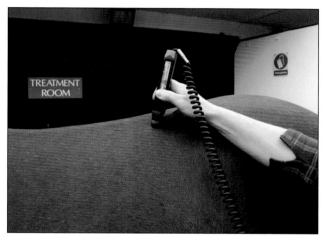

Figure 14.4 Laser acupuncture

- Injection of vitamin B12, local anaesthetic or homeopathic medicines into acupuncture points with hypodermic needles.
- Implantation of gold beads or wire into an acupuncture point to give long-lasting stimulation.
- Moxibustion. Selected acupuncture points are warmed by burning a herb, *Artemesia vulgaris* above the skin. This is especially useful for chronic muscular or arthritic conditions in cold weather (Figure 14.3).
- Laser acupuncture. The acupuncture points are stimulated by a laser. This has the advantage that there is no risk of infection and the treatment is pain free. It is believed by some practitioners to be less effective than needling. However, it is useful for superficial sites directly over joint capsules where needling is potentially hazardous (Figure 14.4).

What are acupuncture points?

Acupuncture points are areas on the skin that have high concentrations of free nerve endings and blood vessels. They have a higher electrical conductivity than the surrounding skin.

What conditions can acupuncture treat?

Acupuncture can be used as part of a treatment protocol for almost any medical condition with the exception of malignant tumours, irreparable fractures and end-stage organ failure. It is often used in conjunction with conventional veterinary treatment and so the patient experiences the benefits of their combined effects.

In equine practice, acupuncture is commonly used for the relief of chronic musculoskeletal pain and to influence the function of internal organs. An example of the latter is the stimulation of intestinal motility in some cases of colic.

Acupuncture is especially useful for treating the following.

- Any type of muscle soreness, particularly of the neck, shoulders, back and hindquarters. Clinical signs that may be alleviated by acupuncture include:
    - cold backs, i.e. resentment of saddling and girthing, dipping on mounting
    - general stiffness, inability to bend on one or both reins
    - head tilt, inability to flex from the poll
    - shortness of stride, not going forward from the leg
    - disunited or 'bunny-hopping' at canter
    - moving unlevel behind
    - 'hopping' in the transition from walk to trot
    - bucking in the transition from trot to canter
    - irritability and bucking
    - soreness experienced during grooming.
- Digestive problems including poor appetite, diarrhoea, some types of colic.
- Respiratory problems.
- Reproductive problems.
- Post-viral lethargy.
- Poor immunity.
- Horses that are just 'under the weather' where a specific diagnosis has not been made despite investigations including blood tests.

How does acupuncture work?
WESTERN SCIENTIFIC EXPLANATION

Inserting an acupuncture needle causes a very small amount of trauma to the tissue. This causes the release of many chemical mediators, each of which plays a role in repairing the damage. As a result of this stimulation, the blood supply and immune status of the tissues is increased and they are better able to deal with any problems.

The acupuncture needles also stimulate sensory nerve endings which transmit impulses to the spinal cord and the brain. This leads to the release of opioid neurotransmitters such as endorphins and enkephalins that have an action similar to morphine and reduce the amount of pain experienced by the horse. This is achieved in two ways. For a horse to experience pain, nerve impulses travel from the site of injury to the spinal cord and thence to the sensory area of the cerebral cortex of the brain, where the sensation of pain is perceived. Acupuncture can stimulate inhibitory nerve pathways that block the transmission of pain at the spinal cord, thus preventing the impulses reaching the brain. Secondly, acupuncture stimulates descending pathways between the brain and the spinal cord which also block incoming pain signals, preventing them travelling from the spinal cord to the brain.

Acupuncture can influence the function of internal organs. This is because the nerve supply to and from the organs travels between the spinal cord and the brain in pathways very close to those from the muscles and the skin and there are connections between them. The acupuncturist can influence the function of the internal organs by placing the needles at specific sites on the body surface.

Finally, the pathways stimulated by acupuncture influence a part of the brain called the hypothalamus. This accounts for the effect of acupuncture on homeostatic regulatory mechanisms such as the control of blood pressure, pulse, respiration, intestinal motility, hormone secretion and white blood cell production. This is important as the purpose of an acupuncture treatment is to restore the patient to a state of balance or homeostasis.

Traditional Chinese Medicine

An acupuncturist who practises Traditional Chinese Medicine (TCM) will look at the whole animal rather than just the diseased part. Consideration will be given to why the disease developed in the first place. Health is defined as a state of harmony of an animal within its internal environment and with its external environment. There is complete physical, mental and social wellbeing and not merely the absence of disease. In TCM a great deal of consideration is given to environmental factors such as Wind, Heat, Cold and Damp and their role in causing disease. Other factors include poor nutrition, lack of exercise, physical strain, traumatic injuries and emotional stress. Extremes of emotion such as joy, worry, grief, fear and anger, all play a part in causing disease.

The patient is given a physical examination which includes 'looking, asking, palpating, listening and smelling'. Inspection of the tongue and feeling the pulse are important parts of the examination. A detailed history is taken and the diagnosis and treatment are determined using the traditional Chinese Five Element theory (Wood, Fire, Earth, Metal and Water) and the Eight Principles (Yin, Yang, Interior, Exterior, Cold, Heat, Deficiency and Excess). Further information can be obtained from the text recommended in the reading list at the end of the book.

The shortened muscle or myofascial pain syndrome

Many horses are chronically stiff and sore because they have **myofascial trigger points** in their muscles. (Myo = muscle, fascia = the dense white fibrous tissue that surrounds muscles.) Myofascial trigger points (MFTPs) are small, circumscribed exquisitely tender areas that may be found in taut bands within a muscle. They may develop from:

- a direct injury
- chronic over-use of a muscle
- chilling
- repeated microtrauma (repetitive strain injury).

They are classified as **active** if they hurt all the time or **latent** if they are painful only when pressure is applied. Firm pressure over any trigger point may cause the muscle to jerk involuntarily. This is known as the **jump sign** and it happens because the nerve endings in the muscle have become abnormally sensitized. These trigger points cause chronic muscle pain in horses and are very commonly found in the lower neck, the abdominal wall and the hamstrings. They cause muscle shortening which is not under voluntary control. This myofascial pain syndrome is responsible for many of the chronically sore backs we see in horses.

The pain experienced by the horse has several characteristics:

- it often develops days or weeks after the original injury appears to have healed
- it can manifest as a deep aching pain or a brief powerful shooting or stabbing pain
- if left untreated, mild stimuli to the affected muscle can generate extreme pain out of all proportion to the stimulus.

Unfortunately it does not end there because pain may be experienced elsewhere in the body due to the muscle shortening. Shortened muscles:

- limit the range of movement of a joint; the horse's gait will become increasingly short and choppy
- may pull on their tendons and their attachments causing tendonitis and tenosynovitis
- can lead to increased pressure on the cartilage of joint surfaces, thus the chronic pull of shortened muscles can lead to degenerative changes within the joint, leading to osteoarthritis; this in turn leads to more pain, further muscle shortening and thus the vicious cycle is perpetuated.

THE 'BUTE' TEST

A feature of this type of pain is that it may not respond to non-steroidal anti-inflammatory drugs including phenylbutazone (bute). Unfortunately this leads people to mistakenly believe that the horse is not experiencing pain and it is forced to carry on working without treatment.

HOW DOES ACUPUNCTURE AFFECT MYOFASCIAL TRIGGER POINTS?

When a needle penetrates a trigger point, the muscle will often contract and then relax and lengthen almost immediately. Sometimes the needle is 'grasped' by the muscle and the relaxation and lengthening take place over a period of 20–30 minutes. It may be hastened by twirling the needle. As soon as the trigger point is released, the pain and tenderness disappear and the blood supply to the muscle improves immediately.

HORSES, STRESS AND CHRONIC PAIN

We tend to keep horses stabled for many hours of the day and so prevent expression of their natural behaviour and grazing patterns. Stress and anxiety can lead to the development of chronic pain in the horse. When a horse becomes anxious, the body tone is increased and this can cause the muscle groups to become tense and shortened, leading to myofascial pain. It is important not to underestimate the stress that can be caused by stabling, isolation, rehoming, transport and competition schedules.

Acupuncture examination and point selection

Examination of a horse to be treated with acupuncture is no different from any other veterinary examination, apart from including a careful palpation of the whole horse. The selection of points to be treated is determined following a full clinical examination. With a horse suffering from musculoskeletal pain, this will include assessment of the horse in hand, on the lunge and where appropriate, under saddle. It is important not only to identify the problem area but also to ask why it developed and to deal with the causes.

The routine veterinary tools used in establishing a diagnosis may include:
- clinical examination including flexion tests
- nerve blocks
- radiography
- ultrasonography
- scintigraphy
- thermography
- MRI scans.

Also included in the examination is:
- a dental examination: a sore or dysfunctional mouth will quickly lead to myofascial pain elsewhere in the body
- an assessment of foot balance: mediolateral imbalance or 'long-toe, low-heel' syndrome can lead to chronic lameness
- a bridle and saddle examination: it is important to check that the bridle, bit and saddle are correctly fitted and suitable for the horse

- an assessment of the rider's ability: unfortunately, some riders are unwittingly the cause of their horse's discomfort; it is important to identify this and arrange for professional help in this area if necessary.

Taking a good history is essential as chronic pain may be the result of an injury that occurred and appeared to heal many months or even years ago. Temperament changes are important as the horse only has a limited number of ways to express discomfort. Certain behaviour patterns may be classified as 'resistance', when what the horse is really saying is 'I can't' or 'This hurts'.

Taking the history in the stable gives the horse some time to become accustomed to the vet before the examination begins.

PALPATION

The acupuncture point examination involves careful palpation of the horse to find areas of abnormal sensitivity to either light or deep pressure. It is important for the horse to be relaxed and comfortable so the horse is usually examined in the stable wearing just a headcollar.

The individual points are tested using fingertips or a blunt probe such as the rounded end of a pen. The pressure is gentle to begin with and gradually increased. The reaction of the horse is observed carefully as it may be a tiny muscle twitch, a slight movement away from the pressure or a change of facial expression. Alternatively, the horse may swish its tail, turn round and bite or lash out when a sensitive area is palpated.

THE TREATMENT

When the acupuncturist has selected the points to be treated, they are collectively called a 'treatment formula'. This is worked out after considering the findings of the clinical examination, the sore areas, which nerves supply them and the principles of Traditional Chinese Medicine. Between 1 and 20 needles are commonly used.

Will the horse or pony object to treatment?

This depends on the condition being treated and the temperament of the horse. Ill horses and those with colic are usually very tolerant and many become profoundly relaxed and appear to enjoy the experience. Most horses with musculoskeletal pain accept the treatment and show little discomfort when the needles are inserted (Figures 14.5 and 14.6). Acupuncture definitely works best if the horse, the owner and the vet are calm and relaxed.

The treatment of trigger points and chronic back pain can be uncomfortable and while many horses will stoically stand for the treatment, others may need a little sedation and analgesia for effective treatment to be given. The safety of the horse, its handler and the vet are of paramount importance.

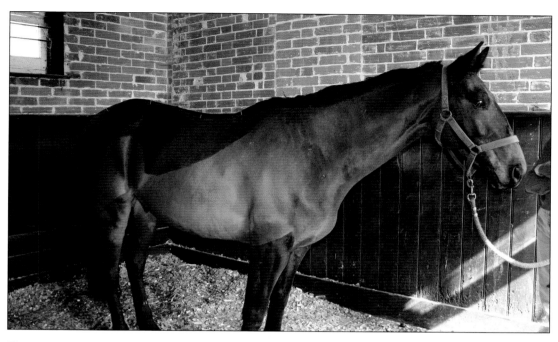

Figure 14.5 Most horses tolerate acupuncture well and are happy and relaxed with the needles in place

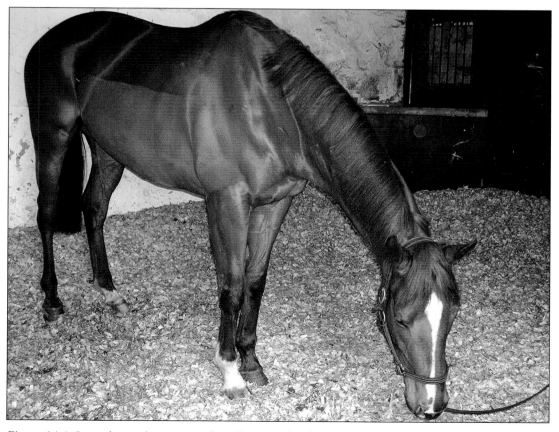

Figure 14.6 Some horses become profoundly relaxed and sleepy

How many treatments will the horse require?

With musculosketetal problems, the number of treatments is variable, depending on the severity of the symptoms and how long the horse has been experiencing the pain. Acute injuries may only require one or two treatments. Realistically, a horse that has been experiencing back pain for months or years is likely to need four or five treatments at weekly intervals to start with, followed by a couple more at fortnightly intervals.

It is important to be realistic in one's expectations. When the problem has developed owing to the horse's conformation, acupuncture is likely to be needed at regular intervals as the underlying problem remains. The aim of treatment in these cases is to enable the horse to continue to perform without pain and so lengthen and improve the quality of its working life.

When acupuncture is used to stimulate gut motility and reduce the pain associated with colic, a single session usually suffices.

Acupuncture as a preventative treatment

Acupuncture has a valuable role as a preventative treatment. Fit competition horses taking part in a wide range of disciplines are prone to developing minor injuries that often go unnoticed. Eventually these build up and cause the horse to compensate by altering its way of moving and this makes it susceptible to more serious injury. Regular examination and treatment throughout the season can catch these injuries at an early stage. By restoring normal blood supply and function to the muscles, they heal quickly and competition schedules are uninterrupted.

How will the horse feel following acupuncture?

Most horses and ponies are very relaxed following treatment. Owners are always warned that the horse may feel better, worse or the same following the first session. Most horses treated for musculoskeletal problems will show some improvement. Very often the owners report that the horse seems much happier in himself. Subsequent treatments tend to give longer remissions until the horse remains pain free.

Occasionally, those being treated for very sore backs experience tenderness for up to 48 hours following the first treatment. The vet will usually advise against brushing or ridden exercise for that period of time. A horse should never be worked hard immediately following acupuncture.

It is important to realize that, as with every treatment, there will be failures as well as successes.

Are there any risks?

As acupuncture can only be done by a vet who will have a good knowledge of anatomy, the risk to the patient is minimal. By far the greatest risk is that the vet will be kicked or bitten!

The very small risks include:

- haematoma
- infection
- 'stuck' needles
- needle breakage.

These risks can be minimized by ensuring that the horse is:

- suitably restrained with a good headcollar and an experienced handler
- clean and dry
- in a stable with a non-slip floor: rubber matting is ideal so that any dropped needles are easily retrieved
- calm and relaxed.

Rehabilitation

When a horse is treated with acupuncture, it is important that it is re-examined prior to each treatment. Where possible, factors which contributed to the problem should be addressed and removed. If appropriate, the horse's owner should be given an exercise programme and advice on rehabilitation.

Summary

Acupuncture can be used to achieve a therapeutic or homeostatic effect. It stimulates nerves, increases local blood flow, relieves muscle spasm and causes the release of a number of neurotransmitters. We still do not know all of the pathways involved, but increased interest is stimulating new research into the neurophysiological basis of acupuncture.

Acupuncture provides an exciting new tool for veterinary surgeons to use. It may be used in conjunction with conventional treatment or as a primary therapy. It works well with manual therapies including chiropractic and osteopathy. Acupuncture provides another option when the results of conventional treatment have been disappointing.

MANIPULATIVE THERAPIES: OSTEOPATHY AND CHIROPRACTIC

Introduction

Osteopathic and chiropractic medicine share many of the same treatment principles and mechanisms of action as acupuncture. Practitioners of each of these disciplines usually adopt a holistic approach and recognize that health is a state of harmony of an animal both within its body and with its external environment. Healthy people and animals have physical, mental and social wellbeing and not merely the absence of disease.

The body is finely tuned and each part is in communication with every other part through the flow of body fluids and nerve impulses. All the organs and tissues in the body are joined and held together by connective tissue called fascia. This takes the form of tough sheets of fibrous tissue covering muscles and the protective tissues surrounding the brain and internal organs. It supports and links all of the bones, muscles, internal organs, blood vessels and nerves.

The body relies on circulation of blood for the distribution of nutrients, oxygen supply and hormones to all parts of the body and also for the removal of wastes. An intact nervous system is necessary for the transmission of information from the environment and within the body to all other parts of the body so that appropriate responses can be generated. Any mechanical injury can interrupt the flow of body fluids and nerve impulses, ultimately causing pain and dysfunction. A local injury can have far-reaching effects due to alteration in the patterns of nerve signals and by affecting blood flow and lymphatic drainage. The body has a great capacity to adapt to the environment and heal itself when problems occur. Disease results when this ability is overwhelmed.

Osteopaths treat not only the area of dysfunction but the interactions of the entire spine. Treatment is aimed at restoring the function of the animal as a whole by re-establishing the body symmetry and normal range of movement of the joints and associated tissues. Chiropractic treatment is similar but the emphasis is on manipulation of the vertebrae to correct local positional changes of the skeleton that have occurred as a result of muscle tension. The goal of treatment is to reduce musculoskeletal pain and restore joint mobility, normal muscle function and neurological reflexes.

Tissue injury and the concept of 'facilitation' or 'wind-up'

When a horse is injured, chemicals are released from the inflamed tissues. These stimulate nerve endings which carry signals to the spinal cord. The spinal cord sends these signals on to the brain where they are perceived as pain. Sometimes the nerve cells in the spinal cord become sensitized to the incoming pain messages and send increased pain signals to the brain. Initially this is a normal response which prevents the horse from using the affected area and aggravating the injury. However, sustained overactivity of these nerve cells, known as **facilitation** or **wind-up**, is harmful as the sensation of pain can be generated from stimuli such as light touch. Pain may also continue to be felt after the injury has healed.

It is believed that tissue has a **pain memory** and that repetitive insults can lead to a lower threshold to the perception of pain and faster onset of wind-up which can occur after just 45 minutes of painful stimulation.

An example may help you to understand the concept of wind-up, which can occur with sensory nerve endings in the skin as well as within the spinal cord. Have you ever purchased a new garment and been slightly irritated by a label contacting the skin? The initial sensation is one of mild irritation rather than pain. However, if the label is not removed, the stimulus is perceived as increasingly painful and the area will become inflamed. The stimulus itself has not changed but sensitization of the nerve endings in the skin due to repeated stimulation make it feel very sore. This soreness can remain some time after the garment is removed. Imagine then the discomfort of the horse that has to tolerate an uncomfortable saddle or numnah.

Facilitation of the spinal cord also influences the outgoing nerve signals to skeletal muscles, causing alteration in muscle tone. This in turn affects the range of motion of the joints and the way the horse moves.

Nerves from the musculoskeletal system share common pathways from the spinal cord to the brain with nerves from the organs of the body. As a result, pain from the internal organs can influence the muscles and vice versa. This is why practitioners of acupuncture, osteopathic and chiropractic treatments undertake a complete and holistic examination of their patients, rather than focusing immediately on the apparent problem.

What happens during the examination?

- A detailed history will be taken. Consideration will be given to previous injuries as well as the current complaint.
- The horse will be examined at rest. The practitioner will assess the conformation, stance and muscle development of the horse. Any abnormal wear pattern on the shoes will be noted.
- The horse is examined at exercise. While the horse is walked and trotted in hand, its movement, stride length and foot placement is assessed. The horse is then observed turning in a small circle. If it is considered necessary, the horse will be seen on the lunge or ridden.
- The patient will be palpated all over. The osteopath or chiropractor will be looking and feeling for changes in tissue texture, areas of increased sensitivity to touch and areas of muscle spasm or discomfort. The range of motion of individual joints is tested to identify the problem areas.

Treatment

The aim of osteopathic and chiropractic treatments is to restore symmetry and freedom of movement to areas affected by injury, thereby improving flow of body fluids and modifying the activity of the nervous system. In this way, the body is allowed to restore itself to a healthy state.

Manipulative techniques

Once the musculoskeletal system of the horse has been thoroughly evaluated, a treatment plan is made. This may include a variety of manipulative techniques to mobilize the joints, stretch the skin, fascia and muscles and ease the pain.

HIGH-VELOCITY, LOW-AMPLITUDE THRUSTS

The aim of this treatment is to restore the lost range of motion or at least to improve it. In humans, the restricted joint is taken to the point where it resists further movement and then subjected to a quick, short thrust in that direction. A clicking sound may be heard and if the manipulation is successful, an increased range of movement and reduction of pain will be experienced. In horses, high-velocity, low-amplitude thrusts are used to relieve muscle tension by activating reflexes within the tense muscles.

SOFT TISSUE THERAPY

This may involve any of the following techniques which can encourage relaxation of tense muscles and tight fascia:

- tissue stretches
- traction (Figure 14.7)
- deep pressure
- massage
- myofascial or sustained positional release: the tissues are taken to a point where they restrict further movement and held in that position until they relax (Figure 14.8).

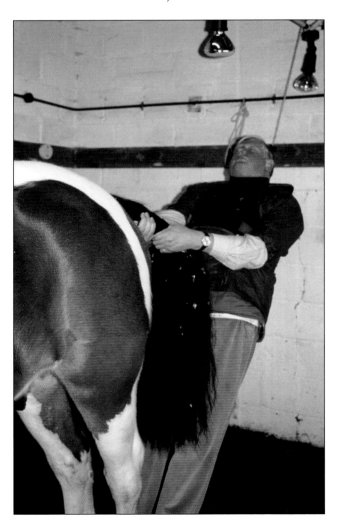

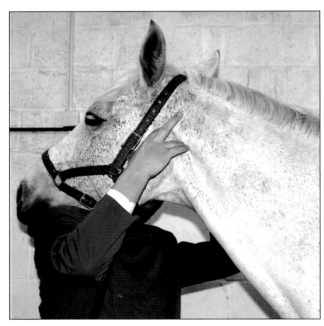

Figure 14.7 Traction applied to the horse's tail (left)

Figure 14.8 Horse undergoing osteopathic treatment for a stiff neck (above)

The treatment will vary according to the needs of the individual patient and the particular skills and experience of the therapist who will constantly reassess the tissues and monitor their response to treatment. An immediate relaxation of tissues is often seen.

THE USE OF SEDATION

If the horse is anxious or in pain, treatment may be helped by light sedation of the horse. Occasionally, horses with long-standing problems are examined and treated under general anaesthesia.

Combining manipulation with acupuncture

The combination of manipulative therapy with acupuncture can sometimes give a better response than either treatment on its own. Both techniques release tension in the muscles and fascia, thus allowing the circulatory, lymphatic and nervous systems to function optimally to restore homeostasis.

They also reduce the sensation of pain by:

- activating nerve pathways that block or 'gate' the ingoing pain signals and prevent them reaching the brain and being perceived as pain
- activating descending nerve pathways from the brain that act in the spinal cord to prevent transmission of pain signals
- releasing endorphins.

Environmental influences

Physical injuries often affect the mental status of an animal. Altered behaviour such as withdrawal from social interaction is a common consequence of injury. It also reduces the ability of the horse to obtain food and protect itself. Horses and people tend to heal faster if they are comfortable with their environment, so attention should be paid to keeping the horse relaxed and happy as well as seeing to its physical needs.

Aftercare

Following treatment, advice will be given on aftercare. This will include advice on:

- the period of rest
- rehabilitation
- injury prevention
- exercise and training programmes
- tack.

What conditions can be treated with manipulation?

Manipulation may be an appropriate treatment for horses with reduced mobility or range of movement of the spine which is causing stiffness or muscle tension and discomfort.

384 THE VETERINARY CARE OF THE HORSE

Some examples include the following.

- Stiffness of the neck. Many horses have a reduced range of neck movement following a fall or pulling back while tied up.
- Back pain. There are numerous causes of back pain. This may be primarily due to a fall or poor saddle fit, or it may occur as a consequence of compensating for pain elsewhere, e.g. hock pain. In either case, muscle spasm is usually a feature and this can often be relieved by manipulation. The cause of the pain must also be addressed where appropriate or else the relief will only be temporary.

Veterinary permission

Prior to any treatment, the horse should be examined by a veterinary surgeon. This is so that any underlying problems requiring veterinary attention can be identified and treated at the same time. The horse will be examined to ensure that manipulative techniques are appropriate and not likely to cause further damage or exacerbate the problem. Sometimes back, neck or limb radiographs or other clinical investigations are undertaken prior to commencement of the treatment.

HOMEOPATHY

Homeopathic medicines made from plant, mineral and animal sources are used to treat a wide range of conditions. This branch of medicine was founded by the German doctor Samuel Hahnemann in the nineteenth century. He observed that if a homeopathic substance causes a number of specific symptoms in a healthy person, a very dilute form of the same substance may be used to stimulate the immune system and assist healing of an ill person showing the same symptoms.

Homeopathy is unusual in that the more dilute the medicine, the stronger the remedy. The original substance is serially diluted and shaken vigorously (the shaking is called succussion). The remedies are dispensed as pills, powders, granules, drops and creams.

Exactly how homeopathy works is not fully understood as in many cases the original homeopathic substance is so dilute that no molecules are left in the preparation. It has been suggested that the remedy has an energy of its own which is 'imprinted' on the water molecules and is responsible for activating the immune system and stimulating healing of individual patients.

Nevertheless, an increasing number of vets are successfully using homeopathic medicines in their practices. Vets with the letters VetMFHom after their names have undertaken a three-year training course in veterinary homeopathy and passed examinations admitting them as members of the Faculty of Homeopathy. This faculty provides training in homeopathy for doctors, dentists, vets, nurses and pharmacists.

Homeopathic medicines are prescribed following a very thorough clinical examination of the horse and a detailed discussion about the animal's character, environment and lifestyle. They are selected for the individual patient so horses with similar symptoms may receive different remedies. They are used to treat a wide range of acute and chronic conditions including allergies, skin problems, digestive problems, hormone imbalances, behavioural problems, viral infections, respiratory disease, degenerative joint disease and traumatic injuries. On occasions, the clinical signs may temporarily become aggravated before a beneficial response is seen.

Homeopathic medicines need to be handled and stored with care. The oils in one's hands can spoil the medication so the remedy should be placed directly into the animal's mouth or onto a piece of apple. They must be stored away from bright light, extremes of temperature and substances with a powerful smell, e.g. aromatherapy oils, peppermint and garlic. Electromagnetic radiation from mobile phones, computers and televisions can also reduce their potency. When stored correctly, many homeopathic medicines have a shelf life in excess of 5 years.

Most vets practising homeopathy do not use it to replace conventional medicine, rather to add an extra dimension to the treatment options available to their patients.

HERBAL MEDICINE

In many parts of the world there is still a great dependence on plant-based medicines. In some cultures, remedies have been passed down from one generation to the next as the healing properties of certain plants were recognized. Many early veterinary remedies were made from plant material and a considerable number of our modern medicines have been manufactured from plant or fungal extracts. A few examples include:

- salicylic acid (aspirin) from meadowsweet or white willow
- digoxin from the foxglove
- morphine from the opium poppy
- quinine (an anti-malarial drug) from the bark of the cinchona tree
- penicillin from moulds.

As herbivores, horses in the wild have the opportunity to selectively graze the plants that have a particular therapeutic effect. However, with only restricted access to limited pasture, this opportunity is lost with modern horse management systems. In the last few years there has been revived interest in herbal medicine and an increase in the number of herbal supplements available. A wide range of these are offered as dietary supplements by feed manufacturers.

In the pure form, however, some herbal substances are toxic to the horse. Herbal medicines must only be prescribed by a vet who has specific training in this area. The vet will carry out a thorough examination of the horse, its environment and the history before prescribing a particular remedy. These medicines come in a variety of forms including:

- freshly cut or dried herbal preparations
- infusions (made by adding boiling water and allowing to stand for 15 minutes) and decoctions (made by simmering for 15 minutes)
- tinctures
- ointments
- compresses and poultices.

When prescribed at the correct dose, it is thought that these herbal medicines work in a gentler way than manufactured pharmaceutical products. It may be that inclusion of the whole plant rather than purified extracts enhances the therapeutic value of the plant in ways that we do not fully understand and has fewer side effects than concentrated drug extracts. Vets who prescribe herbal medicines do so as part of their approach to the treatment of a particular individual. Herbal medicines cannot replace conventional veterinary treatment in every situation.

Warning

Some herbal medicines are licensed for veterinary use but many are not. Their use can lead to risks from unknown withdrawal times which may cause a problem for the competition horse. Do consider this when using herbal medicines and supplements.

HEALING

Whilst conventional veterinary treatment is very important, the overall wellbeing of the horse should not be forgotten and this section by Margrit Coates is included to highlight this.

HANDS-ON HEALING

Margrit Coates MNFSH, MBRCP
Author of *Healing for Horses*, *Horses Talking*, and *Hands-on Healing for Pets*.

The history of healing
The therapy of healing using hands to channel beneficial energy into the spirit or soul of a human or an animal is many thousands of years old. In fact it is the oldest form of

medicine and, as well as historical documents from numerous cultures, there are ancient drawings and paintings showing people laying their hands onto others. Two thousand year old Vedic texts also describe how universal energy is channelled deep into the body's cells through energy centres called chakras. Priests in Egyptian temples are known to have used their hands to give healing to the sick and the Ebers papyrus which dates from 1550 BC mentions that healing by laying on the hands was given for pain relief.

The ancient Greeks practised healing for medical conditions, and followers of the Greek philosopher Pythagoras believed that energy comprised negative and positive states, the positive being used for healing. Pythagoras also coined the term 'pneuma' for the energy associated with healing which is similar to the Chinese Yin and Yang dual energy states that need to be in balance for mind, body and soul harmony. This applies as much to our horses as it does to us.

Another famous Greek philosopher Hypocrites noticed that sensations of heat and tingling were produced by healers, and were accompanied by relief of a patient's symptoms. Later, throughout Europe, kings practised healing, and around the world today, the touch of the hand to comfort sick or troubled humans and animals has continued.

Studies and efficacy

Many scientific studies into healing have now been conducted and reported★. Owing to the known benefits, registered healers in the UK are now working in NHS hospitals. Doctors may also refer patients to healers. The Royal College of Veterinary Surgeons (RCVS) has stated it has no objection to healing by the laying on of hands as long as a vet has been consulted about the animal's problems and permission for healing has been given.

Registered healers

The largest and leading organization in the UK for healers is the National Federation of Spiritual Healers (NFSH - www.NFSH.org.uk). To become a full healer member and be accepted for the professional referral register, people have to undertake at least two years of training and a panel assessment. Once accepted, members adhere to a strict code of conduct including working within the Veterinary Act. Professional healers also carry insurance.

What is healing energy?

The understanding of life force or soul energy is not new and many long-established medical philosophies share this concept for helping recovery and rebalance. Disruption of the balance of vital energy adversely affects wellbeing.

With our horses, inner harmony is vital to enable them to both function and perform

---

★ *Healing Research Volume 1, Spiritual healing: Validation of a healing revolution* by Daniel J. Benor MD, Helix, ISBN 1 886785 11 2. *Professional Supplement to Volume 1*, Helix, ISBN 1 886785 12 0. *Energy Medicine – the Scientific Basis* by James L. Oschman, Churchill Livingstone, ISBN 0 443062 61 7.

to the best of their ability. The state of 'optimum balance' will of course vary, depending on the age of the horse and the types of trauma or lifestyle changes they have experienced, or are experiencing.   Horses in their natural state were intended to roam free, with the opportunity to run and interact with nature and the elements. Man has imposed unnatural constraints on horses' behaviour and in many cases they have no outlet for the frustration that these may cause.

Healing is often called spiritual healing because it works deeply in the spirit, or essence, of the individual, whatever the species. Healing energy aims to help recovery and this may take place on a mental, emotional or physical level, or a combination of these. Because healing reaches the soul, hands-on healing is a true holistic therapy for horses.

Hands-on healing energy should never be used as a substitute for, or alternative to, veterinary care, but alongside it. It is a natural therapy that anyone can offer to their horse at anytime. It can be used not just for problems, but also to strengthen the bond between human and horse. It is not necessary to know that there is anything wrong with a horse to give healing. This is because when signs of illness or emotional depletion show, the root cause may have been brewing for some time.

In some trials with animals, healing was shown to have a positive benefit: a number of animals who received healing prior to injury or surgery recovered more quickly than those in the studies who did not receive healing. Thus healing is also useful for treating a horse post injury or surgery.

Hands-on healing is not exclusive to a chosen few, but is accessible to everyone at anytime, no matter what their beliefs or backgrounds. Horses do not have a faith in the religious sense, yet they readily understand cosmic healing energy because they are so in tune with the natural world around them. Everything on earth is connected and every life is part of the whole, meaning that we all share a common energy that links to a universal source of life. Each of us, including our horses, has an individual energy signature which is affected by the subtle vibrations of all living creatures around us. Throughout our lives we are affected by numerous factors including education, upbringing, diet, genetic inheritance, climate and environment. All of these influences are reflected in our energy fields, thus we can affect the behaviour or wellbeing of horses as we reflect either harmonious or chaotic energy, which the horse can absorb. Unlike us, horses do not have the freedom to walk away from disturbing situations and people. They become a mirror of our inner being and this is a good reason to calmly send out positive loving thoughts when offering healing to them.

Thoughts are a powerful language and they create energy of their own, affecting everything around us. What we are thinking is therefore vitally important when giving healing. The intent to help and a true empathy with horses is very important for the healer to activate a strong energy connection. The ego must also be set aside, as must be thoughts of what we want from the horse. Instead, they should be offered unconditional love, thus allowing the horse the opportunity to work with the healing energy. In this way we allow healing to flow at the level that is most beneficial for the horse, rather than trying to manipulate it for our own gain.

It can take only a split second to upset or even harm a horse, but repairing the damage can take a long time. With healing, we should therefore be generous with our offer of help when the horse tells us that things are not right for him. Even with healing communication, it can take quite a while to unravel disturbances deep within a horse and allow him to find harmony. If the horse is not at peace in his soul he does not stand the best chance of emotionally being able to cope with whatever life brings, and can become more prone to physical disorders.

What can healing be used for?

With horses and other animals there is no placebo effect as sometimes occurs with humans, whereby someone in great need may feel better simply due to the reassuring manner or words of a practitioner. Through healing, the horse can let go of chaotic and disturbed energy that humans may release as tears. As a result, there have been good responses reported when healing is used with horses, and there can often be dramatic improvements. This, of course, is provided that any lifestyle and management issues have been addressed.

Healing can be offered for any condition, and can be used alongside all types of veterinary treatment or complementary therapy. Healing can safely be given to any horse including pregnant mares, newborn foals, and the elderly. Conditions for which healing is used in horses include pain, distress, grief and other emotional issues, chronic illnesses and diseases, tumours, wounds, shock and trauma, toxicity, stress, boosting cellular repair and general wellbeing.

Healing can also be offered to the horse who has no known problems, given simply as an expression of love. We need to listen to, and respond to, the needs of the horse and that which he is communicating to us. Healing helps us to take a step forward in this.

Healing is also communication

Animal behaviourists have concluded after extensive research that animals have an inner world similar to that of the human, including thoughts, fears, worry about the future as well as an ability to experience happiness. Scientists have also concluded that animals have a highly developed telepathic sense through which they communicate with each other and the world around them. The 'sixth sense' is something of which horses and other animals appear to have a strong awareness. Through healing we become sensitive and 'energy aware'. We can activate and rediscover our sixth sense and then healing becomes a form of communication. Through this we receive feedback from the horse about issues of the present. Horses also have an emotional and physical energy memory existing at cellular level. It is possible therefore to communicate about past issues and how they play a part in what is troubling the horse in the present.

From the horse's standpoint, communication from him to humans is clear, but many a time it is misunderstood by us. Communication from humans to the horse is not always clear, and they frequently have little idea of what we want, or why we want to do something. We need to explore different ways of communicating with them. As healing and the sixth sense work on the same energy wavelengths, this is another good reason to practise the art of hands-on healing because it opens up the powerful, deep communication channels. Tuning in on a healing vibration activates the mind-to-mind communication levels and helps us to listen deeply to the horse and what he is trying to say to us.

How to give healing to a horse

Healing treatments can be planned ahead, selecting a time when the environment is quiet for the horse and the healer will not be disturbed. The horse should be standing on a soft bed and not be tied up. This allows the horse to relax and stretch out if he feels the need to do so. Healing can also be given without prior planning in an acute situation, as a first-aid help, whilst waiting for the vet to arrive. In all cases the methods are the same: either one or both hands, are gently laid on the body, or held just above it (Figure 14.9). Wounds and sensitive areas should not be touched. The healer then focuses on sending positive thoughts of wanting to help at soul level, which activates the universal healing source to connect with the energy field of the horse, allowing beneficial energy to flow. The horse takes what he or she needs, at whatever level is possible, at any given time. The healer may feel heat or tingling under the hands or fingertips and the horse can become very relaxed.

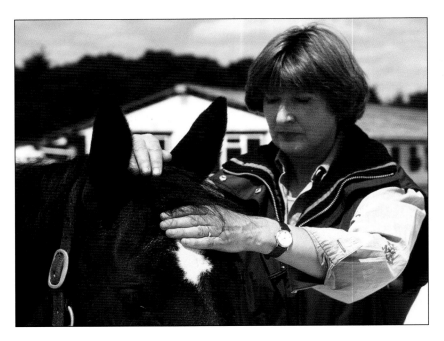

Figure 14.9 Pony receiving hands-on healing

15

RESPIRATORY CONDITIONS

THE RESPIRATORY SYSTEM

The function of the respiratory system is to draw air into the lungs so that oxygen can be absorbed from the air sacs into the bloodstream and carbon dioxide can be eliminated. When a horse breathes in, contraction of the muscles between the ribs and in the diaphragm causes the chest cavity to expand and the lungs to fill with air. When these muscles relax, air is exhaled. The normal respiratory rate is 8–16 breaths per minute.

The exchange of gases

Air enters the nostrils and passes through the nasal passages. It is drawn into the nasopharynx and through the larynx into the trachea. The trachea runs down the underside of the neck in the midline and into the chest cavity where it divides into two main bronchi. The bronchi divide into progressively smaller tubes; the finest airways are called bronchioles. (Figures 15.1a, b and c.)

Each bronchiole ends in a cluster of air sacs known as alveoli. The thin, elastic walls of the alveoli are in close contact with a network of capillaries. Capillaries are tiny, thin-walled blood vessels. Oxygen in the inhaled air diffuses from the alveoli into the blood. Here, it combines with haemoglobin in the red blood cells and is transported to the tissues. Carbon dioxide diffuses in the opposite direction and is exhaled.

During its passage from the nostrils to the lungs, air is warmed, moistened and filtered. Inhaled dust and spores are trapped in a thin layer of mucus which lines the airways. The mucus is continually moved towards the pharynx by tiny hair-like projections (called cilia) on the epithelial cells. This is known as the mucociliary escalator. On reaching the pharynx, the debris is swallowed.

The effects of respiratory disease

When a horse succumbs to infectious or allergic respiratory disease, the quiet, relaxed pattern of breathing is disturbed. This is because the diameter of the airways is reduced by:

- excessive production of mucus or pus

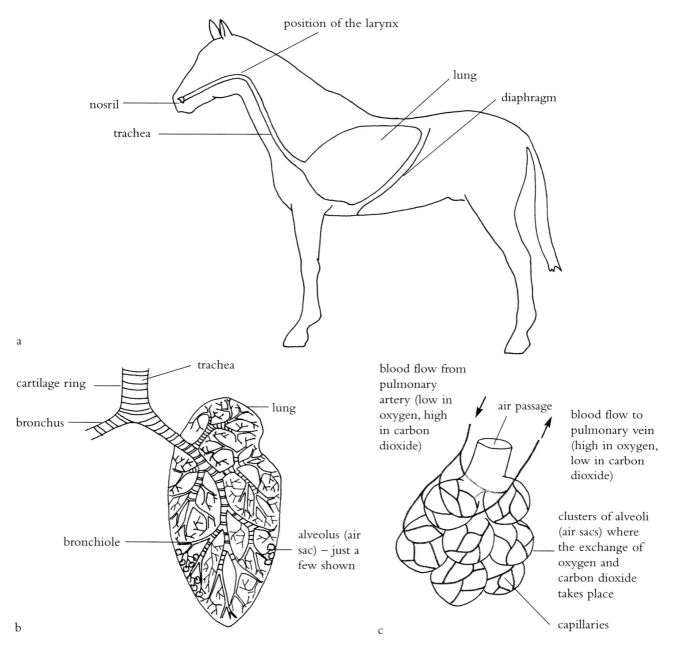

Figures 15.1a, b and c a) the respiratory system; b) the airways of the lung; c) the air sacs of the lung

- inflammation and swelling of the epithelial cells lining the airways
- spasm of the smooth muscles in the airway walls.

More effort is needed to draw the same volume of air through the narrowed tubes and gas exchange is less efficient. The smallest airways may become completely blocked. Prompt treatment is required to prevent permanent damage occurring to the delicate lung tissues.

Diseases of the respiratory system include:
- viral infections
- bacterial infections
- fungal infections
- allergic respiratory disease
- parasitic infections.

Veterinary examination

When you call a vet to examine a horse with respiratory disease, the vet will need information about the horse's management, including details of the:
- diet, e.g. type of concentrate, quality of forage
- type of bedding
- grazing and worming history
- vaccination status
- nature of work the horse performs
- recent exposure to respiratory disease, e.g. attendance at shows, sales etc.

The vet's clinical examination of the horse may include:
- observation of the rate and character of breathing while the horse is resting and relaxed
- taking the temperature
- listening to the chest with a stethoscope (known as auscultation) for any abnormal wheezing or crackling sounds
- checking the heart
- feeling for enlarged lymph nodes (glands) under the mandible
- observation of any nasal discharge: a small volume of watery nasal discharge is normal
- a discussion of the symptoms such as coughing and altered exercise tolerance
- percussion may be done on occasions; this involves tapping the chest to see if any areas sound less air-filled than normal, e.g. owing to fluid in the chest cavity
- the respiratory tract may be examined with an endoscope.

Where appropriate, samples will be taken for examination in the laboratory, eg:
- blood
- swabs
- faeces
- tracheal wash
- bronchoalveolar lavage.

ENDOSCOPIC EXAMINATION

The flexible fibreoptic endoscope is used for visual examination of the upper respiratory tract. These instruments provide the vet with a clear, bright image of the tissues from the nostrils all the way to the point where the trachea divides into the two main bronchi. The nasal passages, nasopharynx, soft palate, gutteral pouches, larynx and the trachea can be closely inspected. It is a valuable tool in the diagnosis and management of equine respiratory disease.

PROCEDURE

The horse is restrained in a stable or stocks with a headcollar and sometimes a twitch. Mild sedation may be necessary, although this can affect structures such as the larynx. Two assistants are required, one to hold the horse and the other to hold the endoscope at the horse's nostrils (Figure 15.2). The long, flexible endoscope is introduced into the nostrils and slowly advanced. A viewing screen or video camera can be attached allowing the images to be more clearly seen and/or recorded.

Tracheal wash

The endoscope can be used to collect respiratory secretions for bacteriology and cytology (examination of the cells under a microscope).

PROCEDURE

A long, sterile catheter is inserted into the biopsy channel of the endoscope and advanced part of the way along the channel. The endoscope is introduced into one nostril and carefully guided through the larynx and into the trachea. The catheter is then pushed in further so it protrudes from the end of the endoscope and is positioned at the lowest point of the trachea. If there is a pool of discharge, this may be sucked up through the catheter with a syringe. If a sample cannot be obtained in this way, 50–100 ml of warmed saline is introduced via the catheter. This runs down the wall of the trachea and washes epithelial cells, discharges and bacteria from the lining of the airway. The fluid pools at the entrance to the chest and this can be retrieved through the catheter. The scope is then withdrawn.

Samples of tracheal secretions can also be obtained by making a skin incision over the trachea at the bottom of the neck and passing a catheter between adjacent cartilage rings.

EXAMINATION OF THE SAMPLES

- **Cytology** The sample is examined under a microscope. It will contain epithelial cells, macrophages, neutrophils, lymphocytes, eosinophils and possibly red blood cells. The numbers of these are compared with those from the tracheal secretions of a normal horse. The degree of inflammation can be assessed (graded 1–3). A high number of eosinophils may be indicative of parasitic infection. Lungworm larvae can sometimes be seen in the washes from infected horses.

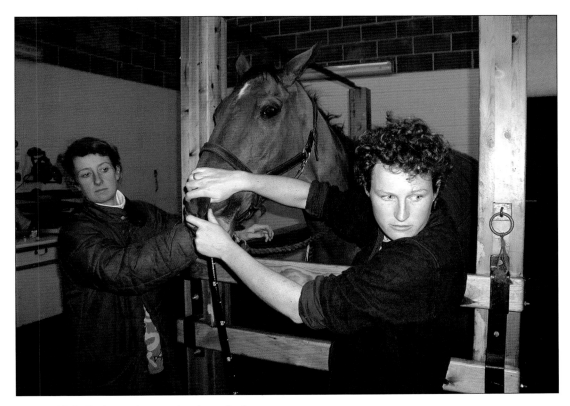

Figure 15.2 Endoscopic examination of a horse

- **Bacteriology** The wash may contain large numbers of pathogenic bacteria. These are cultured in the laboratory and their sensitivity to different antibiotics is tested. This helps the vet choose the correct antibiotic to eliminate the bacteria.

Bronchoalveolar lavage (BAL)

Bronchoalveolar lavage (BAL) is used to investigate diseases of the lower respiratory tract. The advantage over tracheal washes is that cells from the lower airways are aspirated and these tend to reflect more accurately the disease processes in the alveoli (air sacs) and small airways. The technique is particularly valuable in the diagnosis of:

- small airway inflammatory disease
- recurrent airway obstruction
- summer pasture associated obstructive disease.

PROCEDURE

The technique may be performed through a long endoscope and catheter or by insertion of a special BAL tube into the small airways via the nostril. It is essential that the horse stays still for this procedure, so sedation and a twitch are routinely used. A bronchodilator may be administered to reduce coughing or more commonly local anaesthetic is instilled into the airways before the endoscope or tube is passed to minimize coughing.

The endoscope or BAL tube is inserted until resistance is encountered. Once the BAL tube has lodged in a small airway, an inflatable cuff just behind the tip is blown up with air to secure it in position and prevent the escape of fluid. If an endoscope is used, a catheter is now passed along the biopsy channel. Between 150–250 ml of warmed sterile saline is instilled into the airway and immediately aspirated. All of the equipment used is sterile.

The aspirated samples are centrifuged and the cells obtained are smeared onto a slide and examined under the microscope. Cultures can also be performed if infection is suspected.

Following the procedure, the horse should not be allowed to eat until the effects of the sedation and local anaesthesia have worn off, to ensure that it can swallow safely.

EQUINE INFLUENZA

Equine influenza (flu) is a disease that affects the upper and lower respiratory tract of horses, donkeys and mules. It is caused by several strains of the equine influenza virus. The disease is very infectious and spreads rapidly through groups of horses. The incubation period is 1–3 days. People cannot be infected with equine flu.

Clinical signs
These may include:
- a temperature of 39–41 °C (103–106 °F) which lasts for 1–3 days
- a harsh, dry cough that can last for 2–3 weeks
- a clear, watery nasal discharge that may become thick and yellow or green (Figure 15.3)

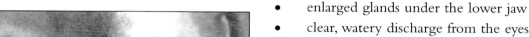

- enlarged glands under the lower jaw
- clear, watery discharge from the eyes
- depression
- loss of appetite
- oedema of the lower limbs.

The disease usually lasts for 1–3 weeks. Vaccinated horses may be affected, but the illness is generally less severe.

When to call the vet
If you suspect your horse has equine influenza you should call your vet immediately. Steps can then be taken to limit the spread of the disease.

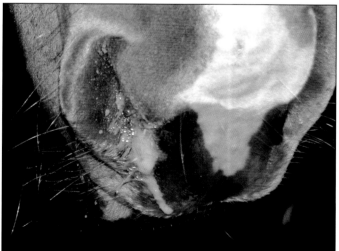

Figure 15.3 The nasal discharge may become thick and yellow or green

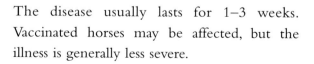

Diagnosis

The diagnosis is made on:

- the clinical signs
- isolation of the virus from nasopharyngeal swabs
- a number of other laboratory tests which identify the virus
- rising antibody levels in blood (serum) samples taken early in the course of the disease and 2–3 weeks later
- history of recent contact with a confirmed case of the disease.

How does the virus cause the illness?

The disease is spread by inhalation of virus released into the atmosphere as an aerosol by coughing and blowing. Once inhaled, the virus invades the lining epithelium of the trachea, bronchi, bronchioles and alveoli. The airway lining becomes swollen and inflamed, resulting in tracheobronchitis. Patches of the epithelium slough off and these changes disrupt the clearance of mucus and other debris from the airways.

Complications

- Adult horses sometimes develop a secondary bacterial infection.
- Young foals are at risk of developing pneumonia which can be fatal.
- Occasionally, the virus spreads from the respiratory tract and can cause damage to the liver or the muscle of the heart.

Treatment and management

There is no specific treatment for respiratory viruses in the horse. If the horse develops a secondary bacterial infection, antibiotics are given. All horses with respiratory infections should be given complete rest. Ideally, they should not recommence any strenuous exercise until two weeks after apparent recovery.

STABLE MANAGEMENT

Good stable ventilation and management are essential. Exposure to dust and spores should be minimized as horses with respiratory infections are susceptible to developing recurrent airway obstruction (RAO). If hay is fed, it should be of good quality and soaked. If weather conditions permit, affected horses benefit from being turned out into a small paddock for at least part of the day once their temperatures have returned to normal. This is especially important in the recovery stages.

Control

Since the disease is spread by inhalation of virus released into the atmosphere as an aerosol by coughing and blowing, equine flu is highly infectious within a group of horses. As soon as a horse shows any symptoms, strict hygiene and isolation procedures should be applied. Any horses that have been in contact with the affected animals should be carefully monitored and not attend shows, lessons etc., as they may be incubating the disease.

Prevention

Regular vaccination is the key to the prevention of outbreaks of equine influenza (see Vaccination on page 23).

- A vaccination programme should be established for *every horse* in the yard. Do not overlook youngstock, donkeys and elderly companions.
- Pregnant mares should be given a booster one month before foaling to give maximum protection to the foal.
- In the event of an outbreak, horses should not attend shows or any other equine gathering. Exposure to the virus combined with the stress of travelling will make infection more likely.
- When the disease occurs locally, it is advisable to give a booster to any horse that has not been vaccinated in the previous 6 months, provided they are not thought to be incubating the disease. Maximum immunity is not reached until 2 weeks after the vaccination.

Every now and then an outbreak of equine influenza occurs. Vaccinated horses may show symptoms but these are usually milder than those experienced by unvaccinated horses. The reason that vaccines do not always provide 100% protection is because the virus can change slightly with time and different strains develop. The vaccines are regularly updated in order to provide maximum protection.

EQUINE HERPESVIRUS

There are four types of equine herpesvirus.

- **Equine herpesvirus–1 (EHV-1)** can cause respiratory disease, abortion and paralysis.
- **Equine herpesvirus–2 (EHV-2)** can cause respiratory disease with pharyngeal lymphoid hyperplasia and ulceration of the pharynx.
- **Equine herpesvirus–3 (EHV-3)** causes venereal disease with lesions on the external genitalia.
- **Equine herpesvirus–4 (EHV-4)** is also known as equine rhinopneumonitis virus. It usually causes respiratory signs but occasionally results in abortion.

EHV-1 and EHV-4 are the most common strains.

Clinical signs

Respiratory disease caused by EHV-1 and EHV-4 can affect any horse, but tends to occur in groups of weaned foals and yearlings. The signs include:

- a raised temperature
- swollen glands under the mandible
- depression and lethargy
- loss of appetite
- watery nasal discharge which becomes purulent if secondary bacterial infection occurs
- coughing
- conjunctivitis.

Additional signs that can occur particularly with EHV-1 include the following.

- Equine infectious abortion, which can occur at any time between the 5th and 11th months of gestation but most commonly occurs in late pregnancy and may be responsible for single or multiple abortions; these often occur in the absence of any other clinical signs. This can result in a so-called 'abortion storm' with several in-foal mares slipping or losing their foals.
- The birth of weak, jaundiced foals that show respiratory distress and usually die within three days.
- Swollen limbs.
- The paralytic form of equine herpesvirus presents as progressive incoordination and weakness, sometimes leading to paralysis and a total inability to stand. These horses are often unable to lift their tail or pass urine as a result of degenerative changes in the brain and spinal cord caused by the virus. These signs often follow respiratory disease.

With EHV-4, young animals may develop a secondary pneumonia. Abortion occasionally occurs in a single mare.

Transmission

Infection with EHV-1 and EHV-4 occurs by inhalation of the virus released into the atmosphere as an aerosol from the respiratory tract of infected horses. This occurs when a horse coughs or snorts. EHV-1 infection can be also acquired by ingestion of material released onto the pasture from the foetus, foetal membranes and fluids when a mare aborts. The mare will be infectious for a month after the abortion occurs. Sick foals with EHV-1 are also a source of infection.

It is possible for a horse to carry and spread the virus without showing any symptoms. The virus may be shed at times of stress, such as weaning, following transportation or when new animals are introduced into an established group.

When to call the vet

Call your vet as soon as symptoms are observed. Measures to prevent the spread of the disease can then be implemented straight away. The owners of any 'in-contact' horses should also be notified immediately.

Diagnosis

Diagnostic tests include the following.

- Isolation of the virus from naso-pharyngeal swabs taken early in the course of the disease. Swabs taken from other horses in the group that have a temperature can be helpful in making a diagnosis.
- Isolation of the virus from fresh tissues of the aborted foetus, dead foal or paralysed horse (following euthanasia).
- Laboratory examination of tissues from the dead foal, aborted foetus and membranes.
- Measurement of antibody levels in the blood. As soon as a horse is challenged by a virus, antibody levels begin to rise. Blood is taken when the symptoms first appear and again 3 weeks later. A marked rise in antibodies present indicates recent infection. A high reading from a single blood test may indicate recent exposure to the virus. This test is not useful in cases of abortion as there may be a considerable time lapse between infection of the mare and the abortion occurring.

Treatment

Treatment of horses with respiratory signs includes:

- complete rest
- dust free management
- antibiotics as necessary if secondary bacterial infection occurs.

Horses with neurological signs require:

- careful nursing in a stable, covered yard or small, flat paddock as appropriate
- good bedding
- catheterization if they are unable to pass urine
- regular turning or support with slings if they are unable to stand
- regular provision of food and water which may involve intravenous fluids and other supportive treatment.

Mares that have aborted do not usually appear ill or require any specific treatment. However, they **must be isolated** as they can shed virus for up to one month.

In some recent outbreaks of paralytic herpes, horses have been treated with antiviral medication such as acyclovir. However, it is expensive and has to be given by mouth several times a day. Currently it is not certain how beneficial it is for affected horses.

Control measures

If a pregnant mare aborts or a foal is ill or dies within a few days of birth, the cause should be investigated. Early diagnosis of EHV-1 infection is essential to prevent the spread of infection. If abortion occurs:

- contact the vet immediately
- isolate the mare in a stable
- put the foetus and membranes in a leak-proof container and send to an approved laboratory for examination
- disinfect any areas likely to be contaminated by foetal fluids with a disinfectant recommended by your vet
- burn any bedding
- if the mare aborted in the field it should be left empty for a period of four weeks.
- the person looking after the mare should not have any contact with pregnant mares
- sick newborn foals should be isolated with the mare and tested for EHV-1; nasopharyngeal swabs and blood samples should be taken and sent to an approved laboratory.

Until the results are available, no horses should be moved on or off the premises. All in-contact mares should be managed as though infected.

If the tests are positive for EHV-1, the movement restrictions must be enforced for a minimum of 28 days. Any other pregnant mares should remain on the premises to foal. There is a Code of Practice to reduce the spread of the disease which is published by the Horserace Betting Levy Board (HBLB) and is available from the HBLB (www.hblb.org.uk), the Thoroughbred Breeders' Association and the Welfare Department of the British Horse Society. It offers guidelines on many aspects of disease control and the movement of non-pregnant mares on and off the premises.

Prevention
VACCINATION

There is a vaccine available which gives some protection against EHV-1 and EHV-4. Pregnant mares are vaccinated during the 5th, 7th and 9th months of pregnancy.

Foals may be vaccinated from 5 months of age. Following the primary course where the first and second injections are given 4–6 weeks apart, boosters are recommended every 6 months. Immunity following vaccination and natural infection is relatively short-lived. However, it may help to prevent infection by increasing herd immunity and reducing the spread of the virus.

MANAGEMENT

Wherever possible, pregnant mares should foal at home.

On a stud, they should be kept in small groups, preferably with other mares due to foal at the same time. They should be kept separate from young animals. The introduction of new animals into the group should be minimized.

As horses can harbour the virus without showing any signs and shed it into the environment if they are stressed for any reason, pregnant mares should be kept away from horses regularly attending competitions or that have recently been in training.

HYGIENE

- The virus can survive in the environment for several weeks but is susceptible to disinfectants and heat. Thorough cleaning of foaling boxes, equipment and vehicles is essential.
- On studs, attention should be paid to hygiene at foaling. Disposable gloves should be used routinely.
- If the same people handle different groups of horses, the pregnant mares should be handled first.

Prognosis

Once a mare has aborted, the virus does not remain in the genital tract and she may be covered on her second heat. She should be kept away from pregnant mares for 8 weeks.

The prognosis is reasonable for animals that develop neurological signs of weakness and incoordination. However, once they are unable to stand up, the chances of recovery are very small and the outlook is grave.

EQUINE VIRAL ARTERITIS (EVA)

Equine viral arteritis is a flu-like disease that affects horses, ponies and donkeys worldwide. It is caused by the equine arteritis virus (EAV) and the incubation period is between 2 days and 2 weeks. There have been a few isolated positive horses and an occasional outbreak in the UK, but (at the time of writing) the UK has remained relatively free from EVA. This means that the horse population has little immunity to the virus, so it is important to maintain our disease-free status and prevent this virus infecting the UK horse population. All possible precautions should be undertaken to prevent the virus from becoming endemic.

In other parts of the world, particularly continental Europe, it is more widespread and horses have some immunity. The situation on this disease may change and current information should be checked with your own vet.

Clinical signs

These are variable and many mildly affected animals may not show any obvious signs. Possible signs of disease may include:

- fever
- lethargy
- conjunctivitis: the conjunctiva may become swollen and the disease is sometimes referred to as 'pink eye'
- oedema (swelling) of the lower limbs, the ventral abdomen, the scrotum or udder
- nasal discharge
- abortion or the birth of weak foals: 50–70% of in-foal mares will abort their foetuses
- EVA can occasionally be fatal.

Transmission

The disease is transmitted via:

- inhalation of the virus released into the atmosphere as an aerosol during coughing or snorting
- the teasing or mating process: the virus localizes in the accessory sex glands and is shed in the semen
- artificial insemination with semen from infected stallions
- contact with aborted foetuses or foetal fluids and membranes.

Following the incubation period (which is an average of 7 days), the virus is excreted in all body secretions. Once a stallion has been infected, he may continue to shed the virus in his semen for weeks, months or the rest of his life. His fertility is not affected once he has recovered from the early stage of the disease. If he infects mares during mating, they may then spread the virus via the respiratory route.

Diagnosis

It is not always possible to identify the disease from the clinical signs, so laboratory tests are essential. The diagnosis is made by detecting the virus (virus isolation test) in:

- nasopharyngeal swabs
- blood
- semen
- urine
- the tissues and fluids from the placenta and aborted foetuses.

Blood is also tested for antibodies to the virus. If there are no antibodies, the horse is **seronegative**. If antibodies to equine arteritis virus are present, it is **seropositive**. If rising levels of antibodies are seen in consecutive samples, this indicates recent infection.

Characteristic changes are seen in infected foetal tissues such as lymph nodes, spleen, lung and liver when they are examined under the microscope.

Treatment

As with most viruses there is no specific medical treatment available and none is usually necessary apart from general nursing. Non-steroidal anti-inflammatory drugs may help to bring down the horse's temperature and alleviate some of the discomfort caused by the disease.

Vaccination

A vaccine (Artervac) is available for protection against equine arteritis virus. The vaccine is not available to everyone and a special application has to be made for each individual animal. In the UK, stallions and teasers are vaccinated annually. The vaccine is not given to mares.

All vaccinated horses become seropositive and it is not possible to determine from a blood test whether the antibodies are due to the vaccination or to infection. This information is important if the horse is going to be used for breeding or be exported. For this reason, a blood test is taken prior to vaccination to establish that the horse is seronegative. A second test is taken 3 weeks later to measure the stallion's response to the vaccine. The date of testing, the test result and the vaccination date must be recorded in the horse's passport.

Notification

Under the 1995 Equine Viral Arteritis Order, **EVA is a notifiable disease**. This means that if the disease is even suspected in a stallion or in a mare that has been mated or artificially inseminated in the previous 14 days, the Divisional Veterinary Manager (DVM) in the local Animal Health Offices of DEFRA (Department for Environment, Food and Rural Affairs) must be notified. The DVM will immediately prohibit the use of the suspect stallion or its semen for breeding and take samples to determine if the disease is present. If the disease is confirmed, further samples will be taken from other horses to see how far it has spread. The relevant breeder's association should be informed.

If you are suspicious that a horse in your care may have EVA, call your vet immediately.

Prevention

For detailed instructions and advice, refer to the Code of Practice published by the Horserace Betting Levy Board (www.hblb.org.uk). The aim is to prevent horses with active infection from being used for breeding or being imported into this country.

ROUTINE TESTING OF BREEDING ANIMALS

It is important to establish whether an animal is infected at the beginning of each breeding season. *The blood of all unvaccinated stallions and teasers should be tested after 1st January every year for antibodies to EAV.* They must not be used for breeding activities until the results are available.

All mares used for breeding should be tested after the 1st January and within the 28-day period before mating is planned.

With both stallions and mares, if the result of the blood test is negative, the horse is not infected and may be used for breeding. If the horse is seropositive, further tests are carried out (see Code of Practice).

Horses that are imported from countries known or suspected to have cases of EVA should be tested prior to import. If the test results are satisfactory, they are isolated for a minimum of 21 days on arrival in the UK and further tests are carried out. This is as important for a horse going abroad for a single competition and then returning as it is for a new horse being imported into the country: *any horse can bring EVA into the UK at any time.*

The Code of Practice also contains guidelines for prevention of EVA transmission during artificial insemination and embryo transfer.

Control of infection

If EVA is suspected:

- stop all breeding activities and contact your vet straight away
- DEFRA should be notified immediately
- stop all movement of horses on and off the premises
- isolate the horse concerned
- if possible, a different person should look after each group of horses, this reduces the risk of infection being spread.

If EVA is confirmed, your vet will advise you on the steps necessary to control infection. Current recommendations can be found on www.hblb.org.uk.

Infected shedder stallions

There is no proven effective treatment for infected shedder stallions. However, due to the fact that several quality stallions in Europe are infected, efforts are being made to find some way of managing the disease in the breeding horse. Currently, the only safe options for stallions that continue to shed the virus are:

- castration
- euthanasia.

STRANGLES

Strangles is a highly contagious disease affecting the upper respiratory tract of horses. It is caused by the bacterium *Streptococcus equi*. It affects horses of all ages but young animals are particularly susceptible. The incubation period is usually between 3–14 days.

Clinical signs

Strangles is characterized by swelling of the lymph nodes (glands) below the horse's throat and a thick yellow nasal discharge from one or both nostrils (Figure 15.4).

First signs may include:

- raised temperature up to 40.5 °C (105 °F)
- watery discharge from one or both nostrils
- dullness and lethargy
- slight enlargement and tenderness of submandibular and retropharyngeal lymph nodes; the region below the horse's throat may appear slightly swollen
- a soft, moist cough
- slight increase in respiratory rate
- loss of appetite.

As the disease progresses:

- the nasal discharge becomes thick and yellow
- there may be a purulent discharge from the eyes
- painful abscesses form in the lymph nodes under the throat and at the back of the pharynx (submandibular and retropharyngeal lymph nodes)
- swallowing is uncomfortable leading to depressed appetite and possible loss of condition
- saliva may drool from the horse's mouth
- the horse may intermittently show choke-like symptoms
- over the next few days the abscesses increase in size and eventually burst to release large amounts of pus (Figure 15.5); this generally occurs around 10–14 days after the start of the disease and at this stage the horse begins to feel better.

Some horses are only mildly affected and show only mild respiratory signs such as a runny nose or slight cough. This may allow the disease to spread unnoticed.

Pathophysiology

- The bacterium is inhaled or ingested.
- It colonizes the mucosa of the pharynx and tonsils and spreads to the lymph nodes of the head and upper neck.
- Toxins and enzymes are released which cause severe tissue damage resulting in pain and abscessation.
- The toxins cause the high temperature, depression and anorexia.
- The bacterium is surrounded by a capsule containing a special protein which prevents it from being ingested and destroyed by white blood cells.
- Occasionally, the bacterium spreads via the bloodstream to other sites in the body resulting in 'bastard strangles'.

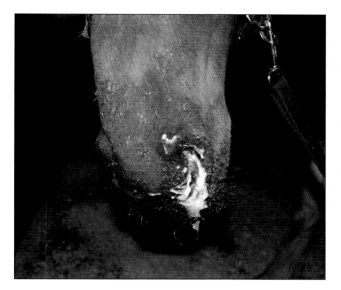

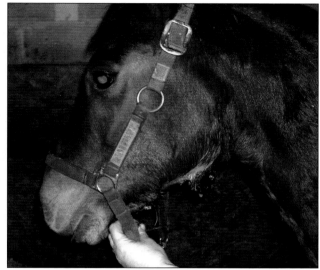

Figure 15.4 Thick nasal discharge typical of strangles

Figure 15.5 A burst strangles abscess

Which horses are particularly susceptible?

- The disease is particularly common in situations where groups of young horses are kept together and new individuals are introduced regularly to the group.
- The resistance of the individuals to infection is decreased by poor management factors such as inadequate feeding and parasite control measures. Mortality in these situations can be 5–7%.
- Any factor causing chronic stress will make a population susceptible to strangles and other diseases.
- Any situation in which many horses are in close proximity with a number moving on and off the premises, e.g. racing stables, studs and livery yards, facilitates the spread of disease.

When to call the vet

If you suspect strangles infection, contact your vet immediately. Early diagnosis and prompt action reduces the risk of a large outbreak occurring.

Diagnosis

Diagnosis is made on the clinical signs. It is confirmed by isolation of *Streptococcus equi* from swabs taken from the nasopharynx or burst abscesses. Blood tests are not usually necessary. If they are taken they reveal a high total white cell count with a marked neutrophilia. Serum fibrinogen and globulins are also likely to be raised.

Differential diagnosis

Abscesses of the lymph nodes can occur due to bacteria other than *Streptococcus equi*. Foreign bodies or dental problems can also cause submandibular swellings.

Treatment
ISOLATION

The affected horse should be isolated if possible and not allowed to come into contact with healthy horses. The stable should be well ventilated but draught free with a warm, dry bed. Dust levels should be kept to a minimum.

FEEDING

- Soft, moist, palatable food should be offered while swallowing is difficult.
- Hand-cut grass may tempt a horse to eat.
- Feeding from the ground encourages the discharges to drain.
- Horses unable or unwilling to eat at all can be fed by nasogastric tube or intravenously.
- Good quality hay should be soaked for 20 minutes to soften it and reduce airborne dust.

WATER

Affected horses may play with their water. They want to drink but are discouraged by the discomfort of swallowing. As the head is lowered, pus may drain into and around the bucket. The water should be changed frequently and buckets kept clean to encourage drinking.

GRAZING

If the horse is well enough, it can be turned out to graze provided the paddock is away from other horses. However, this will contaminate the paddock for several weeks as the bacteria can live for a long time in lumps of discharged pus.

ABSCESSES

- Warm poultices or hot fomentations may be used to speed up maturation and rupture of the abscesses.
- Ruptured abscesses and those which the vet has lanced should be flushed out twice daily with a dilute povidone-iodine solution or dilute hydrogen peroxide.

NURSING CARE

Good nursing is essential. Nasal discharge should be wiped away with cotton wool and warm water as often as necessary. It may help to apply petroleum jelly (Vaseline®) around the nose or abscess after cleaning to prevent the skin becoming sore.

Medication
NON-STEROIDAL ANTI-INFLAMMATORY DRUGS

Non-steroidal anti-inflammatory drugs such as flunixin meglumine, phenylbutazone or ketoprofen may be used early in the course of the disease. These lower the horse's temperature and reduce the pain and soft tissue swelling associated with the abscesses.

THE USE OF ANTIBIOTICS

Antibiotics are not normally used once the abscesses are forming. If given at this stage, they can delay the maturation and rupture of the abscesses and so prolong the course of the disease.

However, antibiotics may be used in the following situations.

- Horses that have been exposed to the infection but are not showing any signs are sometimes treated prophylactically. This strategy is only effective if the horse can then be kept away from potential sources of infection. However, the efficacy of this is debatable, especially as antibiotics should only be given when strictly necessary. If the infection is already being incubated, it may prolong and complicate the course of the disease.

- Where large numbers of horses are kept in close proximity and blanket medication is impractical, temperatures should be taken twice daily. If horses are given antibiotics as soon as their temperature begins to rise, this may limit progression of the disease to full blown strangles, but again may complicate the course of the disease.

- If the horse has a very high temperature, is depressed and anorexic or has difficulty breathing, then antibiotics are likely to be used. Each case will be considered individually.

- Any horse developing life-threatening complications will be treated with antibiotics. Their use will also be considered in any situation where factors such as the age of the horse and the severity of the condition give cause for concern. Thus horses in the same yard may receive different treatments.

Penicillin is the antibiotic of choice but others are also effective. When the diagnosis is confirmed by culturing the bacterium from discharges, the sensitivity to different antibiotics is usually tested. Horses that are known to be allergic to penicillin can be treated with potentiated sulphonamides.

Owner's responsibilities

As soon as the disease is suspected, inform the owners of any in-contact horses so they can take temperatures twice daily, keep their horses in quarantine and be prepared to take immediate action.

Management of an outbreak

Bacteria are released into the environment when the horse coughs and in the discharges. Flies can spread the disease, but it is most likely to be spread by direct contact. Since the disease is acquired by inhalation and ingestion of the bacteria, isolation and hygiene are of paramount importance.

HYGIENE MEASURES

- Isolate all infected horses.
- Where possible, a separate groom should nurse the sick animals.

- Protective clothing such as overalls, boots and disposable gloves should be worn and used only in the infected stables.
- A bucket of disinfectant, e.g. Virkon®S, and brush should be positioned outside each stable for cleaning boots when leaving the box. The bacterium is not killed by bleach.
- Separate feed and water buckets should be used and not taken outside the infected area (not into the feed shed or to taps used for filling buckets of healthy horses). The buckets should be scrubbed regularly as water troughs, buckets and damp areas are sites where infection may persist in the environment. Feed and hay for the ill horses should be kept separately.
- Contaminated bedding and swabs from cleaning up the discharges should be burned.
- Rugs, headcollars and the stable should be cleaned with an approved disinfectant (your vet will recommend one) once the horse has recovered.
- Recovered animals should not be turned out into the same field as healthy horses for 6–8 weeks after the symptoms have resolved as they could still be a source of infection.

CONTROL MEASURES

- When an outbreak occurs, any horse developing a temperature or a nasal discharge should be segregated from unaffected horses.
- Horses recovering from the infection may shed bacteria for some time following apparent recovery. To test for this the horse should have three nasopharyngeal swabs taken within a 2-week period. If none grow *Streptococcus equi* then the horse is unlikely to be a source of infection to others.
- The whole yard should be treated as an isolation area until 4 weeks after the last abscess has healed. No new horses should be allowed into the yard and no horses should go to public events such as shows or lessons, or visit other yards until they have had three negative nasopharyngeal swabs.

CARRIERS

The strangles story is further complicated by carriers: the apparently healthy horses harbouring the disease. Some horses can remain as carriers or shedders for a year or even longer. This makes disease control and elimination of the infection difficult and is the usual explanation for a spontaneous outbreak. Although the vet can test if a horse is a carrier by taking swabs from the nasopharynx or by collecting samples via an endoscope, some horses only shed the bacteria intermittently. Thus in most, but not all, cases if three swabs are negative, the horse is clear. As it cannot completely guarantee a horse is free from infection, vigilance is still required.

THE GUTTURAL POUCH

Some animals can become chronic carriers and intermittent shedders of the bacteria due to a low-grade persistent infection of the guttural pouch. This may occur if the retropharyngeal lymph nodes burst and drain into the guttural pouch. Such infections require drainage and flushing of the guttural pouches as they do not respond to systemic antibiotic therapy alone.

Possible complications
'BASTARD STRANGLES'

Most cases of strangles recover with careful nursing. Occasionally, the infection spreads to lymph nodes in other parts of the body. This is known as 'bastard strangles'. The symptoms depend on the site of infection. The affected animal may show general malaise and unthriftiness. There may be chronic weight loss and intermittent periods of colic, raised temperature and abnormal breathing.

Some of these animals remain below par for several months following apparent recovery. Death may follow from eventual maturation and rupture of undetected abscesses into:

- the lungs causing pneumonia
- the abdominal cavity leading to a fatal peritonitis.

If the abscesses are in superficial sites on the body, they burst and drain without complications.

If 'bastard strangles' is suspected, antibiotic therapy will be started and continued for 4–6 weeks. The white blood cell count and fibrinogen may be monitored regularly. Samples of peritoneal fluid may be examined.

RESPIRATORY OBSTRUCTION

Occasionally, the swollen retropharyngeal lymph nodes can cause a life-threatening respiratory obstruction. In these cases the vet will drain the abscesses and may perform a temporary tracheotomy to relieve the airway.

PURPURA HAEMORRHAGICA

Purpura haemorrhagica is a possible sequel to infection with strangles (see next section).

Prevention
VACCINATION

A new vaccine which helps to protect horses against strangles became available in September 2004. It is injected into the mucosa on the inside of the horse's upper lip. The primary course is two injections given 4 weeks apart. Foals can be vaccinated from 4 months of age. Horses in high-risk situations (e.g. new horses regularly being introduced into the group, regular attendance at competitions or being close to an outbreak of strangles) should be given boosters every 3 months. Those in medium-risk situations (e.g. horses kept at home but with occasional outings) should be vaccinated every six months.

If an outbreak occurs, any horse that has not had a booster within 3 months should be re-vaccinated. Provided the last injection was less than 6 months ago, a single dose is sufficient. Horses that are kept in a group with other horses that do not attend shows etc., are generally low risk and may not need vaccinating. Pregnant or lactating mares should not be vaccinated, and this vaccine should not be administered at the same time as other vaccines. Some horses experience temporary swelling of the upper lip and muzzle following vaccination.

In conclusion

Strangles can have huge cost implications as the activities of affected equine establishments may be restricted for a considerable period of time. Early diagnosis and good management are essential for prompt control of an outbreak.

PURPURA HAEMORRHAGICA

Purpura haemorrhagica is an immune-mediated condition that can develop as a sequel to strangles and other respiratory infections including equine influenza, equine herpesvirus 1 and *Rhodococcus equi*. Occasionally it develops following a wound infection or without any obvious cause. The symptoms occur 1–4 weeks after the horse appears to have recovered from the original infection.

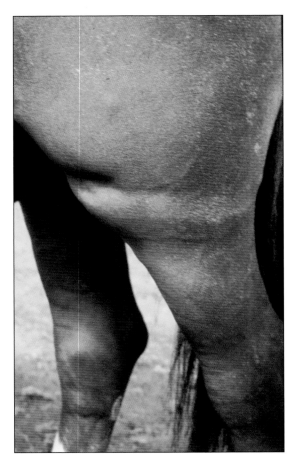

Figure 15.6 Swollen limbs and sheath of a horse with purpura haemorrhagica

Causes

The disease is caused by an allergic reaction to the streptococcal or viral antigens which circulate in the bloodstream. The blood vessels become inflamed and blood cells and serum leak through the capillary walls into the tissues. All of the major organs, i.e. heart, lungs and kidneys, may be affected.

Clinical signs

Some or all of the following signs may be seen:
- oedema (swelling) of the nostrils, eyes and lips
- oedema of one or more limbs which may become very swollen (Figure 15.6)
- soft, oedematous plaques of variable diameter on the neck, chest and thighs
- oedema of the ventral abdomen
- stiffness and reluctance to move
- leaking of clear or blood-stained fluid through the skin of the swollen areas (Figure 15.7)

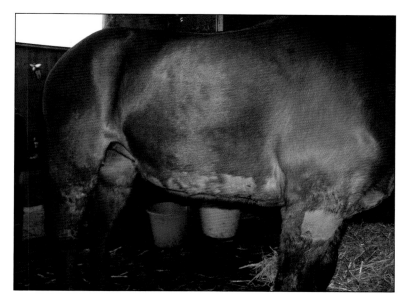

Figure 15.7 Serum may leak from the skin of the swollen areas

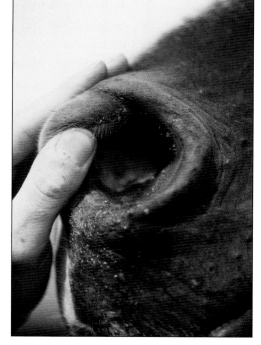

Figure 15.8 Small haemorrhages on the nasal mucosa

- affected areas may be very painful to touch
- small haemorrhages on the lips, gums and nasal mucosa (Figure 15.8)
- raised temperature
- secondary bacterial infection of skin lesions
- colic and blood-stained diarrhoea due to intestinal oedema
- respiratory distress if fluid accumulates in the lungs or larynx
- fatal circulatory collapse may occur.

Diagnosis

Diagnosis is made on the clinical signs and, if necessary, confirmed with the results of blood tests and a skin biopsy.

Treatment

The aim of treatment is to:
- eliminate any underlying infection
- reduce the immune response
- reduce the inflammation of the blood vessels
- provide supportive therapy and good nursing care.

This is achieved by using:
- antibiotics which are continued for several days after the patient appears to have recovered

- corticosteroids to dampen the exaggerated immune response
- non-steroidal anti-inflammatory drugs to reduce the pain and the inflammation in the blood vessel walls
- diuretics may be given at the start of treatment.

NURSING CARE

Good nursing is essential. The horse should be kept in a warm dry stable with a clean, comfortable bed. Shavings tend to stick to the weeping sores more than other bedding materials. Weeping areas should be gently cleaned. Rugs should be avoided if possible as they can cause pressure sores. The limbs may be lightly bandaged to reduce oedema and prevent bedding sticking to the exudate. Gentle exercise in hand may help to decrease the swelling.

Horses that experience difficulty eating and drinking should be given fluids intravenously or by nasogastric tube.

Prognosis

With early diagnosis and prompt treatment, the prognosis is fair. However, in severe cases, even with the best of care, 30–50% of affected horses and ponies will die. Respiratory distress, diarrhoea and a poor response to initial treatment are all poor prognostic signs.

SINUSITIS

In the horse's head there are several air-filled spaces which are collectively called the paranasal sinuses. These are lined with mucous membrane which continually secretes mucus. This is cleared by mucociliary flow and drains via small holes called ostia into the nasal passages. From here it evaporates, runs from the nostrils or is swallowed. Sinusitis is the term used for inflammation of the sinuses. It is usually caused by bacterial infection.

Causes

Infection of the paranasal sinuses may be the result of the following.

- **An upper respiratory tract infection** Viruses can damage the lining of the sinuses and this can interfere with the normal clearance of mucus. Initially there is a nasal discharge due to overflow of mucus or pus. As the lining becomes thickened as a result of inflammation, the drainage ostia may become partially blocked and mucus collects within the sinuses which then become infected by bacteria. This is called primary sinusitis.
- **Tooth root infection** The roots of the back four molar (cheek) teeth of the upper jaw lie within the maxillary sinuses. If a tooth root becomes infected the sinus is also involved.

- **Trauma** If the horse is kicked and the bone overlying the sinus is fractured and contaminated, secondary infection of the sinus may develop.
- **Cysts, tumours or an ethmoid haematoma** (see page 437) Any of these within the sinus can block the drainage of mucus and cause sinusitis.
- **Fungal infection** This can occur after sinus surgery if the horse is given hay and bedded on straw. Primary fungal infections are uncommon.

Clinical signs

These will include some of the following.

- **A unilateral nasal discharge** This may be mucopurulent, purulent or bloody depending on the cause of the sinus infection. A thick, foul-smelling discharge is likely to be secondary to tooth root infection. A yellow discharge without an unpleasant odour may be the result of primary sinusitis or a sinus cyst (Figure 15.9). Bloody discharges arise from trauma, a haematoma or a tumour. It is uncommon but possible for the discharge to come from both nostrils.
- **Localized facial swelling on one side** This occurs at the front or side of the face when there is an enlarging mass, e.g. a cyst or tumour within the sinus. Occasionally the swelling can block the flow of tears along the nasolacrimal duct causing tear overflow.

- **A dull sound on percussion of the sinuses** If an air-filled sinus is tapped with the fingers or knuckles the sound is hollow. This becomes dull if the sinus is filled with fluid, pus or a mass.
- **Abnormal respiratory noise** If the sinus is distorted it can obstruct the nasal passages and restrict air flow. This causes a noise which is present when the horse inhales and exhales and is constant from day to day. If the noise is present at rest, the obstruction is severe.
- **Evidence of tooth root infection** If the mouth is inspected with a gag in place, there may be evidence of a dental problem affecting one of the back molars in the upper jaw, e.g. a loose, broken or missing tooth. The gum surrounding a particular tooth may be inflamed or separated from the tooth. There may be a foul-smelling discharge from a draining sinus near the tooth and the horse's breath may smell unpleasant. The horse may experience pain on eating. However, in many cases of sinusitis secondary to dental disease, there is no obvious abnormality visible in the horse's mouth.

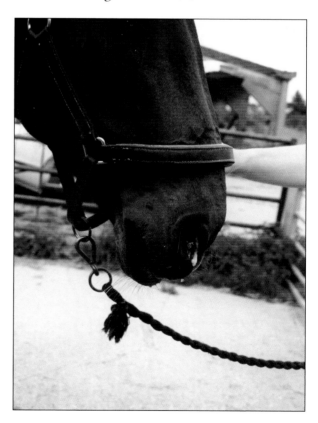

Figure 15.9 This horse with sinusitis has a persistent, thick yellow discharge from one nostril

- **Enlargement of the submandibular lymph node** This may occur on the affected side.
- **The presence of air under the skin** This sometimes occurs if the horse has experienced facial trauma, e.g. a depression fracture caused by a kick or polo ball. This is usually accompanied by soft tissue swelling and pain.
- **Poor performance and behaviour changes** A horse with sinusitis may well have a headache which is more painful with athletic activity, especially jumping or galloping.

Diagnosis

Diagnosis is usually straightforward. The history is often suggestive of sinusitis and the diagnosis is confirmed by radiography and endoscopy.

RADIOGRAPHY

The sinuses of normal horses are filled with air and appear black on radiographs. If there is an accumulation of liquid pus within the sinus, an obvious horizontal line can be seen. This is because the pus is denser than air and looks grey. Soft tissue masses such as mucus-filled cysts and tumours are also visible on the radiographs.

When a tooth root is infected, it may be possible to see erosion of bone or areas of increased bone density around the apex of the tooth. The affected root may have been eroded by the infection and have an altered outline. With dental disease a fluid line may or may not be visible.

ENDOSCOPY

This is done in two ways. By passing the endoscope up the nasal passages, the vet will try to locate the source of the discharge. The drainage opening (ostia) of the sinuses can be seen and checked for abnormalities. Sometimes pus or blood can be seen trickling from them. The vet will also check for any narrowing or ulceration of the nasal passages. If an ethmoid haematoma is the cause of the sinusitis, it can usually be seen with an endoscope.

Alternatively, sinus endoscopy may be performed. The endoscope is inserted directly into the sinus through a hole (trephine) drilled in the overlying bone. The sinus cavity can then be inspected.

BIOPSY

The results of the radiography and endoscopy may suggest the presence of a cyst or tumour. In this case, exploratory surgery and biopsy may be performed. If the sinus cavity has not already been opened, a small hole is made in the overlying bone. Samples of the pus or abnormal tissue can be taken for culture and examination under the microscope. This can be done under sedation using local anaesthetic.

Treatment

- A sinus infection that develops following an upper respiratory tract infection usually responds well to antibiotics if treated promptly. Mucolytics and steam inhalation can help to shift the mucopus and restore the normal mucociliary clearance mechanisms. Light exercise should be continued. If the nasal discharge returns when the antibiotics are finished, further investigation is necessary.

- If the discharge persists, an in-dwelling catheter may be inserted into the sinus through a small hole. The sinus is flushed regularly for 1–2 weeks with large volumes of lukewarm saline, dilute antiseptics and/or antibiotics to clear the mucus and eliminate infection. During this time, light exercise is beneficial

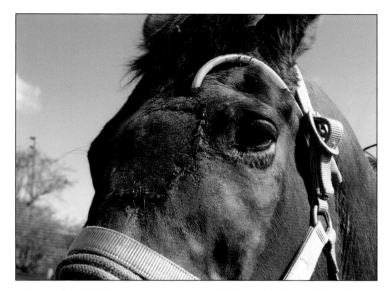

Figure 15.10 A sinus cyst was removed through a bone flap; the sinus is flushed regularly with an in-dwelling (Foley) catheter

- In chronic cases where the pus has become very solid, surgery may be necessary to remove it. This is done through a bone flap made in the horse's face while under general anaesthesia. In order to assist subsequent drainage, a hole (fistula) may be artificially created between the sinus and the nasal cavity.

- Cysts and ethmoid haematomas are surgically removed through a bone flap (Figure 15.10).

- Infected cheek teeth should be removed. The hole which is left between the sinus and the mouth is then filled with dental wax to prevent food material entering the sinus cavity. The sinus is flushed for a few days post operatively. Complications are relatively common following dental extraction.

- Tumours are rare and they are usually malignant. As they tend to occur in older animals, euthanasia is often the kindest option.

- Fungal infections are treated with twice daily flushing with an antifungal drug through an in-dwelling catheter.

- Traumatic injuries may be treated conservatively with antibiotic cover in some cases. Surgery may be necessary to remove bone fragments and foreign material from the sinuses if there is an open fracture. With depression fractures, surgery can be carried out to lift the bone into more normal alignment for a better cosmetic result.

Prognosis

With appropriate treatment, most cases of sinusitis resolve and carry a good prognosis. The occasional horse continues to show intermittent, low-grade signs that temporarily respond to antibiotics. The cost of treatment can be high.

PNEUMONIA

Pneumonia is a serious condition caused by bacterial infection of the lungs or inhalation of foreign material. The bacteria cause severe inflammation, and pus accumulates within the lung tissue and the airways. Large abscesses may form. These are difficult to treat and the mortality rate is high. Even if the animal survives, there may be permanent damage to the lung tissue. Bacterial pneumonia is uncommon in adult horses and tends to affect foals and young animals.

Causes

- Viral infections can damage the respiratory epithelium and weaken the horse's immune system allowing secondary bacterial infection. These bacteria are usually inhaled.
- The bacteria most commonly involved are *Streptococcus spp, Pasteurella spp, Actinobacillus spp, Mycoplasma spp, Rhodococcus equi, E. coli* and *Pseudomonas*.
- Inhalation of food or liquid, e.g. in any disease where the horse has difficulty swallowing. It may follow careless drenching or a severe episode of choke.
- Stress can predispose to pneumonia, e.g. long journeys or strenuous exercise, before an animal has fully recovered from an upper respiratory infection.
- Bacteria may enter the navel of a newborn foal, enter the bloodstream and reach the lungs or the joints.

Clinical signs

These include:
- fever, 39–41 °C (103–106 °F)
- fast, shallow breathing
- coughing
- abnormal lung sounds
- lethargy and depression
- loss of appetite and condition
- chest pain
- enlargement of the lymph nodes under the mandible
- in advanced cases, young animals may have flared nostrils and experience severe respiratory distress.

When to call the vet

If you suspect your horse or foal has pneumonia, call the vet immediately.

Diagnosis

- The condition is diagnosed on:

- the clinical signs
- auscultation of the lungs (listening with a stethoscope)
- endoscopy
- tracheal wash or bronchoalveolar lavage – a sample of the mucopus is taken from the trachea or bronchi and smeared onto a slide and stained so the type of bacteria involved can be identified; the secretions are also cultured for identification of the bacteria and to determine their sensitivity to different antibiotics
- in foals and young animals, radiography and ultrasonography are useful diagnostic tools; in advanced cases, abscesses can be seen in the lung tissue
- blood tests are likely to show increased white cell counts and raised fibrinogen and globulins.

Treatment

This depends on the severity of the condition. Affected individuals should be isolated as the disease can be spread to other animals from direct contact or from the discharges that are released into the environment by coughing.

- Antibiotics are always administered. The choice of antibiotic will be determined from the results of the culture and sensitivity. These may be given for a period of 4–6 weeks.
- Mucolytics to help thin the mucus and pus and/or bronchodilators to relieve any bronchospasm can help to clear the airways and make breathing easier.
- Non-steroidal anti-inflammatory drugs help to reduce the fever and pain.
- In severe cases oxygen is administered by a face mask.
- Intravenous fluids may be necessary.

NURSING

The horse must be nursed in a well-ventilated box with a deep, clean bed. Soft palatable food, e.g. warm mashes, should be offered and fresh drinking water must be available. If necessary, a rug should be used to keep the animal warm.

Prognosis

This is extremely guarded. In some cases the condition is rapidly fatal. Once abscesses have formed in the lungs, the mortality rate is high. Early diagnosis and immediate treatment give the horse the best chance of survival.

PLEUROPNEUMONIA AND PLEURISY

The surface of the lungs and the inside of the chest cavity are lined with a membrane called the pleura. Inflammation of these membranes is known as pleuritis or pleurisy. It is caused by bacterial infection. Pus forms and collects at the bottom of the chest cavity. If the pleural effusion develops secondary to pneumonia or a lung abscess, the condition is known as pleuropneumonia.

Causes

- Stress, e.g. prolonged travelling is considered to be a major factor in triggering the disease. When pleuropneumonia occurs following long journeys it is known as 'Transit or Shipping Fever'. During transport, horses may be exposed to warm temperatures and high humidity. This combined with the fact that the horse has his head tied up for long periods, compromises the immunity of the respiratory tract. As the horse is unable to lower its head, the secretions of the airways are unable to drain and bacterial invasion readily occurs.
- It may develop following viral or bacterial respiratory disease.
- A penetrating injury to the chest can cause pleurisy.
- The disease may develop after inhalation of foreign material into the lungs.
- Over-exertion, e.g. during racing, can predispose to pleuropneumonia.

CLINICAL SIGNS

The early signs include:

- raised temperature
- fast, shallow breathing
- a soft, painful cough
- +/- nasal discharge; if present, this can be watery, purulent or haemorrhagic, and it may have an unpleasant smell
- poor appetite
- moving stiffly with small steps and a general reluctance to move
- abnormal posture with the elbows held outwards, away from the chest wall
- the condition is painful and affected animals are very miserable.

As the condition progresses:

- respiration becomes even more of an effort
- pus collecting in the lower part of the chest cavity may prevent the lungs from expanding fully; the patient becomes short of oxygen and may grunt with the pain and effort of breathing
- adhesions may form between the surface of the lung and the chest wall and this makes breathing and moving even more painful
- the horse may become toxic
- swelling may develop under the skin of the lowest part of the chest or abdomen (ventral oedema)
- the horse may sweat and look very anxious
- there is usually significant weight loss.

Diagnosis

The history and the clinical signs are enough to make the vet consider a diagnosis of pleuropneumonia or pleurisy. The examination is likely to include the following.

- Taking the horse's temperature. However, fever is not a consistent sign and the temperature may fluctuate.
- Listening to the chest with a stethoscope. Wheezing and crackling sounds may be heard in the upper part of the chest and there is usually an absence of normal respiratory sounds in the lower part of the chest. Sometimes there are 'rubbing' sounds due to the friction between pleura on the chest wall and the surface of the lungs.
- Percussion (tapping) of the chest wall to determine the extent of the fluid in the chest. Where the lungs are surrounded by pus or fluid, the sound generated will be dull. Where they are surrounded by air, the sound will be hollow. This procedure is rarely resented by a normal horse but is very uncomfortable for a horse with pleural inflammation.
- Ultrasonography. This is very useful for showing the presence, extent and nature of an effusion. Adhesions and abscesses can also be identified.
- Taking a sample of fluid from the chest for microscopic examination and culture. The ultrasound examination will show the best place to insert the cannula to obtain a sample. This procedure is known as **thoracocentesis**.
- Performing a tracheal wash or bronchoalveolar lavage to identify the bacteria causing the pneumonia and their antibiotic sensitivity.
- Blood tests. The total white cell count and fibrinogen will be raised.
- If radiographs are taken, the pus may show up as a horizontal line. This is only suitable for foals and small horses.

Treatment

The aim of treatment is to:

- eliminate the bacterial infection
- remove the fluid and pus from the pleural cavity
- provide good nursing and supportive care to minimize the risk of complications.

Treatment includes:

- complete rest
- drainage of the chest cavity (Figure 15.11)
- flushing of the pleural cavity if pus and debris are present
- antibiotics for a long period of time including metronidazole to eliminate anaerobic bacteria
- analgesics as the condition is very painful
- intravenous fluids as necessary
- careful nursing to make the horse as comfortable as possible and minimize stress; the horse should be tempted to eat

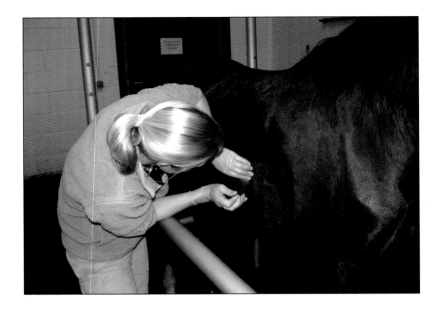

- if there is a discrete abscess in the pleural cavity, a portion of rib may be removed under local analgesia with the horse standing.; the abscess is drained and flushed, then the chest is left open to drain and heal by second intention
- surgical drainage under general anaesthesia is occasionally carried out as a salvage procedure to try and save, for example, a valuable mare for breeding.

Figure 15.11 Inserting a chest drain

The treatment requires hospitalization and the costs are considerable. The risk of complications is high.

Prognosis

If the condition is diagnosed in the early stages and the correct treatment is started at once, then the horse has a reasonable chance of recovery. If the disease is more long standing and adhesions have formed, the prognosis for recovery and return to the previous level of performance is poor.

Prevention

- If long journeys are unavoidable, horses should be allowed to rest, eat and drink regularly. Their heads should not be tied up for lengthy periods.
- They should be allowed to recover fully from respiratory conditions before travelling or competing.
- Unnecessary stress should be avoided.

GUTTURAL POUCH DISEASE

The guttural pouches are a pair of air-filled sacs which lie between the roof of the nasopharynx and the base of the brain. They are outpouchings of the Eustachian tubes connecting the middle ear with the nasopharynx. They are lined with mucous membrane and drain into the nasopharynx via ostia (openings) which are covered by flaps of cartilage. These only open when the horse swallows. A number of important nerves and blood vessels run through and around the guttural pouches.

There are three main diseases of the guttural pouch:

- tympany
- empyema
- mycosis.

Guttural pouch tympany

This is a quite rare congenital condition whereby an anatomical or functional defect allows one (or occasionally both) pouches to fill with air but not to empty. Young foals are the most likely to be affected. The pouch becomes distended and a swelling is visible in the parotid region behind the mandible. This is not painful but affected foals may have difficulty breathing and eating as a result of the swelling. Milk may return down the nostrils after attempts to swallow. The normal drainage of mucus may be obstructed leading to secondary bacterial infection and a mucopurulent nasal discharge.

The condition is diagnosed on the clinical signs and can be confirmed by radiography and endoscopy. Treatment involves creating a window in the thin septum between the two pouches so the air from both can drain from the normal pouch into the nasopharynx. The outcome is usually good. Complications include inhalation pneumonia and guttural pouch empyema.

Guttural pouch empyema

This is when the guttural pouch(es) fill up with pus. It can occur as a sequel to strangles or other upper respiratory infections. The retropharyngeal lymph nodes can form abscesses which burst and drain into the guttural pouches. The disease usually affects one gutteral pouch but is occasionally bilateral. The main symptom is a unilateral purulent nasal discharge which occurs especially when the horse has its head down, e.g. when grazing. The discharge may have an unpleasant smell. Sometimes the pus forms hard lumps called chondroids which are like pebbles and cannot drain from the pouch(es). The horse's pharynx may be swollen, causing difficulty with breathing and swallowing and the pouches may be visibly distended (Figure 15.12). Horses with a chronic, less severe infection may show loss of performance.

The condition is diagnosed on the clinical signs and confirmed by radiography and endoscopy. Pus

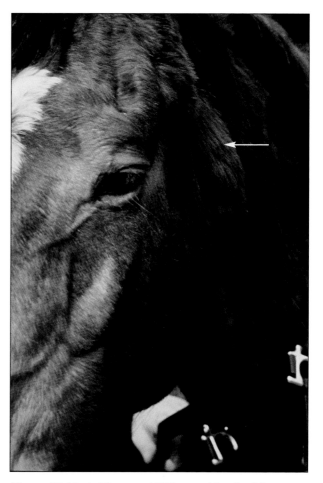

Figure 15.12 A 20-year-old Thoroughbred with guttural pouch empyema; the pus-filled guttural pouch is visibly distended

can often be seen draining from the guttural pouch opening(s) into the pharynx when the horse is examined with an endoscope. A small endoscope can be inserted into the guttural pouch allowing the pus or chondroids to be seen. When radiographs are taken, a fluid line or pebble-like chondroids may be visible. Fluid can be aspirated from the guttural pouches for bacterial culture.

Treatment involves draining and flushing the pouches. Chondroids cannot be flushed out and must be removed surgically. The horse is given antibiotics. If the horse is in pain or generally ill, non-steroidal anti-inflammatory drugs are also administered. Feeding the horse from the ground encourages drainage of the pouches.

Hygiene precautions are taken as the infection is likely to be due to the same bacterium that causes strangles. In some horses it is impossible to eliminate the infection altogether and they remain chronic carriers. The prognosis is guarded in all cases as recurrent episodes of nasal discharge are common.

Guttural pouch mycosis

This is potentially the most serious of the conditions which affect the gutteral pouch. The fungus, *Aspergillus spp,* found in straw and hay is able to colonize the roof of the gutteral pouch, leading to destructive changes and secondary bacterial infection. The clinical signs depend on which nerves and blood vessels have been damaged.

CLINICAL SIGNS

These include:

- bleeding from one nostril which is not related to exercise; this can vary from a trickle of bright red blood to a profuse and rapidly fatal haemorrhage (Figure 15.13)
- a foul-smelling nasal discharge
- neurological signs due to cranial nerve damage, e.g. Horner's syndrome (drooping eyelid, sunken eye, protrusion of the third eyelid), facial paralysis, laryngeal paralysis and pharyngeal paralysis leading to difficulty eating
- headshaking.

DIAGNOSIS

The diagnosis is easily confirmed by endoscopy of the guttural pouches. Plaques of fungal growth which may be black, grey, white or yellow are visible in the roof of the pouch or on folds of mucosa which

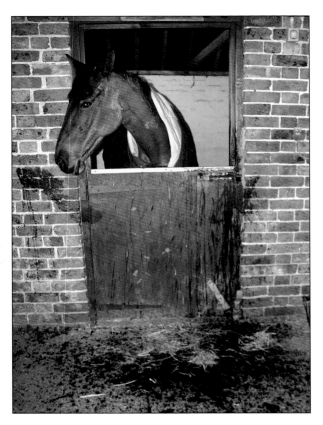

Figure 15.13 With guttural pouch mycosis bleeding can be profuse and rapidly fatal; urgent surgery is needed

contain nerves and blood vessels. Blood or pus may be seen within the pouch or escaping from the opening of the pouch into the pharynx. Fluid lines within the pouch are sometimes seen on radiography.

TREATMENT

If the horse has experienced a severe bleed, surgery should be done as soon as possible to tie off the affected artery. Any delay could result in the horse dying from a fatal haemorrhage. Following the surgery, antifungal powders are sprayed onto the roof of the pouch through in-dwelling catheters for at least a week.

PROGNOSIS

This depends on the extent of any nerve damage. Although the fungal plaques can be treated, some horses have permanent nerve damage and have to be destroyed. Where there is no nerve damage and the damaged artery is successfully ligated, the prognosis is good.

RECURRENT AIRWAY OBSTRUCTION (RAO)

Recurrent airway obstruction (RAO) is one of the names given to a common respiratory disease syndrome that affects horses and ponies. It is also known as chronic obstructive pulmonary disease (COPD), recurrent airway disease (RAD) and 'heaves'.

Causes

It is caused by inhalation of dust from the environment when a horse is stabled. Hay and straw contain fungal spores which trigger an allergic response which causes inflammation and narrowing of the lower airways.

When hay is baled with a high moisture content (above 20%), the bales heat up and the growth of moulds such as *Aspergillus fumigatus, Faenia rectivirgula* and *Thermoactinomyces vulgaris* occurs. Inhalation of spores of these fungi triggers the airways to become hypersensitive. It has now been shown that inhaled endotoxin from bacteria present in the environment triggers airway inflammation in normal horses. This is also likely to be a contributory factor in causing the disease. The sources of these bacteria have not yet been identified but they are likely to be from faeces, the horse's coat and the forage.

It is thought that some horses have a genetic susceptibility to RAO and are more easily sensitized than others.

FREE RADICALS AND OXIDATIVE STRESS

The horse's respiratory system is constantly exposed to external irritants. This can cause the release of abnormal amounts of **free radicals** which can attack cell membranes.

What are free radicals?

A free radical is a molecule or atom that has one or more unpaired electrons. It is unstable and tries to attract electrons from other molecules to pair up with these. This can start a chain reaction with increasing amounts of free radicals being released. If the production and removal of these is not controlled, tissue damage may occur, leading to inflammation. This is known as **oxidative stress** and may be an important factor in the development of RAO.

In a normal horse, the production of free radicals is controlled and those produced are 'neutralized' by well-developed antioxidant defence mechanisms. Experimental work has shown that the major antioxidant in the fluid lining of the lungs is ascorbic acid (vitamin C) and horses suffering from RAO or airway inflammation often have reduced levels of this vitamin.

Predisposing factors

- Repeated exposure to hay and straw dust containing moulds, forage mites, endotoxins and inorganic material.
- Dusty feeds.
- Long hours in the stable.
- Poor stable hygiene.
- Inadequate ventilation.
- A respiratory virus, e.g. equine influenza which damages the epithelial surface of the respiratory tract. This adversely affects the clearance of inhaled allergens and may alter the immune response of the horse.

Clinical signs

The disease usually develops over a period of time. Affected horses do not have a temperature and they appear well in themselves. The first signs include:

- reduced exercise tolerance
- increased respiratory rate
- increased expiratory effort – the abdominal muscles are used to force the air from the lungs; this results in a characteristic biphasic expiratory movement
- an occasional cough, usually at the start of exercise
- milky-white nasal discharge from both nostrils, especially first thing in the morning and after exercise (Figure 15.14)

As the condition progresses:

- breathing out requires even more effort and there is considerable movement of the abdominal muscles; this is known as 'heaving'
- the abdominal muscles become overdeveloped and a 'heave line' is seen (Figure 15.15)
- the respiratory rate increases further

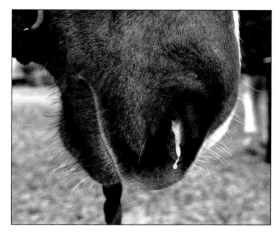

Figure 15.14 Milky white nasal discharge may be seen especially first thing in the morning or after exercise

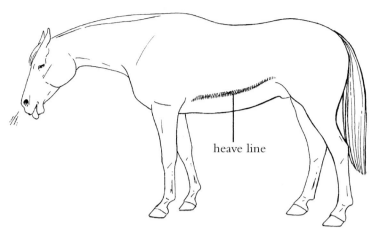

Figure 15.15 A 'heave line' is seen as the abdominal muscles become overdeveloped from the effort of breathing out

- expiratory airflow at the nostrils is biphasic
- the horse's anus moves in time with the respirations
- the nasal discharge may become thick and yellow
- the horse coughs at rest in the stable
- lumps of mucus are coughed up (Figure 15.16).

Once a horse has become sensitized, it may suffer acute attacks of the disease and develop severe respiratory difficulties in a short period of time. The animal breathes with flared nostrils and heaving flanks and has spells of continuous paroxysmal coughing. Wheezing sounds may be heard at the nostrils.

The incidence of the disease increases with age.

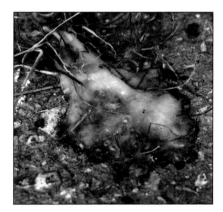

Figure 15.16 Lumps of mucus are commonly found on the ground outside the stable door

Why does this develop?

The expiratory difficulty is caused by obstruction of airflow in both the large and small airways. This is due to spasm of the smooth muscle (bronchospasm) in the larger airways and inflammation and the accumulation of mucus in the bronchioles. Both lead to a reduction in airway diameter so breathing requires more effort. These changes occur within a few hours of a susceptible horse being placed in a stable environment.

If the disease is not controlled, structural changes occur in the lungs over a period of time. The chronic inflammation leads to thickening of the mucosal lining of the bronchiolar walls and proliferation of the smooth muscle in the airway walls. In severe, long-term disease, the alveoli become over-inflated and emphysema can develop. The horse is colloquially described as '**broken-winded**'.

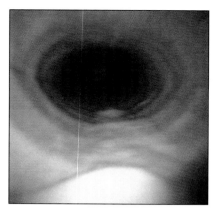

Figure 15.17 A stream of mucopus in the trachea with a large pool in the foreground

When to call the vet

Call the vet at the first sign of the disease. Early diagnosis, treatment and management changes often prevent it from developing into a serious problem.

Diagnosis

The diagnosis is made on the history and the clinical signs. In mild cases the vet may not hear any abnormal sounds with the stethoscope. In severe cases, a wide range of lung sounds including crackles and wheezes may be heard.

If the upper respiratory tract is examined with an endoscope, a stream of mucopus may be seen in the trachea (Figure 15.17). Examination of airway secretions taken by bronchoalveolar lavage reveals large numbers of neutrophils when compared with secretions obtained from an unaffected horse.

Treatment and control

Once a horse has developed a hypersensitivity to stable dust, there is no cure. If treated promptly, the changes are reversible but the horse remains more sensitive to respiratory allergens than normal. Treatment involves:

- environmental control
- administration of bronchodilators to relieve the bronchospasm
- corticosteroids to reduce the inflammation
- antioxidant supplementation.

Management

The key to both treatment and prevention of the disease is good stable management and stable design.

TURNING OUT

All horses should have plenty of fresh air with minimal exposure to dust and fungal spores. Wherever possible, they should be turned out for a few hours each day. The first step in treatment of horses with RAO is to turn them out completely for a period of at least 2–3 weeks. The field should be well away from the muck heap and the hay store. Bringing the horse into a stable for even a short period, e.g. for grooming or for the farrier will cause further inflammatory changes to take place in the lungs and prolong the period of recovery. The best management for a horse with RAO is to keep it permanently out at grass with no access to hay or straw.

STABLE DESIGN

In mild cases, changes in stable management and design may be all that is required to control the symptoms. Good ventilation is essential for the horse's health. Many modern boxes have low roofs and insufficient air vents to achieve the recommended ventilation rate of 8–10 complete air changes per hour. The ventilation of most boxes can be improved with relatively little expense. These improvements could include the following.

- Additional air inlets and outlets. To avoid draughts, air inlets should be positioned at the same height as the eaves. Ideally, each stable should have an outlet in the roof.
- An extra window at the back of the box can improve the air quality and considerably reduce the incidence of the disease.
- Top doors should be routinely left open.
- Wherever possible, each horse should have its own air space and the side walls should reach the roof of the stable. Management changes are still of value if the horse has to share the same air space as a horse with dry hay and straw, although this is far from ideal.

BEDDING

Straw is not the most suitable bedding as it has higher levels of fungal contamination than a well-managed peat, dust-extracted wood shavings, cardboard or paper bed. All beds need to be kept clean with the urine and droppings removed each day to prevent mould growth. Deep litter is not recommended as high levels of noxious gases such as ammonia and hydrogen sulphide may be produced. These are irritant to the respiratory tract as are some disinfectants, pesticides and preservatives. Rubber matting may be helpful if used with a small amount of bedding material. However, good drainage and management are required with rubber mats to prevent pooling of urine and an unhealthy atmosphere.

MUCKING OUT

It is essential that *all* the bed is removed and replaced at regular intervals. Wood shavings and paper beds that look clean can develop high levels of fungal growth after several months in the stable especially if the environment is damp.

During normal mucking out, the number of fungal spores and the dust levels in the stable are increased three to sixfold and they remain airborne for many hours. It therefore makes sense to muck out as soon as the horse is turned out so the spores and dust have a chance to settle before the horse is brought in again.

Ledges and window sills should regularly be cleared of dust and cobwebs to remove dust, fungal spores, bacteria, endotoxins etc.

THE MUCK HEAP

The muck heap should be sited as far from the stables as practical and preferably downwind.

TRANSPORT

When travelling, horses are often exposed to high dust levels. Straw and shavings in lorries and trailers quickly become musty and mixed up with old hay. The best solution is to use rubber matting and avoid feeding hay inside the vehicle.

RESPIRATORY INFECTIONS

Horses with RAO should avoid contact with others suffering from respiratory viruses. The symptoms may be exacerbated following a respiratory infection.

Diet
FORAGE
Hay

Wherever possible, hay should be excluded from the diet altogether as even well-made, good-quality hay has very high levels of dust and fungal spores. Grass, silage or vacuum-packed forage such as Horsehage® are suitable alternatives.

Buying and storing hay

It is always worth buying the best quality hay that is available. When a bale is opened it should have a fresh, sweet smell with no visible mould or dust. Hay should be stored in a separate building from the horse because millions of fungal spores are released into the atmosphere when hay nets are filled. In order to minimize fungal growth, the bales should be raised from the floor on wooden pallets.

Soaking hay

The area within 30 cm (1 ft) around the horse's nose is called the 'breathing zone'. When a horse pulls dry hay from a net, large numbers of fungal spores and dust particles (up to 63,000 per litre of air) become airborne and are inhaled. Soaking the hay prior to feeding significantly reduces the amount of dust inhaled provided it is all eaten before it dries out. Total immersion in clean water for between 30 minutes and 2 hours is recommended.

Ideally the hay net should be positioned by the door or a window. If the stable is large enough, it should be tied so there is minimal mixing with the bedding and any that is not eaten can be swept up and removed.

Vacuum-packed forage

Vacuum-packed forage has been developed as an alternative to hay. Grass is cut and allowed to wilt before being baled and compressed. The bales are sealed in bags to exclude air and a mild fermentation process begins. Under these conditions mould growth is inhibited and the feed will keep for up to 18 months.

Vacuum-packed forage has a higher nutritional content than most hay. It should be introduced into the diet over a period of 2–3 weeks and concentrates may need to be reduced. Opened packs should be used within 5 days. If the bag is accidentally punctured it should be fed immediately. A feeding guide can be obtained from the manufacturers. Hay nets with small holes slow down the intake of this forage.

CONCENTRATES AND GRAINS

A complete cubed diet or molassed mix has considerably less dust and fungal spores than rolled grains such as oats or barley.

ANTIOXIDANT SUPPLEMENTATION

Antioxidants are sometimes known as 'free-radical scavengers'. They are able to donate an electron and neutralize free radicals without becoming a free radical themselves. Some antioxidants occur naturally in the body but their capacity may be overwhelmed in the face of challenge. Horses and ponies suffering from RAO often have low natural antioxidant defences. Dietary supplementation with a balanced antioxidant mix has been shown to improve lung function and reduce inflammation in horses with RAO. Vitamin C is the most important antioxidant in the fluid lining of the lungs.

Exercise

Horses with moderate to severe breathing difficulties should not be worked. Mildly affected horses should have their exercise restricted to a level they can manage comfortably. During a bout of coughing, the horse should be allowed to extend its head and return to walk.

With good management, a definite improvement should be seen in mildly affected horses within 3–4 weeks. However, moderate and severely affected horses require medication to alleviate the respiratory distress and aid recovery.

Medication

The most useful medications are bronchodilators and corticosteroids.

BRONCHODILATORS

Bronchodilators are used to relieve the respiratory distress from bronchospasm experienced by horses during acute episodes. They relax the smooth muscle in the airways. The commonly used ones include the following.

- Drugs such as clenbuterol (Ventipulmin®) relieve bronchospasm and increase the speed of clearance of mucus from the airways. The drug can be given intravenously or orally. Some horses require up to four times the normal dose of this drug for it to be effective. At higher doses, side effects including sweating and trembling, and the horse's heart rate may be raised.
- Inhaled bronchodilators such as salmeterol are sometimes administered using an Equine Aero Mask™ or other inhalation devices but their duration of action is relatively short.

- Atropine which may be given once by intravenous injection at the start of treatment to relieve acute respiratory distress. If bronchospasm is a contributory factor, the drug will be effective and provide relief within 15–20 minutes. However, atropine can cause colic as a side effect and so is not safe for regular use.

If there is no response to bronchodilators then inflammatory changes are involved and corticosteroids are often prescribed.

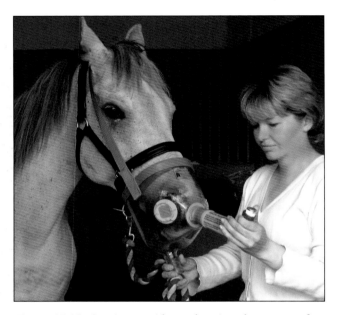

Figure 15.18 Corticosteroids can be given by means of a face mask with an attached spacer and metered dose

CORTICOSTEROIDS

Corticosteroids are the drug of choice for reducing inflammation in the lungs of horses with RAO. They can be administered by injection, orally or by inhalation. A horse with severe disease needs the treatment to be given by injection or orally to start with as they are unable to breathe in enough of the drug. Dexamethasone and prednisolone are commonly used. Once the symptoms are controlled, inhaled medication is preferable as there is less risk of side effects which include laminitis, Cushings-type signs and suppression of the immune system. Immunosuppression increases the risk of the horse succumbing to bacterial infection. The inhaled corticosteroids include beclomethasone dipropionate and fluticasone propionate. The horse is treated twice a day using a metered dose canister. A number of systems for delivering the drug are now available including face masks with an attached spacer and metered dose canister (Figure 15.18).

OTHER MEDICATION

Disodium cromoglycate is sometimes used as a prophylactic treatment to prevent the disease occurring when a horse that is known to be susceptible to RAO is unavoidably exposed to allergens. It is administered by nebulization. The response to this treatment is not consistent. It appears to work for some horses but not for others.

Mucolytics are drugs that help to break up the mucus so it is more easily cleared from the airways. The efficacy of these drugs in horses has not been proved.

Antibiotics are rarely necessary as secondary bacterial infection is uncommon.

Prognosis

If managed correctly, the changes in the lungs are reversible. However, once a horse or pony has been sensitized, the symptoms will recur if it is exposed to environmental allergens. The airways also become hyper-responsive to other irritants in the atmosphere such as noxious gases. The condition tends to become worse with age and causes reduced exercise tolerance. The prognosis is therefore guarded.

SUMMER PASTURE ASSOCIATED OBSTRUCTIVE PULMONARY DISEASE (SPAOPD)

A number of horses and ponies develop the signs of recurrent airway obstruction (RAO) while out at grass with no exposure to hay and straw. The condition tends to occur between the spring and early autumn months, with complete remission of symptoms during the winter, and is known as summer pasture associated obstructive pulmonary disease (SPAOPD). A number of affected animals also have RAO so they experience respiratory problems all year round. Once affected, the symptoms tend to recur in subsequent years. The incidence of SPAOPD increases with age.

Causes
The cause is thought to be a hypersensitivity of the lungs to inhaled pollens and moulds. The symptoms are often worse when conditions are hot and dusty. Once the airways become hyper-responsive, non-specific triggers such as cold or dry air, irritant dust and exercise may exacerbate the condition. Harvesting of crops in nearby fields is a common trigger.

Clinical signs
These include:
- severe respiratory distress with fast, shallow breathing
- breathing out is particularly laboured as the airways are obstructed
- there is a marked abdominal lift on expiration as the muscles are used to help force air out of the lungs
- a 'heave line' develops in the muscles on each side of the ventral abdomen
- coughing
- flared nostrils
- nasal discharge
- anal movements in time with respiration due to extra abdominal effort
- crackling and wheezing sounds if the condition is severe.

Mildly affected horses and ponies have a normal appetite and demeanour. In a severe case the animal will have a bluish tinge to the mucous membranes due to receiving insufficient oxygen. If the condition is chronic and severe, the affected animal is likely to experience some weight loss. If left untreated, SPAOPD can be life-threatening.

WHY DOES THE HORSE DEVELOP THESE SIGNS?

As with RAO, the respiratory tract is hyper-responsive to inhaled allergens. The end result is inflammation and swelling of the airway walls, excessive production of mucus and bronchospasm, all of which cause narrowing of the airways.

Diagnosis

Diagnosis is made on the history and the clinical signs. If bronchial secretions are examined under the microscope they have an abnormally high percentage of neutrophils.

Treatment

The treatment consists of changing the environment of the horse to remove it from the source of the inhaled allergens. This is combined with the administration of bronchodilator and anti-inflammatory drugs. Oxygen is used in an emergency if the horse has severe breathing difficulties.

ENVIRONMENT

Some animals show an immediate improvement if they are moved to another location. However, this is not always possible. Provided the horse does not also suffer from RAO, it may improve if stabled in an environment that is as dust-free as possible (see Recurrent Airway Obstruction).

BRONCHODILATORS

Drugs such as clenbuterol (Ventipulmin®) sometimes help but often provide only temporary relief.

CORTICOSTEROIDS

Corticosteroids are the most useful treatment as they reduce the inflammation in the airways. They may be given intravenously in the emergency situation and then orally. As soon as the respiratory distress is under control, inhaled corticosteroids are used instead if possible to reduce the risk of side effects such as laminitis.

ANTIOXIDANT SUPPLEMENTATION

The addition of a balanced antioxidant supplement to the diet can improve respiratory function and reduce inflammation (see Recurrent Airway Obstruction for more information)

Prognosis

The prognosis is guarded as the condition tends to recur in subsequent years and effective management is often very difficult.

EXERCISE-INDUCED PULMONARY HAEMORRHAGE (EIPH)

When horses undertake strenuous exercise, bleeding can occur from the blood vessels in the lung tissue. This is known as exercise-induced pulmonary haemorrhage (EIPH). The uppermost lung lobes at the back of the chest, i.e. those under the back of the saddle are affected.

Clinical signs

- Bleeding from the nostrils is seen in severe cases (Figure 15.19). Most affected horses do not bleed from the nostrils, but haemorrhage can be seen in the airways when the horse is examined with an endoscope (Figure 15.20).
- Reduced performance.
- Coughing after exercise.
- Swallowing more than usual after exercise.
- Slower recovery from the exertion than normal.
- Some horses have recurrent episodes that become worse with age.

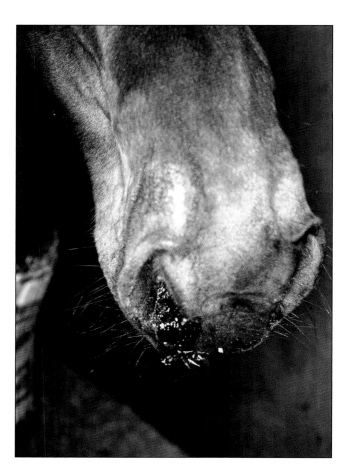

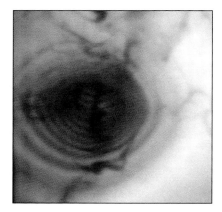

Figure 15.19 Bleeding from the nostrils is seen in severe cases of exercise-induced pulmonary haemorrhage (left)

Figure 15.20 Streaks of blood in the trachea of a horse with EIPH (above)

Up to 75% of Thoroughbreds have some blood in their windpipe after racing. It also occurs in other sport horses that perform at speed such as polo ponies and eventers.

Causes

The condition is not fully understood. It is thought that the high pressures that develop in the lungs during racing are sufficient to rupture the small capillaries that surround the alveoli (air sacs). Horses with underlying airway inflammation from infection or recurrent airway obstruction (RAO) are more likely to bleed. Poor air hygiene from dust, fungal spores and ammonia are all contributory factors. Laryngeal hemiplegia may also predispose to the condition.

Diagnosis

The diagnosis is made on the history, clinical examination and endoscopy. Endoscopy is essential to determine the source of the bleeding and rule out conditions such as guttural pouch mycosis. If there is no blood at the nostrils and EIPH is suspected, the horse should be scoped shortly after the end of a race. The amount of bleeding is variable. If it is severe, blood is visible in the trachea for several days. Tracheal washes and bronchoalveolar lavage samples contain an abnormally high number of red blood cells. Macrophages containing pigment (haemosiderin) from degenerating blood cells may also be present, indicating previous pulmonary haemorrhage.

Severe bleeding also results in the affected part of the lung appearing denser than normal on radiographs.

Treatment

There is no proven treatment for EIPH. The haemorrhage into the lungs causes inflammation which becomes worse with successive episodes. Various remedies have been tried but most are not permitted under the rules of racing.

- Corticosteroids may be used to try and settle the inflammation.
- Bronchodilators may be helpful if the horse is suffering from RAO.
- The use of diuretics during training and prior to racing is controversial. These drugs increase the amount of urine produced and lower the blood pressure.

Fresh air and good stable hygiene are important for all horses. Affected animals should be allowed sufficient rest after severe episodes of bleeding.

Prognosis

Some horses have the occasional bleed with no obvious loss of performance. However, the prognosis is guarded if a horse experiences repeated episodes of EIPH.

NOSEBLEEDS IN HORSES

The veterinary term for a nosebleed is **epistaxis**. Nosebleeds are common in horses; they can look alarming but usually stop on their own. However, there are one or two serious causes of nosebleeds and it is crucial to know which ones are worth worrying about.

Causes

A nosebleed occurs when any part of the nasal passages (which are richly supplied with blood vessels), throat, lower airways or lungs, are injured to such a degree that blood vessels are damaged and blood leaks out. Possible causes include the following.

- A simple knock on the head may cause blood to pour from one nostril. These nosebleeds usually stop within fifteen minutes.
- Passage of a stomach tube may cause a nosebleed if the delicate nasal tissues are inadvertently knocked, e.g. if the horse moves at the wrong moment. The flow of blood can appear alarming but again the bleeding usually stops within 10–15 minutes.

More serious causes of nosebleeds are listed below.

- Guttural pouch mycosis. This is a condition that may cause severe nosebleeds unrelated to exercise or trauma. It is unusual for the horse to die as a result of the first nosebleed associated with this, but more than 50% will succumb, usually within days or weeks if they do not receive the appropriate surgical treatment to control the bleeding. The diagnosis and treatment of this disease is discussed in more detail on pages 422–5.
- Progressive ethmoid haematoma. This is a growth that develops on the tissues at the back of the horse's nose, sometimes within the sinuses. One of the first signs is a unilateral (one-sided) blood-tinged nasal discharge, but as it enlarges it may obstruct the airflow and cause abnormal respiratory noise, facial swelling and neurological signs. The condition is diagnosed by endoscopy and sometimes radiography. The treatment options include surgical excision, laser treatment, injection with formalin or freezing with liquid nitrogen. The recurrence rate following surgery is around 25%. Fortunately the condition is rare.
- Exercise-induced pulmonary haemorrhage (EIPH). This occurs when the tiny thin-walled blood vessels in the lungs are damaged by the high pressures that develop within the lungs of the galloping horse. Bleeding is sometimes seen at both nostrils and may be accompanied by coughing and poor exercise performance. The bleeding may remain within the airways rather than appear at the nostrils and requires endoscopy to detect it. It varies from slight to severe but is only very rarely fatal. Affected horses are sometimes known as 'bleeders' or described as having 'burst a blood vessel'. The condition is described in more detail on pages 435–6.

Less common causes of nosebleeds include:
- a foreign body wedged in the nose or throat
- inflammation/infection of the sinuses
- a tumour in the respiratory tract
- some types of heart disease.

How to decide if a nosebleed is serious
- How much blood is being lost? It is important to estimate the blood loss as a small bleed down the front of a grey horse can look dramatic while a large bleed may be concealed under straw bedding. Would the drips slowly fill a teacup or would the flow rapidly amount to several litres (half a stable bucket)? Most minor bleeds stop within 15 minutes but if you are concerned, seek immediate veterinary advice.
- Is the blood coming from one nostril or two? This is important as bleeding from guttural pouch mycosis (which can be rapidly fatal) usually occurs from one nostril.
- Is there any obvious reason for the bleed? Has the horse just had a knock or fall? Has the vet just passed a stomach tube up the nose?
- Is it a one-off nosebleed? If it has happened repeatedly then it definitely needs investigation.
- Has the horse just been exercising hard and therefore be likely to have an EIPH?

Diagnosis
In order to determine the cause of recurrent or persistent nosebleeds, the vet may use the following techniques.
- Endoscopy.
- Sinoscopy – the endoscope is inserted directly into the sinus cavity through a small hole drilled in the skull.
- Radiography.
- Magnetic resonance imaging (MRI).
- Computed tomography (CT).

Treatment
Once the source of the nosebleed has been identified, the most appropriate treatment can be given.

First aid for nosebleeds
- With any nosebleed the horse should be kept as calm as possible. Confining it to a stable may help.
- The nose should never be packed as horses breathe through their noses so this would prevent them breathing properly and cause distress.
- If the bleeding is profuse or continues for more than 15 minutes, request urgent veterinary help.

Remember that the average Thoroughbred horse has approximately 50 litres of blood, so although the horse appears to be losing a lot of blood, it may not be critical.

RECURRENT LARYNGEAL NEUROPATHY (RLN)

This condition is also known as laryngeal paralysis, idiopathic laryngeal hemiplegia and idiopathic laryngeal paresis.

Recurrent laryngeal neuropathy is a condition in which affected horses make a characteristic whistling or roaring sound due to obstruction of inhaled air as it passes through the larynx. It occurs in Thoroughbreds, Warmbloods and draught horses over 16 hh and rarely affects horses under 15.2 hh. It may be an inherited condition that is usually apparent by the time the horse is 6 years old.

Structure and function of the larynx

The larynx (voice box) is situated in the horse's throat at the top of the trachea (windpipe) where it opens into the pharynx. It is made up of several cartilages and ligaments, joined in such a way that it can open and close. The opening and closing of the larynx is controlled by several small muscles. Most of these are innervated by the right and left recurrent laryngeal nerves which run from the chest area along the trachea to the larynx.

NORMAL MOVEMENTS OF THE LARYNX

When the horse swallows, the larynx closes to prevent inhalation of food. During strenuous exercise, the larynx opens fully to allow maximum air flow to the lungs. During respiration while the horse is at rest, the larynx is in an intermediate position. It opens a little wider during inspiration and narrows during expiration. In normal horses, the opening of the larynx is symmetrical and the movement is smooth and equal on both sides.

Causes

For reasons that are not fully understood, the left recurrent laryngeal nerve degenerates in some horses. It is thought that the considerable length of the nerve may be a factor and that viruses could possibly exacerbate any pathology. The muscles supplied by the damaged nerve waste away and the left side of the larynx is no longer capable of the normal range of movement. There is incomplete opening of the left side of the larynx resulting from loss of function of the dorsal cricoarytenoid muscle. During fast exercise the flow of air is obstructed (Figure 15.21).

The right recurrent laryngeal nerve is shorter than the left nerve and is rarely affected. Neuropathy of the right recurrent laryngeal nerve is a rare and unfortunate consequence

normal larynx   *paralysed larynx*

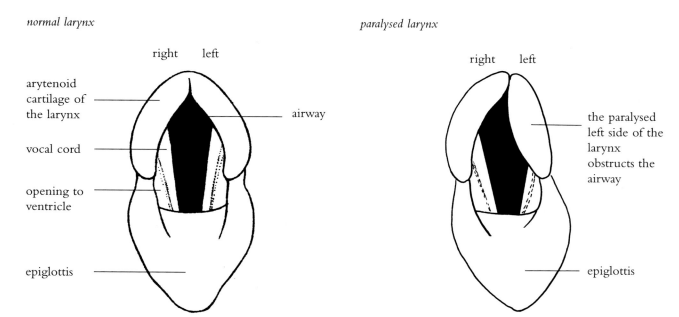

Figure 15.21 A normal and a paralysed larynx

of intravenous injections given on the right side of the neck where some of the drug is accidentally deposited outside the vein.

Clinical signs

- The horse makes an abnormal noise when it *breathes in* at canter and gallop. This is due to turbulence in the air stream as the air passes through the obstructed laryngeal opening. The tissue on the affected side vibrates and causes a noise. It may be a high-pitched whistle (in mild cases) or a harsh roaring sound. In severe cases it can be heard at trot. The noise should not be confused with normal expiratory (breathing out) sounds such as 'high blowing' which is caused by air turbulence at the nostrils.
- The horse may show reduced performance at exercise as the tissues receive less oxygen.
- The horse's voice may change.
- As the muscles on the left side of the larynx atrophy (waste away), the process on the left arytenoid cartilage where the wasted muscle attaches becomes more prominent and may be palpated through the skin.

These signs can develop anytime up to 6 years of age and the condition is often progressive. Thoroughbred yearlings destined for racing are frequently wind tested prior to sale.

Diagnosis

Diagnosis is made on the clinical findings.
- Abnormal inspiratory noise. The horse is examined at canter. At this gait, the horse's

stride pattern and the respiratory cycle are linked. The horse breathes out as the leading foreleg contacts the ground and so by careful observation it can be determined whether the noise occurs on inspiration or expiration,

- Laryngeal palpation.
- Endoscopy.

ENDOSCOPIC FINDINGS

The larynx is examined at rest and usually immediately following strenuous exercise. Endoscopy is necessary to assess the degree of paralysis as well as to confirm the diagnosis. To make a full assessment, the horse may be examined with an endoscope whilst working on a treadmill. Since the degree of laryngeal dysfunction is variable, it is graded according to the endoscopic findings.

Grade 1 Normal (Figure 15.22). All movements of the larynx are equal and occur at the same time on both sides. The larynx opens maximally after strenuous exercise.

Grade 2 The opening of the left side of the larynx may occur fractionally after the opening of the right side during inspiration. The movement of the left side may have a slight 'flutter' or else open in two stages. However, when the horse exercises, the larynx opens fully. This is not considered to be significant as it occurs in many horses and their performance is not affected.

Grade 3 There is definite asynchrony of movement between the right and left sides of the larynx. Following exercise there may be slight asymmetry.

Grade 4 There is marked asymmetry of the laryngeal opening at rest and after exercise.

Grade 5 There is no active movement of the left side of the larynx. The opening appears markedly asymmetrical and the left arytenoid cartilage and vocal cords obstruct the airway (Figure 15.23).

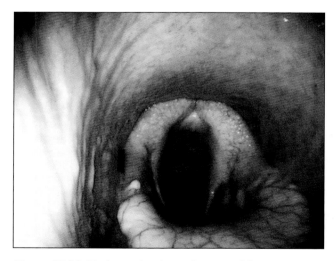

Figure 15.22 Endoscopic view of a normal larynx

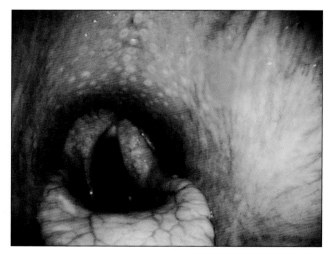

Figure 15.23 Endoscopic view of a paralysed larynx; this is a severe case of recurrent laryngeal neuropathy, note the marked asymmetry of the laryngeal opening

Treatment

Once the condition has developed it cannot be reversed. The nerve and muscle activity will never return. There are several treatment options.

No treatment Many horses perform satisfactorily with a degree of laryngeal dysfunction despite making a noise.

Management changes Many horses apparently improve with increased fitness and being kept in a dust-free environment.

Hobday operation (ventriculectomy) and vocal cord resection On each side of the vocal folds which form the lower margin of the laryngeal opening, there is a small opening called the lateral ventricle. This leads into a small blind sac of mucous membrane. Removal of both ventricles or the left ventricle and the edge of the left vocal fold may help reduce the noise. It is unlikely to enlarge the airway sufficiently to improve the horse's performance.

Abductor muscle prosthesis (prosthetic laryngoplasty or 'tie-back' operation) In cases of severe or complete paralysis, the wasted dorsal cricoarytenoid muscle is replaced by a prosthesis. A band of material is used to tie the left side of the larynx in the open position. This may be combined with a ventriculocordectomy (described above). The operation is usually successful in relieving the obstruction of the airway and may improve exercise tolerance but it is not without complications. With the larynx held permanently open, food material sometimes enters the trachea during swallowing. For a small number of horses this is a serious problem and the horse is left with a persistent cough. Aspiration pneumonia is a rare complication. Other complications include:

* post-operative infection
* failure of the prosthesis to open the airway sufficiently
* collapse of the left side of the larynx post-operatively due to the prosthesis cutting through the cartilage.

Nerve and muscle grafting Techniques have been tried where a branch of the first cervical nerve and pieces of the omohyoideus neck muscle are transplanted as a nerve-muscle pedicle into the wasted dorsal cricoarytenoid muscle. If the surgery is successful the function of the larynx continues to improve for up to a year following the surgery. This operation is not widely available.

Prognosis

Recurrent laryngeal neuropathy is not life threatening. If the above techniques are not successful, a tracheotomy is sometimes performed as a last resort.

Tracheotomy and tracheostomy

A **tracheotomy** is used as a temporary or emergency treatment if the upper airway is obstructed. A tracheotomy tube is inserted into the trachea at the junction between the upper and middle third of the underside of the neck. The tube can be removed and the wound left to heal when it is no longer needed. The shorter the time the tube is in position, the lower the risk of healing complications resulting in tracheal stricture when it is removed. While it is in place, the tube needs to be checked and cleaned twice daily to prevent the build up of mucus.

A **tracheostomy** is a more permanent operation involving removal of a piece of several tracheal rings to create an opening directly into the trachea. The disadvantage of these procedures is that the air that enters the trachea has not been filtered and humidified by passing through the nasal passages. Combined with the disruption to the normal mechanisms for clearance of mucus from the trachea, this may have an adverse affect on lung function. Care must be taken to keep these horses in an environment that is as dust-free as possible and to avoid foreign material (bedding and water) from entering the trachea.

Bilateral laryngeal paralysis does occur but is very rare. It may occur as a result of lead or organophosphate poisoning, severe liver disease or severe electrolyte imbalances.

DORSAL DISPLACEMENT OF THE SOFT PALATE (DDSP)

This condition is often referred to as 'gurgling', 'choking up' or 'swallowing the tongue'. It occurs most in 2-year-old Thoroughbred racehorses during fast work or just after they have pulled up.

Clinical signs
- During a race, the horse may suddenly slow down or stop in its tracks.
- This is usually accompanied by a loud gurgling or choking sound as the horse struggles to breathe.
- The horse recovers as soon as it swallows.

Why does this happen?
The horse is an obligate nose breather. This means that he can only breathe efficiently through his nose and not through his mouth. Air passes through the nostrils, along the nasal passages and into the nasopharynx. From there it passes through the larynx, down the trachea and into the lungs.

The pharynx of the horse is separated into two parts by a flat sheet of muscular tissue called the soft palate. The upper part is the nasopharynx which is part of the horse's airway. The lower part, the oropharynx is continuous with the back of the mouth.

The larynx opens into the nasopharynx through a hole in the soft palate, rather like a button that is done up, and the epiglottis lies on top of the soft palate. The seal is sufficiently tight that neither air nor food passes between the two parts of the pharyngeal cavity. Gurgling occurs when this anatomical relationship is disrupted. For a short period of time during maximal exercise, the soft palate is displaced above the epiglottis. This obstructs the flow of air and causes turbulence leading to loss of performance and loud inspiratory and expiratory noise. As soon as the horse swallows, the soft palate and larynx return to their normal position and the horse can breathe properly again.

Causes

There are numerous factors that may predispose the horse to dorsal displacement of the soft palate. These include the following.

- Lack of fitness.
- Exhaustion.
- The presence of blood or mucus in the pharynx, e.g. from recurrent airway disease, or exercise-induced pulmonary haemorrhage.
- Airway obstruction, e.g. if the horse has a degree of laryngeal hemiplegia the reduced airway diameter causes a high negative pressure in the nasopharynx during inspiration which may cause the soft palate to be sucked upwards into the airway.
- Inflammation of the pharynx, e.g. pharyngeal lymphoid hyperplasia.
- Ulceration or cysts on the soft palate or epiglottis.

The larynx and tongue are joined by the hyoid apparatus which is important in the process of chewing and swallowing. Anything that pulls the tongue or larynx backwards may cause 'unbuttoning' of the larynx from the soft palate. It is thought that the powerful muscles on the underside of the neck could sometimes be responsible for pulling the larynx backwards. The horse's bit may also be a factor for the following reasons.

- It breaks the airtight seal of the lips and air entering the mouth could elevate the soft palate.
- If it causes pain it may trigger a gagging reflex.
- When a horse tries to evade the bit, the base of the tongue pushes upwards onto the soft palate and may elevate it.
- Using the bit to ask for excessive neck flexion, e.g. in dressage horses, can cause a mechanical displacement of the soft palate and obstruct the airway.

Where no specific reason can be found, it may be that during severe exertion the larynx is pulled backwards and waves of movement in the soft palate allow it to slip upwards from under the epiglottis and block the airway. Alternatively there may be an abnormality in the functioning of the nerves and muscles of the soft palate.

Diagnosis

This is usually made from the history as the horse will appear normal at rest. It is difficult to confirm by endoscopic examination as many horses only experience the condition during racing. These conditions can be reproduced by scoping the horse while on a high speed treadmill. However, this requires training of the horse to familiarize it with the treadmill and the facilities are not universally available.

A routine endoscopic examination is essential to detect other abnormalities of the respiratory system which could predispose to DDSP.

Treatment

The first step is to make sure that the horse is fit enough for the work being asked of it. Sometimes the condition goes away as the horse reaches peak fitness. Other horses grow out of the condition with no treatment.

The next step is to treat any medical problems that may predispose to DDSP, e.g. lung disease, pharyngeal inflammation and epiglottic cysts.

TACK CHANGES

The following may be used to stop the horse opening its mouth and to prevent the tongue or larynx moving backwards.

- A drop, flash or grackle noseband can be used to prevent the horse opening its mouth. This discourages swallowing.
- An Australian noseband holds the bit high in the mouth and reduces the likelihood of the horse getting his tongue over the bit which increases the risk of DDSP.
- Tongue straps are used to tie the tongue down into the interdental space and hold them forward in the mouth. These are considered to be effective and are permitted on the racecourse. They should be fitted just before the race and removed immediately afterwards. In order to ensure they are correctly fitted, the Jockey Club Rules require that every horse fitted with a tongue strap is checked by a vet before going down to the start.
- Special tongue bits are available that put pressure on the top of the tongue and discourage swallowing.
- Another external device known as a laryngohyoid support has recently been tested in America, where it has been shown to have some effect in supporting the larynx in a more forward position. However, it is not permitted under the Rules of Racing in the UK.

SURGICAL TREATMENTS

Surgery is only considered if the above methods fail. There are a number of procedures that are performed with variable success rates.

- **Staphylectomy** This is the name given to an operation in which a strip of tissue is removed from the caudal border of the soft palate. The operation is carried out under general anaesthetic through an incision in the horse's throat. The theory is that with healing, the scar tissue contracts and tightens the seal between the larynx and the soft palate. If dislocation does occur, there is less soft palate to obstruct the airway. The success rate is reported to be approximately 60%.

- **Myectomy** A portion of the strap muscles on the underside of the neck is removed with the horse sedated under local anaesthesia. This operation is often done in combination with a staphylectomy.
- **Thermocautery** The palate is 'fired' with a hot instrument. The scarring is thought to make the palate firmer and less liable to dislocate.
- **Soft palate thermoplasty** Staphylectomy and myectomy may be combined with laser treatment of the soft palate. The fibrosis and scar tissue reduce the potential for displacement.
- **Injection of Teflon® into the epiglottis** If part of the problem is considered to be an unusually small or floppy epiglottis, Teflon® can be injected into the underside of the epiglottis to make it firmer.
- **Surgical tightening of the soft palate** To tighten a particularly floppy soft palate, a piece of tissue can be removed from either side. This reduces the chance of it obstructing the airway.
- **Laryngeal tie-forward** This is a relatively new procedure whereby the larynx is sutured in a forward position so it cannot be pulled backwards.

Prognosis

The prognosis is variable. In many horses the condition is successfully controlled with changes of management. For some animals it is a temporary condition that goes away with time or with treatment of underlying problems.

The results of surgery are unpredictable and for a number of horses DDSP is a performance-limiting condition. Removal of too much of the soft palate breaks the seal between the nasopharynx and oropharynx and can lead to difficulty eating and inhalation of food into the airway.

16
THE HORSE'S HEART AND THE CIRCULATORY SYSTEM

THE CIRCULATORY SYSTEM

Blood is continuously pumped around the body by the heart. It carries gases, essential nutrients and hormones between the various organs. The normal heart beats in a regular and co-ordinated manner to ensure smooth and efficient passage of the blood around the body.

The heart has four chambers known as the left and right atria and ventricles (Figure 16.1). Deoxygenated blood from the body collects in the right atrium and then flows into the right ventricle. The ventricle pumps it through the pulmonary artery to the lungs where it takes up more oxygen and releases carbon dioxide. The oxygenated blood from the lungs is carried by the pulmonary vein to the left atrium and ventricle. It is pumped by the powerful left ventricle into the aorta which branches into a network of arteries and smaller arterioles that carry it to all the tissues of the body. The finest arterioles branch into networks of very thin walled vessels called capillaries where gas exchange occurs. After leaving the capillary beds in the tissues, the now deoxygenated blood is taken by veins back to the right side of the heart. A large vein called the vena cava drains into the right atrium. From here, the blood flows into the right ventricle and then back to the lungs. The equine heart beats on average between 30 and 40 times per minute. To ensure maximum efficiency, it is important that blood flows in a one-way direction. There are 4 valves which prevent the blood flowing backwards.

1   The **tricuspid valve** is positioned between the right atrium and the right ventricle.
2   The **mitral valve** separates the left atrium and ventricle.

The tricuspid and mitral valves are sometimes known as the right and left **atrioventricular (AV) valves**.

3   The **aortic valve** is situated inside the aorta where it leaves the left ventricle.
4   The **pulmonary valve** is located at the origin of the pulmonary artery where it leaves the right ventricle.

The aortic and pulmonary valves are together known as the **semilunar valves**.

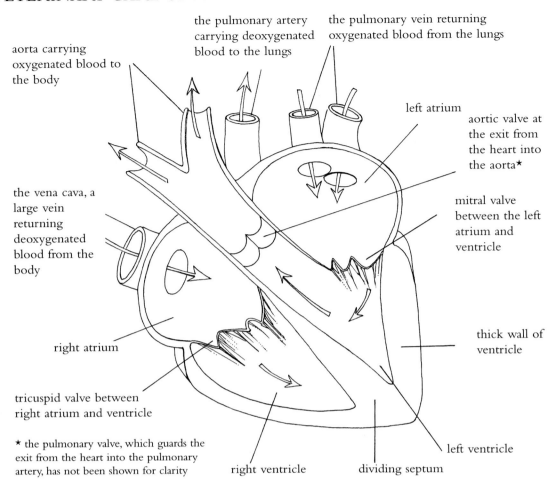

the pulmonary artery carrying deoxygenated blood to the lungs

the pulmonary vein returning oxygenated blood from the lungs

aorta carrying oxygenated blood to the body

left atrium

aortic valve at the exit from the heart into the aorta★

the vena cava, a large vein returning deoxygenated blood from the body

mitral valve between the left atrium and ventricle

thick wall of ventricle

right atrium

tricuspid valve between right atrium and ventricle

★ the pulmonary valve, which guards the exit from the heart into the pulmonary artery, has not been shown for clarity

right ventricle

dividing septum

left ventricle

Figure 16.1 The horse's heart

The control of heart rate and rhythm

The heart is made up of specialized cardiac muscle cells. The stimulus for the heart to contract is an electrical impulse that is received by the specialized cells of the sinoatrial node (SA node) in the wall of the right atrium. This causes a wave of contraction to spread across the atria, pushing the blood into the ventricles. The electrical stimulus then reaches the atrioventricular node (AV node) at the bottom of the septum between the two atria. The signal is briefly delayed here so atria empty and the ventricles fill with blood. Then the signal is conducted down specialized fibres which cause the ventricles to contract in a regular and co-ordinated fashion. The regular beating of the heart is known as **sinus rhythm**. Any deviation from the normal rhythm of the heart is known as an **arrhythmia**.

The heart rate is controlled by the **autonomic nervous system** which makes adjustments all the time without the horse being aware of it. The **sympathetic** branch of the autonomic nervous system is responsible for speeding up the heart rate to meet the increased demands for oxygen, e.g. when the horse is exercising. The **parasympathetic** nerves restore the heart rate to the resting level.

The normal heart sounds

We tend to think of each heartbeat as having two sounds: 'lub dup'. However, in most resting horses it is possible to hear four different sounds when listening carefully with a stethoscope: 'le lub dup dup' making up each heart beat or **cardiac cycle**. Each of these sounds corresponds to a particular event, e.g. the closing of valves or acceleration or deceleration of blood that occurs as the blood flows through the heart. By positioning the stethoscope at different sites on the chest wall, the vet is able to listen to the sounds coming from each of the four valves individually. The mitral, the aortic and pulmonary valves are heard best on the left side of the chest. Sounds from the tricuspid valve are listened to from the right side.

Each cardiac cycle can also be divided into:

- **systole** which is the part of the cycle where the ventricles contract
- **diastole** during which the ventricles relax and refill with blood.

Many heart abnormalities are detected at a routine veterinary examination for another reason, e.g. during a prepurchase examination. The significance of detected heart abnormalities can be difficult to evaluate and the horse may need more than one examination and/or referral to a cardiologist.

Examination of a horse with suspected heart disease

The vet will need to know the following details.

- The horse's age – congenital defects may cause symptoms in young foals or when the horse first starts work.
- How long the horse has been known and its use or intended use.
- Whether the horse has shown any signs of possible heart disease and when they first started.
- Its general health and any previous medical problems including viral and bacterial infections.

THE CLINICAL EXAMINATION

This will include the following.

- Examination of the horse or pony while undisturbed at rest to assess its condition, stance and demeanour. The respiratory rate should be noted.
- Checking for any oedema or swelling of the head or along the lower part of the abdomen.
- Taking the heart rate.
- Examination of the mucous membranes. This is easily done by gently lifting the upper lip of the horse or pony (Figure 16.2). Normal mucous membranes are a healthy salmon pink colour. If the animal is anaemic, the membranes may be unnaturally pale and in severe heart disease they may have a bluish tinge. However, this is not a very sensitive or reliable test.

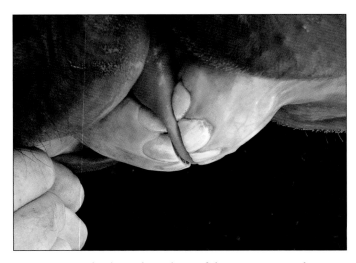

Figure 16.2 Checking the colour of the mucous membranes

- Measurement of the capillary refill time. This is the time taken for the colour to return if the mucous membrane is pressed firmly for a couple of seconds. In a healthy animal it should return to normal within three seconds.
- The pulse rate and character will be assessed. The easiest place to feel this is where the facial artery crosses the lower part of the jaw. It should be strong and regular.
- The jugular veins will be checked on both sides of the neck to ensure they are patent (not blocked). Any abnormal filling will be noted together with the time it takes for the jugular to fill and distend fully when it is occluded with a finger or thumb. It is normal to see a pulse in the jugular vein at the bottom of the neck.
- Checking that the horse is not dehydrated. In a healthy horse, a gently pinched together fold of skin on the neck or shoulder will spring back into position immediately it is released. If it remains elevated or 'tented', the horse is dehydrated.

Examination of the horse's heart

There are many reasons for examining a horse's heart. It may be done:

- as part of an annual health check, for example with vaccination
- during an examination for purchase or insurance

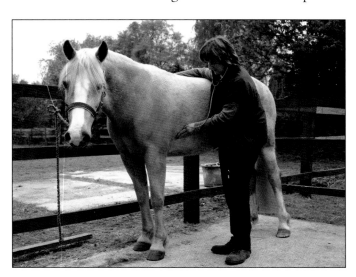

Figure 16.3 Listening to the horse's heart with a stethoscope

- if the horse is not performing as well as expected
- prior to sedation or anaesthesia
- if cardiac or lung disease is suspected.

The horse's heart can be examined using the following techniques:

- palpation
- listening with a stethoscope; this is known as **auscultation** (Figure 16.3)
- electrocardiography
- echocardiography
- exercise tolerance test.

PALPATION

The heartbeat can be palpated through the chest wall by placing the flat of the hand behind the elbow. The point of maximum intensity of the heart beat is found where the heart lies in contact with the chest wall.

AUSCULTATION

This should be carried out in a quiet environment with the horse resting and relaxed. The vet will listen to:

- the heart rate: this is measured over a minimum of 30–60 seconds; the horse has to be allowed to settle to the presence of the stethoscope at the start of the examination as any anxiety or excitement will elevate the heart rate
- the heart rhythm: the vet will be listening for any missed or extra heartbeats and any irregularities of rhythm
- the normal heart sounds (see page 449)
- any abnormalities of the above.

ELECTROCARDIOGRAPHY

An electrocardiogram (ECG) is a recording of the electrical activity of the heart. It is a useful tool for measuring the heart rate and recording any arrhythmias. Deviations from the normal pattern of electrical activity can also be seen if there is damage to the cardiac muscle.

ECHOCARDIOGRAPHY

Echocardiography is a specialized ultrasound examination of the heart. It is used to assess the size, structure and motion of the heart. It may be helpful in identifying any changes such as enlargement of a heart chamber or congenital defects. A special (Doppler) technique may be used to investigate the flow of blood through the heart. It can help to identify the source of a murmur. The function of individual valves and the degree of regurgitation (back flow from leaky valves) can be determined.

EXERCISE TOLERANCE TEST

The horse's heart is examined at rest and immediately after moderate exercise. The time taken for the heart to return to the resting rate is recorded. The amount and type of exercise will depend on the age and type of horse, its level of fitness, co-existing health problems, the state of the going etc. Moderate exercise for a fit racehorse would be completely unrealistic for a Shetland pony! In general, ten minutes of brisk exercise at trot and canter is sufficient for most fit, working horses.

Immediately following the exercise, the heart rate is likely to be between 60 and 110 beats per minute. (The maximum heart rate following a fast gallop is around 225 beats per minute.) Rates of greater than 125 may indicate that the heart is not functioning as it should. As a general rule, it should return to close to the resting rate within 20 minutes if the horse is left undisturbed and not excited in any way. This test is obviously not performed if the horse is considered to be unfit for any kind of exercise.

The results of these tests are interpreted together with the findings of the full clinical examination. Some of the most common conditions will now be considered.

Heart murmurs

Abnormal 'whooshing' sounds are sometimes heard between the normal heart sounds. These sounds are known as murmurs and they vary in their significance. They may be the result of turbulence in the blood flow due to a leaky heart valve. They are classified according to the following.

- Whether they occur in systole or diastole and also their timing within this period, e.g. can the murmur be heard throughout the whole of systole or just in the early, mid or late part of it?
- Whether the murmur is very localized, i.e. heard in only a small area or can it be heard over a wide area of the horse's chest?
- The location on the chest wall where the murmur is most easily heard. This helps the vet decide which valve is leaking.
- Some murmurs can actually be felt as a vibration through the chest wall. This is known as a 'thrill'. The area over which this thrill can be felt is noted.
- Their intensity. Murmurs are graded as follows:

   Grade 1: the murmur is very faint and can only be heard with very careful listening in a localized area

   Grade 2: the murmur is faint but can be readily heard after a few seconds of auscultation

   Grade 3: the murmur is obvious as soon as the stethoscope is placed on the chest but is restricted to a localized area

   Grade 4: the murmur is loud and can be heard over a large area of the chest

   Grade 5: the murmur is loud, radiates widely and there is a palpable thrill

   Grade 6: the murmur can often be heard without a stethoscope or with the stethoscope lifted off the chest wall and there is a palpable thrill over a wider area of the chest wall.

- The response to exercise. Murmurs may be more obvious when the horse is exercised because the flow of blood through the heart increases. Some murmurs are less audible or disappear after exercise.

CAUSES

Murmurs may be caused by the following.

- Normal blood flow. In fit horses, the sound of blood accelerating as it is pumped out of the heart can often be heard. This is known as a **physiological, or flow, murmur** and it is of no clinical significance.

- Turbulence as blood escapes and flows in a backward direction through a leaking valve. This may result from degenerative changes on the atrioventricular valves or nodules forming on the semilunar valves.

- Deposits on the heart valves caused by bacterial infection are fortunately uncommon in horses, but when they are present, a significant murmur is often heard.

- Anaemic horses have an abnormally low number of red blood cells to carry oxygen to the tissues. To compensate for this, the heart rate may speed up. The increased flow of blood with possibly reduced viscosity and density may lead to a murmur being heard.

- Narrowing of any valve as this restricts blood flow and causes turbulence.

HOW DOES THE VET TELL IF A MURMUR IS SIGNIFICANT?

Sudden collapse and death due to heart failure is uncommon in the horse. A horse rarely has a heart attack in the same way as a person. When horses collapse and die during or immediately after exercise, it is usually due to rupture of a major blood vessel. Significant heart disease usually causes a loss of performance or reduced exercise tolerance, rather than sudden collapse and death. Many horses with murmurs continue to perform normally throughout their working lives. When a possible abnormality is discovered, the vet needs to decide whether it is affecting the current performance of the horse or is likely to cause a problem in the future. The following may indicate significant heart disease.

- The resting heart rate is often elevated with severe heart disease. A resting rate of 50 or more is usually significant.

- A raised resting respiratory rate or uncharacteristic respiratory distress after exercise needs further investigation.

- Unexplained loss of performance, apparent weakness or unsteadiness on their legs. These horses should have a cardiac examination without delay.

- Abnormal distension of the jugular vein or ventral oedema are serious signs.

- With severe heart disease the horse may cough and have breathing difficulties at rest. Weight loss is common if they reach this stage.

As a very rough guide, loud murmurs with a palpable thrill that can be heard and felt over a wide area of the chest are likely to be significant. They are associated with serious abnormal flow and even if there are no obvious clinical signs, these horses should be checked regularly. However, there are no hard and fast rules. A minor lesion can cause a loud murmur and the murmur from a serious lesion may be very faint.

The vet may be confident that the murmur is not of any significance following auscultation and clinical examination. However, if there is any doubt, further investigations including electrocardiography (ECG) and echocardiography will be recommended.

Cardiac arrhythmias

Cardiac arrhythmias arise from:

- abnormalities of conduction of the electrical impulse, e.g. as a result of damage to the SA or AV node
- damage to the muscle of the heart wall leading to abnormal impulse conduction and contraction
- electrolyte imbalances.

There are a number of recognized arrhythmias in the horse and they are not all of clinical significance. Indeed, some are considered to be 'normal' in the resting horse. ECG traces are essential for the accurate identification of arrhythmias.

ATRIAL FIBRILLATION

This is a relatively common arrhythmia in the horse. There is no regularity of rhythm at all and the heartbeat is often described as 'irregularly irregular'. Instead of contracting in a synchronized fashion, the cardiac muscle cells of the atria contract in a random and inefficient manner. Consequently, the amount of blood entering the ventricles and pushed out by the heart is significantly reduced.

Causes

When a wave of muscle contraction passes through the atria of a normal heart, the muscle cells do not respond to nerve impulses for a short period afterwards. This is known as the **refractory period**. In horses such as Thoroughbreds that have large hearts, some of the cells may have a shorter refractory period than the others and be ready to contract again before the previous wave of contraction has died out. If there is a disturbance to the normal conduction of nerve impulses, the muscle fibres can contract individually, rather than in a co-ordinated fashion. Any event or underlying heart disease that interferes with the normal electrical activity of the atria can predispose to atrial fibrillation. It occurs in horses which have enlarged atria as a result of valvular disease, especially mitral regurgitation. It may be triggered by extreme physical exertion. The condition is much more common in large horses; it is not seen in ponies.

Clinical signs

These include the following.

- In a horse that is used for light exercise there may be no signs at all.
- Loss of stamina and performance in horses that work at speed, e.g. racehorses, point-to-pointers, hunters and endurance horses. When maximally exerted, the horse may suddenly pull up with breathing difficulties and a staggering gait.
- Longer than normal recovery time after exercise.

- In some cases the first sign is a sudden onset of ataxia, i.e. the horse becomes uncoordinated and slightly wobbly during exercise.
- Some affected horses have exercise-induced pulmonary haemorrhage and bleed from the nostrils following moderate work.
- On auscultation the heartbeat is irregular and often faster than normal. If it is more than 50 beats per minute, there is likely to be underlying heart disease.
- During fast work the heart rate may increase to around 300 beats per minute in an attempt to pump sufficient blood around the body to meet the requirements of the horse.

Diagnosis

This is made on the results of the clinical examination and confirmed by taking an ECG. The horse will have completely irregular heartbeats of different intensity and variations in the rate and quality of the pulse. Only three of the four normal heart sounds are present. The fourth sound, which is heard when the atria contract, is absent in horses with atrial fibrillation.

Some horses develop atrial fibrillation for a short period of time during the last stages of a race. This may cause the horse to pull up or slow down. The fibrillation may persist for up to 48 hours, but some horses spontaneously convert back to sinus rhythm immediately, making it very difficult to diagnose. When this occurs, it is known as **paroxysmal atrial fibrillation**.

Treatment

When atrial fibrillation is diagnosed, treatment should be delayed for 48 hours as a number of horses spontaneously convert back to normal.

It is also important to establish whether there is any sign of co-existing heart failure before treatment begins. Ideally, an ECG and echocardiography should be performed to determine this. In the absence of heart failure, atrial fibrillation is most commonly treated using a drug called quinidine sulphate. This is given by stomach tube every 2 hours until the heart returns to its normal rhythm. During treatment the horse is closely monitored for any signs of toxicity and a maximum dose of 60–80 g is not exceeded. Symptoms such as anorexia, depression and swelling of the nasal mucosa are quite common during the treatment period. Other side effects are diarrhoea, colic, laminitis, increased heart rate, reduced blood pressure, weakness, difficulty breathing and even death. The treatment is successful in 82–88% of cases. Of these, 20–30% will have a recurrence of the condition. Treatment is most successful in horses that have only just started to fibrillate. In one study, 5% of treated horses died as a result of treatment.

Owing to the small risk of serious side effects, horses used for light work that have no symptoms may not be treated. Atrial fibrillation on its own is unlikely to cause collapse during light exercise. However, if at all possible these horses should have an ECG taken while exercising to rule out the possibility of additional problems.

Subsequent management

Following successful treatment, the horse is usually given a few days off work so the heart can adjust to the normal rhythm. If the condition has been present for some time, a longer period of up to 2 months off work is recommended.

The horse should be monitored regularly as the condition may recur. Most owners of horses that have experienced atrial fibrillation purchase a stethoscope and listen to the heart at regular intervals. The vet will explain how to distinguish between atrial fibrillation and a normal rhythm.

Prognosis

The prognosis is good for horses that have no murmurs or other signs of underlying heart disease. The earlier they are treated, the greater the chance of a successful outcome. If there are other heart problems, the prognosis is poor.

Horses that do not respond to treatment and remain in atrial fibrillation may perform successfully in less demanding activities. If no other heart conditions are present, they do not necessarily develop them at a later date.

THE COMPOSITION AND FUNCTION OF BLOOD

Blood is composed of red blood cells, white blood cells and platelets suspended in fluid called plasma. It is estimated that an average-sized Thoroughbred horse has over 50 litres (88 pt) of blood in its body. It is pumped by the heart through the tissues in a network of arteries, capillaries and veins. Its many functions include the transport of oxygen and nutrients to all the tissues, defending the body against infection and carrying hormones and other chemical messengers between the organs.

Red blood cells

Red blood cells are also known as **erythrocytes** or **red blood corpuscles**. They are very small cells that are unusual in having no nucleus. They are made up of water (60%) and a pigment called haemoglobin (33%) within a cell membrane. They have a flattened shape which is concave on both sides to increase the surface area for gas exchange. In the lungs, the haemoglobin combines with oxygen to form oxyhaemoglobin which is then circulated to the tissues. The tissues use oxygen and produce carbon dioxide as a waste product of metabolism. This is collected by the haemoglobin and taken back to the lungs for excretion.

The red blood cells are made in the bone marrow and have a lifespan of approximately 120 days. When they die, they are removed from the circulation by the liver and the spleen. Approximately 30% of the red blood cells of a resting horse are stored in the spleen. These are released into the circulation if the horse is exercised or excited.

White blood cells

White blood cells or **leucocytes** defend the body against infection and help to clear up any damaged tissue or foreign matter in a wound. There are 5 cell types.

1 **Neutrophils** migrate from the bloodstream into the tissues and engulf and digest invading bacteria.

2 **Eosinophils** are involved in allergic reactions and parasitic disease. Relatively small numbers circulate in the blood, most migrate into the skin, the gut and the mucosal lining of the bronchi.

3 **Basophils** are only present in very small numbers. Their numbers increase in allergic and parasitic conditions.

4 **Lymphocytes** are important for recognizing antigens such as viruses, bacteria and fungi. B lymphocytes produce antibodies which help to protect the horse from infectious diseases. T lymphocytes recognize and destroy cancer cells.

5 **Monocytes** are important cells in the immune system. In the presence of inflammation from tissue damage or infection, they migrate from the blood into the tissues and transform into macrophages. They engulf and digest bacteria, viruses, dead tissue and foreign bodies.

Platelets

Platelets play an important part in the clotting mechanism of blood. This helps to ensure that damaged blood vessels are quickly plugged and sealed to prevent serious haemorrhage.

Plasma

Plasma is the fluid in which the above cells are suspended and circulated around the body. It is 93% water and approximately 6% protein and 1% minerals and salts. In the healthy horse it is a clear straw colour. Whereas the blood cells and large protein molecules remain in the circulation, the water component of the plasma with dissolved nutrients and gases can pass freely through the thin capillary walls into the tissues where it forms **tissue fluid**. At the arterial end of the capillary network, the pressure within the capillary from the pumping action of the heart encourages the escape of fluid into the tissues. At the venous end the pressure in the capillaries is smaller and most of the fluid is drawn back into the capillaries due to an osmotic gradient caused by the large blood proteins such as albumin. Some of the tissue fluid drains into a second network of vessels that form the **lymphatic system**. Once it enters these vessels, it is called **lymph**.

BLOOD DISORDERS

Anaemia

Blood is made up of red blood cells, white blood cells and platelets, suspended in fluid called plasma. If a horse has fewer red blood cells than considered normal for its breed and type, it is said to be **anaemic**.

Red blood cells contain a pigment called **haemoglobin**. This pigment combines with oxygen in the lungs to form **oxyhaemoglobin**. As the blood circulates around the body, the oxygen is given up and used by the various tissues to produce energy.

There are several laboratory tests used to check whether a horse is anaemic.

- A measurement of the number of red blood cells per litre of blood. (This is expressed as x 10^{12}/litre.)
- The **haematocrit** or **Packed Cell Volume (PCV)**. This is the percentage volume of red blood cells in a sample of whole blood.
- Haemoglobin concentration. This is measured in g/dl.

The expected 'normal' values vary according to the type of horse and its level of fitness. A fit Thoroughbred in training would be expected to have more red cells and a higher haemoglobin concentration than a child's pony or a cob. These can be measured from a blood sample.

CAUSES

The red blood cells have a lifespan of approximately 120 days. They are produced in the bone marrow and released into the circulation. When they reach the end of their life, they are removed and destroyed by the liver and spleen. Anything that upsets the balance between red cell production and their removal from the blood is likely to lead to problems.

Anaemia occurs if:

- fewer red blood cells are produced than normal
- blood cells are lost from the circulation due to injury or disease.

Reduced red cell production

This occurs if there is a problem with the bone marrow. Examples include lymphoma and leukaemia. These types of cancer are uncommon in the horse.

Increased red cell loss

Examples include:

- severe haemorrhage, e.g. from trauma, uterine haemorrhage post foaling and gutteral pouch mycosis
- intestinal parasites, e.g. redworm
- external parasites, e.g. *Haematopinus asini*, the sucking louse

- any other condition where there is chronic blood loss such as a tumour that is bleeding internally, e.g. certain tumours affecting the spleen will do this.

Clotting disorders and haemophilia are rare in the horse.

CLINICAL SIGNS

If the horse is slowly losing blood over a long period of time, there may not be any obvious clinical signs. In many cases the bone marrow increases red cell production and makes up the additional loss. It is possible for horses that are moderately anaemic to remain a good colour.

Clinical signs associated with acute or significant, longstanding blood loss
- Shock (acute, life-threatening haemorrhage).
- Pale mucous membranes.
- A raised heart rate.
- Development of a heart murmur.
- Increased respiratory rate.
- Exercise intolerance.
- Weight loss.
- Other signs of parasitism or trauma.

DIAGNOSIS
- Measurement of the red cell count, PCV and haemoglobin from a blood sample.
- A bone marrow biopsy if reduced red cell production is suspected.

TREATMENT OF ANAEMIA CAUSED BY BLOOD LOSS
- Control of the bleeding.
- A blood transfusion if the PCV has dropped dramatically.
- Parasite control.
- A balanced supportive diet.
- Vitamin K or a plasma transfusion may be given if the horse has a clotting problem (Figure 16.4).
- An iron supplement may be necessary if the horse has been losing blood over a long period of time. Special tonics containing iron, B vitamins, cobalt and folic acid are available.

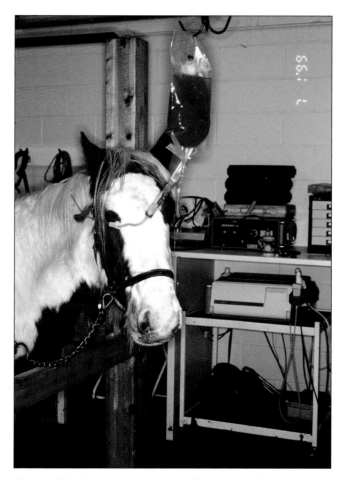

Figure 16.4 A horse receiving a plasma transfusion

PROGNOSIS

The prognosis is good providing the cause of the blood loss is eliminated.

Chronic lethargy syndrome

There is a well-recognized syndrome that is frequently diagnosed when competition horses that look well and have a good appetite perform in a disappointing manner. Blood tests show a persistently low white cell count despite a programme of rest, vitamin supplements and conventional veterinary therapy.

CAUSES

It is often suggested that the horse is suffering from a postviral lethargy syndrome. This may be the case for some horses, but a significant number have no history of recent bacterial or viral infection. Other possible causes include:

* chronic exposure to stressful situations such as transport and competitions causing high levels of corticosteroids to be released into the circulation
* over-exertion in the training period.

TREATMENT

A number of horses will recover with rest, good management and time. Two treatments are used with reasonable levels of success.

1   Levamisole is an immune stimulant. It is added to the feed for a period of 2 weeks.
2   A good quality aloe vera oral gel can be added to the feed at a high dose for 3–5 weeks. This preparation which is extracted from aloe plants has been shown to be effective in a number of cases.

Many horses that have failed to respond to other treatments respond well to the oral aloe vera medication. The white cell count improves and this coincides with improved performance and general vitality.

PREVENTION

It is difficult to make recommendations when the condition is not fully understood. However, it makes sense to:

* take care not to work the horse too early after a bacterial or viral infection
* take it easy for a couple of days following a vaccination
* try to reduce the stress levels of the horse.

THE LYMPHATIC SYSTEM

The lymphatic system is a branching network of lymphatic vessels. Tiny, blind-ending lymph vessels are found in the tissues. These drain into progressively larger vessels which eventually empty into the large veins near the heart. Their function is to drain excess fluid from the tissues. In contrast to the circulation of blood, the movement of the lymph is assisted by the action of muscles rather than being pumped by the heart. Valves in the vessels prevent backflow and ensure one-way flow of the lymph.

The lymphatic system plays a vital role in removing inflammatory products from injured or infected sites. The fluid is filtered by the **lymph nodes** (glands) along the course of the larger vessels before draining into the bloodstream. These can become swollen and painful or form abscesses in the presence of infection.

Conditions of the lymphatic system
OEDEMA AND FILLED LEGS

Most of the time, the production of tissue fluid and the drainage of lymph are kept in balance. However, if for any reason the flow of lymph slows down, the tissues become swollen with accumulated tissue fluid. This is known as **oedema.** Oedematous tissues are not normally hot or inflamed, but if pressed firmly with a finger a deep impression of the finger (or 'pit') remains for some time.

Oedema can be caused by the following.

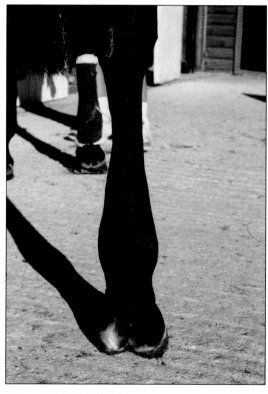

Figure 16.5 A filled leg

- Obstruction to the flow of blood in the veins. This can be localized due to an injury or generalized if the horse is in heart failure.

- Obstruction to the flow of lymph in the vessels.

- Reduced levels of protein in the blood so there is insufficient osmotic pressure to draw the tissue fluid back into the blood vessels. This can occur with severe kidney, liver or gut disease or as a result of severe parasitic problems.

- Restricted exercise. In the horse, the tissue fluid in the lower limbs may accumulate if there is insufficient activity to massage the flow of lymph back to the heart against the pull of gravity. This is why some horses develop **filled legs** at night when they are stabled (Figure 16.5). This can be exacerbated by overfeeding of concentrates which interferes with the protein and electrolyte balance. The filling is more common in the hind limbs, but the front legs may also be affected. The lower limb becomes rounded in shape and the definition

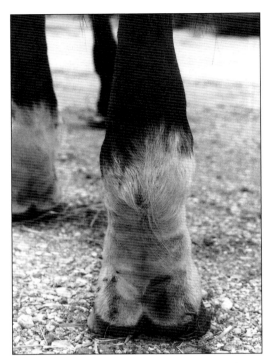

Figure 16.6 This horse's infection entered through the small wounds on its heel

between the tendons and the suspensory ligament is lost. The swelling is not painful but may cause stiffness at the start of exercise. Both the swelling and the stiffness usually resolve within a few minutes when the horse begins to move. The condition can be managed by turning the horse out for longer periods and by applying stable bandages when the horse comes in.

LYMPHANGITIS

Inflammation of the lymphatic vessels is known as **lymphangitis**. It causes painful swelling of the limbs and one or both of the hind limbs are most commonly affected.

Causes

The legs swell due to restriction of lymphatic drainage which occurs as a result of inflammation of the lymphatic vessels. Extra fluid collects in the tissues under the skin. The condition is usually caused by bacterial infection which has entered through a small skin wound on the lower leg (Figure 16.6). It can develop secondary to cellulitis which is inflammation of the loose tissues beneath the skin.

Clinical signs

These depend on the severity of the condition. It may result in the following.

- Variable degrees of swelling of the lower limb. In a severe case this can spread above the hock or knee to as far as the stifle or elbow. The upper limit of the swelling may be clearly demarcated as a prominent ridge. Over a period of 24 hours, the limb may become 2–3 times its normal size.
- Stiffness or mild to severe lameness. The horse may be reluctant to move or bear weight on the affected limb.
- In severe cases, yellow serum may ooze from the limb which is hot, firm and painful to touch.
- The pain may cause the horse to become very distressed.

Additional symptoms may include:
- sweating
- trembling
- fast breathing
- a raised temperature
- loss of appetite.

When to call the vet

The vet should be called as soon as the condition is suspected.

Diagnosis

The diagnosis is made on the clinical signs. Ultrasonography may be used to check for any damage to the ligaments and tendons.

Treatment

Prompt, vigorous treatment is required as any delay can result in permanent thickening of the leg. Treatment is likely to include:

- broad spectrum antibiotics to control the infection
- non-steroidal anti-inflammatory drugs, e.g. phenylbuta-zone, to reduce the soft tissue swelling and relieve the pain
- gentle exercise in hand or at grass to improve the circulation and reduce the swelling
- if the horse is not too sore, bandaging is used to prevent further swelling and stop the bedding sticking to the weeping areas
- a low protein diet, e.g. poor grass or hay
- physiotherapy may be helpful in some cases.

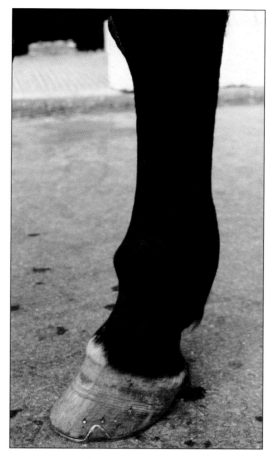

Figure 16.7 This leg is permanently thickened following several attacks of lymphangitis

Prognosis

The prognosis is variable. Some horses have recurrent episodes and the swelling may take a long time to resolve. In many of these cases the legs remain thickened as a result of fibrous tissue forming in the tissues under the skin (Figure 16.7).

17
THE DIGESTIVE SYSTEM

INTRODUCTION

The horse is a herbivore, meaning that its diet is made up of plant material. The digestive tract of the horse is designed to cope with the digestion of protein, fat and carbohydrates. The large intestine acts as a fermentation vat where bacteria are involved in breaking down the fibre component of grass, hay and grain (Figure 17.1).

The stages of digestion
MOUTH

Horses use their incisor (front) teeth and lips to take food into the mouth. Here it is thoroughly chewed and mixed with saliva. The mucus content of saliva lubricates the passage of food down the oesophagus into the stomach. When food material becomes lodged in the oesophagus, it causes the condition known as **choke**. The teeth must be kept in good order so that food is sufficiently broken down before entering the stomach.

STOMACH

The stomach of the horse is relatively small with a capacity of some 7–8 litres. The horse should therefore be fed little and often to avoid digestive upsets. Horses are unable to vomit because there is a powerful muscular sphincter between the stomach and the lower end of the oesophagus. Food reflux occurs only when very high pressure builds up in the stomach. This can occur in horses with **grass sickness** and **obstructions of the small intestine**.

The lining of the stomach is divided into glandular and non-glandular parts. The glandular region secretes digestive enzymes and acid. Horses exposed to high levels of stress and inappropriate feeding may suffer from **gastric ulcers**.

SMALL INTESTINE (DUODENUM, JEJUNUM, ILEUM)

The food passes out of the stomach into the duodenum, where it is mixed with pancreatic enzymes and bile secreted by the pancreas and liver. The digestive enzymes break down protein, carbohydrate and fat. Digestion and absorption occur along the length of the small

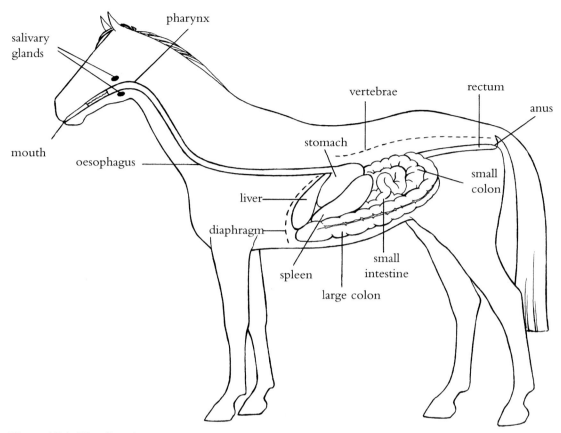

Figure 17.1 The digestive system

intestine, which is more than 20 m (65 ft) in the average Thoroughbred-sized horse.

The food material is moved along by contraction of smooth muscle in the gut wall. The waves of muscular activity are called **peristalsis**.

LARGE INTESTINE (CAECUM, COLON)

Undigested food and fibre now enter the large intestine where bacteria continue the digestion of protein, carbohydrate and fat. They also:

- ferment and digest cellulose
- form essential amino acids
- produce B vitamins and vitamin K.

The bacterial population varies according to the nature of the diet. Horses fed on grass and hay will have a different microbial population from those fed on high-concentrate diets. If the diet is suddenly changed, the fermentation process is disturbed and the horse may suffer from **colic, constipation** (known as **impaction**) or **diarrhoea**.

In order to avoid such problems, changes to the diet should be made slowly over a period of two weeks. This allows the bacteria time to adapt to the different food.

Wild horses graze almost continuously, whereas domesticated horses have their food intake controlled. This can lead to problems, especially if the horse eats large volumes of roughage in a short period of time. **Impactions** may develop at any of the three U-bends (known as flexures) in the large intestine. A horse normally passes droppings every couple of hours.

Water is absorbed as the food passes through the large intestine.

RECTUM

Undigested residues from the food eaten by the horse pass into the rectum and are expelled as faeces through the anus.

CHOKE

Choke occurs when food material becomes impacted in the oesophagus (gullet) and does not pass into the stomach.

Clinical signs

These include:

- coughing
- holding the head and neck in an extended position
- retching and difficulty swallowing: the horse often flexes and then stretches its neck during an attempt to swallow; at the same time it may grunt or squeal in pain
- trickling of green/brown fluid or clear saliva and food material from the nostrils (Figure 17.2)
- saliva drooling from the mouth
- a swelling may sometimes be seen along the line of the oesophagus on the left side of the neck
- some horses become very distressed.

Causes

- Bolting of food. Greedy, tired or anxious horses may swallow food before it is adequately chewed. Irregular feeding increases the likelihood of this.
- Sharp teeth or other dental abnormalities may prevent normal chewing.

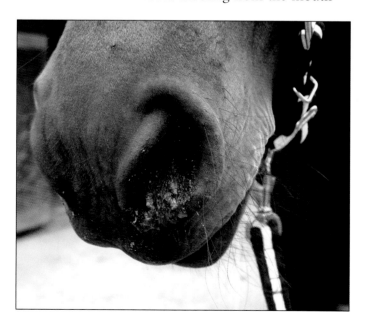

Figure 17.2 Food material and saliva may trickle from the nostrils of a choking horse

- Cubes and odd-shaped lumps of food such as carrots and apples can become lodged in the oesophagus.
- Inadequately soaked sugar beet can continue to swell and cause an impaction.
- Local tumours outside the digestive tract may obstruct the oesophagus – this is very rare.

Immediate action

- Do not panic.
- Move the horse to a stable.
- Do not offer any food or water.
- Keep the horse under observation.

Many cases of choke clear spontaneously in 5–10 minutes. If the condition does not resolve rapidly or if the horse is distressed, call your vet.

Diagnosis

The diagnosis is made on the clinical signs and confirmed by passage of a nasogastric (stomach) tube. The tube will not pass any further than the level of the obstruction. In more long-standing cases or if oesophageal damage is suspected, an endoscope may be passed to inspect the oesophageal mucosa and the impaction.

Treatment

The vet usually administers a sedative and muscle relaxant to reduce both the horse's anxiety and the spasm of the oesophageal wall. A stomach tube is sometimes passed into the oesophagus to try to relieve the obstruction by gently pushing the food into the stomach. This is done with care as forcing it may cause tissue damage.

MANAGEMENT OF HORSES WITH UNRELIEVED CHOKE

In some cases, the obstruction does not clear immediately. In these cases the horse should be:

- kept in with an inedible bed such as shavings, paper or peat
- deprived of food and water
- kept under observation but left as undisturbed as possible.

The vet may pass the stomach tube at regular intervals to see if the obstruction has been relieved or can now be dislodged into the stomach. The vet may use an endoscope to see how severe the obstruction is and the amount of damage in the area of the blockage. **Most horses recover within 24 hours**.

If the impaction shows no sign of shifting or is suspected to have been present for some time, it can be gently irrigated with warm water. The horse is sedated to keep its head low so all the fluid and food can drain back out of the mouth rather than entering the trachea (windpipe). In some cases this is performed under general anaesthesia with an endotracheal tube in the horse's trachea and careful positioning of the head to prevent aspiration pneumonia.

MEDICATION

Initially this is likely to include:

- a sedative

- a muscle relaxant.

If the choke persists for any length of time:

- antibiotics are given to treat or help prevent aspiration pneumonia
- tetanus antitoxin is administered if the horse's vaccinations are not up to date
- non-steroidal anti-inflammatory drugs help to control the pain and inflammation
- intravenous fluids keep the horse hydrated while it is unable to drink.

Complications

These include:

- aspiration pneumonia due to inhalation of food material
- oesophageal ulceration: if this is severe, scar tissue may cause permanent narrowing of the oesophagus (known as a stricture), predisposing to future episodes of choke
- rupture of the oesophagus: this is very rare but is a potential complication if a stomach tube is used too forcefully in attempts to clear the obstruction.

Aftercare of the patient

Once the obstruction has been relieved, the horse should be allowed to graze or offered small, soft, moistened feeds several times a day. Cubes should be thoroughly soaked or avoided altogether for a few days. If the obstruction took some time to clear, grazing is preferable to consuming large quantities of hay. Small quantities of *soaked* hay can be re-introduced after 48 hours.

If the choke was prolonged and damage occurred to the oesophageal wall or food inhalation is suspected, antibiotics and non-steroidal anti-inflammatory drugs are given.

The horse should be monitored for any signs of inhalation pneumonia. These include a raised temperature and respiratory rate, coughing and general malaise.

Prognosis

The prognosis is generally good. By far the majority of horses make a full recovery without complications.

Horses with inhalation pneumonia and oesophageal strictures have a guarded prognosis.

Prevention

- Regular feeding in a relaxed environment is helpful as the horse is less likely to bolt its food.
- Avoid feeding cubes to horses that choke regularly.
- Make sure that apples and carrots are cut up into small pieces.
- Dampen all feeds.
- Soak sugar beet as directed prior to feeding.
- Have the horse's teeth checked regularly.

GASTRIC ULCERS

The stomach of the horse is located in the upper part of the abdominal cavity behind the diaphragm and the liver, mostly on the horse's left side. The inside of the stomach can be divided into two areas. The oesophagus opens into the upper, non-glandular region. This area is white in colour and lined with squamous epithelium (Figure 17.3a). The lower, glandular area which produces hydrochloric acid and digestive enzymes is reddish brown in colour and opens into the small intestine though the pyloric sphincter. Between the glandular and non-glandular areas is a raised ridge of tissue (the margo plicatus).

The squamous part of the stomach is very sensitive to acid and this is where most ulceration occurs (Figure 17.3b). The glandular region has a bicarbonate-rich mucous lining which protects it from the harmful effects of acids most of the time.

The incidence of gastric ulcers

Gastric ulceration is very common in performance horses and is the most common

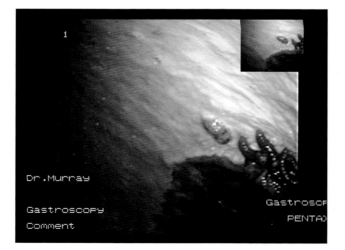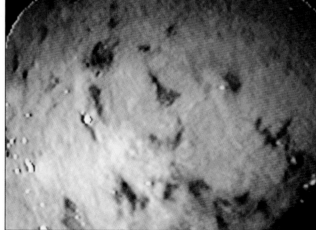

Figures 17.3a and b (Courtesy of Dr M. J. Murray): a) normal gastric squamous mucosa adjacent to margo plicatus; several *Gasterophilus spp.* larvae are attached; b) mild multifocal erosions in the gastric squamous mucosa adjacent to the margo plicatus

disorder of the equine stomach. As many as 90% of Thoroughbreds in training have gastric ulcers, together with up to 60% of horses competing and working in other disciplines. It can also be a significant problem in foals. The incidence is very low in horses that are turned away at grass.

Most ulcers occur close to the margo plicatus, in the squamous part of the stomach which does not have a protective mucus layer on its surface. However, they can also occur in the glandular portion. There is a wide spectrum of severity ranging from mild inflammatory changes to deep, bleeding erosions of the stomach lining. In severe cases, the ulceration extends to the oesophagus and duodenum. Fatal perforation occasionally occurs.

Causes and predisposing factors
DIET
Horses continually produce acid in their stomachs. In the wild, when a horse is grazing for up to 16 hours a day, the acidity is reduced by the forage and also by bicarbonate in the saliva. If horses are stabled, however, and fed high-concentrate diets with only limited access to hay and grazing, the acidity in the stomach increases. Any period without forage intake, whether due to management practices or illness leads to increased gastric acidity and risk of ulcers.

EXERCISE
Training and racing at fast speeds is associated with a high incidence of gastric ulceration. This may be due in part to the various stresses associated with training. Another consideration is that the high abdominal pressures that occur in the galloping horse may be sufficient to squeeze the acid stomach contents into the upper, acid-sensitive non-glandular portion of the stomach. Intensive exercise may have a number of adverse effects on gastric physiology, e.g. by reducing blood flow to the stomach, increasing the acid secretion or delaying emptying of the stomach contents into the duodenum.

STRESS
Stress factors that may play a part in the development of gastric ulcers include:
* intensive exercise
* insufficient time in the field
* injury
* other illnesses
* disruption to the horse's normal routine.

A combination of these predisposing factors can affect the gastric mucosa allowing the acid and enzymes to erode the stomach wall and form ulcers. The temperament of the horse is an influential factor.

NON-STEROIDAL ANTI-INFLAMMATORY DRUGS

In some horses, as in humans, administration of non-steroidal anti-inflammatory drugs, e.g. phenylbutazone and flunixin meglumine, increases the risk of gastric ulceration, particularly in the glandular part of the stomach. They do this by decreasing blood flow to the stomach lining, increasing acid secretion and disrupting the protective mucus-bicarbonate barrier.

Clinical signs

It is possible for a horse with gastric ulceration to show no obvious clinical signs. However, treatment of these horses may result in improved performance.

The clinical signs can be vague and non-specific but they include:

- poor appetite
- loss of condition or difficulty maintaining weight
- teeth grinding
- depression
- a dull, rough coat
- poor performance
- behavioural changes, e.g. cribbing
- lying down more than normal
- intermittent colic
- excessive salivation
- change in attitude, e.g. increased sourness and irritability
- back pain.

Foals with ulcers are frequently colicky and spend periods of time lying on their backs (Figure 17.4). Regular suckling helps to reduce gastric acidity; anything that interrupts this leads to increased acidity. Foals are especially sensitive to non-steroidal anti-inflammatory medication. Extensive gastric ulceration in foals can cause diarrhoea.

Diagnosis

A diagnosis of gastric ulceration may be suspected from the clinical signs or response to treatment, but can

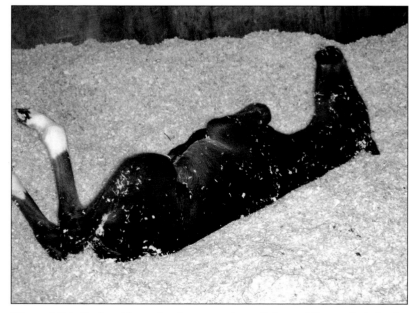

Figure 17.4 Foals with gastic ulcers may be colicky and lie on their backs

only be confirmed by endoscopy. A long endoscope is needed and the horse has to be starved for at least 6 hours beforehand so that the ulcers are not obscured from view by food material in the stomach. As this type of endoscopy is not universally available, a good response to treatment is often taken as support of the clinical diagnosis.

Treatment

Treatment involves management changes and medication.

MANAGEMENT CHANGES

Management changes are an essential part of the treatment for horses with gastric ulceration. Affected horses need:

- plenty of time at pasture
- continuous access to forage if stabled
- reduced levels of grain and concentrates in the diet
- minimal stress
- a reduced level of training.

Unfortunately these recommendations are hard to achieve for racehorses and other elite equine athletes, so medication is needed to help heal the ulcers and prevent recurrence. The primary aim is to reduce gastric acidity, either by changing the management or instigating medical treatment.

MEDICATION

- Omeprazole (GastroGard®) is the drug of choice. It is administered once daily as an oral paste. It works by reducing acid production in the stomach. Horses with ulcers are treated once daily for 4 weeks, then at a reduced dose for another 30 days. It can also be used as a preventative measure if a period of stress is anticipated, e.g. travelling of competition horses. Its use is not permitted in some disciplines so this must be checked for each individual sport. Unfortunately it is expensive.
- Cimetidine and ranitidine also act by inhibiting acid secretion. However, these drugs are not licensed for horses and the dose required varies between individual animals. They are generally considered to be less effective than omeprazole.
- Sucralfate is a medicine sometimes used as a protective coating for the ulcerated stomach as it binds to the damaged tissue and helps to prevent further damage from digestive juices. It is used for horses and foals with ulcers in the glandular part of the stomach and the duodenum.
- Other treatments such as aluminium hydroxide have been used.

ADDITIONAL TREATMENTS

It is common for horses with gastric ulceration to experience back pain. This may be the result of abnormal posture caused by the gastric discomfort or due to the fact that pain from internal organs can be referred to specific sites on the body wall. Acupuncture is an effective supportive treatment for these horses.

Complications
Complications are uncommon but they include:

- perforation of a gastric or duodenal ulcer with fatal peritonitis
- scar tissue narrowing the lumen of the oesophagus or duodenum, predisposing the horse (especially foals) to subsequent bouts of choke or colic.

Prevention
Gastric ulceration can be prevented in many cases by good management and sensible feeding. However, this can be challenging in certain horses that are prone to the condition.

COLIC IN THE ADULT HORSE

Colic is the name given to a number of conditions where the horse shows characteristic behavioural signs as a result of abdominal pain. It is usually caused by a problem with the digestive tract and can be mild or severe. Pain can arise from:

- disturbances to the normal motility of the gut, e.g. intestinal spasm
- stretching of the gut wall by accumulated gas or food
- damage to the mucosal lining of the intestines
- increased tension on the mesentery (which is the thin fold of tissue that carries blood vessels and attaches the gut to the dorsal wall of the abdomen)
- loss of blood supply to the intestines.

Many horse owners fear the worst when their horse has colic. However, the majority of cases respond well to medical treatment and will make a full recovery if correctly and promptly treated.

Clinical signs
The *earliest signs* may include some or all of the following. The horse may be:

- less enthusiastic about its feed than normal or not eating at all
- passing fewer droppings than normal
- quiet and lethargic
- looking around at its flanks, kicking at its belly or pawing the ground

As the pain increases, there may be:

- patchy sweating

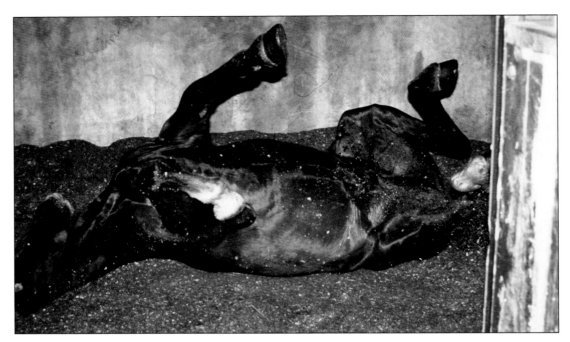

Figure 17.5 Horse with colic

- attempts to lie down and roll
- lying on the back
- fast, shallow breathing that develops into blowing with flared nostrils
- spasms of severe pain which cause violent rolling and groaning (Figure 17.5)
- distension of the abdomen.

In the terminal stages the horse may become very quiet and depressed as a result of developing toxaemia.

When to call the vet

If the horse exhibits anything more than mild abdominal discomfort for a few minutes, the vet should be consulted. Even if the horse is better when the vet arrives, discussion of the case may help to avoid future recurrences.

Immediate action

- Stay calm and keep spectators away.
- Remove the hay net but allow access to water.
- If the signs are mild, keep the horse in a stable and ensure there is plenty of bedding.
- If the horse is lying down quietly, do not force it to get up, it will be in the position it finds most comfortable. Remove buckets and any fixtures and fittings which could cause injury if the horse starts rolling.
- A *few minutes* of quiet walking may distract the horse and stop it from rolling. Gentle exercise encourages normal gut motility. *Do not* walk the horse to the point of exhaustion.

- When the horse is rolling violently and continually in a stable, it is likely to become cast. In these cases it is often safer to move it to a field or riding arena. Take care to keep the horse well away from hazards such as ditches and fences.

Note the following information for your vet.
- Has the horse passed any droppings? If so, when and what consistency, i.e. firm, loose?
- Are there audible stomach rumbles and noises?
- Is the pain intermittent or continuous?
- Have there been any changes in the diet?

Do not:
- offer the horse any food
- administer any kind of colic drench; these old-fashioned remedies are unlikely to do any good and may accidentally enter the lungs with serious consequences
- risk injury to yourself or other people in your attempts to help the horse.

How to help the vet
- Make sure the horse is adequately restrained in a bridle or headcollar whilst the vet examines it.
- Provide a bucket of clean, warm water.
- At night, have the horse in a well-lit stable when the vet arrives. Examination is more difficult when carried out by torch or car headlights.

The examination
The vet will carry out a thorough examination of the horse. This serves two purposes. Firstly to establish whether the horse really has colic or whether it is suffering from some other condition causing colic-like symptoms. Amongst the more common false colics are:
- laminitis
- exertional rhabdomyolysis syndrome
- foaling
- liver disease.

Secondly, the examination and history will sometimes reveal the cause of the abdominal pain. Specific medical treatments may then be prescribed or a decision made that surgery is necessary. The examination includes the following tests.

TAKING THE PULSE AND TEMPERATURE
The pulse rises in response to pain and cardiovascular shock. With spasmodic colic, the pulse may rise to as high as 90 beats per minute during the bouts of pain, but then return

to close to normal. A pulse that remains above 60 in the quiet periods despite the administration of painkillers, is a cause for concern.

In many cases the temperature is normal but it may be raised if colitis or peritonitis is developing. Sub-normal temperatures occur in horses that are toxic.

LISTENING TO THE GUT SOUNDS

The vet will listen to the chest and abdomen with a stethoscope to establish whether the gut noises (known as borborygmi) are greater or less than normal. On the whole, an absence of gut sounds is more worrying than a noisy abdomen.

OBSERVATION OF THE RESPIRATORY PATTERN

Fast, shallow breathing often accompanies severe colic.

EXAMINATION OF THE MUCOUS MEMBRANES

The gums of a healthy horse are a pale salmon-pink colour. In a serious colic they change colour, becoming redder, bluish purple or greyish white. The conjunctival membranes turn from salmon pink to brick red as the horse becomes toxic and circulatory changes occur.

MEASUREMENT OF CAPILLARY REFILL TIME

Pressing firmly on the horse's gum blanches the mucous membrane. The pink colour should return within three seconds. Failure to do so indicates circulatory shock.

CHECKING IF THE HORSE IS DEHYDRATED

This will be assessed from the skin tone and inspection of the mucous membranes.

ASSESSING IF THE ABDOMEN IS DISTENDED

Accumulation of gas and food material in the intestines may lead to painful abdominal distension.

RECTAL EXAMINATION

A lot of valuable information can be obtained by the vet performing a rectal examination. The vet will feel for:

- droppings in the rectum, to see if digested food material is still passing through the horse
- the consistency of the droppings, to see if the horse has diarrhoea or is constipated
- impaction of the large bowel
- loops of small intestine (normally not palpable) distended by gas
- tight bands of tissue and sites of acute pain indicating bowel displacement
- with a severe displacement, the rectum may be so tight that internal examination is not possible.

PASSING A STOMACH TUBE

A warmed, flexible stomach (nasogastric) tube may be passed up one nostril, into the pharynx. When the horse swallows, the tube is pushed down the oesophagus, into the stomach (Figure 17.6). This procedure may be helpful in establishing a diagnosis. For example, reflux of a large amount of gas or fluid suggests that the problem lies in the stomach or first part of the small intestine. Reflux of more than 2 litres of fluid is significant. It can indicate a small intestinal obstruction or functional abnormalities of the gut, e.g. grass sickness. Draining the fluid decompresses the stomach and makes the horse more comfortable.

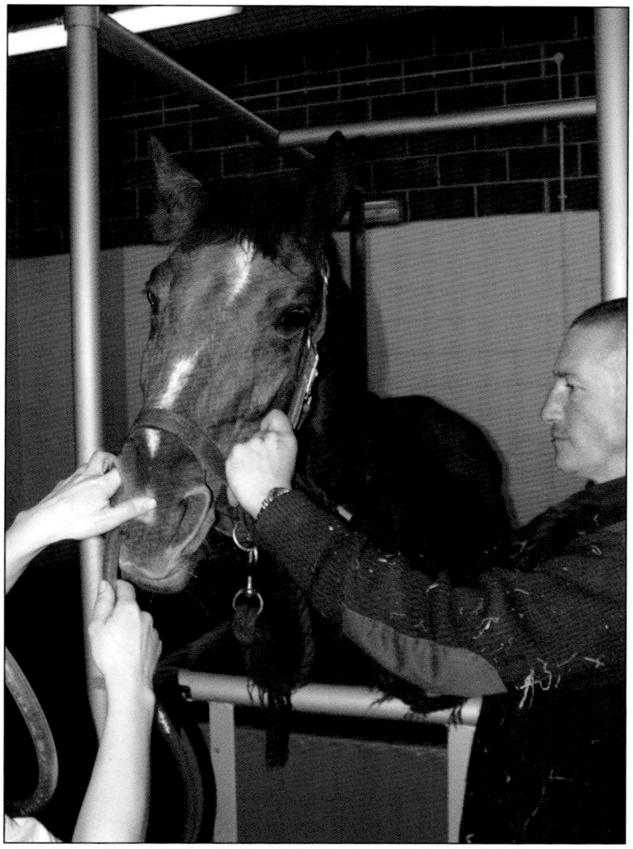

PERITONEAL TAP

This test involves obtaining a small sample of peritoneal fluid from the horse's abdominal cavity. The lowest part of the abdomen is clipped and scrubbed, and then a needle is inserted through the ventral midline. A fluid sample is collected for examination.

Normal peritoneal fluid is a clear, pale straw colour (Figure 17.7). Horses with grass sickness and those with medical colics usually have darker yellow fluid due to dehydration or increased bilirubin. If the horse has a problem and the blood supply to the gut is beginning to be affected, the fluid may be orange. Where severe ischaemia (loss of blood supply) has occurred, the fluid may be dark reddish brown and turbid. When a horse has developed peritonitis, the fluid will be a cloudy, yellowish colour. A ruptured gut will yield greenish brown fluid with visible debris in it.

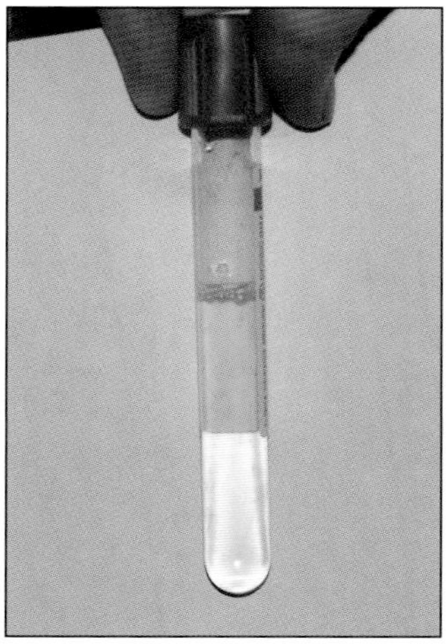

This test can be helpful and is routinely carried out if the colic persists or more serious problems are suspected. However, a normal peritoneal tap does not rule out the possibility of a serious problem developing. The protein content and specific gravity may also be measured. These are often normal in medical colics but increased in horses with inflamed and ischaemic intestines.

If peritonitis is suspected, the fluid will be cultured to try and identify the bacteria involved and their antibiotic sensitivity.

Figure 17.6 Stomach-tubing a horse

Figure 17.7 Normal peritoneal fluid is a clear, pale straw colour

BLOOD TESTS

A number of blood tests may be taken. The ones most commonly used to monitor a patient are:

- packed cell volume (PCV)
- white cell count
- total protein.

ULTRASONOGRAPHY

Ultrasonography can be helpful for identifying some small intestinal problems including obstruction and lack of motility.

HISTORY

The history may provide clues to the possible cause of the colic. The vet will want to know:

- the age of the horse
- if the horse has had colic before
- when the first problems were observed
- what were the first signs
- if the horse has had any recent dietary changes
- when it was last treated for worms and which preparation was used
- if any dental problems are present and when the teeth were last inspected
- if the horse is taking medication for any other condition.

Types of colic and their causes

In the following sections, brief descriptions of the types of colic most commonly treated in practice are given. They can be divided into those that can be treated medically and those which require surgery or euthanasia.

Medical colics
SPASMODIC COLIC

Spasmodic colic occurs when the smooth pattern of peristalsis is disrupted. The peristaltic movements become uncomfortable, irregular and ineffective at moving the food along the gut. The horse shows periods of acute pain interspersed with periods of calm. Causes include:

- worms
- sudden change in diet, e.g. access to lush spring grass
- irregular feeding
- drinking a lot of cold water
- stress, anxiety, transport
- unaccustomed hard exercise

and

- it may accompany diarrhoea.

Signs include intermittent abdominal pain with elevation of the heart and respiratory rates. Droppings continue to be passed. Overall, the gut sounds are increased.

These horses are starved for a few hours and they usually respond rapidly to various medications with spasmolytic, analgesic and sedative effects. On some occasions a second dose is required. Food is normally withheld for a few hours and gradually reintroduced. The prognosis is good.

TYMPANITIC COLIC

Highly fermentable or unsuitable food, e.g. grass cuttings, clover and apples, can lead to abnormal fermentation and accumulation of gas within the intestines. There may be visible abdominal distension and the pain can be very severe. Distension in one part of the gut can cause other parts of the bowel to contract, further increasing the pain. The heart rate may rise to around 80 beats per minute. The gut sounds can be increased or decreased. Gas may intermittently be passed from the rectum. If the stomach is distended with gas, the passage of a stomach tube can give immediate, albeit sometimes temporary relief.

Treatment includes painkillers and muscle relaxants. Liquid paraffin and other treatments may be administered by stomach tube. This helps to reduce further fermentation. If gas accumulates in the colon there is an increased risk of torsion so these horses should be closely monitored and discouraged from rolling.

Gas accumulations also occur when the lumen of the gut is obstructed. This is discussed under surgical colics.

FOOD IMPACTIONS

When at grass, the horse grazes for many hours of the day, so food passes through the gut at a steady rate. The stabled horse has its diet artificially regulated and impactions may develop. The pelvic flexure is the commonest site of impaction as the gut narrows and does a 180 degree turn at this site.

Other factors which may play a part in the development of impactions include:

- redworm damage affecting the normal motility of the gut
- neglected teeth
- unsuitable diet
- eating the bedding
- insufficient access to water, e.g. in winter if the water supply is frozen
- change in diet and management, e.g. box rest
- stress.

In the early stages, the pain is less acute than in the other types of colic discussed. The symptoms may develop over a couple of days. They include:

- adopting a urinating stance and straining intermittently

- passing fewer droppings than normal or none at all; those that are passed may be firm, dry and covered with mucus
- walking backwards into the corner of the box
- teeth grinding
- lying flat out (Figure 17.8) or sitting up, often groaning at the same time
- looking round at the flanks
- getting up and down, rolling and stamping the feet
- the horse may be unusually quiet and off its food
- the gut sounds are reduced
- the horse may become dehydrated as the disease progresses.

This type of colic is normally diagnosed following rectal palpation. Treatment includes:
- withholding hay and concentrates until the impaction is relieved
- then feeding small meals of grass or bran mashes to keep the gut moving
- gentle exercise may encourage peristalsis
- administering laxatives such as liquid paraffin by stomach tube (Figure 17.9)
- in some cases osmotic laxatives such as Epsom salts which draw water into the lumen of the gut and soften the impaction are helpful
- oral fluids
- intravenous fluids may be used in horses that are dehydrated or do not improve as expected
- painkillers as necessary.

Most cases respond to medical management and the horse passes a large volume of droppings. Surgery is only occasionally required. The prognosis is good provided there is no underlying cause of the impaction such as grass sickness.

TREATMENT OF MEDICAL COLICS

Every horse with colic is treated individually, taking into account the history and the clinical signs. The aims of treatment are:
- pain relief
- elimination of the cause of the discomfort
- restoring normal gut motility and function
- preventing secondary problems such as infection and toxaemia.

Treatment may include the following.

Pain relief

Analgesics are administered to all cases of colic. Some medications also relax the muscle in the gut wall and help to relieve painful spasm and re-establish normal peristalsis. In each case the vet will choose the medication with care so as to make the horse feel more comfortable without masking signs of any serious problems that may be developing.

Sedatives

These help to reduce anxiety. Some sedatives also have analgesic and muscle relaxant properties.

Passing a stomach tube

This may be done regularly to decompress a distended stomach since a horse cannot vomit. If the stomach keeps filling up, surgery may be indicated.

Laxatives and oral fluids

Several litres of a mixture of liquid paraffin and warm water may be given by stomach tube to a horse with an impaction. In some cases, salt or electrolytes may be added. The mixture helps to soften the faeces and break up the mass of accumulated material. Alternatively, osmotic laxatives such as magnesium sulphate may be given.

Anthelmintics

These are given when worms are suspected as a contributory factor. *Strongylus vulgaris,* cyathostomes and tapeworms can all cause colic.

Intravenous fluids

Theses are sometimes necessary for medical colics. Horses with impactions that persist for more than a couple of days may benefit from their administration to prevent dehydration.

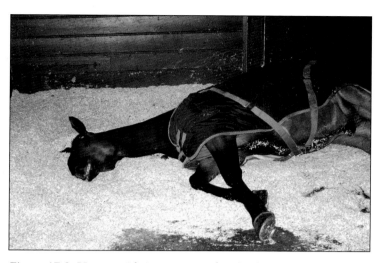

Figure 17.8 Horses with impactions often lie flat out

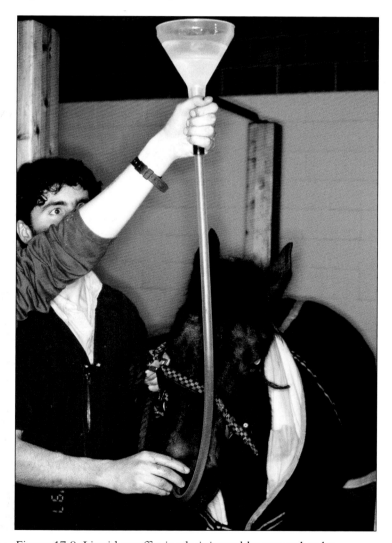

Figure 17.9 Liquid paraffin is administered by stomach tube

Antibiotics

Antibiotics are given at the discretion of the vet, depending on the clinical and laboratory findings. They are rarely necessary but may be given if the bowel wall is damaged and bacteria and toxins are released into the circulation. They are used for cases of peritonitis.

Acupuncture

Acupuncture can be useful as a supportive treatment for medical colics. It helps with pain relief, restoration of normal gut motility and relaxation of the horse.

CARE OF THE PATIENT

Your vet will advise on:

- how often you need to check the horse following treatment
- the signs to look for
- feeding including grazing
- exercise and return to work
- prevention of further attacks.

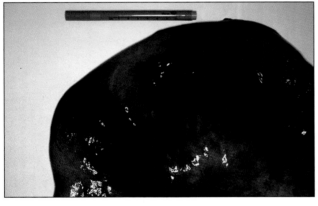

Figure 17.10 This section of small intestine has changed colour due to loss of its blood supply

Surgical colics

Approximately 7% of colic cases are caused by conditions that require surgery for the horse to have any chance of survival. For a variety of reasons (see below), a portion of the gut may lose its blood supply and die. This is known as **infarction**. The normally pink intestine goes through a series of colour changes from red to purple, bluish black or grey-green (Figure 17.10). Bacterial poisons which are called toxins, leak from the damaged gut wall and the horse goes into shock. Unless surgery is carried out promptly, the horse will die.

INDICATIONS FOR SURGERY

Horses with colic that do not respond well to medication should be regularly re-examined as the horse may be taking a turn for the worse. The earlier any serious signs are recognized and the horse is referred to an equine hospital, the better the chance of successful surgery.

The signs that surgery may be required that your vet will be looking for include:

- continued severe pain despite the use of painkillers
- a heart rate that is persistently above 60 beats per minute
- deterioration in the colour of the mucous membranes and capillary refill
- a rising PCV

- rectal findings that give cause for concern, e.g. gas-filled loops of small intestine that can indicate an obstruction
- changes in the peritoneal fluid
- spontaneous gastric reflux from the nostrils
- reflux of 2 litres or more on passage of a stomach tube
- progressive abdominal distension and decrease in gut sounds.

Sometimes the decision is not clear cut. In these cases, it is better for the horse to be referred at an early stage rather than waiting until its condition has deteriorated to a state that is inoperable. If the horse becomes quiet and depressed but the colour and pulse continue to deteriorate, a portion of gut may have died, necessitating immediate surgery or euthanasia.

EXAMPLES OF SURGICAL COLICS

Intussusception

This is most common in foals and yearlings. A piece of gut becomes folded inside an adjacent piece of gut, causing a partial or total obstruction and disruption to the blood supply. Intussusceptions tend to develop if the peristaltic activity of the gut increases, e.g. secondary to diarrhoea in foals. It is also associated with high ascarid and tapeworm burdens.

Torsions (twisted gut)

The large and small intestine can rotate so that the bowel is obstructed or trapped in the wrong area of the abdomen. Consequently the blood supply to that section of the gut wall is either partially or completely cut off. Bacteria and toxins leak into the bloodstream and peritoneal cavity resulting in the rapid development of toxic shock. The pain is severe and unrelenting. Unless surgery is carried out in the early stages, death is inevitable. The outcome depends on the location of the lesion and how much of the gut is involved. It may be possible to remove the damaged portion of gut, but not all lesions are operable.

Strangulation by a pedunculated lipoma

In older animals, particularly ponies, benign fatty balls of tissue (lipomas) may develop and attach to the mesentery by long pedicles of stringy tissue. Unfortunately, these have the potential to wrap around a loop of bowel, occluding its lumen and cutting off its blood supply (Figure 17.11). Affected horses may

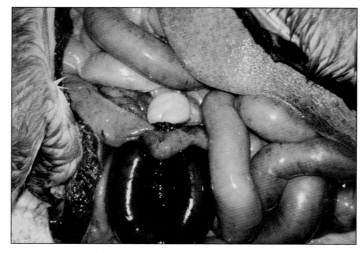

Figure 17.11 The lipoma (yellow tissue) has strangulated the loop of small intestine (black) in the foreground (found at post mortem)

present with sudden onset of severe and acute colic or with a mild discomfort that gradually increases in severity as the lipoma tightens. Surgery is the only treatment.

Worm damage

Larvae of *Strongylus vulgaris* migrate from the gut to the arteries supplying the gut. This can cause inflammation of the vessels and portions of the gut may lose their blood supply. If just a short segment of gut is involved, the horse can sometimes be saved by surgical removal of the affected piece of gut. This is less common with the use of modern worming treatments.

SURGERY OR EUTHANASIA?

When a surgical colic is diagnosed, the horse should be operated on as soon as possible or humanely destroyed. This is not an easy decision for many owners. You should be guided by your vet; some abdominal catastrophes develop so quickly that by the time the horse is examined, the horse has deteriorated too much for surgery to be a realistic option.

Some of the factors that may be considered include the following.

Distance to the nearest operating facilities

If the horse is seriously distressed and the nearest equine hospital is some distance away, it may be kinder to destroy the horse than to subject it to a long and painful journey.

The age of the horse or pony

Provided they are well in every other way, horses in their early twenties can have a similar survival rate to younger horses. Horses in their mid to late twenties have a reduced survival rate. One needs to remember that full recovery from colic surgery can take up to 6 months and it is important to consider what benefit colic surgery will be to a very elderly horse or pony.

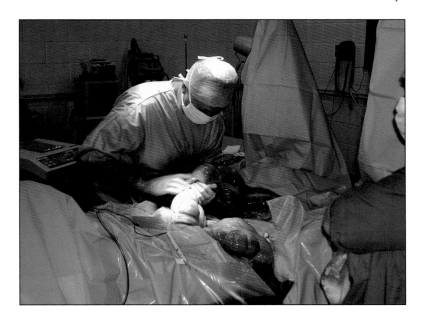

The financial implications

Colic surgery requires several vets for a period of several hours and a whole back up team to help before and after the surgery (Figure 17.12). The intensive care and fluid therapy that follows is also expensive and the cost can be several thousand pounds.

Figure 17.12 Colic surgery

The survival rate

Thanks to early diagnosis and improved anaesthetic and surgical techniques, the survival rate has trebled over the last 20 years. Around 75% of horses now survive the surgery, but 10–15% of these die of post-operative complications.

MEDICATION

Once the decision to operate has been made, the horse may be treated with:

- flunixin meglumine, a non-steroidal anti-inflammatory drug to relieve the pain and protect against the effects of endotoxin
- antibiotics
- an in-dwelling stomach tube may be sutured in place for the journey to the hospital; this prevents painful distension of the stomach in horses with intestinal obstructions
- intravenous fluids usually via a jugular catheter in the neck.

PROGNOSIS

The survival of an individual horse is influenced by the degree of endotoxaemia prior to surgery. The vet will have an idea of this from monitoring the horse. Some examples of poor prognostic indicators include:

- a heart rate of more than 100 beats per minute
- an accompanying weak pulse
- a PCV of more than 60%
- dark red or purple-blue mucous membranes
- dark red peritoneal fluid
- a horse that has been in severe pain for several hours.

Horses that have long anaesthetics and portions of gut resected have a worse prognosis than those where displacements and early twists are corrected before the gut becomes ischaemic (loses its blood supply). Some cases are found to be inoperable when the intestines are examined and the horse is euthanased on the operating table.

Of those horses surviving the surgery, between 10–15% will die in the next few days. An increase in PCV, total plasma protein and a sustained heart rate of over 60 beats per minute in the post-operative period are poor prognostic signs. A poor colour and slow capillary refill rate are also bad signs as is a lack of gut motility (known as **ileus**).

A longer-term complication of surgery is the formation of adhesions within the abdomen. These are the main cause of recurrent colic and mortality in horses that have previously undergone successful surgery.

PREVENTION

- Avoid sudden dietary changes. Make any changes to the feed gradually over a period of two weeks.

- Use only fresh, good quality food. Discard anything that is mouldy or suspect.
- Do not work the horse for at least an hour after feeding, or feed immediately following strenuous work.
- Have your horse's teeth inspected regularly.
- Worm your horse regularly. Faecal worm egg counts and blood tests to detect tapeworm can be used as a guide to how often it is necessary, together with advice from your vet.
- Make sure fresh water is always available.
- Know your horse well, so you can tell if it is off colour. If in doubt, keep it under close observation.

Unfortunately, despite excellent management and meticulous care, many horses will experience a bout of colic. When it does occur, prompt treatment and close monitoring of the horse are essential.

DIARRHOEA

Diarrhoea may be defined as the passage of faeces with a higher water content than normal. In most horses, the faeces consist of firm balls that break on contact with the ground. Those of a horse with diarrhoea may resemble a sloppy cow pat or pour out like dirty water. Diarrhoea may be mild and self-limiting or serious and life-threatening. It can be sudden or gradual in onset.

Causes

The causes include the following.

- Excitement or nervousness.
- Sudden dietary changes, e.g. access to lush grass or a change of hay.
- Grain overload, e.g. if a pony gains access to the feed store.
- Worms, e.g. cyathostomosis.
- The use of antibiotics which lead to overgrowth of harmful bacteria such as *Clostridium spp.* This is sometimes known as colitis X.
- Infection by bacteria, e.g. *Salmonella spp.*
- Viruses in foals, e.g. rotavirus.
- Tumours, e.g. lymphoma/lymphosarcoma.
- Infiltrative/inflammatory bowel diseases, e.g. granulomatous enteritis, eosinophilic enteritis and lymphocytic/plasmacytic enteritis. In these conditions the intestinal wall becomes thickened by infiltration of abnormal cells and this reduces its capacity to absorb water and other nutrients.
- Poisoning, e.g. acorns, non-steroidal anti-inflammatory drug toxicity.

- Sand accumulation. This can occur when horses and ponies graze on sandy land or eat hay in a sand school. It may also be a consequence of drinking from streams that reduce to a trickle in the summer. The sand accumulates in the large colon and irritates the gut lining.
- Peritonitis.

Clinical signs

These are variable, depending on the cause of the disease. They can include:

- increased gut sounds which may be audible from some distance
- weight loss
- depression
- loss of appetite
- dehydration
- colic
- faecal contamination and staining of the tail and hind limbs (Figure 17.13)
- a raised temperature
- increased heart rate
- a change in the colour of the mucous membranes
- reduction in capillary refill time
- sweating
- muscle fasciculation
- weakness
- ventral oedema
- laminitis (from grain overload).

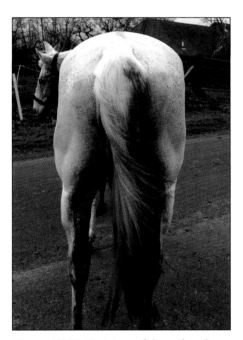

Figure 17.13 Staining of the tail and hind limbs of a horse with diarrhoea

When to call the vet

Diarrhoea is a sign of many conditions. It may be the consequence of a dietary change and last for a couple of days or it may indicate that something is seriously wrong. The following guidelines are offered.

- If the horse is off colour or has a temperature, the vet should be called immediately.
- Foals with diarrhoea should also be examined by the vet urgently. The exception is the mild self-limiting diarrhoea seen in a foal when it is about 10 days old. This is foal-heat diarrhoea associated with the mare coming into season.
- If the horse seems fine in itself but has loose droppings for more than a day or two, it should be checked over by the vet.

Diarrhoea due to dietary changes is usually short-lived and requires sensible management rather than veterinary treatment. However, diarrhoea caused by *Salmonella spp.* or *Clostridia spp.* infections may be severe and debilitating and is potentially fatal. The absorption of bacterial endotoxins leads to severe clinical signs and affected horses need urgent treatment.

> **Caution**
>
> *Salmonella* is a **zoonosis** which means it can be transmitted to humans. Up to 20% of horses carry the bacterium without showing any clinical signs and only excrete it during times of stress. Your vet will decide if the *Salmonella* is the cause of the diarrhoea or whether it is being excreted due to the stress of another illness. *Salmonella spp.* may be cultured from a horse with diarrhoea but there is often another underlying cause. All animals shedding *Salmonella* should be isolated from other horses as they are a potential source of infection. Overalls and disposable gloves should be worn when dealing with infected horses and great care must be taken not to accidentally ingest the microorganism. Your vet will advise you on suitable disinfectants and hygiene precautions.

Diagnosis

The first step with either acute or chronic diarrhoea is to try to find the cause through clinical examination and discussion of the history. The vet may take:

- blood samples to check for evidence of infection, inflammation, dehydration, anaemia, toxaemia or worm infestation
- a dung sample to look for worm eggs, pathogenic bacteria and viruses, sand.

SAND SEDIMENTATION TEST

A sample of faeces is suspended in water in a clear plastic container and shaken well. If sand is present, it forms a layer of sediment at the bottom of the container.

FURTHER DIAGNOSTIC TESTS

If the horse does not respond to treatment and management changes or the vet is concerned about the possibility of a tumour or other infiltrative disease leading to malabsorption, various tests may be carried out including:

- a peritoneal tap (see page 477)
- glucose absorption tests
- ultrasonography
- small intestinal biopsy
- a rectal biopsy.

Glucose absorption tests

These tests assess the ability of the small intestine to absorb glucose. The horse is starved overnight on inedible bedding and a blood sample is taken the next morning to measure the glucose concentration in the blood at the start of the test. The horse is then given a solution of glucose by stomach tube. Further blood tests are taken at regular intervals and a graph is made to show the change in the blood glucose concentration over the time of the test (usually 4 hours). In a normal horse the blood glucose concentration peaks at approximately double the starting level after 2 hours and then declines. A reduced peak or no change indicates malabsorption by the small intestine.

Ultrasonography

Ultrasonography may be helpful in detecting tumours, abscesses and thickening of the intestinal wall as well as signs of peritonitis and other problems.

Small intestine and lymph node biopsy

On occasions it is necessary to anaesthetise the horse and examine the intestines and lymph nodes. A biopsy may be taken from any suspicious-looking tissues. Sometimes it is possible for biopsies to be done in the standing patient at laparoscopy (see Castration on page 571), which is a safer technique than subjecting the horse to a full general anaesthetic. However, only a limited region of the intestine is accessible this way (Figure 17.14).

Rectal biopsy

Biopsy forceps are introduced into the rectum and a fold of the rectal wall is positioned between the jaws. The sample is then taken and sent off for histology to look for abnormal cells.

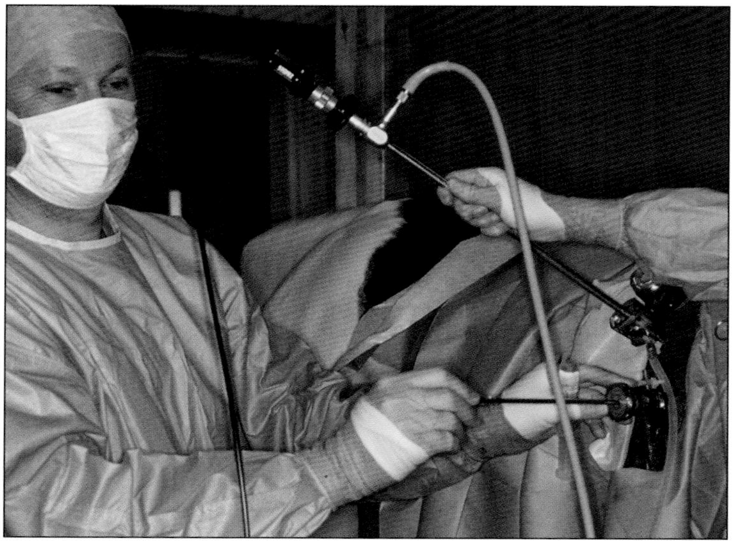

Post mortem

In some cases, the costs of the more specialized investigations are prohibitive, so the vet will provide symptomatic treatment. If the treatment is not successful, the diagnosis may be made at post mortem.

Figure 17.14 Laparoscopy

Treatment

The aims of treatment are to:

- remove the cause wherever possible
- replace fluids and electrolytes
- minimize the absorption of endotoxin
- restore the normal population of gut microorganisms
- provide suitable food.

In some cases treatment will be given to reduce inflammation of the gut wall or to slow down the passage of food through the gut, allowing more time for water absorption. The treatment will depend on the cause of the diarrhoea and the clinical assessment of the horse.

MEDICATION
This may include some of the following.
- Anthelmintics.
- Intravenous fluids – volumes of 40–80 litres may be required to rehydrate a horse.
- Oral electrolytes.
- Codeine phosphate to slow the passage of food through the gut.
- Antibiotics if the diarrhoea is caused by harmful bacteria.
- Administration of substances to coat and protect the irritated gut lining and reduce the absorption of endotoxin, e.g. activated charcoal, bismuth subsalicylate, kaolin and pectin.
- Flunixin meglumine to relieve pain and inflammation, also to reduce the effect of endotoxin.
- Spasmolytic and analgesic drugs to ease the pain.
- Corticosteroids to reduce the inflammation of the gut.
- Psyllium, a bulk laxative, to help move sand through the colon.

FEEDING AND MANAGEMENT
This again will depend on the cause of the diarrhoea and your vet will advise you of the most appropriate management and diet. In most cases:
- the horse should kept off fresh grass and fed good quality hay and alfalfa
- succulent feeds such as carrots and sugar beet should be limited or avoided
- a vitamin B supplement is recommended as this is normally produced by bacteria within the gut
- a broad spectrum vitamin and mineral supplement is beneficial
- small feeds should be offered several times a day
- fresh water should be freely available: horses with diarrhoea need to drink more water than usual to replace the lost fluids
- probiotics help to re-establish a normal gut flora: a probiotic is a specially prepared supplement that contains a mixture of the bacteria that are important for digestion in the horse.

NURSING
- Horses with severe diarrhoea must be kept clean to prevent scalding of the skin under the tail and down the back legs. These areas should be washed and dried, then protected with a thick layer of petroleum jelly.

- It is helpful to wrap the tail in a protective plastic sleeve.
- The bedding must be kept clean and dry.

SURGERY

If a large amount of sand has accumulated in the colon, this may have to be removed surgically. This is not always straightforward and there is quite a high risk of complications.

Prognosis

The prognosis depends on the cause of the diarrhoea and how quickly it is treated. With the exception of grain overload which may lead to severe laminitis, most cases of diarrhoea caused by dietary changes have an excellent prognosis. They usually improve spontaneously or with good management and non-specific treatment.

Horses with diarrhoea or colic caused by the accumulation of sand in their colons may be successfully treated if the disease is recognized and treated early. However, large accumulations of sand can damage the gut and lead to endotoxaemia and death.

Diarrhoea caused by severe cyathostomosis or bacterial infection has a guarded prognosis and fatalities are not uncommon. This is also the case with inflammatory bowel diseases such as eosinophilic, granulomatous and lymphocytic or plasmacytic infiltrations of the gut. Many of these horses are euthanased.

The prognosis for horses with neoplastic (cancerous) diseases such as lymphoma (also known as lymphosarcoma) is usually hopeless.

GRASS SICKNESS

Grass sickness, also known as **equine dysautonomia**, is a disease in which degenerative changes occur to the nerves of the autonomic nervous system. This results in dysfunction of the whole of the digestive tract, from the pharynx (at the back of the mouth) all the way to the rectum. It usually affects young, adult horses between 2 and 7 years. Although Scotland still has the highest incidence of grass sickness, it is seen throughout the UK and in other northern European countries.

Cause

The cause is unknown. It is thought to be either:
- the result of ingesting a neurotoxin (nerve poison) from the pasture, or
- bacteria in the digestive tract producing a toxin.

The possibilities currently under investigation include:
- ingestion of toxins produced by moulds on the pasture
- production of specific toxins (type C) by the bacterium *Clostridium botulinum* in the gut

- the influence of cyanogenic glycosides found in white clover on the susceptibility of the horse to the disease.

Grass sickness is not thought to be contagious. If the causative toxin is confirmed to be associated with *Clostridium botulinum,* it is hoped that a vaccine will be developed.

Predisposing factors

The disease is associated with the following.

- It occurs in animals that spend all or part of their time at grass. Grass sickness has been reported in fully stabled horses but this is rare and may develop because grass has been picked for them.
- Sporadic outbreaks occur and some premises or individual fields have a higher risk than others.
- Soil type may be influential. The disease appears to occur less frequently on chalky ground than it does in areas with loam or sandy soils or those with a high nitrogen content.
- Affected horses have often been moved to a new pasture within the preceding 2 months or had dietary changes made in the 2 weeks prior to succumbing to the disease.
- Horses in good condition are most commonly affected.
- The disease tends to occur on premises with a large number of horses.
- There is a seasonal incidence. In the UK, most cases occur between April and July, with a peak in May.
- Outbreaks tend to follow periods of cool, dry weather, with temperatures of 7–11 °C
- Mechanical removal of droppings and disturbance of the soil by cultivation appears to increase the risk.
- Stress such as castration, being sold, breaking, travelling long distances, moving premises and meeting new horses may be a significant factor.

Horses which have grazed, and been in contact, with other horses succumbing to grass sickness seem to be resistant to the disease. This may be due to high antibody levels to *Clostridium botulinum* type C.

Clinical signs

The toxin in the intestine is absorbed and causes damage to the nervous system. This reduces the motility of the gut and leads to the symptoms described below. There are three forms of the disease and many of the signs are common to all three forms.

ACUTE FORM

The symptoms include the following.

- Depression.

- Difficulty swallowing (known as **dysphagia**).
- Drooling of saliva from the mouth.
- Distension of the stomach and abdomen.
- Reflux of a foul-smelling greenish-brown fluid from the nostrils.
- Reduced or absent gut sounds.
- Colic due to abdominal pain.
- Raised pulse rate (70–120 beats per minute)
- Muscle tremors.
- Generalized or patchy sweating.
- Constipation (impaction).
- Severe dehydration.
- The temperature may be normal or raised.
- On internal examination, the rectal wall is abnormally dry. The rectum may be empty or contain small, dry faecal balls with a thick covering of mucus. The large colon is often impacted and loops of distended small intestine may be felt.

Horses with acute grass sickness die or are destroyed on humane grounds within two days.

SUBACUTE FORM

Horses with this form show many of the above signs but they are not quite as severe. Their appetite is usually reduced and attempts to eat and drink may be slow and clumsy. Chewed food and water may drop from the mouth or drain through the nostrils. Thirsty horses that have difficulty swallowing often stand over the trough and 'play' with the water. The stomach is less distended so reflux of the stomach contents down the horse's nose is less common. These horses may stand with all four feet drawn closely together under the body. They rapidly lose weight and have a 'tucked up' appearance.

Horses with subacute grass sickness either die or are put down within 3–7 days or they enter the chronic phase.

CHRONIC PHASE

In the chronic phase of the disease the signs may develop slowly over a period of time or follow on from a subacute episode. They include:

- slow eating and a reduced appetite
- weight loss and 'tucked up' appearance (Figure 17.15)

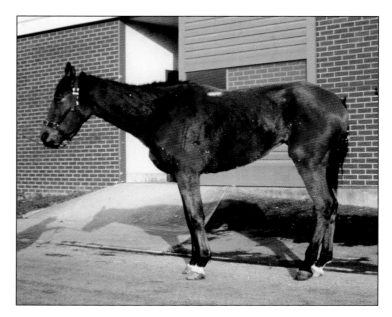

Figure 17.15 A case of chronic grass sickness

- standing with all four feet close together
- muscle tremors
- mild, intermittent colic
- patchy or generalized sweating
- dry and inflamed nasal passages with accumulation of thick mucous material causing the horse to 'snuffle' when breathing
- weakness and exercise intolerance
- drooping of the eyelids giving them a sleepy expression
- reduced gut sounds and motility
- no impaction but reduced amounts of dry, firm droppings.

Diagnosis

The vet will be suspicious of grass sickness from the clinical signs, but confirming the diagnosis is not straightforward. A number of blood tests support the diagnosis but are not conclusive. A sample of peritoneal fluid taken from the abdomen is often a deeper yellow colour than normal.

PHENYLEPHRINE EYE DROPS

A relatively new test involves applying 0.05% phenylephrine eye drops to the conjunctiva of one eye. If the eyelid of the treated eye is less droopy 30 minutes later, this increases the suspicion that the horse is suffering from grass sickness.

BIOPSY

Conformation of the diagnosis is made by identification of characteristic degenerative changes in the nerve cells of either:

- a piece of ileum removed from the horse under general anaesthesia or during a laparoscopy performed on the standing, sedated horse, or
- in autonomic ganglia obtained after the horse has died.

RADIOGRAPHY

Radiographs of the oesophagus have been used to help diagnosis but are not always conclusive. In a normal horse, a bolus of swallowed liquid takes between 4 and 10 seconds to reach the stomach. If radiographs are taken immediately after the horse has swallowed some barium contrast medium, pooling of the barium may be seen along the length of the oesophagus or at the thoracic inlet.

Treatment

Treatment of acute and subacute cases with impactions and nasogastric reflux is not attempted as the nerve damage is too great for any prospect of recovery. These animals should be euthanased on humane grounds.

Some chronic cases respond to treatment but others do not. For treatment to be considered the horse should be:

- capable of swallowing
- reasonably free of pain
- bright and alert.

Treatment includes the following.

- Offering frequent small meals that are palatable, high in energy and protein and easy to swallow. Chopped fresh grass (from a 'safe' field) and soaked high-energy concentrates with added molasses are suitable. Apples and carrots can be added to improve palatability.
- Probiotics.
- Pain relief as required, e.g. flunixin meglumine.
- Cisapride. This is a drug that increases the motility of the whole of the intestinal tract and helps emptying of the stomach. It is expensive and can cause colicky signs. It must not be given to horses that have impactions and is not necessary in every case.

NURSING CARE

Excellent nursing care is essential. The horse should:

- be rugged to prevent it getting cold as these animals often have a subnormal temperature; rugging sometimes reduces the sweating
- have plenty of human company and attention, i.e. regular grooming to remove the sweat and short walks in hand 2–3 times daily
- fresh water should always be available.

Prognosis

Acute and subacute cases have a grave prognosis and some chronic cases continue to deteriorate despite treatment. Of those horses considered suitable for treatment, between 50% and 70% survive, but recovery may take many months. Many are able to return to work. Some horses experience residual problems, e.g:

- mild swallowing difficulties which cause them to eat more slowly than before
- increased sweating
- coat changes including colour change, greasiness, patches where the hair stands on end.

Prevention

- Stable the horse all the time or avoid using fields where the disease has occurred, especially in the spring and summer.
- If this is not practical or possible, horses should be offered hay or haylage during the high-risk period.
- Stable horses in affected areas following a 7–10 day period with temperatures of between 7–11 °C.

- Stable horses moving onto high-risk premises for the first 2 months.
- Remove droppings from the pasture by hand.
- Minimize stress of horses kept in high-risk areas.
- There may be an association between frequent use of certain anthelmintics and grass sickness in susceptible horses; however, more work needs to be done on this; check with your vet for current advice.

LIVER DISEASE

The liver has many important functions. These include:
- storage and metabolism of carbohydrate, protein and fat
- production of bile which is important for the digestion of fat
- synthesis of proteins, e.g. albumin, globulin and blood clotting factors
- breakdown of excess protein to urea (which is excreted by the kidneys)
- storage of vitamins and minerals
- detoxification of poisonous substances.

The liver filters blood from the intestines and plays an important part in regulating the levels of fat, glucose and amino acids in the bloodstream. The horse does not have a gall bladder to store bile as it is continuously secreted because the horse eats for many hours of the day.

Causes
The causes of liver disease include:
- plant toxins, e.g. ragwort
- viruses
- bacteria
- parasites
- tumours
- severe energy deficiency
- chemical toxins.

When damaged, the liver has enormous capacity for regeneration. When this capacity is exceeded, the damaged cells (called hepatocytes) are replaced by non-functional fibrous tissue. Signs develop when more than 70% of the cells have been replaced and there are insufficient healthy hepatocytes to cope with the functions listed above.

Clinical signs
The clinical signs are variable. They arise due to one or more of the following.

- Destruction of the liver cells.
- Obstruction to bile flow.
- Excessive accumulation of fats.

Some of the following will be seen.
- Chronic weight loss.
- Lack of appetite.
- Abdominal pain leading to colicky episodes.
- Diarrhoea.
- Ventral oedema (collection of fluid under the skin of the lowest parts of the abdomen).
- Photosensitization of non–pigmented skin, which results in areas that are inflamed and sore in response to exposure to sunlight (see page 549). The horse may be itchy and uncomfortable. (Figure 17.16 and see Figures 18.21 and 18.22)
- Jaundice (Figure 17.17). The whites of the eyes and the mucous membranes of the mouth and eyes have a yellowish tinge due to abnormal accumulation of bile pigment. However, this is not a definitive sign and it can also arise if the horse is starved for 24 hours or the horse experiences abnormal destruction of red blood cells.

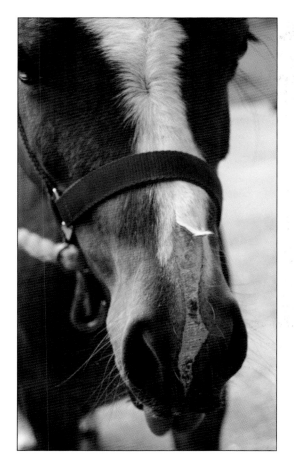

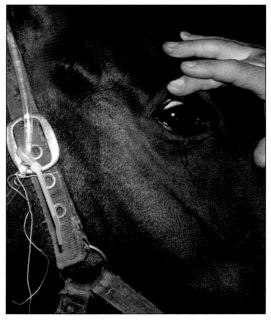

Figure 17.16 Photosensitization in a pony with liver disease (left)

Figure 17.17 Jaundiced mucous membranes (above)

Behavioural signs include:

- depression
- sleepiness
- excessive yawning
- restlessness and aimless wandering.

In the advanced stages of the disease, the liver dysfunction leads to accumulation of abnormal metabolites in the blood, e.g. ammonia, which affects the brain. This is known as **hepatic encephalopathy.** The behavioural signs listed above may be seen together with some of the following.

- Lack of awareness of the surroundings.
- Circling (repeatedly walking in a circle).
- Head pressing against solid objects.
- Jerky movements.
- Compulsive walking.
- Blindness.
- Incoordination.
- Excitement.
- Maniacal behaviour.
- Coma.
- Death.

Specific liver diseases
TOXIC HEPATITIS

A number of plant and fungal toxins cause liver disease in horses. Ragwort is one of the commonest causes of liver disease in the UK. This is discussed in some detail in the section on poisonous plants on page 510.

CHOLANGIOHEPATITIS

This disease is caused by bacteria entering the bile ducts of the liver from the small intestine, causing inflammation of the bile ducts and the adjacent liver tissue. It can also be caused by migrating liver fluke (see below). Stones may form and obstruct the bile ducts. Signs include fever, recurrent colic, jaundice, photosensitivity, loss of appetite, weight loss and depression. Treatment includes supportive therapy and antibiotics. Surgery to remove the biliary stones is possible as a last resort. The prognosis is reasonably good provided treatment is started early before significant fibrosis develops.

THEILER'S DISEASE

This disease which affects adult horses is sometimes associated with the administration of tetanus antitoxin in the preceding 4–10 weeks. For this reason, it is also known as **serum sickness**. However, the cause is uncertain; it may be associated with a viral infection. The acute hepatitis can lead to liver failure and hepatic encephalopathy. Some horses do survive with supportive treatment and early diagnosis but the mortality rate is over 50%. The disease is fortunately rare.

TYZZER'S DISEASE

This is an acute bacterial infection caused by the bacterium *Bacillus piliformis* that occurs in foals between 1 and 6 weeks of age. The disease is rapidly fatal and the foal is usually found dead. Symptoms include a high temperature, depression, diarrhoea and convulsions. The foals die of septic shock and liver failure. Treatment includes antibiotics, intravenous fluids and nursing. The prognosis is extremely grave.

LIVER FLUKE (*Fasciola hepatica* and *Fasciola gigantica*)

Liver fluke is a serious problem for sheep and cows grazing on marshy pastures, but it is rarely diagnosed in horses. However, horses sharing these pastures with cattle or sheep have the potential to be infected. They are fairly resistant to infection so signs are not always seen. Indications of a possible problem can include abdominal pain, loss of appetite, anaemia and poor performance.

The adult flukes live in the bile ducts and lay eggs that are excreted in the faeces. The diagnosis is confirmed by finding the eggs in the faeces of infected horses. However, this is unreliable and not all of the flukes develop into egg-laying adults. The migrating flukes cause local damage to the liver tissue, so liver enzyme levels are raised.

Treatment involves removing the horse from the infected pasture and treatment with a suitable medication supplied by your vet. The disease may be prevented by draining marshy pastures so conditions are no longer favourable for the fluke larvae or the snail intermediate hosts.

OTHER CAUSES OF LIVER DISEASE

Other possible causes of liver disease have been investigated. Viral hepatitis has been shown to exist in other species and is suspected in horses. Equine herpesvirus–1 (EHV-1) damages the liver cells of the developing foetus and newborn foals.

Diagnosis

The diagnosis may be made on the clinical signs and confirmed by blood tests. In many cases, however, the signs of general malaise are too vague to be diagnostic in themselves but the blood tests may show raised liver enzymes and bile acids (see page 680).

A liver biopsy may yield further information on the cause and extent of the disease, but this only samples a small part of a large organ. The use of ultrasound is helpful when taking a liver biopsy and it may provide additional information. The degree of fibrosis of the liver sample can be used as a prognostic guide. Biopsy samples are cultured for bacterial growth so the most appropriate antibiotic can be selected if infection is present.

Treatment

Unless the disease is caused by an acute bacterial infection, there is no specific treatment. All therapy is aimed at supporting the liver, in the hope that cell regeneration will occur. In cases of liver disease caused by ingestion of poisonous plants, removal from the pasture or a change of forage supply is essential.

Supportive treatment includes the following.

- A high energy, low protein (10% or less) diet.
- Supplementation with B vitamins.
- Reducing exposure to sunlight.
- Complete rest.
- Antibiotics if bacterial infection is present.
- If the horse is showing signs of hepatic encephalopathy, sedation may be needed as well as medication to reduce further ammonia production and absorption. The oral antibiotics neomycin and metronidazole decrease ammonia-producing bacteria in the large intestine, and lactulose limits absorption.
- Corticosteroids may be prescribed for specific types of liver problem.
- Intravenous fluids may be administered.

Progress can be monitored by regular blood tests.

THE DIET

The aim of dietary management is to give the liver the minimum amount of work to do whilst still supplying adequate energy and nutrients. Some general guidelines are given below. However, it is important that you discuss the diet with your vet and/or qualified nutritionist. Individual requirements vary; for example, the recommendations for a thin horse will differ from those for a fat pony.

The general principles include:

- offering small feeds 4–6 times daily (less work for the liver than 2 larger ones)
- avoid alfalfa as it is high in protein (one of the liver's functions is to breakdown excess protein)
- avoid feeds and supplements that are high in fat or oil
- flaked maize and molassed sugar beet are useful energy sources for horses with liver disease
- provide a vitamin B supplement
- allow the horse access to pasture and hay as a forage source; rapidly growing spring grass and recently fertilized pastures should be avoided.

Prognosis

The prognosis depends on the cause of the liver disease and the stage at which treatment is started. On the whole, the prognosis is guarded. Horses that have apparently recovered may relapse as soon as they go back into work.

Once the terminal stages have been reached, the horse may behave in a dangerous manner and have to be humanely destroyed. In many cases, the liver damage is irreversible by the time the signs are seen.

HYPERLIPAEMIA (FATTY LIVER SYNDROME)

Hyperlipaemia is a disease where an abnormal amount of fat is carried in the blood and deposited in the liver and kidneys. The disease is seen primarily in ponies and donkeys. It tends to occur when there is insufficient intake of food energy to meet their nutritional requirements. The disease leads to liver and kidney failure. It has a mortality rate of up to 70%.

Causes and predisposing factors

The main causes of hyperlipaemia are insufficient food intake and stress. Overweight female ponies and donkeys are particularly susceptible. Other predisposing factors include:

- pregnancy and lactation (which require additional energy)
- insufficient provision of food, e.g. starvation of laminitic ponies
- any disease that reduces the food intake, e.g.
    - severe dental disease
    - a heavy parasite burden
- stress, e.g.
    - transport
    - severe weather conditions.

Why does the disease occur?

The liver plays an important part in maintaining the horse's energy balance. When food is plentiful, the plasma glucose is stored in the liver as glycogen. This process relies on the action of the hormone insulin. At times when the energy intake is reduced or the nutritional demands increase, glycogen stores are used up and fatty acids are released into the blood from fat stores in the body as an alternative source of energy. This release of fatty acids is normally inhibited by insulin and glucose. Most of these fatty acids are taken up by the liver and used to produce glucose or changed into triglycerides which are either stored in the liver or released back into the blood as very low density lipoproteins (VLDLs). The VLDLs in the blood are normally cleared from the circulation and deposited in fat stores (adipose tissue), skeletal or heart muscle; their removal is promoted by insulin and heparin.

Many obese ponies and donkeys with large, internal deposits of fat are 'insulin resistant' (see page 611) and this causes severe disruption to the normal energy metabolism. The combination of insulin resistance and insufficient energy intake or stress leads to overproduction of triglycerides which build up to dangerously high levels in the circulation. Fatty infiltration of the liver and kidneys can lead to liver or kidney failure. This disease can progress rapidly. If any fat pony or donkey goes off its food, it is one of the first things to consider.

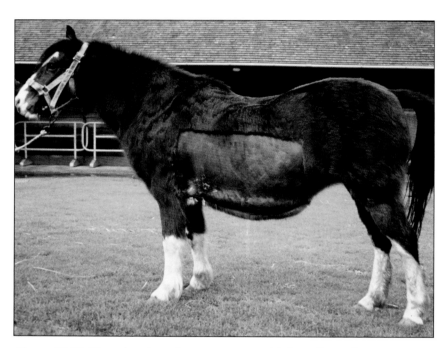

Figure 17.18 Ventral oedema in a pony mare with hyperlipaemia

Clinical signs

These include:

- anorexia
- depression
- lethargy
- weakness
- ataxia (they are unsteady on their legs)
- ventral oedema (Figure 17.18)
- mild abdominal pain due to swelling of the liver.

If they progress to liver failure, signs may include:

- weight loss
- extreme depression
- playing with water rather than drinking it
- fatty, foul-smelling diarrhoea
- jaundice
- bad breath
- abortion
- head-pressing, convulsions, coma and death.

Diagnosis

The diagnosis is confirmed by taking a blood sample. The plasma looks milky instead of the normal clear yellow colour (Figure 17.19); this is due to the high amount of triglyceride present. A normal pony has a triglyceride level of less than 0.35mmol/litre. Animals with levels of 1–5mmol/litre are at risk and anything above 5mmol/litre is considered to be hyperlipaemic. Severe cases have levels between 20–80mmol/litre.

Blood tests are also taken to assess the degree of liver damage and any developing kidney problems.

Treatment

Early diagnosis and treatment are essential for any chance of a successful outcome. The majority of affected ponies and donkeys do not recover.

The most important considerations are to:

- increase the energy intake
- treat any underlying illness
- reduce the circulating triglycerides
- reduce any stress.

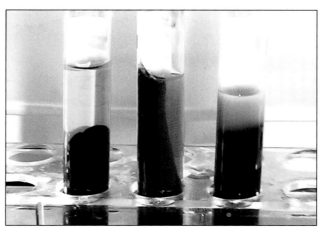

Figure 17.19 Lipaemic blood samples: the sample on the left is normal; the sample in the middle is slightly lipaemic; the sample on the right is very lipaemic

INCREASING THE ENERGY INTAKE

This prevents further quantities of fat being mobilized into the bloodstream. It can be achieved in 3 ways.

1 Every effort should be made to encourage the patient to eat. Small, palatable, high-energy feeds and freshly cut grass should be offered. Tempt them with treats like apples, mints or even ginger biscuits. If the pony will not eat, high energy gruel can be administered regularly through a stomach tube that is sutured in place. The gruel is made by soaking complete cubes in water. Fat should not be added as an energy source.

2 Glucose may be administered by stomach tube together with insulin injections.

3 If the intestine is damaged as a result of disease, intravenous feeding may be used. This is very expensive.

TREATING UNDERLYING DISEASE

This may involve:

- worming the horse, pony or donkey to reduce the parasite burden
- remedial dentistry
- treating any other conditions
- weaning any foals.

MEDICATION

- Intravenous fluids may be given to correct the electrolyte imbalance and dehydration.
- Insulin is used to reduce the release of fatty acids into the bloodstream from adipose tissue and to encourage the uptake of VLDLs from the blood into adipose tissue, skeletal and cardiac muscle. It also assists with the uptake of glucose from the blood.

If the animal is insulin resistant, the effect will be reduced.

- Heparin is sometimes used to promote uptake of VLDLs but its efficacy has been questioned.
- Low doses of non-steroidal anti-inflammatory drugs such as flunixin meglumine may be used to help control the inflammation and pain.

REDUCING THE STRESS

Stress is reduced by immediate treatment of any other condition. The stress of lactation is eliminated by early weaning of the foal. Aborting the foal of pregnant mares is not ideal due to the risk of complications such as a retained placenta and subsequent laminitis. Occasionally it is carried out if it is considered to be the mare's only hope of survival.

Prognosis

The prognosis is poor unless the condition is diagnosed early in the course of the disease and treated vigorously.

Prevention

- Good management is needed to prevent ponies and donkeys from becoming obese in the first place.
- Regular exercise helps with weight loss and improves insulin sensitivity.
- Care should be taken to ensure that the energy intake of susceptible animals is adequate all year round. This is especially important for pregnant and lactating mares.
- When mares are transported long distances to and from stud, stop regularly and allow them to rest and eat.
- Take care when restricting the diet of laminitic ponies. Do *not* starve them; ask your vet or a nutritionist for advice.
- Animals that live out should be provided with shelter and additional food when the weather is particularly bad.
- Regular blood tests can be used to monitor the triglyceride levels of at-risk animals, together with close observation of their appetite, behaviour and condition.

PERITONITIS

Peritonitis is inflammation of the peritoneum. The peritoneum is a single layer of cells that lines the abdominal cavity and the organs contained within it. It overlies a thin layer of connective tissue with blood vessels, lymphatic vessels and nerves. The abdomen contains a small amount of peritoneal fluid which is continually produced and absorbed. It minimizes friction between the abdominal organs which is essential for normal functioning of the gastrointestinal tract and when the animal moves.

Causes

There are many causes of peritonitis. In horses, it is usually widespread throughout the abdomen and secondary to some other condition. The peritoneum can become inflamed following mechanical damage or exposure to toxins and bacteria. This occurs in a number of ways.

- As the result of penetrating external injuries, e.g. a stake wound.
- Following an episode of colic when the blood supply to the gut is reduced and bacteria and toxins leak into the abdomen.
- Following perforation of a gastric ulcer or rupture of any part of the gut allowing intestinal contents into the abdomen.
- Rupture of any other abdominal or pelvic organ, e.g. the spleen, uterus or bladder, exposes the peritoneum to bacteria and chemical irritants such as urine.
- Rupture of abdominal abscesses, e.g. from *Streptococcus equi* (strangles) infection.
- Septicaemic foals may develop peritonitis.
- Castration complications.
- Following abdominal surgery.
- Through migration of intestinal parasites.

WHAT ACTUALLY HAPPENS WITHIN THE ABDOMEN?

Once the peritoneum becomes inflamed, the blood vessels dilate and more peritoneal fluid is produced. Neutrophils migrate into the abdomen to help the peritoneal macrophages clear up the bacteria. Fibrin clots are deposited on the surfaces of organs and fibrous adhesions begin to develop (Figure 17.20).

With a minor perforation, fibrin may seal it off very quickly and the fibrous tissue helps to localize the infection. If this is successful, the affected organ repairs and the fibrin clots are dissolved. However, with an overwhelming infection, it quickly spreads throughout the abdominal cavity. Affected animals become toxic from absorption of bacterial endotoxins and show signs of shock.

Clinical signs

The clinical signs are variable, depending on whether the peritonitis develops in response to an abdominal catastrophe such as rupture of the gut or develops slowly over a period of time, for instance in response to migration of parasitic worm larvae.

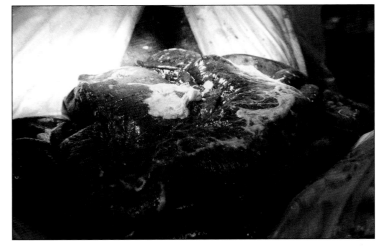

Figure 17.20 Large yellow fibrin clots on the intestines of a horse with peritonitis

ACUTE PERITONITIS

The signs develop very rapidly and include:

- a rapid heart rate with a weak pulse
- fast, shallow respirations
- high temperature
- sweating
- severe depression
- loss of appetite
- abdominal pain
- reduced gut sounds
- diarrhoea
- fewer droppings than normal
- very congested mucous membranes that may be brick red or bluish in colour
- increased capillary refill time
- dehydration
- distension of the abdomen
- muscle fasciculations
- cold extremities
- collapse
- sudden death
- rectal examination may be painful.

These horses are often reluctant to move and walk uncharacteristically slowly and stiffly. Death may occur within hours.

CHRONIC PERITONITIS

The symptoms are less acute in onset and can develop over a period of days or weeks. They include:

- depression
- poor appetite
- intermittent low-grade colic
- gradual weight loss
- temperature fluctuations
- increased heart and respiratory rates
- reluctance to move and a stiff, slow gait
- ventral oedema
- diarrhoea and reduced passage of faeces.

Diagnosis

Diagnosis is made on:

- the clinical signs
- analysis of peritoneal fluid
- blood tests
- rectal examination.

TAKING A PERITONEAL TAP

The vet will collect a sample of peritoneal fluid from the horse's abdomen. The lowest part of the abdomen is clipped and scrubbed, and then a hypodermic needle or teat cannula is inserted through the ventral midline. It is slowly advanced until fluid drips from the hub. A sample is collected for analysis.

ANALYSIS OF THE SAMPLE

Appearance

Normal peritoneal fluid is a clear, pale straw colour. If the horse has peritonitis, the fluid may be a cloudy, cream colour. Dark, blood-stained fluid is indicative of loss of blood supply to an area of gut and is a serious sign. Green or brown fluid with visible vegetable matter is obtained if the gut has ruptured.

Measurement of the protein content and white cell count

The peritoneal fluid from a horse with peritonitis has raised protein and white blood cell counts when compared with the peritoneal fluid taken from normal horses.

Culture and microscopic examination of the fluid

The sample is examined under the microscope and also cultured to confirm the presence and type of bacteria. This helps the vet to decide which antibiotic to use for treatment.

BLOOD TESTS

The blood test results depend on the stage of the disease and the cause. There may be a low neutrophil and total white cell count in the early stages as the cells migrate from the blood into the abdomen to help fight the disease. Later on, the neutrophil count may be raised. The vet will assess the degree of dehydration and monitor the protein levels (see Blood Tests, page 679). These results will be interpreted together with the clinical signs.

RECTAL EXAMINATION

This may be uncomfortable for the horse but is necessary to help make the diagnosis and rule out other problems.

ULTRASONOGRAPHY

This may be helpful in establishing or confirming the diagnosis especially in young foals.

Treatment

The aims of treatment are to:

- deal with the identified cause
- stabilize the horse's condition
- control the pain
- eliminate infection
- correct the dehydration and electrolyte imbalances.

MEDICATION

This is achieved by:

- intensive intravenous fluid therapy
- long courses of antibiotics
- anti-endotoxin drugs (very expensive)
- administration of plasma in some cases
- flunixin meglumine to control the pain and provide protection against the endotox-aemia
- anthelmintics if migrating worms are suspected as the cause.

PERITONEAL DRAINAGE AND LAVAGE

Once the horse's condition has stabilized, this may be performed to try to remove bacteria, toxins and fibrin from the abdomen. It can be done during surgery or in the standing, sedated horse (Figure 17.21). A catheter is placed in the midline of the lowest part of the abdomen and between 10 and 20 litres of warmed saline is introduced into the abdomen. The horse is gently walked around for 20 minutes to disperse the fluid around the abdomen and the fluid is then drained. This may be done 2–3 times daily for 2–3 days.

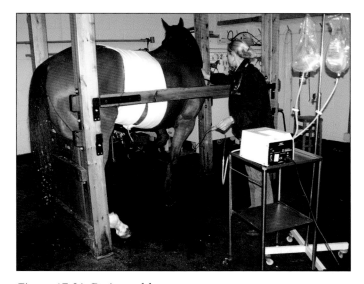

Figure 17.21 Peritoneal lavage

SURGERY

If a recent rupture of the gastrointestinal tract or the uterus is suspected, exploratory surgery may be carried out. This allows identification of the problem and repair or euthanasia as appropriate. Any abscesses or foreign material can be removed. Peritoneal lavage can be carried our more effectively than in the standing horse.

Surgery may also be performed if the horse is not responding to medical management or is experiencing severe, unrelenting pain. In many cases the horse is euthanased on the operating table.

Prognosis

Cases of gut rupture have a hopeless prognosis. In other cases, the prognosis depends on the cause of the peritonitis and how quickly the appropriate treatment is given. Unfortunately there is no laboratory test that is helpful in determining which cases are likely to survive and treatment is very expensive. A good response to the initial treatment is a hopeful sign. The reported mortality rate is between 25 and 70%. Horses with postoperative peritonitis are reported to have a high mortality rate.

POISONOUS PLANTS

There are a large number of plants that are potentially poisonous to horses in Britain. Horses and ponies at pasture are especially at risk at those times of year when grass is in short supply. The degree of toxicity varies, some being dangerous in small doses and others requiring consumption of larger amounts over longer periods of time. Fortunately poisoning is rare, but tends to be blamed as the cause of any mystery illness. To minimize risks as far as possible, poisonous plants should be identified and removed from the pasture.

Some of the poisonous plants found in Britain

Alder buckthorn	Flax	Lily of the valley
Black bryony	Foxglove	Linseed
Black nightshade	Fritillaria	Lupin
Bluebell bulbs	Greater celandine	Meadow saffron
Bog asphodel	Ground ivy	Monkshood
Box	Hellebore	Oak
Bracken	Hemlock	Pimpernel
Broom	Hemlock water dropwort	Poppy
Buckthorn	Hemp	Potato
Buckwheat	Hemp nettle	Privet
Buttercup	Henbane	Ragwort
Chickweed	Herb Paris	Rhododendron
Clover	Horseradish	Sandwort
Columbine	Horsetail	Snowdrop bulbs
Corncockle	Hyacinth bulbs	Soapwort
Cowbane	Iris	Sowbread
Cuckoo pint	Kale	St John's wort
Daffodil bulbs	Laburnum	Thornapple
Darnel	Larkspur	White bryony
Deadly nightshade	Laurel	Yew

A number of the commonest poisonous plants are discussed in more detail below.

Ragwort (Senecio jacobaea – tansy ragwort, and Senecio vulgaris – groundsel)

The tansy ragwort plant has a 2-year life cycle. In its first year, it has a dark green rosette form that grows amongst the grass. In the second year it flowers and grows to between 30 cm and 1 m (1 ft and 3 ft) high. The characteristic yellow flowers of the ragwort plant are a common sight on horse-sick pastures and roadsides during the summer months (July–September) (Figure 17.22). The plant contains toxic pyrrolizidine alkaloids which cause irreversible liver damage. In the UK, the spread of this plant is meant to be controlled by law.

The growing plant tastes very bitter and horses usually avoid it unless other grazing is scarce. However, once it is cut and dried, the plant becomes palatable. It is most dangerous when baled with the hay or if pulled up and left to wilt where horses are able to eat it.

CLINICAL SIGNS

The effects of the alkaloids are cumulative and signs are not usually seen until some time after consumption of the plant begins. In some cases the signs are delayed and may not appear until up to 1 year later, by which time the horse may have no exposure to the plant. The signs of ragwort poisoning include any of those listed in the chapter on liver disease, e.g:

- anorexia and weight loss
- depression
- yawning
- abdominal pain
- diarrhoea or constipation
- head pressing against fixed objects
- circling or aimless wandering
- ventral oedema
- jaundice
- incoordination.

In the terminal stages the horse may go into a coma and die quietly or become delirious and suffer convulsions.

DIAGNOSIS

The diagnosis is made on:

- the clinical signs
- blood tests
- liver biopsy.

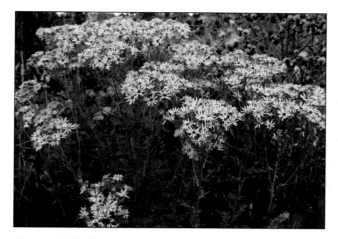

Figure 17.22 Ragwort

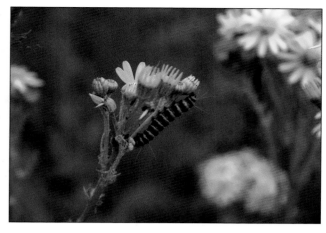

Figure 17.23 Caterpillar of the cinnabar moth feeding on ragwort

TREATMENT

There is no specific treatment. Supportive therapy is as described for liver disease.

PROGNOSIS

The prognosis is always guarded.

PREVENTION

Familiarize yourself with the appearance of ragwort and check the pasture regularly. Pull up any plants and *remove* them from the field. The plant becomes palatable (and therefore dangerous) after spraying with a selective weed killer so horses should be removed from the pasture until all traces of the plant have disappeared. Attempts have been made to control the plant biologically by introducing the cinnabar moth Their caterpillars only eat ragwort, starting at the top of the plant and working down towards the roots (Figure 17.23). However, the number of moths and caterpillars decrease as the plant is controlled.

Yew (Taxus baccata)

The yew is an evergreen tree that prefers chalky soils (Figure 17.24). It is often found in churchyards. All parts of the tree except the flesh of the red berries contain toxic alkaloids, e.g. taxine. These are rapidly absorbed from the digestive tract and affect the heart. *One mouthful is enough to kill.*

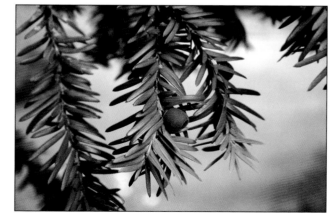

Figure 17.24 Yew with berries

CLINICAL SIGNS

Signs are rarely observed as the horse may die within minutes of ingesting the poison. They include:

- muscle tremors
- staggering
- convulsions
- difficulty breathing
- collapse
- rapid, weak pulse
- heart failure.

TREATMENT

The speed of death means that treatment is rarely possible. There is no antidote.

PREVENTION

It is essential to check hedges for the presence of yew. When discovered it should be fenced off or removed. The dried, dead leaves and twigs are just as poisonous as the fresh plant so they should be disposed of carefully.

Oak and acorns (Quercus spp.)

Oak leaves and acorns contain tannic acid which is poisonous to horses. Poisoning may occur in the spring when the young leaves are eaten or due to the ingestion of acorns in the autumn. Acorns can be addictive; some horses will actively search for them once they have acquired the taste. Small amounts do not usually cause problems but some horses have a greater tolerance to oak leaves and acorns than others. When it occurs, oak poisoning causes gastroenteritis. Gastric impactions also occur. In severe cases, death is caused by kidney failure.

CLINICAL SIGNS

These include:

- depression
- loss of appetite
- mouth ulcers
- abdominal pain (colic)
- constipation followed by diarrhoea which may contain blood
- blood in the urine
- weakness
- incoordination
- kidney damage and death.

THE DIGESTIVE SYSTEM 513

TREATMENT

There is no antidote. The horse is treated with medication to reduce the pain and control the diarrhoea. Fluid therapy and antibiotics may be prescribed.

PREVENTION

Fence off oak trees – either permanently or with an electric fence.
Pick up the fallen acorns daily.

How many acorns is it safe for my horse to eat?

Individual animals have different levels of tolerance. It is therefore not possible to say how many acorns can be eaten in a given period of time without causing symptoms. However, many horses, ponies and donkeys die from acorn poisoning each autumn. The only way to keep the horse safe is to ensure that it has no opportunity to consume acorns or large quantities of foliage.

Bracken (Pteridium aquilinum)

The bracken fern is common in moorland or woodland areas in Britain. It has large triangular fronds and grows up to 2 m (6ft) in height. The leaves grow from spreading underground roots in the spring and die back in the autumn.

The plant contains the enzyme thiaminase which breaks down thiamine (vitamin B1), leading to symptoms of thiamine deficiency. Horses usually eat the bracken for a couple of months before symptoms occur.

CLINICAL SIGNS

These include:

- muscle tremors
- an unsteady gait (known as 'bracken staggers')
- more obvious muscle twitches resulting in jerky movements of the body
- seizures
- death.

TREATMENT

Treatment is usually successful if caught in the early stages. The horse is given thiamine injections and disturbed as little as possible to reduce the likelihood of convulsions.

Buttercups (Ranunculus spp.)

The meadow buttercup is commonly seen in horse pastures during the late spring and summer. It contains a toxic, irritant substance called protoanemonin.

CLINICAL SIGNS

Buttercup poisoning is rarely seen, even when horses graze in pastures full of them. This is because large amounts need to be ingested for them to have an effect and they are less palatable than fresh grass. When signs do occur they include:

- inflammation of the lips and mouth
- blisters
- increased salivation
- abdominal pain.

Death from buttercup poisoning may be preceded by convulsions, but this is very rare.

TREATMENT

Affected horses should be removed from the pasture. Treatment is symptomatic.

Clover (Trifolium spp.)

There are many types of clover found in the UK. These include red clover (*T. pratense)* and white clover *(T. repens)*. They may be introduced into pasture to enrich the grazing and to increase the nitrogen content of the soil when ploughed in. Clovers contain a number of toxic substances including:

- oestrogens
- cyanogenic glycosides
- nitrates
- goitrogens.

These can cause a number of problems in animals including reproductive problems, laminitis, photosensitivity and blood coagulation disorders. A possible association between the cyanogenic glycosides in white clover and grass sickness is currently under investigation.

St. John's wort (Hypericum perforatum)

St John's wort is found in meadows, grassland and open woods. It is usually 30–80 cm (1 ft–2 ft 6 in) high and has clusters of bright yellow flowers. All parts of the plant are poisonous as they contain hypericine. It loses some of its toxicity when baled with hay but is still dangerous.

CLINICAL SIGNS

- Photosensitization. Skin lesions develop when unpigmented skin is exposed to sunlight. The affected areas are itchy and sore.
- Loss of appetite.
- General debility.
- Staggering gait.

- Blindness.
- Coma.

TREATMENT

Horses with low-level poisoning usually make a full recovery if they are removed from the affected pasture. Treatment involves:

- antibiotics
- good wound management
- keeping the horse in a darkened stable during daylight hours.

Laburnum (Laburnum anagyroides)

Laburnum is an ornamental tree with bright yellow flowers, commonly planted in gardens. It is very poisonous as all parts of the plant contain the alkaloid cytisine, especially the seeds and bark.

CLINICAL SIGNS

- Fever.
- Diarrhoea.
- Incoordination.
- Muscle spasms.
- Unsteady gait.
- Colic.
- Recumbency.
- Seizures.
- Death.

Treatment is symptomatic. Fatal poisoning is uncommon.

Privet (Ligustrum spp.)

Poisoning by privet usually occurs when horses and ponies eat garden hedges or gain access to compost heaps containing hedge clippings.

CLINICAL SIGNS

Clinical signs may include:

- intestinal disturbances
- a rapid pulse
- staggering
- paralysis
- death.

Treatment is symptomatic.

Linseed (Linum usitatissimum)

Linseed is grown commercially for its oil and also the fibrous stem. It contains a substance called linamarin which releases a cyanide-containing substance after being digested. It is destroyed by heat which is why linseed should always be thoroughly cooked before being fed to horses.

CLINICAL SIGNS

These may include:

- salivation
- rapid pulse
- gasping
- staggering
- convulsions.

Death may occur very rapidly with no opportunity for treatment.

18
THE HORSE'S SKIN

THE STRUCTURE AND FUNCTION OF SKIN

Skin is the outer, protective covering of the body. It has a complex structure which allows it to perform many important functions. For descriptive purposes, the skin can be divided into two layers: the outer epidermis and the inner dermis. These sit on a layer of subcutaneous fatty tissue which allows the skin its mobility (Figure 18.1).

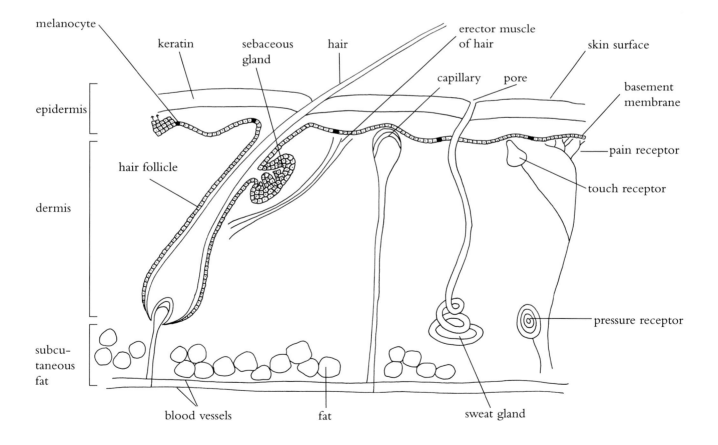

Figure 18.1 Diagrammatic section through the skin

Epidermis

The **epidermis** is composed of several layers of cells which are separated from the dermis by a thin basement membrane. The cells of the deepest layer divide all the time and are pushed up towards the surface to replace those that continually wear away or flake off.

As the cells are pushed up to the surface, they die and become transformed into a tough protein material called **keratin**. Keratin is virtually waterproof. It prevents water evaporating from the living tissues underneath. It also prevents the skin from absorbing water.

The cells also receive pigment called **melanin** from special cells called **melanocytes** in the deepest layer of the epidermis. This determines the colour of the skin and protects the body from the harmful effects of ultraviolet light.

Another function of the tough epidermis is to act as a barrier, preventing bacteria from entering the body.

Dermis

The underlying **dermis** consists of loose connective tissue, containing strong collagen fibres and elastic fibres. These give the skin its properties of strength and elasticity so it keeps its shape and is resistant to tearing.

Within the dermis are **hair follicles**, **sweat** and **sebaceous glands**, **blood vessels** and **nerve endings**.

Most of the horse's body is covered by **hair**, which protects the skin from injury and keeps the horse warm. Each hair grows from a hair follicle. Attached to this is a small band of muscle. When the weather is cold, the muscle contracts, causing the hair to stand up. The extra air trapped between the hairs is a poor conductor of heat and acts as a warm insulating layer.

Opening into the hair follicle is a sebaceous gland which produces an oily substance. This coats the hair, preventing it from becoming dry and brittle. It also helps to waterproof the skin surface.

Sweat glands consist of long, coiled tubes which open onto the skin surface. When sweat evaporates, the skin surface is cooled.

The skin's blood vessels bring oxygen and nutrients to the living cells. They also play an important role in temperature regulation. On a very cold day, the vessels near the skin surface constrict. The reduced blood flow lessens the heat lost to the atmosphere by radiation. Conversely, when a horse is warm, these vessels dilate and more heat is lost from the body.

Skin has numerous nerve endings. These supply the brain with continuous information about touch, pressure, cold, heat and pain. Perception of these sensations allows the horse to move away from unpleasant stimuli. In addition to these numerous functions, the skin synthesises vitamin D in sunlight.

As the largest and most exposed organ in the body, the skin is subject to a variety of ailments.

RINGWORM

Ringworm is a fungal infection of the skin which can affect both horses and people. It is caused by two groups of fungi, *Trichophyton spp. and Microsporum spp.* The fungal spores can survive for a long time in the environment, e.g. in stables, horse boxes and on wooden fences; they can also live on tack, grooming kit, rugs and clippers. Horses become infected through small abrasions in the skin. The fungus colonizes the superficial layers of the skin, the hair follicle and the hair shaft. This causes the hair to break off resulting in unsightly stubble. Despite the name, the lesion is not always ring-shaped.

The incubation period is usually between 4 and 14 days but can be up to 1 month. Ringworm is very contagious so outbreaks often occur. Young horses are particularly susceptible, especially when kept in groups in the damp conditions of the UK winter.

Clinical signs (Figures 18.2a–f)

- Ringworm can occur anywhere on the body but usually affects regions abraded by tack, e.g. the head, neck, girth and saddle regions.
- The lesions are very variable in appearance. In the early stages, tufts of hair may stand up from the rest of the coat. Affected areas vary from a couple of millimetres up to 4–5 cm ($1\frac{1}{2}$ –2 in). They are often round but can be any shape.
- The tufts of hair then fall out leaving an area of grey, scaly skin. The patches may enlarge as the fungus spreads outwards from the edge of the lesion.
- Some horses react to the fungal toxins and the skin becomes inflamed. A crust of exudate forms under the hair tuft. The lesions are not generally itchy unless secondary bacterial infection occurs.

Diagnosis

A diagnosis is made on the following.

- The clinical signs.
- The response to treatment.
- Microscopic examination of hair plucks to confirm the presence of a fungus.
- Culture of the fungus which can take up to 10 days.
- The history which can be helpful. If the horse is known to have been in contact with an infected horse or a number of animals are affected, then ringworm infection is likely. Young horses that have been through sale rings and transported recently often pick up ringworm on their travels.

Treatment

If the disease is not treated it is self-limiting and most horses recover in 4–12 weeks. However, prompt treatment can reduce the severity and duration of the disease. Good hygiene reduces contamination of the environment and the risk of spread to other horses.

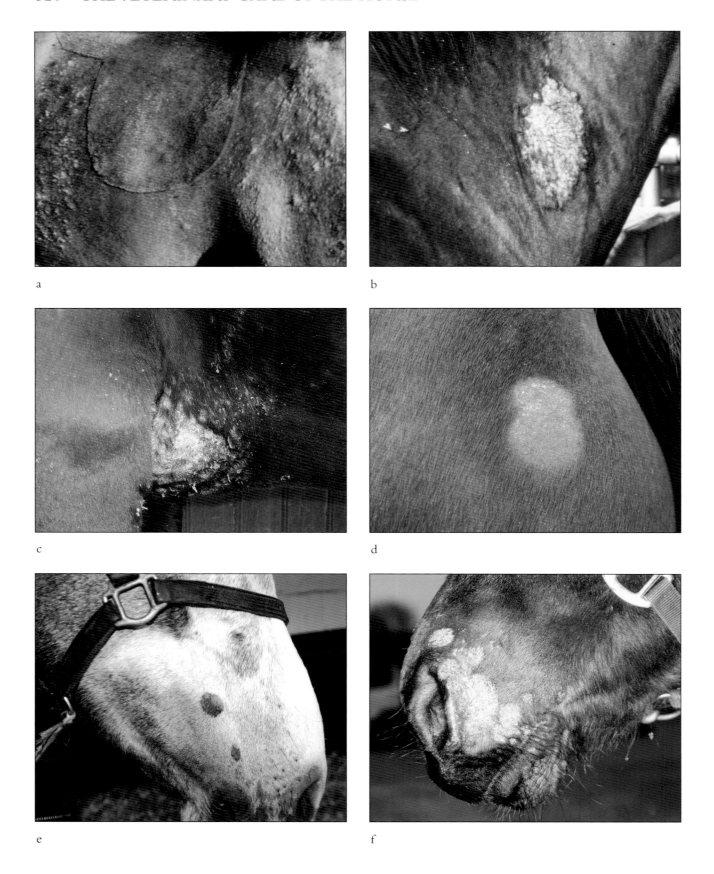

a

b

c

d

e

f

ISOLATION AND HANDLING

The disease is spread by direct contact and so infected horses should be isolated wherever possible. Since the fungus can spread between horses, on clothing and hands, one person should handle only the infected animals, or, the infected animals should be handled last. Individual owners of an infected horse in a yard should not touch the other animals.

Ringworm is transmissible to humans, so overalls should be worn to protect clothes from contamination. Avoid touching the lesions and always wash your hands with an appropriate wash, e.g. Pevidine®, after handling an infected horse.

While the lesions are active, the horse should not travel or mix with other horses. The lorry or trailer will be contaminated and the disease will be spread.

TOPICAL TREATMENT

There are a number of antifungal shampoos, washes and sprays on the market for spraying or sponging onto the horse. These should be used as advised by your vet.

SYSTEMIC TREATMENT

On occasions an antifungal medication, griseofulvin may be prescribed. This is added to the horse's feed and may help prevent further fungal invasion. However, there is some doubt about the efficacy of this treatment in the horse. It must be handled with care by women of childbearing age and should not be given to pregnant mares as it is teratogenic which means it can cause abnormalities in a developing foetus. Impervious gloves should be worn when handling the product.

MANAGEMENT

Once in the environment, the fungus can live for months or years. Measures should be taken to reduce environmental and equipment contamination. These include the following.

- Starting treatment and taking hygiene precautions as soon as the condition is suspected.
- Not grooming infected horses as this is likely to spread the infection.
- Soaking brushes, rugs, tack, clippers etc in a fungicidal wash, e.g. Virkon®. Equipment and grooming kit should not be shared between horses in the event of an outbreak.
- Remember to treat your riding boots as these can be a source of infection.
- Avoid clipping an infected horse as this is likely to spread the infection. The exception is if the horse has a very thick coat preventing effective treatment of the lesions.
- Contaminated stables and wood may be treated with pressure washing and an antifungal wash or dilute bleach. Bedding should be removed and burned if possible.

18.2a–f Ringworm: a) lesions may be distributed widely over the horse; b) a large lesion on a horse's neck; c) a severe case affecting the girth area; d) the hair has fallen out leaving a patch of grey, scaly skin; e) lesions on a horse's face; f) extensive lesions on a horse's muzzle

EXERCISE

If the lesions are under the girth or saddle, the horse should not be ridden. The pressure could irritate the skin and cause a severe reaction.

Prevention

New horses introduced to the yard should be regularly inspected and isolated if lesions occur. As soon as the disease is suspected, all the hygiene measures discussed above should be implemented. The condition and fit of each horse's tack should be regularly checked so the skin does not become chafed.

Prognosis

The prognosis is good and most horses recover in 1–3 months. Re-infection is possible, but the signs are usually milder. Occasionally a horse is hypersensitive to the infection and has a more serious skin reaction. Debilitated animals or those with weak immune systems may be more severely infected and take longer to recover.

The cost of ringworm

An outbreak of ringworm can be very disruptive and costly in terms of lost days of work. Competition schedules, training programmes and planned activities are interrupted.

MUD FEVER

Mud fever is a common condition that affects horses living or working in wet, muddy conditions. The skin over the pasterns and heels becomes infected, resulting in scabby or exudative lesions which can be very painful (Figure 18.3). Sometimes the infection extends to the skin further up the legs. White limbs are particularly susceptible (Figure 18.4). It occurs mainly in the winter months.

In fact, mud fever is not a single disease but a collection of clinical signs associated with a number of different causes. To manage the condition successfully, one needs to be able to recognize the signs and identify their underlying cause. Although very common, it appears in various forms and is not limited to horses that are literally paddling knee deep in mud.

Clinical signs

Mud fever can range from a mild skin irritation to very painful, infected sores. The disease can actually affect the whole body and is given different names depending on the part of the horse affected.

- When it occurs along the backs of horses that are kept outside without rugs, it is known as **rain scald** or **rain rash** (this is discussed on page 528).

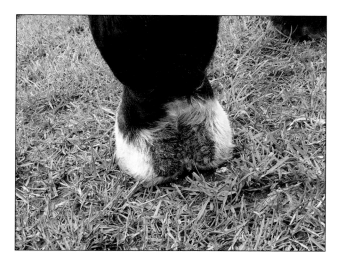

Figure 18.3 Mud fever lesions like this can be very painful

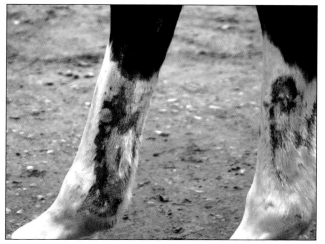

Figure 18.4 Infection can extend up the legs especially on white limbs

- **Mud fever** is the term used to describe the condition when it involves the lower limbs, most commonly the back of the pastern and the heels, where it is seen as crusty scabs (Figure 18.5). The inflamed skin may discharge serum, causing the hair to matt, giving the coat a rough, ungroomed appearance.
- With severe cases, the skin at the back of the pastern may split open producing deep horizontal cracks, commonly called **cracked heels** (Figure 18.6).

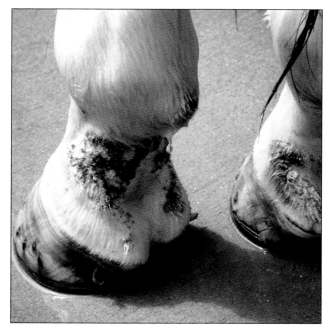

Figure 18.5 Crusty scabs on the back of the pastern and the heels

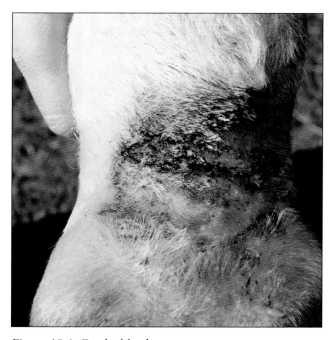

Figure 18.6 Cracked heels

Infection can enter these areas of damaged skin, resulting in a hot, swollen and painful leg and cause severe lameness. In the summer months, a less severe but equally persistent form of the disease occurs. Firmly adherent scabs are found in the pastern and heel regions.

Causes

There are many factors which can be divided into the predisposing and infectious causes.

PREDISPOSING CAUSES

These include the following.

- The horse's own genetic make-up. Any horse with white hair on the lower limbs and/or a long shaggy coat around the lower limbs (known as feathers) may be prone to mud fever. Thus the heavy horse with long white feathers is a high-risk candidate for the disease.
- Environmental conditions. Anything that irritates, softens or breaks the skin so that infection can enter, makes mud fever more likely to develop. Typically in the UK it is due to the cold, wet, muddy conditions experienced by the outdoor horse in winter. It can also be a problem in horses whose skin is irritated by the sand in some riding arena surfaces. These environmental factors damage the skin so it is more vulnerable to infection, in exactly the same way as we develop chapped hands and lips.
- Physical and chemical irritants which damage the skin. These include contact allergies, insect bites and injury (rubs) from dirty overreach or brushing boots.
- Other infections, e.g. ringworm and chorioptic mange mites, can damage the skin and allow secondary infection to occur. In these cases it is important that the underlying cause is identified as neither the mites nor the fungus will be sensitive to antibiotics. This is one of the reasons why antibiotics do not always cure the condition.

INFECTIOUS CAUSES

Certain infections are able to invade the skin when it is compromised by the factors discussed above. These include bacteria such as *Dermatophilus congolensis* and *Staphylococcus spp.* These are opportunists, i.e. they take advantage of the sore skin and would not produce infection if the skin was healthy.

Diagnosis

Diagnosis of the disease is usually straightforward. The diagnosis is made on:
- the clinical signs
- identification of the microorganisms under the microscope and occasionally culture of the microorganisms in the laboratory.

Identifying the factors that caused the irritation is not always easy. While muddy paddocks are often the cause, skin trauma from working in fields of stubble or irritation from harvest mites can be contributory factors.

Treatment

There are many treatments for mud fever. It has to be remembered that with any condition for which there are a large number of possible treatments, it is often because nothing is a guaranteed success.

CHANGING THE ENVIRONMENT

The first step is to remove the horse from the cause, e.g. the wet and the mud. Unfortunately, the solution of moving horses to better land or stabling them is not a practical option for many horse owners, so they try to manage the problem where they are, often without success. Undoubtedly, there are cases where the only hope of a cure is to change the environment and this usually means stabling. However, if the horse is kept in all the time and not exercised, the legs will tend to swell. Walking exercise in hand several times a day is helpful initially. Once any lameness has resolved, working on a dry surface which does not scratch the legs further will help the circulation and encourage healing. Roadwork is often best for these horses.

STABLE MANAGEMENT

The horse should be stabled with a clean, dry bed. Dirty bedding will increase the risk of infection. Straw may be abrasive to the damaged skin and shavings are best avoided as they adhere to the wounds. Cardboard or paper bedding are suitable and protective bandages can be useful.

Treating the lesions
PREPARATION

- The affected area should be carefully clipped, taking care not to traumatize the skin further. This may be done with clippers or a good pair of curved scissors.
- Then use an antiseptic wash such as chlorhexidine (Hibiscrub®) to remove as many of the unhealthy, crusty scabs as possible. Clipping and cleaning may be easier said than done as the horse is often very sore. You may need your vet to help by sedating the horse and giving painkillers.
- Next, gently rinse and then blot the skin dry with clean, absorbent tissue. Rubbing it with a towel will be painful for the horse and could cause further damage to the skin. A hairdryer with a circuit breaker may be used, taking care not to burn the delicate skin.

TOPICAL TREATMENTS

There are numerous topical treatments that can be used as an emollient to maintain hydration of the skin. These include soothing ointments, gels and creams, some of which contain antibiotics. Recent additions to the range of treatments include an ointment containing an antibiotic and silver and also a dressing impregnated with silver which has been shown to have strong antibacterial properties. Early trials with these products look promising. Your vet will recommend the most suitable for your horse. An inexpensive option to start with is E45 Cream®.

DRESSINGS

In the early stages, open wounds resulting from the removal of the scabs should be covered with a non-stick dressing applied under cotton wool or gamgee, held in place with bandages. This keeps the lower limb warm, clean and dry. It may help to leave the legs unbandaged for at least an hour a day to allow the area to 'breathe'. The horse may be stood in an empty box for this short period of time. Treatment of the sore areas needs to be repeated daily until the condition is under control.

ANTIBIOTICS

Severe cases with obvious infection often need a long course of antibiotics. These may need to be continued for 7–10 days after the soreness has settled down. Your vet may also prescribe non-steroidal anti-inflammatory drugs such as phenylbutazone to reduce the pain and swelling.

AFTERCARE

Once the infection has resolved and the lesions have dried up, the bandages may be removed. The legs should be protected from moisture, mud, abrasions and flies as the newly healed skin may be tender and susceptible to injury or re-infection.

Prognosis

Mud fever is a difficult condition to treat and it may take many weeks for the lesions to heal completely. If the case is straightforward and the causes are treated or removed, then the disease will usually resolve quickly. However, if the condition has been ongoing for some time, the skin itself will have developed chronic changes which are harder to treat.

Treatment is time-consuming and may be difficult if the horse is sore and reluctant to allow it. It is therefore sensible to catch the disease early and start treatment as soon as the tell-tale scabs appear. Lesions which do not heal may have an underlying unidentified cause such as mites, or the treatment may not be thorough enough. As mentioned earlier, some horses are genetically predisposed to the condition and the infection may recur many times despite good management.

Prevention

Prevention and early recognition and treatment are the keys to success in the management of mud fever. Susceptible horses should be carefully inspected each day. There are different schools of thought on whether muddy legs should be left to dry or hosed off when the horse is brought in. High pressure hosing and use of a coarse brush on muddy skin should be avoided as it could damage the skin and introduce infection. Some horse owners find that application of barrier creams such as zinc and castor oil help prevent infection in susceptible horses. The legs must be clean and dry when these are applied or moisture will be sealed in, creating an environment where the harmful bacteria thrive.

Protective boots and bandages may be used during turnout (Figure 18.7). These can be very helpful as long as mud does not work its way underneath and rub the horse's skin. Bandages can be applied when the horse is stabled to help dry the lower limbs.

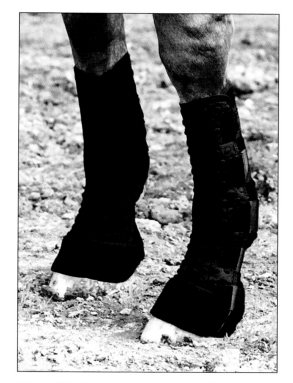

Figure18.7 Protective wraps may help prevent mud fever

Hygiene measures

The following points should be noted.

- *Dermatophilus congolensis* can survive in crusts of scab and exudate for up to $3\frac{1}{2}$ years. Chronically infected animals are a source of soil contamination.
- The infection can be spread on shared grooming kits and clippers. These should be cleaned and sterilized after use on an infected animal.
- Scabs that have been removed from infected legs should be disposed of carefully. The bedding should be removed and the stable disinfected, e.g. with Virkon®, after the horse has recovered.

In conclusion, mud fever is one of those conditions that can be very difficult to control. Unfortunately many horses will have a bout of mud fever at some time in their lives, despite all efforts at prevention.

RAIN SCALD

Rain scald is a skin infection that occurs in horses and ponies kept at grass during spells of warm, moist weather.

Causes

Prolonged or driving rain can lead to excessive wetting of the skin. The bacterium, *Dermatophilus congolensis* is able to penetrate the skin through small abrasions and cause an exudative (oozing) dermatitis. This is the same bacterial infection that causes mud fever and cracked heels.

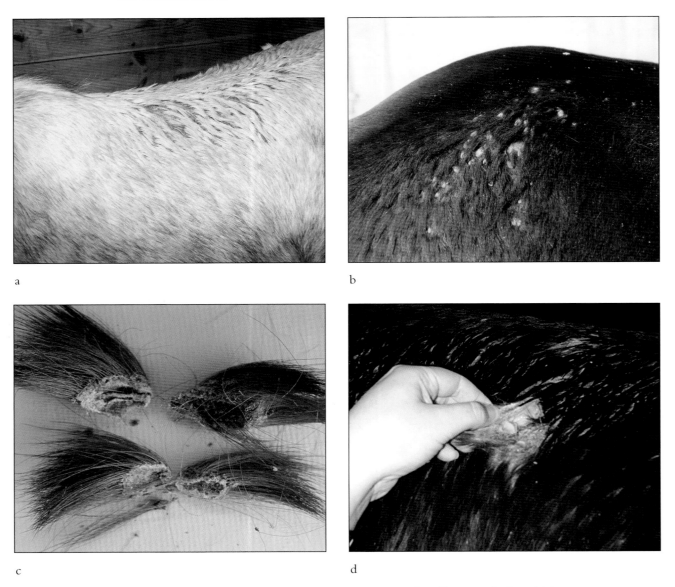

a

b

c

d

Figures 18.8a, b, c and d a) and b) rainscald on the back and quarters; c) tufts of hair attached to thick scabs; d) thick layer of pus under the scabs

Clinical signs

- The most commonly affected areas are the face, shoulders, back, loins and quarters (Figures 18.8a and b). Tufts of hair begin to lift away from the skin. These can be lifted off together with a thick crust of exudate. The undersurface of the scab is concave and the removed tufts look like the head of a paintbrush (Figure 18.8c).
- The underlying skin may be dry and flaky or exude serum. If secondary infection is present, a thick layer of pus is found under the scabs. (Figure 18.8d)
- The lesions may be patchy, giving the horse a moth-eaten appearance or joined up to cover large areas of the horse's body.

Treatment

- Stable the horse until the lesions have healed. It is difficult to clear the infection if the horse is still exposed to rain.
- Gently tease off the scabs. Where these are small and widespread throughout the coat, careful use of a fine-toothed metal comb removes them very effectively.
- If exudate is present under the scabs, clean the skin with cotton wool and an antibacterial wash, e.g. Hibiscrub® or Pevidine®. In severe cases, consult your vet as an antibiotic ointment may be necessary. Systemic antibiotics are occasionally prescribed.
- The horse should remain stabled with a clean bed until the skin is dry and healthy. It can then be turned out in a waterproof rug.

Hygiene measures

- The scabs should be disposed of carefully as *Dermatophilus* can live for up to $3\frac{1}{2}$ years in infected crusts.
- Grooming kit, tack, rugs, clippers and stables should be cleaned with a suitable disinfectant recommended by your vet.

Prevention

- Provide shelter or bring in susceptible animals during wet periods.
- Use a protective outdoor rug.

SWEET ITCH

Sweet itch is an allergic skin condition causing horses and ponies to feel very itchy and uncomfortable. It is more common in ponies and the condition can be hereditary. The disease can be very disfiguring.

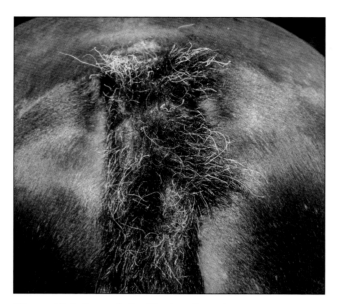

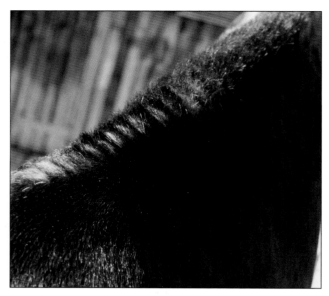

Figure 18.9 Sweet itch affecting the tail

Figure 18.10 Ridges of thickened skin at the base of the mane

Causes

Affected animals are hypersensitive to the saliva of the biting *Culicoides* midge. There are over 100 species of this midge. Some horses develop a similar allergy when bitten by stable flies (*Stomoxys spp.*) and black flies (*Simulium spp.*).

Clinical signs

- Affected animals rub themselves against trees, fences and stables in an attempt to relieve the irritation.
- The condition varies in severity from occasional rubbing with some broken mane and tail hairs to almost complete loss of the mane and tail (Figure 18.9). Initially the horse or pony has patches where the hair has obviously been rubbed. This may progress to bald patches or weeping sores.
- Lesions occur most commonly on the face, forelock, poll, mane, neck, withers, rump, tail head and dock. Some animals experience irritation along the ventral midline especially on the soft skin in front of the udder or sheath.
- Secondary bacterial infection can develop.
- With time, the repeated trauma causes thickening and ridging of the skin at the base of the mane, especially near the withers (Figure 18.10).
- Some ponies are so bothered by the condition that their behaviour becomes erratic and unpredictable. They can be miserable and bad-tempered, swishing their tails and kicking their bellies.

The condition tends to be seasonal, with symptoms occurring in the UK between late

March and early November when the insects are prevalent. In a mild winter (or warmer climates), a sensitized pony may be affected all year round. The flies are very small and are not strong fliers. They feed less on windy days when the wind speed is more than 7 km/hour (4 miles/hr).

Diagnosis

Diagnosis is made on the clinical signs. Intradermal skin tests or a biopsy can confirm the diagnosis, but these are rarely necessary.

Prevention

With horses or ponies that suffer every year, the aim should be to *prevent* the signs by careful management, rather than waiting for them to develop. This is done by reducing their exposure to the midges.

- The midges breed in standing water and damp, rotting vegetation so wherever possible, the pony should be moved away from these.
- Drainage of marshy fields and ponds may help.
- Any stagnant troughs or water containers near the stable should be removed.
- The flies feed primarily at dawn and dusk and may continue during the night. The pony should be stabled from an hour before sunset until at least an hour after sunrise the next morning. The safest period for grazing is mid-morning to mid-afternoon.
- Screening the stable windows, door and also air spaces that communicate with the next stable with a fine mesh to stop midges entering will help.
- The use of a large ceiling-mounted electric fan may help to drive the midges away.
- When the pony is in the stable or turned out, a special Boett® Blanket and hood which prevents midges biting and covers as much of the pony as possible affords considerable protection (Figure 18.11) This is made of a breathable material and can be worn for up to 24 hours a day.

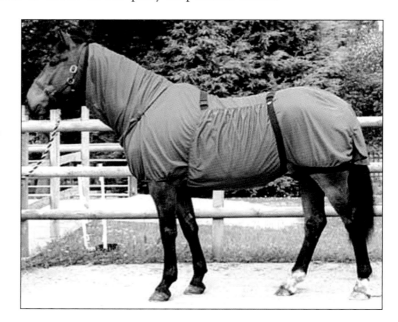

- Regular application of a fly repellent, e.g. pyrethrin, is likely to help.
- Benzyl benzoate may give some relief by making the midges less likely to bite, but it is an irritant and should not be applied to skin that is already broken and sore. Benzyl benzoate is a weak insecticide that requires daily application.

Figure 18.11 Boett® Blanket

- Oily lotions are messy, but these can provide a mechanical barrier and prevent the flies biting.
- Some owners report an improvement with the inclusion of garlic in the diet.
- If at all possible affected horses and ponies should be moved to a midge-free area such as an exposed hilltop or breezy coastal site.

These measures should be in place *before* the start of the midge season.

PERFORMING A 'PATCH TEST'

It is sensible to carry out a **patch test** for any topical preparation used to deter the midges from biting or to treat the skin. The preparation should be applied to a small area of the horse and observed for 24 hours to check for any adverse reaction (swelling, heat, irritation or soreness) before applying it more extensively. Choose a site least likely to cause a problem if sensitivity occurs. Protective gloves should be worn when applying these products.

Treatment

Treatment to reduce the irritation should be started as soon as the first signs are seen.

TOPICAL PREPARATIONS

- Soothing lotions such as Sudocream® or aloe vera preparations and sprays can reduce the irritation.
- Provided there is no infection, a corticosteroid cream may be prescribed by your vet. Gloves should be worn when applying this and the treatment is only practical for small areas.
- If secondary infection occurs, an antibiotic cream may be necessary.
- Shampooing the horse every 1–2 weeks to remove the scurf and scabs may help to decrease the irritation. A hypoallergenic shampoo should be used.

SYSTEMIC MEDICATIONS

If the irritation is severe and cannot be relieved by topical treatment and good management, then it may be necessary for the vet to prescribe antihistamines or corticosteroids. Corticosteroid tablets, e.g. prednisolone, are usually given daily to start with while the symptoms are severe. As soon as possible, the dose is reduced to a minimum and given on alternate days to reduce the risks of side effects which include laminitis and immunosuppression. Any wound infection should be cleared up with antibiotics before corticosteroids are given. Long-acting corticosteroid injections may help with some cases but these are not recommended as they carry an increased risk of complications such as laminitis.

Prognosis

If the condition is recognized early and the owner has the time and facilities to manage it well, many horses with a susceptibility to sweet itch develop only mild signs with occasional rubbing.

However, in other cases the prognosis is guarded. The disease can be both debilitating and disfiguring. It prevents the animal being used for showing and the sores may limit riding in the summer.

Sweet itch is costly in time, effort and money. Not surprisingly, affected animals may become bad-tempered and unreliable. The condition tends to get worse each year. Moving the horse or pony to another environment may help. However, there are some ponies who reach a state where no treatment is effective and every summer is a time of torment and misery. In these cases, euthanasia may have to be considered.

Warning

Many of these animals are sold during the winter months and the problem is passed on to another unsuspecting owner. Potential purchasers should always be warned about the condition as these horses and ponies require special attention and should go to experienced homes with suitable facilities.

The National Sweet Itch Centre (www.sweet-itch.co.uk) has a helpline and web site providing advice on how to cope with this problem and additional information on the Boett® Blanket.

LICE INFESTATION

There are two types of lice that live on horses. *Haematopinus asini,* the sucking louse, feeds on blood and tissue fluids. *Damalinia equi,* the biting louse, feeds on scurf and other debris on the skin surface. Infestations usually occur in the winter months and early spring when the coat is long. They do not breed when the temperature is above 38 °C (100 °F) and they die if exposed to temperatures of above 50 °C (120 °F). Most lice do not survive the summer months as these temperatures may be reached within the hair coat.

Lice are visible to the naked eye. They are 1.5–3 mm (up to $\frac{1}{10}$ in) long and light brown to dark grey in colour. The cream-coloured eggs, known as 'nits', are firmly attached to the hair. These can often be found in the mane and forelock, close to the skin surface. The lice are 'host-specific' and do not live on humans.

Clinical signs
- Lice cause the skin to become very itchy, especially under the mane, along the back and at the top of the tail.
- Infested horses rub and bite themselves, creating bald patches (Figures 18.12a, b and c) and sometimes sore areas that ooze serum.
- The coat becomes dull and scurfy.

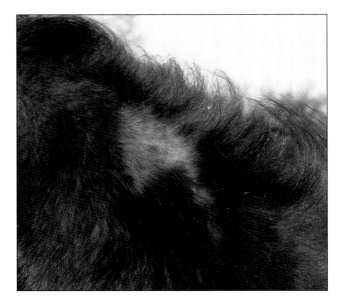

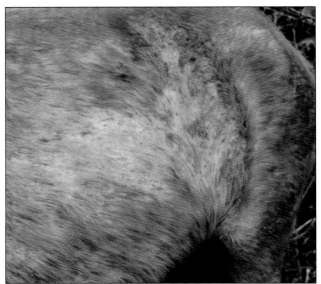

a   b

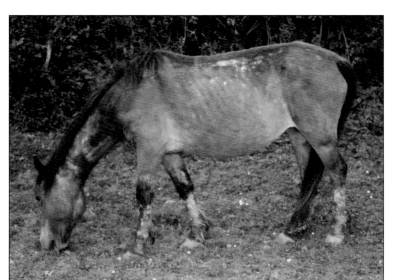

Figures 18.12a, b and c Lice: a) typical appearance of a rubbed mane; b) in severe cases the lesions can be extensive; c) debilitated ponies living out in groups are susceptible

c

- Severely infested animals become restless and lose condition.
- On close inspection, the lice and their eggs can be seen.
- With heavy infestations of sucking lice, the horse may become anaemic.
- Secondary bacterial infection of the lesions can occur.

Diagnosis

The lice can be found in the coat, especially in the mane and at the top of the tail. These can be collected on a piece of clear sticky tape and examined under the microscope. Louse eggs attached to the hair can also be seen.

Treatment and control

The life cycle is between 10 and 21 days. The adult lice lay their eggs on the hair and these hatch and develop into more adults. They pass from one horse to another by direct contact or on rugs, grooming kit and tack. They can also be transmitted via fences and trees on which the animals rub.

Most topical preparations kill the adult lice but not necessarily the eggs. Following treatment, time has to be allowed for the eggs to hatch and the horse is treated again. Three treatments at 10-day intervals are usually sufficient.

TREATMENT OPTIONS

These include the following.

- Topical application of a permethrin spray (Coopers™ Fly Repellent Plus for Horses) to the whole body in accordance with the manufacturer's instructions. It is recommended that this is repeated after 14 days.
- Application of louse powder (Arnolds).
- Deosect® spray; this must be diluted according to the manufacturer's instructions and repeated after 14 days.
- Dermoline shampoo.

The following are not licensed for the treatment of lice in horses but are known to be effective and may be used under veterinary advice.

- Application of 0.25% fipronil spray (Frontline®).
- 1% selenium sulphide (Seleen®) shampoo.
- Ivermectin and moxidectin paste given orally are effective against sucking lice.

Protective rubber gloves and aprons should be worn when using these preparations. Equipment such as tack, brushes and rugs should also be treated. Steam-cleaning of these items is also effective.

Additional treatment is sometimes necessary and may include the following.

- Antibiotics if secondary bacterial infection is present.
- If a horse or pony is severely anaemic, appropriate treatment should be given.

Lice tend to infest groups of young animals living out during the winter. If they are in poor condition, good feeding and management is an essential part of their care. All horses and ponies that have been in contact with infested animals should be treated at the same time.

Prognosis

The prognosis is excellent with proper management and care.

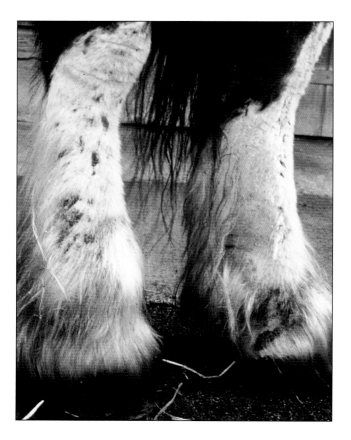

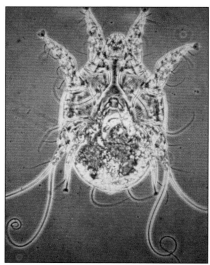

Figure 18.13 Chorioptic mange (left)

Figure 18.14 Chorioptic mange mite
as seen under the microscope (above)

CHORIOPTIC MANGE

Chorioptic mange is caused by a small mite, *Chorioptes equi,* which lives on the skin surface. The mites are less than 1 mm in length and cause irritation by their activity as they feed on the superficial layers of skin. They are frequently found in heavy horse breeds with lots of feathering on the lower limbs (Figure 18.13).

Clinical signs
- The first sign is itchy legs. Infested horses will often be restless, stamping their feet in irritation and nibbling their lower limbs. They frequently scratch below the knee and hock with the hoof of the opposite limb.
- The lesions may be dry and scaly with areas of hair loss and scurfy skin.
- This can progress to small weeping sores and scabs.
- In severe cases it can spread to the upper limbs and trunk.
- If left untreated, the lesions coalesce and become large open sores with matted hair which may become secondarily infected with bacteria including *Staphylococcus spp.* and *Dermatophilus congolensis.*
- Long-standing infestations can lead to thickened skin with a rather greasy appearance.

Diagnosis

Diagnosis is made on the clinical signs and can be confirmed by the presence of mites in brushings of scurf from the skin, or skin scrapes taken by the vet. They are easily visible when examined under a microscope (Figure 18.14).

Treatment

The feathering is clipped and an antiseptic wash is used to remove any crusts of exudate. The most commonly used treatments are:

- a single application of fipronil spray (Frontline®), sufficient to wet the hair and skin surface
- selenium sulphide shampoo every 5th day for 3 treatments
- oral ivermectin paste (200–300µg/kg, i.e. up to $1\frac{1}{2}$ times the worming dose) given once a week for 4 weeks may help to reduce the numbers of mites
- antibiotics are occasionally necessary to control secondary infection.

Control

The mites can live off the host for up to 10 weeks. When the horse is treated, the bedding should be removed and the box sprayed with a suitable parasiticide recommended by your vet. All in-contact horses should be treated, especially those sharing a grooming kit (which should also be treated).

Prognosis

Many horses experience relief as soon as the treatment starts. However, it can be difficult to completely eliminate the mites in heavily feathered animals. Some will need periodic treatment. Other horses can tolerate the mite without showing any obvious symptoms. However, they may experience a low level of discomfort causing them to kick out unpredictably or occasionally stamp their feet.

HARVEST MITES (HEEL BUG)

Harvest mites (*Trombicula autumnalis*) may affect horses that graze on chalky soils between the months of July and September. They cause lesions on the pasterns, heels and muzzles of grazing animals. Stabled horses can be affected on any part of the body if infested hay or bedding is used. The mites can be seen with the naked eye and look like tiny reddish-orange dots on the skin. They feed by biting the horse and injecting saliva containing enzymes into the superficial layers of skin. The horse may become hypersensitive to the enzymes and the affected areas become very itchy and inflamed.

Clinical signs
These include:
- patches of red, inflamed skin which may ooze serum, form scabs and become very sore
- the horse will often rub, bite and scratch the affected areas or stamp its feet in irritation.

Diagnosis
The diagnosis is confirmed by finding the mites and examining them under the microscope.

Treatment
The mites are easily killed by application of:
- topical pyrethroid sprays or washes – ask your vet for advice
- 0.25% fipronil spray (Frontline®) is not licensed for this use in the horse but may be used if recommended by your vet

If the reaction is very severe, anti-inflammatory drugs or antibiotics may be prescribed.

Control
Once a horse has become sensitized, the lesions may recur each year if the horse remains on the same pasture. Ideally, the horse should be removed from the infested pasture during the late summer and early autumn months. If a stabled horse is affected, the bedding and hay should be removed and replaced with supplies from another source.

TICKS

Ticks are often found on horses and ponies during the spring, summer and early autumn months. They climb up on the vegetation and attach themselves to the face, legs, and abdomen of passing horses. They are often found in the relatively hairless areas of the inner elbows and thighs. The ticks penetrate the skin with their mouthparts and suck blood from their host. They are usually grey or brown in colour. They remain attached for several days, gradually swelling up. The horse may develop a hypersensitivity reaction to the tick saliva and develop a weeping sore at the site. Ticks rarely cause serious problems unless they carry the spirochete organism, *Borrelia burgdorferi,* that causes Lyme disease. Both ticks and the incidence of Lyme disease are more prevalent in certain areas of the country.

Ticks can be physically removed from the skin, taking care not to leave the mouthparts in the horse. They may be killed first by the application of petroleum jelly, surgical spirit or with fipronil sprayed onto a piece of cotton wool and applied to the tick.

ONCHOCERCA CERVICALIS

Onchocerca cervicalis is a very thin, filamentous worm that sometimes causes skin lesions in the horse. It is white in colour and may be up to 30 cm (1 ft) long.

Life cycle

The adult worms live in the nuchal ligament in the horse's neck. There may be a fibrous tissue reaction around them and firm, small nodules can sometimes be palpated. The females produce larvae (microfilariae) which migrate to the skin on the face, the underside of the neck, the chest and lower abdomen. Sometimes larvae reach the conjunctiva of the eye. The microfilariae are ingested by *Culicoides* midges when they feed on the horse. Once inside the midges, they develop into infective third-stage larvae. These are then injected into other horses bitten by the midge and migrate to the nuchal ligament where they mature into adult worms.

Clinical signs

Many horses tolerate the parasite with no clinical signs. Occasionally a horse will develop a hypersensitivity to the microfilariae and experience intense pruritis (itchiness) which causes them to rub and bite themselves. They develop bald, sore scabby patches on the face, chest and under their chest and abdomen. When the microfilariae occur in the eye, the conjunctiva may become inflamed and develop raised lesions. They are considered to be one of the causes of equine recurrent uveitis.

Diagnosis

A skin biopsy may confirm the presence of microfilariae.

Treatment

The numbers of microfilariae may be reduced by regular use of ivermectin, but it does not kill the adult worms. There is sometimes a flare-up of signs after treatment as the horse has a reaction to the dying larvae. If this is severe, systemic corticosteroids may help to control the irritation. It is sometimes necessary to use corticosteroid drops in the eyes.

Control

Reducing the horse's exposure to biting midges may help to prevent the spread of the parasite. Stabling the horse at dawn and dusk and the use of fly repellents can be helpful.

HABRONEMIASIS (SUMMER SORES)

Habronema muscae, *Habronema majus* and *Draschia megastoma* are worms that live in the stomach of horses. They rarely cause problems unless the larvae are deposited by flies in the medial canthus of the eye, in wounds or on the male genitalia. These worms are 1–2 cm ($\frac{1}{2}$ –1 in) long and white in colour.

Life cycle

The adult worms in the horse's stomach lay eggs which quickly hatch into larvae. The eggs and larvae pass out of the horse in the droppings. The house fly (*Musca domestica*) and the stable fly (*Stomoxys calcitrans*) lay their eggs on the droppings and these develop into larvae (maggots) which eat the stomach worm larvae. When the adult fly develops, it can contain infective *Habronema* larvae in its mouth parts. When it feeds around the horse's lips and nostrils, the larvae crawl onto the skin and are swallowed. Alternatively, the horse may ingest the flies containing the larvae. Once in the horse's stomach, the larvae mature into adult worms, so completing the life cycle. The infected flies also feed and deposit larvae on moist surfaces such as the conjunctiva, open wounds and the male genitalia. These larvae may produce sores but do not develop into adult worms.

Clinical signs

In the stomach, large numbers of worms can cause a mild gastritis, but this is rarely a problem. However, when larvae crawl into other sites, they cause itchy, granulomatous lesions to develop. These raised patches may be a pink or reddish-brown colour and contain gritty white or yellow nodules. There may be local swelling and discharge from the sheath and eye (Figures 18.15a and b). If the gritty nodules impinge upon the cornea, it may become ulcerated. Infected open wounds often develop exuberant granulation tissue and do not heal as expected (Figure 18.16). Since they occur in the summer months when the flies are around in large numbers, they are often called **summer sores**.

Diagnosis

The diagnosis is made on the appearance of the sores and confirmed by biopsy.

Treatment

The adult worms and larvae are killed by ivermectin and moxidectin. Following treatment, the lesions may become more inflamed due to hypersensitivity of the horse to the dead larvae. This can sometimes be controlled with topical or systemic steroids, but these must be used with care due to the risk of infection or laminitis. The lesions are often removed surgically. Wherever possible, the whole lesion is removed when a sample of tissue is taken for biopsy.

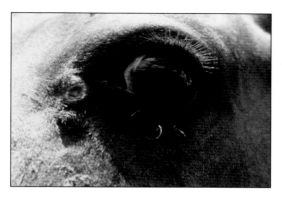

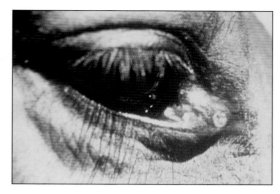

a   b

Figures 18.15a and b a) typical lesion caused by *Habronema* at the medial canthus of the eye; b) lesions on the conjunctiva and eyelid at the medial canthus

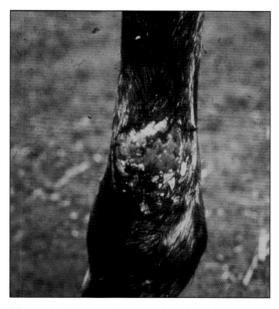

Figure 18.16 Wound infected with *Habronema*

Prevention

Fly control measures (e.g. removing droppings, using fly repellents) will help to prevent re-infection. Wounds should be bandaged where possible. The use of fly masks helps to prevent infected flies feeding on the conjunctiva.

Caution

Some individual horses are particularly sensitive to habronemiasis. Recurrent infection at the medial canthus of the eye can predispose to squamous cell carcinoma.

URTICARIA

Urticaria is an allergic reaction of the skin to something in the horse's environment or diet.

Clinical signs

- The skin develops soft, oedematous wheals that are usually circular or oval in shape, rather like nettle rash (Figures 18.17a and b).
- The wheals are irregularly distributed over the neck, shoulders, chest wall and abdomen.
- They vary from 0.5 cm ($\frac{2}{10}$ in) to the size of a saucer.

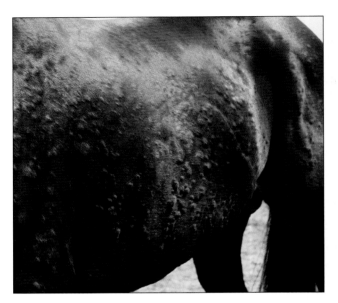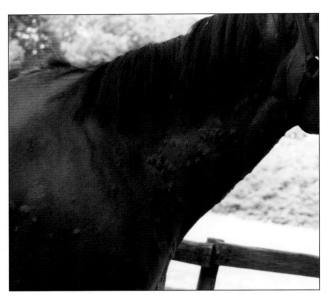

Figures 18.17a and b Urticaria on a) the shoulders and abdomen; b) the neck

- They 'pit' on pressure, i.e. if pressed firmly with a finger, a clearly visible imprint is seen.
- They are usually painless when touched.
- Sometimes they are itchy, causing the horse to rub and bite itself.
- These swellings may resolve very quickly in 1–2 days or be more persistent.
- Occasionally the wheals ooze serum and can become infected.
- Sometimes the horse's head becomes swollen, especially around the eyelids, muzzle and lips.
- If the pharynx or larynx swells, the horse may have difficulty breathing or swallowing.
- The lower limbs may also swell.
- In severe cases, the skin swellings are accompanied by colicky signs and collapse. These horses may become very distressed.

The wheals may become more prominent following exercise, when the horse is warm or if a sedative is administered.

Causes

There are numerous causes of urticaria in the horse. Sometimes the cause is obvious, but in many cases it is very difficult to pinpoint. The various allergens may be ingested (eaten), inhaled, injected or absorbed through the skin. Examples include:

- insect bites and stings, snake bites
- contact allergens, e.g. stinging nettles, topical drugs, chemicals, clipper oil
- medications, e.g. penicillin, phenylbutazone, some sedatives, oxytetracycline

- feeds: the horse may be allergic to a component of mixes and cubes, e.g. wheat, oats, barley, bran, soya and molasses, or to ingredients in dietary supplements
- pasture plants, e.g. some clovers, St John's wort
- inhaled allergens, e.g. pollens, moulds, dust from feedstuffs, feathers
- urticaria may occur following certain infections, e.g. strangles
- it may also develop as a response to the presence of certain parasites e.g. *Onchocerca cervicalis*.

How does this occur?

When a horse is exposed to an allergen for the first time, it produces antibodies (IgE) against it. These bind to mast cells and basophils in the tissues. If exposed to the allergen for a second time, the allergen binds to the IgE and this causes the mast cells to release histamine and other chemical mediators which increase the permeability of the blood vessels, allowing them to leak and form the wheals. This reaction may be almost immediate and occur in minutes, or it may take several hours to develop.

Diagnosis

The diagnosis is usually made on the history and the clinical signs. However, if the lesions are chronic, oozing or infected, skin scrapes may be taken to rule out the presence of parasites. A skin biopsy may also be helpful on occasions. Intradermal skin tests may be helpful but are not always reliable.

When to call the vet

Call your vet if:

- the horse is distressed .
- the eyelids and muzzle are swollen
- the horse is having difficulty breathing or swallowing
- serum is leaking through the skin
- the rash develops while the horse is being treated with medication
- there is no improvement after 2 days and the condition is preventing the horse from taking part in its usual activities.

Treatment

The aim of treatment is to reduce the horse's exposure to the allergen and restore the skin to normal.

MEDICATION

The most effective treatment is **corticosteroids**. In an emergency situation where swelling is obstructing breathing or the horse is very distressed and colicky, these may be given intravenously. If necessary, this is followed up by oral corticosteroids, e.g.

prednisolone given daily to start with. This is then reduced to the lowest dose that prevents recurrence of symptoms when given every other day.

Antihistamines are generally not as effective in the horse as they are with people, but may help in some individual cases. **Non-steroidal anti-inflammatory drugs** and **antibiotics** may be necessary if the horse is colicky or the wheals are oozing and infected.

There are occasions when a horse becomes so distressed after being stung by nettles or insects that sedation is necessary to prevent the horse injuring itself or others. They can squeal, bite themselves and throw themselves violently to the ground in attempts to relieve the irritation. The sedation will prevent any further injury while the other medication takes effect.

Withdrawal of all non-essential medications and supplements should be undertaken if the onset of signs coincides with the administration of any of these.

DIETARY MANIPULATION

Many commercial feed mixes and cubes contain common ingredients, so changing from one food to another is unlikely to be successful in identifying and eliminating the unknown allergen(s). It is often simpler to withhold all concentrates and feed the horse on forage that it has not previously been exposed to, e.g. alfalfa (lucerne) or oat hay. After 3–4 weeks on this diet, additional items may be introduced one at a time at 3–4-week intervals so that it is possible to identify the problem food. During the trial period, fresh rainwater could be used instead of tap water if possible.

ENVIRONMENTAL MANAGEMENT

Dusts, moulds and mites inhaled from the bedding have been known to trigger urticaria, as has contact with feathers. The stable should be thoroughly cleaned and even vacuumed to minimize these challenges. Clean paper or cardboard bedding is recommended for the affected horses.

Every attempt should be made to minimize the horse's exposure to biting flies and midges. This can be accomplished by stabling and the use of cotton summer sheets and fly rugs such as the Boett® Blanket.

CONTACT ALLERGENS

- Irritant weeds, e.g. stinging nettles, should be eliminated from the pasture.
- Avoid riding through dense patches of tall stinging nettles on overgrown bridleways.
- Always test topical preparations such as fly repellent and shampoos on a small area of skin first and wait 24 hours before treating the whole horse.
- Avoid using biological detergents to wash numnahs and girths of sensitive horses.

EXERCISE

The wheals sometimes increase in size if the horse is worked and becomes warm. In these cases, exercise should be avoided especially if the wheals are under the bridle or saddle.

Prognosis

Although the cause often remains undiagnosed, in many cases the signs disappear within a few hours or a couple of days without treatment. However, there are horses that are persistently troubled by this condition and it prevents them from engaging in their normal work. Pinpointing the cause is often difficult and eliminating the allergen may not be possible. In this case the horse can be kept on long-term maintenance corticosteroids, but this has the risk of side effects including laminitis. If the condition is recurrent, the prognosis is guarded although many cases gradually resolve with time, even though the cause is never established.

PEMPHIGUS FOLIACEUS

Pemphigus foliaceus is an autoimmune skin disease. Affected horses and ponies have an abnormal immune reaction and produce antibodies against components of their own skin. Appaloosas may be predisposed; the condition has been identified in both adult horses and those younger than 1 year old.

Causes

Very often there is no obvious cause. On occasions it may be triggered by certain medication, vaccines or stress, e.g. pregnancy.

Clinical signs

These may be mild or severe. They include:

- eruption of vesicles (blisters) or pustules which quickly burst
- patches of skin oozing serum
- areas of crusty, scabby lesions
- hair loss
- the lesions usually begin on the lower limbs or the face (Figures 18.18a and b) but can spread over wide areas of the body
- sometimes the lesions are restricted to the coronary band and lower pastern area (Figures 18.19a and b)
- they are often itchy
- sometimes they are very painful.

Severely affected animals may:

- be depressed
- be lethargic
- have a temperature
- lose their appetite

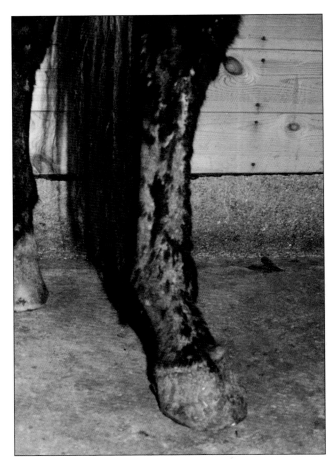 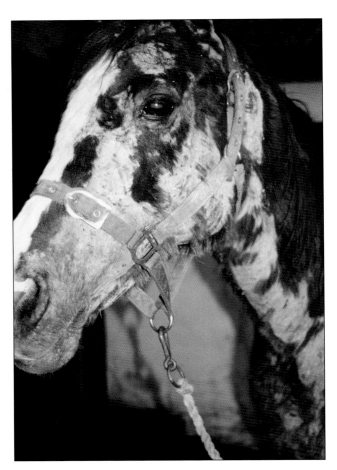

Figures 18.18a and b *Pemphigus foliaceus* often begins on the lower limbs or the face: a) the lower limbs; (b) this mare developed the problem on her face and neck during pregnancy

- lose weight and condition
- develop oedema of their lower limbs or along the ventral midline.

Diagnosis

The diagnosis is made on the history and clinical signs, and confirmed with several skin biopsies, ideally of early blister-like lesions. If blood tests are taken, they may show that the horse is anaemic and has raised neutrophils. It may also have low blood albumin and raised globulins.

Treatment

The most successful treatment for this condition is oral corticosteroids, i.e. prednisolone or dexamethasone. Initially, these have to be given at a high, daily dose. When there is a significant improvement, this is gradually reduced to the lowest dose that stops the lesions recurring, given on alternate days. When the lesions have completely healed and the horse has been fine for a few weeks, the dose may be further reduced and eventually withdrawn altogether.

However, many horses relapse if the medication is reduced beyond a certain level or stopped. Young horses less than 1 year old tend to respond best to treatment and the condition may resolve completely. Most older horses need life-long treatment. Where bacterial infection is present, antibiotics are necessary. Another treatment option is the use of injectable gold salts.

Warning

Laminitis is a well-recognized side effect of corticosteroids. While these patients are on high doses of corticosteroids in the early stages of treatment, they should be carefully monitored for any sign of foot pain or lameness. If this occurs, the vet should be called immediately. While high doses of corticosteroids are being taken, it is sensible to reduce your horse's concentrates and avoid fast work on hard surfaces.

TOPICAL TREATMENT

- The weeping lesions are often contaminated with bedding and dirt. These should be gently clipped and cleaned with an antibacterial scrub, e.g. Hibiscrub® and carefully blotted dry with absorbent tissue. Sedation may be necessary if the skin is very painful.
- Gels, ointments and creams containing corticosteroids and/or antibiotics may help localized lesions, e.g. round the coronary band, to heal. Gloves must be worn when applying these.
- Soothing preparations containing e.g. aloe vera may also help.
- If the condition is made worse by exposure to ultraviolet light, sun screens can be applied to the healed areas of skin.

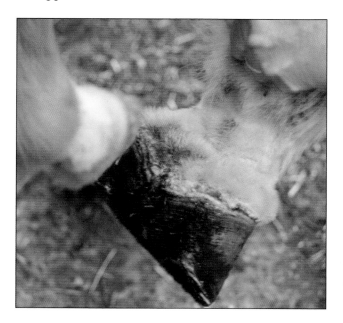 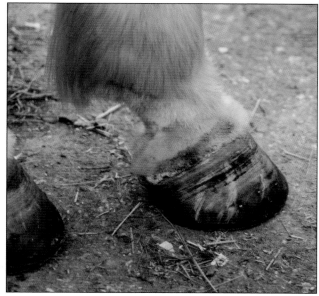

Figures 18.19 a and b Sometimes *Pemphigus foliaceus* lesions are restricted to the coronary band and the lower pastern

Prognosis

The prognosis is reasonable for young animals and guarded for adult horses. Unfortunately management of this condition requires a great deal of effort and commitment on the owner's part. There are occasions when the disease cannot be managed adequately and the horse's life becomes a misery. In these cases, euthanasia must be considered. *Pemphigus foliaceus* is sometimes seen in horses that have other debilitating diseases and weakened immune systems. The condition can be completely overwhelming in these unfortunate animals, necessitating euthanasia.

SUNBURN

Sunburn can occur when horses are exposed to harmful doses of ultraviolet light. This may happen during the summer in the UK.

Clinical signs

The soft, relatively hairless areas of pink skin around the nose and muzzle of some horses are most commonly affected. These have little protective pigment to prevent absorption of the harmful radiation. The signs are:

- redness
- itchiness and irritation
- formation of small blisters
- swelling and tenderness
- oozing of serum
- crusty scab formation.

These symptoms develop because the absorption of light energy in the surface layers of skin causes the release of inflammatory mediators called cytokines. These cause plasma to leak from small blood vessels which then activates a cascade of events leading to inflammation.

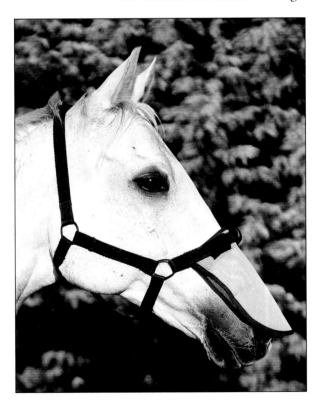

Figure 18.20 This muzzle protector blocks out most of the sun's harmful UV rays

Treatment

Treatment involves:

- stabling the horse on sunny days
- gently cleaning the lesions with an antibacterial scrub, e.g. Hibiscrub®
- applying a soothing gel, cream or ointment; this may contain substances such as aloe vera,

corticosteroid or antibiotic depending on the severity of the reaction
- application of hypoallergenic sun block.

Prevention

On hot sunny days, horses and ponies susceptible to sunburn should:
- be stabled
- have topical sunscreen applied; some of the hypoallergenic sun blocks designed for children when swimming stick well to the skin and are effective
- wear a face mask or muzzle protector to protect the delicate areas (Figure 18.20).

PHOTOSENSITIZATION

This is a condition where pink or lightly pigmented skin with little hair cover reacts abnormally to ultraviolet light, especially on bright sunny days. This is due to photodynamic substances (i.e. compounds that react with light) being deposited in the superficial layers of the skin.

Causes

- **Certain plants**, e.g. St John's wort, perennial ryegrass and some types of clover, contain substances that are absorbed by the horse's gut and deposited in the skin. In areas with little melanin, these photodynamic substances can react with the ultraviolet light and absorb energy, leading to inflammation.
- **Other plants**, e.g. buttercups, cow parsley and hogweed, contain light-reactive substances that can be directly absorbed by contact with the muzzle.
- **Liver disease**: bacteria in the gut of normal horses break down the chlorophyll in plants to a product called phylloerythrin. This is usually removed from the circulation by the liver and excreted in the bile. When a horse has liver disease, e.g. as a result of eating plants such as ragwort, the excretion of bile is reduced and some phylloerythrin remains in the circulation. It is then deposited in the skin causing photosensitization.
- **Certain medications**, e.g. antibiotics such as tetracyclines and sulphonamides can cause photosensitization reactions in the skin.

Clinical signs

- Non-pigmented areas of skin on the face and lower limbs are most commonly affected.
- The skin becomes inflamed, starting with redness and progressing to blisters and oozing of serum (Figure 18.21).
- Thick crusts of exudate may build up with deep cracks and fissures (Figure 18.22).
- In severe cases, the skin dies and begins to slough off.

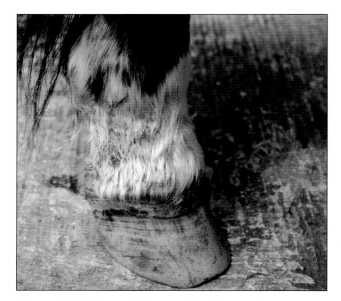

Figure 18.21 Areas of photosensitization can be very sore

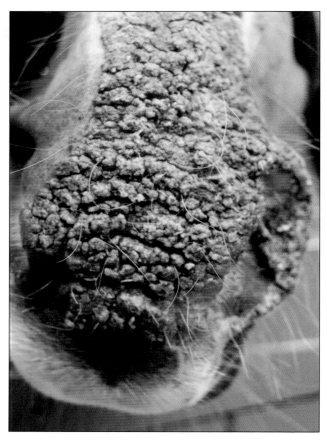

Figure 18.22 Painful crusty lesions on a horse's muzzle

- These areas are uncomfortable and sometimes itchy causing the horse to rub itself and cause raw, bleeding patches which are very sore.
- Affected lower limbs often become very swollen causing the horse to appear stiff or lame.

Diagnosis

Diagnosis is made on the clinical signs and the grazing or medical history. Blood tests should be taken to confirm or rule out the presence of liver disease. The field should be checked for any poisonous plants.

Treatment

- Wherever possible, the cause should be removed. Medication with any suspect drugs should be stopped and plants capable of causing photosensitization should be removed from the grazing. Underlying liver disease should be treated.
- The horse should be stabled during the day so that it is not exposed to sunlight until the condition has resolved.
- Oozing lesions should be gently cleaned with an antibacterial wash, e.g. Hibiscrub® and blotted dry.

- Your vet may prescribe a soothing gel, ointment or cream containing a corticosteroid and/or an antibiotic.
- In severe cases, corticosteroids may be given orally to reduce the inflammation.
- If secondary infection is present, antibiotics are administered.

STABLE MANAGEMENT
Shavings tend to stick to the lesions, so where possible these animals are best bedded on good quality straw, newspaper or cardboard. A horse with a sore, cracked muzzle will find it easier to eat hay from the floor rather than pull it from a net. It should be soaked to reduce dust levels.

Prognosis
With careful management and removal of the cause, the prognosis is good. For horses with chronic liver disease, the prognosis is poor.

SADDLE SORES

In this section, the term 'saddle sores' will be limited to discussion of skin lesions and sensitivity that occur in the saddle area, as a direct result of pressure from the saddle. A more comprehensive discussion of sore backs and saddle fitting can be found in Chapter 12.

Causes
Saddle sores can be caused by:
- incorrectly fitted saddles and numnahs
- failure of the rider to have the saddle checked and adjusted as the horse gains or loses weight or changes shape
- poor saddle maintenance
- unevenly flocked saddles with pressure points
- dirty saddles, numnahs and girths
- over-tightening the girth
- an unbalanced rider sitting to one side
- inadequate grooming
- an itchy animal rubbing itself
- over-tight rollers used to keep rugs in place or rugs that slip back and pull tight over the withers.

Clinical signs
These include the following.
PHYSICAL SIGNS
- Patches of hair rubbed away on the horse's back (Figure 18.23).

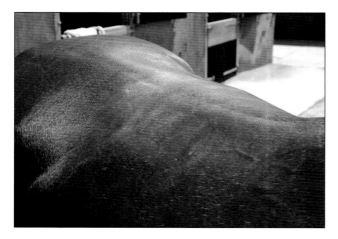

Figure 18.23 Hair has been rubbed away from a large area of this horse's back due to friction from excessive movement of the saddle

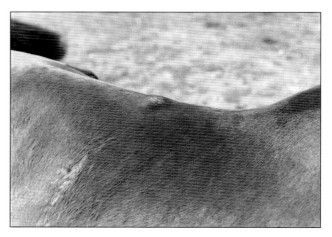

Figure 18.24 Lump on a horse's back caused by saddle pressure

- Raised thickened areas of skin that are sore when pressed (Figure 18.24).
- Swellings that develop shortly after the saddle has been removed (Figure 18.25).
- New patches of white hair (Figure 18.26).
- Raw patches.
- Thickened scar tissue in the skin.
- Atrophy (wasting) of the muscles on either side of the withers.

BEHAVIOURAL CHANGES THAT CAN INDICATE PROBLEMS WITH SADDLE FIT

- A horse with a sore back may become withdrawn or grumpy.
- It may adopt an abnormal posture in the stable or the field in attempts to obtain relief from the discomfort.

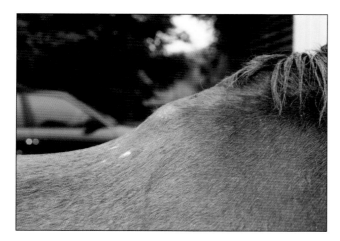

Figure 18.25 Swelling and hair loss caused by an ill-fitting saddle

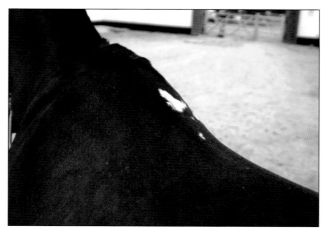

Figure 18.26 White hair often grows in areas where the skin has been damaged by pressure from the saddle

- It may roll or lie down more or less than usual.
- It may become hypersensitive to touch and resent grooming.
- The farrier may report that the horse is uncharacteristically difficult to shoe behind.
- It may object to being saddled or girthed up. Many horses with sore backs will become agitated and put their ears back or fidget and swish their tails when approached with a saddle (see Figure 12.6).
- The horse may have an anxious expression.
- Being 'cold-backed'. Some horses with pain in the saddle region sink down or 'hump' their backs when being mounted or moving off. Others stand still for mounting but run backwards or jump forwards when they start to move.

PERFORMANCE PROBLEMS THAT MAY INDICATE BACK PAIN DUE TO POOR SADDLE FIT

- Being slower than usual to warm up at the start of exercise.
- Demonstrating reluctance to work or respond to the aids.
- Shortening of the stride.
- Working with a hollow back and high head carriage with little engagement of the hindquarters.
- Reluctance to work in an outline and consequent difficulty with collection and impulsion.
- Bucking or rearing. Horses in discomfort will often buck on transitions between trot and canter, especially when working on small circles.
- Reluctance to take a particular lead at canter or change legs.
- Becoming disunited or changing behind at canter.
- Increased resistance as exercise continues.
- Difficulty walking downhill.
- Rushing into fences or rushing off on landing.
- Failure to bascule over fences (jumping flat)
- Refusing jumps or twisting over fences.
- Grinding the teeth and shaking the head from side to side.
- Constant tail swishing.

Treatment

The damaged area must be protected from further trauma. The horse should not be ridden. Exercise may be continued by lungeing the animal or by putting it on a horse walker. If the skin is broken, it should be washed gently using warm water and an antiseptic scrub. If the back is very hot and sore, your vet may prescribe a non-steroidal anti-inflammatory drug, e.g. phenylbutazone, and recommend cold hosing. Acupuncture can stimulate healing and relieve the soreness. Occasionally, antibiotics are necessary if infection is present. A qualified saddler should be called to assess the saddle.

If a poorly fitted saddle or numnah has been used on a horse for any length of time, the soreness can persist for months if it is not treated. Despite being rested and having a new saddle or numnah that is a good fit, many horses remain uncomfortable in their backs. These horses can often be helped with:

- acupuncture
- physiotherapy
- osteopathy
- chiropractic
- any combination of the above.

Prevention
SADDLE FITTING

The fitting of the saddle should be regularly checked by a qualified saddler. Horses change shape as they mature, become fitter and as they gain or lose weight. A well-fitted saddle distributes the weight of the rider evenly over a large area of the horse's back. It must not pinch the horse or have any pressure points. The following checks should be made.

- From the side view the saddle should be level and fit snugly along the contours of the horse's back. It should be positioned behind the shoulder blades but not extend further back than the top of the last (18th) rib.
- With the rider mounted there should normally be three fingers clearance between the withers and the pommel. The withers should not be pinched or bruised.
- The gullet should be approximately 6 cm ($2\frac{1}{2}$ in) wide along the length of the saddle and wider at the front. This is to avoid any of the rider's weight pressing on the dorsal spinous processes in the midline.
- The flocking should be sufficient to allow daylight to be seen along the length of the gullet when the rider is mounted. It must be evenly distributed because lumps or ridges will make the back sore. The panels should not be too hard and must have some 'give' or they can bruise and restrict the back muscles.
- The internal parts of the saddle should be free of lumps and bumps or they will cause pressure points which quickly result in discomfort. This may only be appreciated if your saddler opens up the saddle and checks the inside.
- Numnahs and girths should be of a suitable size and type and correctly fitted.

For more information on saddle fitting, see Chapter 12, pages 335–42.

RIDER PROBLEMS

A rider who is sore and out of balance should seek treatment for themselves as well as their horse. The size of the horse should be appropriate for the rider. Where the problem is caused by the inexperience of the rider, professional help should be sought.

CLEANLINESS

- The horse should be thoroughly groomed before saddling.
- The saddle should be kept clean and supple.
- Sweat should be washed from the saddle and girth area.
- Numnahs should be washed regularly. Some horses react to biological detergents so these are best avoided.

Numnahs and pads

See Chapter 12, pages 341–2.

GIRTH SENSITIVITY AND GALLS

Many horses are very sensitive in their girth regions. There may be no visible lesions but they are uncomfortable when girthed, brushed or touched. They may jump or even collapse when the girths are tightened or immediately afterwards. A girth gall is a sore area that develops under the girth (Figure 18.27).

Causes

These include the following.

- Damage to the ribcage caused by compression during the birth process can cause sensitivity to touch and pressure in the girth area (see Chapter 12)
- Doing girths up too tightly. This can make the horse very uncomfortable and restrict its movement and breathing. It is most likely to happen with elasticated girths. The muscles of the chest wall can become very irritable and jumpy in the girth area.
- Some dressage girths which buckle up behind the horse's elbow actually dig into the soft skin behind the elbow as the horse moves.
- Old or damaged girths.
- Dirty girths with accumulated mud and sweat.
- Loose girths chafing the skin.
- Unusually sensitive skin.
- Girthing over dirt and dried sweat.

Treatment

Girth galls should be cleaned and the horse should not be saddled while the area is healing. Any abrasions on the skin of the girth area should be carefully monitored as they are particularly susceptible to

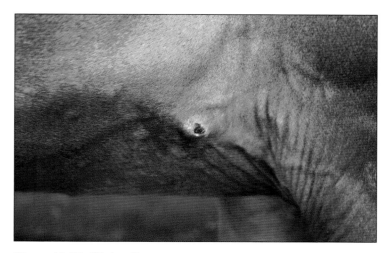

Figure 18.27 Girth gall

ringworm infection. Recently healed skin can be hardened by daily applications of surgical spirit.

Sensitivity of the muscles over the chest wall can sometimes be relieved with chiropractic treatment, physiotherapy and acupuncture or acupressure (see Chapter 12, Cold Backs and Girth Pain, pages 343–6)

Prevention

Consideration should be given to horses with sensitive girth regions. The following may help.

- Soft, supple leather girths are often the most comfortable for the horse.
- The girths should be tightened slowly over several minutes.
- They should not be overtightened. With elasticated girths, the end with the elastic should be attached to the right side (offside) of the saddle and they should be tightened on the left side (nearside).
- Care should be taken that the girth is sitting in the correct position. It should be a short distance back from the elbows where the chest is narrowest. The horse has a natural dip here if you run your hand along the underside of the chest in the midline. This is known as the 'seat of girth'.
- Pulling the forelimbs forwards one at a time will help the girth to sit in the correct position. It also checks that the soft skin in this region is not being pinched underneath the girth.
- Cleanliness of both the girth and the horse are important.

NODULAR SKIN DISEASE

This condition is also known as eosinophilic granuloma, collagen necrosis and nodular collagenolytic granulomata. The disease is characterized by raised nodules on the neck, withers and back, sometimes extending to the chest and abdominal walls (Figures 18.28a and b).

Causes

The cause is unknown but it is thought to be a hypersensitivity reaction. As lesions tend to develop in the spring and summer, insect bites may be a trigger. Pressure from an ill-fitting or poorly flocked saddle may cause the lesions to develop in the saddle region.

Clinical signs

The round, raised nodules are:

- 0.5–1 cm ($\frac{2}{10} - \frac{4}{10}$ in) in diameter
- firm to touch
- usually covered by hair
- painless

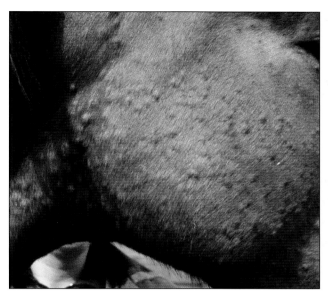 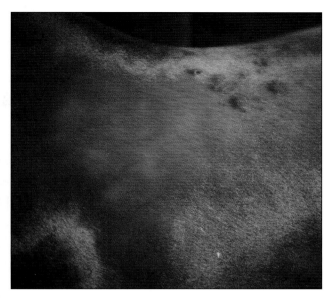

Figures18.28a and b Nodular lesions a) on the head and neck; b) in the saddle area

- non-irritant
- variable in number from one or two to several hundreds
- likely to ulcerate if the lesions are abraded.

Diagnosis

The diagnosis is made on the clinical signs and confirmed by biopsy. The mass consists of degenerative collagen and numerous eosinophils. Calcium deposits may be found in large or long-standing lesions.

Treatment

The treatment options include the following.
- Do nothing (apart from removal of any obvious cause). The nodules sometimes regress without treatment after 3–6 months. In some horses they may come and go for a while before becoming permanent.
- Surgical removal of the nodules is an option where only a small number are present.
- Local injection of corticosteroid under the new lesions may cause them to regress. This is generally not successful for long-standing, calcified nodules.
- Where there are a large number of lesions, a 2–3 week course of systemic corticosteroids, e.g. prednisolone may help.

Care must be taken that lesions under the saddle do not become abraded and sore.

Prognosis

The condition does not always respond to medical therapy and surgical removal is only practical where there are a small number of lesions. The prognosis is guarded for resolution of the nodules. However, the lesions are not painful and they rarely interfere with the horse's work.

PAPILLOMAS

Papillomas are wart-like lesions caused by infection with the equine papilloma virus. There are two different types:
- verrucose warts
- aural plaques.

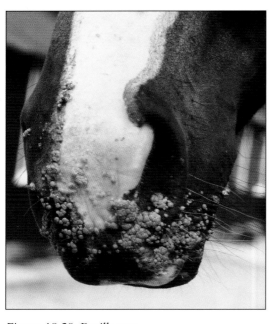

Figure 18.29 Papillomas

Verrucose warts

These warts are also known as grass or milk warts. The small grey or pinky-white lesions tend to occur around the muzzle and on the lips of older foals and young horses at grass. They are also seen on the nose, around the eyes and in the genital region. They may be found in small groups or extensive clusters (Figure 18.29). On close inspection they have a cauliflower-like appearance.

Verrucose warts tend to develop over a period of 2–4 weeks. They can be unsightly but rarely worry the animal. If a wart is knocked and bleeds, it should be cleaned gently. Treatment is rarely necessary as in most cases they spontaneously disappear after 3–4 months. When they drop off, they infect the pasture and the virus can survive from one year to the next. Recovered animals are usually immune to further infection but the virus will infect other young horses through small abrasions on the lips and muzzle. It is also spread through direct contact with an infected animal and on equipment such as brushes and feed buckets. Occasionally, older horses develop papillomas.

PREVENTION AND CONTROL
- Avoid grazing youngsters on infected paddocks.
- Good pasture management should control spiky vegetation which could scratch the soft skin of the muzzle and lips, allowing entry of the virus.

PROGNOSIS
The prognosis for verrucose warts is excellent. There is a congenital form (the foal is born with them) and this can be more persistent, as are those that develop on adult

horses. If the lesions fail to regress, they can be surgically removed or treated with cryosurgery. However, this can lead to scarring and loss of skin pigmentation.

Aural plaques

These occur on the inner surface of the ear and occasionally on the genitalia. They look like grey/white plaques and can be single or multiple, smooth or raised (Figure 18.30). Occasionally they proliferate and the plaques become up to 1 cm ($\frac{1}{2}$ in) thick. They may join up and extend over most of the hairless skin

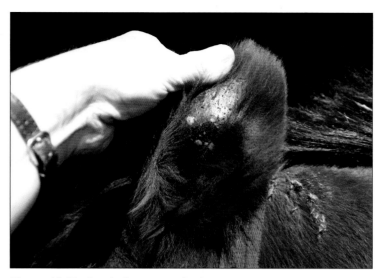

Figure 18.30 Aural plaques on the inner ear

inside the horse's ear. They are thought to be caused by an equine papilloma virus and are transmitted by flies biting and feeding inside the ears. Many horse owners mistakenly think it is a fungus.

Unlike verrucose papillomas, aural plaques do not disappear on their own. Once they have developed they are present for the life of the horse. In most cases they are painless and treatment should be avoided as interference and repeated applications of creams can make a horse or pony very head shy. Occasionally the plaques cause discomfort and have been associated with headshaking.

PROGNOSIS AND PREVENTION

The prognosis for resolution is poor. Many horses and ponies with this condition resent having their ears handled, probably due to previous and inappropriate interference with the lesions.

In areas where horses are bothered by flies in their ears, provision of shelter and use of fly nets can reduce both the irritation and likelihood of infection with the virus. If the horse is tolerant of its ears being handled, careful application of a barrier cream, such as zinc and castor oil, at regular intervals will prevent the skin being penetrated by biting flies.

SARCOIDS

Sarcoids are the commonest type of skin tumour in the horse. The cause is thought to be a papilloma virus but this has not been confirmed. Flies may spread the disease between horses by introducing the infectious agent into wounds, e.g. castration

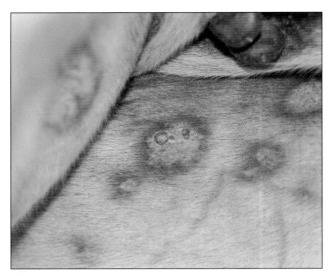

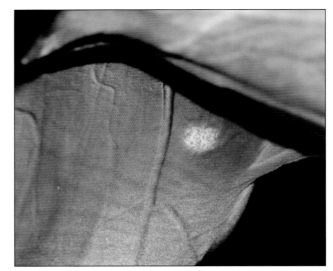

Figure 18.31 A mixture of occult and verrucose sarcoids   Figure 18.32 Verrucose sarcoid

wounds. It is thought that some horses are genetically susceptible to developing sarcoids. Sarcoids consist of fibrous tissue. They may occur singly or in clusters. Sometimes, tiny tumours known as satellite lesions are found around larger growths. Sarcoids are locally invasive; they do not metastasize (spread) to other organs of the body.

Their appearance is very variable and they can be divided into 6 types.

Occult sarcoids (Figure 18.31)

These occur as flat, hairless areas of skin that are quite often round in shape. The skin surface is grey, dry and flaky in appearance, so this can be mistaken for ringworm. Sometimes tiny nodules can be felt within the skin tissue. This type of sarcoid is common on the areas of soft skin of the axilla (between the inside of the elbow and the body wall) and inner thighs. It is also found around the eyes, mouth and on the chest and neck. The lesions tend to grow slowly and may not change over a period of several years.

Verrucose sarcoids (Figure 18.32)

Verrucose sarcoids resemble the occult type, but the skin is much more thickened and irregular. Sometimes they form dry, wart-like lesions on the skin and can have either a broad or narrow base. They may develop from the occult sarcoids, so their distribution pattern is similar. If knocked or abraded, they may ulcerate and develop into a more aggressive, fibroblastic form.

Fibroblastic sarcoids (Figures 18.33a, b and c)

These sarcoids are solid, ulcerated masses that bleed easily and can grow very rapidly. They

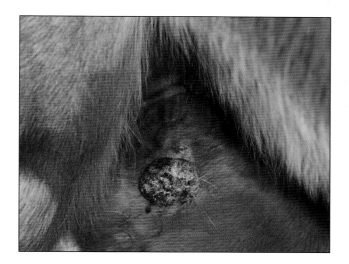

a

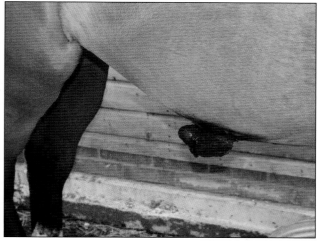

b

Figures 18.33a, b and c Fibroblastic sarcoids:
a) fibroblastic sarcoid on the inner thigh;
b) an 'angleberry'; c) ulcerating fibroblastic sarcoids

may develop from any of the sarcoid types described above or from the proud flesh of a non-healing wound. They may be pendulous, hanging from the horse's body on a stalk of tissue. These are sometimes referred to as 'angleberries'. Fibroblastic sarcoids also occur on the distal limbs where they are easily knocked and may become infected. They are particularly common on the underside of the horse's abdomen, around the sheath of geldings and on the inner thighs.

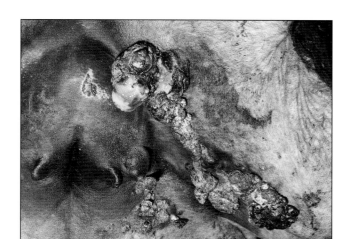

c

Nodular sarcoids (Figure 18.34)

These round, nodular lesions are generally found on the face, especially around the eyes and also on the sheath and inner thighs. In some cases the overlying skin is normal and freely mobile over the lump. In other cases the skin may be attached to the lump and appear thin and shiny. Lesions that grow to larger than 2 cm ($\frac{3}{4}$ in) may ulcerate and develop into fibroblastic sarcoids.

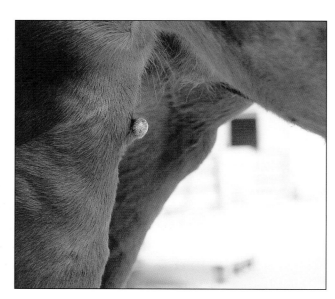

Figure 18.34 Nodular sarcoid

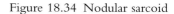

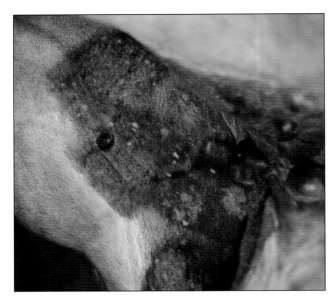

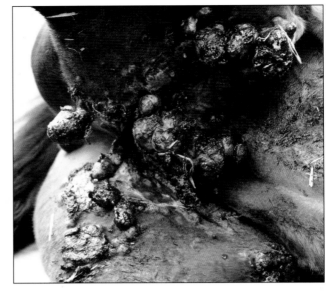

Figure 18.35 A mixture of nodular and verrucose sarcoids

Figure 18.36 Malevolent sarcoid

Mixed sarcoids (Figure 18.35)

Many sarcoids contain a mixture of two or more different types of lesion.

Malevolent sarcoids (Figure 18.36)

Occasionally, fibroblastic sarcoids become very invasive and spread along the lymphatic system to form multiple nodules and ulcerating fibroblastic masses. The most common sites are the face and medial thigh. These are not amenable to treatment and generally result in euthanasia.

Diagnosis

Diagnosis is usually made on the appearance of the lesions. It can be confirmed by biopsy, but this is best avoided as the procedure may cause the lesion to regrow in a more aggressive form. Sarcoid tissue has a characteristic appearance when examined under the microscope.

Management of sarcoids

Care should be taken not to abrade or traumatize sarcoids as this can cause them to ulcerate and grow. Particular care needs to be taken when selecting a girth for horses with lesions in this area. Wherever possible, affected horses should be managed to ensure that their exposure to flies is kept to a minimum.

Treatment

In some cases, it may be best to leave the sarcoids alone. This is especially the case if they are small, not ulcerated and at a site that does not interfere with the use of the horse.

Incorrect treatment can cause the sarcoids to recur and spread. An equine vet who has experience in dealing with these tumours is the best person to ask for advice. The recommendation will depend on a number of factors including the number, location and type of lesions. Consideration will also be given to the availability of equipment and facilities in your area and also the cost.

The treatment options include the following.

TOPICAL TREATMENT WITH CYTOTOXIC DRUGS

Cytotoxic creams are available that can be applied topically or injected into the sarcoid. This is a form of chemotherapy and should only be applied by a vet who will obtain the cream for you. The success rate is reasonably good, especially if the sarcoids have not been previously treated. They usually shrink and drop off over the next few weeks, leaving an obvious scar. Occasionally a horse will react to the cream with considerable swelling and soreness. This usually resolves after a few days and the soreness can be relieved with non-steroidal anti-inflammatory drugs (NSAIDs) such as phenylbutazone or flunixin.

INTRALESIONAL TREATMENT

The following substances can be injected into the sarcoids.

- Cytotoxic cream.
- The drug cisplastin is sometimes injected into small nodular and fibroblastic sarcoids. Repeat injections are often required.
- Other chemotherapeutic agents are currently undergoing trials.
- The human BCG vaccine may be injected into nodular or fibroblastic sarcoids close to the eye. This is repeated 1 week later, then 2 weeks later and again after a further 3 weeks. The injection interval is extended by a week each time until the lesion regresses. The aim is to stimulate the immune system of the horse to reject the tumour tissue. A drawback of this treatment is the risk of the horse developing anaphylactic shock as a result of the foreign proteins. Thus the patient should be carefully monitored for 12–14 hours following each treatment. To reduce the risk of anaphylactic shock, the horse is usually premedicated with a combination of flunixin, a cortiosteroid and an antihistamine before the tumour is injected. Some swelling occurs following the injection.

SURGICAL EXCISION

Surgical removal of small, discrete tumours with a wide margin of healthy skin can be successful. However, there is quite a high rate of recurrence at a variable time (months to years) afterwards. Wound breakdown sometimes occurs following surgical excision.

Incomplete removal of a tumour may cause it to grow rapidly and become even more of a problem.

APPLICATION OF AN ELASTIC BAND OR LIGATURE

Single tumours that have a narrow base may be 'tied off' using a tight, nylon ligature or special elastic band. The blood supply is cut off and after some initial swelling at the site, the tumour usually drops off 2–3 weeks later. Recurrence is common.

CRYOSURGERY

This involves removing the bulk of the tumour(s) surgically and freezing any remaining tissue. It is then allowed to thaw and the procedure is repeated twice more. This is carried out under sedation with local anaesthetic or general anaesthesia. It can be successful but again there is a high recurrence rate afterwards. Cryosurgery is not suitable for tumours close to the eye or over joints due to the risk of damage to these structures.

RADIATION THERAPY

Small tumours around the eye respond well to the use of radioactive implants and the cosmetic result is usually good. However, the cost of the treatment is high and there are radiation safety considerations.

LASER SURGERY

Laser surgery is not universally available, but the results are relatively successful.

Prognosis

The prognosis is guarded as small, benign-looking lesions can develop into large ulcerated tumours. Their behaviour is unpredictable.

The cost of treating sarcoids

Treatment of sarcoids can be costly and is not always successful. They are unsightly and may interfere with the use of the horse, especially those in the girth region. It is common for larger tumours to ulcerate and become infected. Occasionally, horses are euthanased as a result of the condition.

Sarcoids certainly devalue a horse as it is not possible to predict their future behaviour. Many insurance companies will not pay for treatment of sarcoids if they were present at the time of purchase.

Horse owners should be aware that more than one sarcoid may develop in any individual horse, so treatment of one tumour successfully will not prevent the development of another.

MELANOMAS

A melanoma is a tumour consisting of the cells that produce black pigment in a horse's skin. They are most often found in grey horses over 5 years old and their incidence increases with the age of the horse. It is thought that around 90% of grey horses aged over 20 years have at least one melanoma. These tumours are usually benign and grow slowly. Occasionally they transform into a more aggressive form which can be highly malignant and spread rapidly around the body in the blood and lymphatic vessels.

Where do they occur?

Melanomas are commonly found:

- on the underside of the tail (Figure 18.37)
- around the anus (Figures 18.38a and b)
- on the vulva of mares.

They also occur:

- in the parotid salivary gland
- on the ears
- around the sheath
- on the iris of the eye (see Figure 21.28)
- on the neck
- on the limbs
- in lymphatic tissue, internal organs and the guttural pouch.

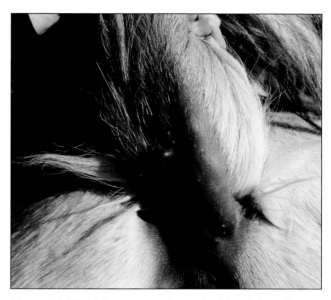

Figure 18.37 Melanoma on the underside of the tail

Appearance

In hairless regions of the horse's skin, melanomas have a raised, smooth, black, knobbly appearance. In other sites, they may be covered with hair (Figure 18.39). They can occur singly or in groups. When they occur in clusters or become very large, melanomas may ulcerate and ooze a thick black fluid.

Diagnosis

Diagnosis is usually straightforward taking into account the site and appearance of the tumour. Occasionally it is necessary to either take a biopsy or perform a fine-needle aspirate. A fine needle is inserted into the tumour and cells are drawn into a syringe for examination under a microscope.

Treatment

Treatment is not always necessary since most tumours are benign and grow very slowly. The options are:

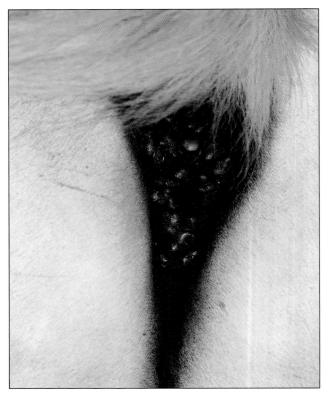

a

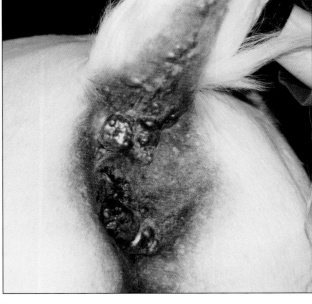

b

Figures 18.38a and b a) Melanomas around the anus;
b) melanomas around the anus and under the tail

- leave alone
- discrete, small tumours in some locations may be surgically removed
- surgery is not attempted when there are multiple lesions around the tail, anus, and vulva due to poor healing and breakdown of the wounds
- when melanomas ulcerate and become infected, they need to be cleaned regularly and treated with antibiotics.

Less commonly used treatments include the following.

- The drug cimetidine which is normally used to treat gastric ulcers. This has been reported to slow the growth of melanomas. The treatment is expensive and has to be given for at least 3 months.
- Injections of a chemotherapy drug, cisplastin, into large tumours can reduce their size. This drug works by binding to the cell DNA and

Figure 18.39 Melanoma partially covered with hair on a pony's neck

causing the dividing cells to die. This is done in a specialist hospital setting as there are important safety considerations when using this drug.

- Cryosurgery (freezing the tumour tissue) is another treatment option.

Problems caused by melanomas

In most cases, melanomas cause no problem apart from being unsightly. When they occur in clusters around the anus, however, they may obstruct the passage of droppings leading to discomfort or impaction colic. Large or multiple tumours around the vulva in mares can interfere with breeding or foaling.

When they occur as a single tumour on the limbs of horses that are not grey in colour, melanomas should be investigated as they have a tendency to be malignant. Such tumours can cause lameness. If they invade the pelvis or spinal cord the horse may develop neurological signs such as weakness and incoordination (ataxia).

If melanomas spread to the internal organs via the bloodstream and lymphatic system, the condition is fatal. It is possible for tumours that have been benign for years to suddenly become malignant in aged horses. Malignant melanomas may spread from the skin to the heart, lungs, liver, spleen, kidney, bone, brain and guttural pouch.

SQUAMOUS CELL CARCINOMAS

The squamous cell carcinoma is the second most common equine skin tumour after the sarcoid. Exposure to ultraviolet light and contact with smegma from the horse's sheath and penis are two possible causes. They tend to occur in areas of unpigmented skin in areas with little or no hair. They are commonest in pale-coloured horses including palomino, cream and coloured animals.

Common sites
These include:

- the penis of male horses and the vulval lips and clitoral region of mares
- the third eyelid, the conjunctiva, the cornea and the sclera (white) of the eye
- lips, muzzles and eyelids.

Appearance
The tumour tissue is pink in colour. Lesions on and around the eye usually develop slowly and look like plaques of

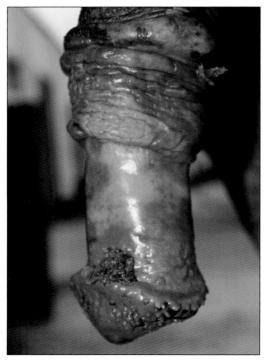

Figure 18.40 Multiple squamous cell carcinoma lesions on a penis

granulation tissue. There is quite often a mucopurulent discharge from the affected eye. Those on the external genitalia start as small, pink nodules but can then develop into larger cauliflower-like lesions which often ulcerate and bleed easily (Figure 18.40) Secondary bacterial infection of these tumours is not uncommon, resulting in a yellow discharge.

Behaviour

These tumours tend to grow slowly but on occasions can be rapidly invasive. On the whole, they are slow to metastasize (spread).

Diagnosis

The characteristic appearance and location of these lesions will immediately alert your vet to the possibility of a squamous cell carcinoma. This is confirmed by biopsy. Sometimes lesions on the penis can be very advanced before they are noticed. Blood dripping from the sheath may be the first symptom noticed by an owner.

Treatment

This depends on the site and the size of the lesion. Surgical removal together with a wide margin of healthy tissue is the treatment of choice. If necessary this can be followed by topical chemotherapy or radiation therapy.

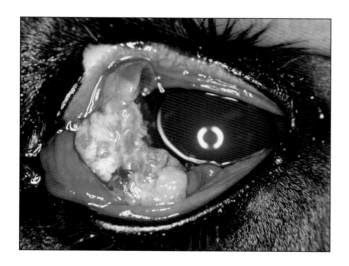

EYES

Lesions on the third eyelid (Figure 18.41 and see Figure 21.26) and conjunctiva can be removed surgically and/or be treated by topical chemotherapy. Squamous cell carcinomas of the cornea and sclera (white) of the eye are surgically removed as far as possible and respond well to radiation therapy using radioactive implants. However, this is expensive and can only be done in specialist centres.

Figure 18.41 Squamous cell carcinoma of the third eyelid (see also Figure 21.26)

PENIS

Small discrete lesions can be treated by a combination of surgical removal and topical application of chemotherapy. Large lesions are dealt with by partial or total amputation of the penis. This procedure is known as phallectomy.

Prognosis

The prognosis is generally good if the tumour is recognized early and can be removed with a wide margin of healthy tissue. Aggressive tumours that are not treated immediately have a guarded prognosis because of local spread. A possible complication of phallectomy is urinary obstruction. If this cannot be relieved, euthanasia is necessary.

VITILIGO

Vitiligo is the name given to the condition where patches of skin lose their pigment and become pink in colour without any obvious explanation.

Causes

The cause is not fully understood. The colour of a horse's skin and coat is determined by the amount and type of melanin it contains. Melanin is a pigment released by special cells in the skin called melanocytes. Its purpose is to protect the skin from harmful ultraviolet radiation. In Appaloosas it is thought that the condition may be hereditary. In other cases, various theories include toxicity, an autoimmune reaction, nutritional or metabolic imbalances.

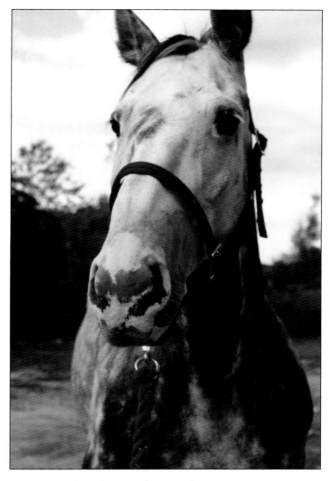

Figure 18.42 Vitiligo on the muzzle

Clinical signs

The patches of pink skin tend to develop in areas where the external skin surface meets a mucous membrane, e.g. around the:

- lips
- muzzle (Figure 18.42)
- eyes (Figure 18.43)
- vulva
- anus
- sheath.

The lesions are often symmetrical in distribution (i.e. occur on both sides of the horse) and gradually enlarge. They most commonly occur in greys, Appaloosas and coloured horses, but can be seen in horses of any colour. These areas are not inflamed or itchy as they develop.

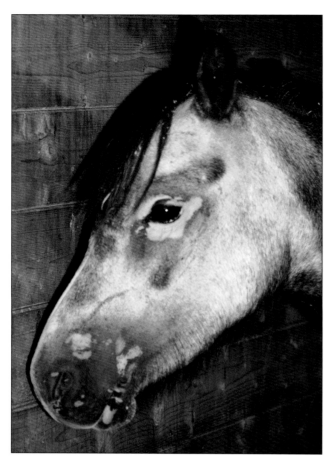

Figure 18.43 Vitiligo around the eye and on the lip and muzzle

Unfortunately, the hypopigmented areas around the eye may be easily irritated by environmental factors such as sunlight and wind. Affected animals can experience sunburn, conjunctivitis and erosions on the eyelid margins. They may then rub their eyes and cause further damage. Exposure to sunlight can ultimately predispose to the development of squamous cell carcinoma of the eyelids.

Diagnosis

Diagnosis is obvious from the clinical signs. If there is any suggestion of cancerous or precancerous changes on the eyelids, a biopsy should be performed.

Management and treatment

There is no treatment for vitiligo. Where the eyelids are irritated by the sun, stabling the horse by day or the use of protective goggles or masks should help. If the skin is inflamed or the horse has conjunctivitis, your vet will prescribe a suitable ointment. Hypoallergenic sun blocks are useful but care should be taken not to put it into the eye itself. A small amount should be applied to a test patch first to check there is no allergic reaction.

Acquired skin depigmentation

It is not uncommon for white hairs to grow when skin has been injured. Common causes include:

- pressure from ill-fitting saddles, rugs, over-tight bandages etc
- cold, e.g. freeze branding, cryosurgery
- chemicals, e.g. blisters
- rubber toxicity from bits and cruppers can lead to depigmentation of the corners of the mouth and the dock.

Such blemishes are often permanent.

19
THE REPRODUCTIVE SYSTEM

CASTRATION

Castration or 'gelding' involves removal of the horse's testicles. This operation is routinely carried out to make the horse:

- unable to breed
- more docile, especially in the presence of mares.

Preparing for the operation

A number of factors should be considered when making the arrangements for a horse to be gelded. These include the following.

TIMING

Horses can be gelded at any age. The most popular time is between 1 and 2 years when sexual behaviour commences. The operation is usually carried out in the spring, autumn or winter when there are relatively few flies. To a certain extent this depends on the available facilities and the local conditions. For example, castration should not be carried out in a waterlogged field.

LOCATION

The horse may be gelded in a stable with a bed of clean straw or paper. Wood shavings are not suitable as tiny chips can enter the wound and cause problems later. The bed should be prepared well in advance of the vet's visit so the atmosphere is not dusty when the operation takes place. Alternatively, the horse can be castrated in a clean field with a good grass cover.

These days many horses are taken to an equine hospital with surgical facilities to be gelded in clean and hygienic conditions. Here there are nurses who are accustomed to the procedure, rather than the vet having to rely on the owner to assist. This may be cheaper for the owner, easier for the vet and safer for the horse.

THE HORSE

The horse should be:

- in good health; if he is off colour or in poor condition, the operation should be postponed
- clean and dry
- calm and relaxed
- well handled
- starved overnight if the operation is being performed under general anaesthesia.

VETERINARY REQUIREMENTS

The vet will need:

- a competent handler to hold the horse
- a clean bucket and a supply of warm water
- two clean towels
- a couple of lead ropes.

Procedure
PRE-OPERATIVE CHECKS

The vet will commence with a pre-operative examination of the horse to ensure it is in good health. The scrotal region is carefully palpated to check that both testicles are present. The vet will also feel the scrotum and inguinal areas to make sure that no gut has herniated through the inguinal ring into the scrotum. The inguinal ring is a slit in the abdominal wall which connects the abdomen to the scrotum. If it is unusually large, loops of bowel may periodically enter and leave the scrotal sac. If a hernia goes undetected, the bowel may prolapse through the castration wound following surgery. In some cases colts may need to be sedated to allow this careful palpation because they are not used to being handled and may object.

RESTRAINT AND ANAESTHESIA

Horses can be gelded under local or general anaesthesia. The vet will discuss this with the owner when the procedure is planned. With local anaesthesia the operation is performed under sedation but the horse remains standing. A twitch is generally applied while local anaesthetic is injected under the scrotal skin and into the testicle prior to the surgery. The advantages of this approach are:

- it is quicker and cheaper than when a general anaesthetic is given
- the risks associated with a general anaesthetic are avoided.

The disadvantages of this method are:

- the operation can be difficult in small ponies with tiny testicles
- there is the risk that the vet will be kicked
- there is also a higher risk of post-operative complications.

Castration under general anaesthesia is more expensive but is safer and easier for the vet. It can be carried out using the 'open' surgical technique as used for standing castrations; this has the advantage of requiring only a short anaesthetic. Alternatively the operation can be performed in a 'closed' fashion which avoids cutting the tough sheet of tissue surrounding the testicle and entering the body cavity. This method is safer as it prevents the possibility of intestinal prolapse following the surgery. Healing tends to be quicker and less aftercare is necessary. It also carries a reduced risk of post-operative problems such as infection and excessive swelling. However, it takes longer and therefore is usually performed at an equine veterinary clinic with proper operating facilities.

If only one testicle has descended or other problems are suspected, the operation will be carried out under general anaesthesia. It is often recommended that stallions over the age of three years are gelded by the closed method under general anaesthesia.

THE OPERATION
- The vet will wash the area thoroughly with an antiseptic solution.
- The scrotum is incised. Emasculators are used to remove the testicles and crush the cord.
- In the open technique performed on the standing horse, the scrotum is left open to allow drainage and prevent excessive swelling.
- In the closed technique the cord is ligated (tied off) and the scrotal incision is closed.

MEDICATION
- Non-steroidal anti-inflammatory dugs are normally prescribed to reduce the pain and inflammation.
- Protection against tetanus is essential.
- Antibiotics are usually given when horses are castrated using the open, standing technique or if any complications have been experienced during the surgery. They are not usually necessary if the horse has been castrated under general anaesthesia in an operating theatre.

AFTERCARE
Exercise is restricted for the first 24 hours following surgery to discourage bleeding. After this time, exercise should be encouraged to prevent swelling. The horse can be turned out onto clean pasture. If turnout facilities are not available or swelling develops, the horse can be walked in hand or trotted on the lunge.

The horse should be checked for complications at regular intervals throughout the day and over the next couple of weeks.

Possible complications
HAEMORRHAGE
In most cases, blood will drip from the wound for a few minutes. This is to be expected and is no cause for concern. However, if the dripping persists or a continuous stream of

blood runs for more than a few minutes, call your vet. The emasculators may need to be reapplied. In severe cases of blood loss, packing of the area or clamping of the bleeding vessels plus intravenous fluids or a blood transfusion may be necessary.

SWELLING/INFECTION

Most horses experience some swelling following castration. It is usually most obvious on the 3rd to 5th day following the operation. This is usually controlled by turning the horse out and giving in-hand or lungeing exercise.

If the swelling seems excessive or the horse is off colour, call your vet. It may be due to an infection and the horse will require a course of antibiotics. Where the scrotal wound has closed and sealed the infection in, it is opened up and flushed. Non-steroidal anti-inflammatory drugs reduce the inflammation and make the horse more comfortable and willing to exercise.

PROLAPSE OF TISSUE FROM THE WOUND

When loops of gut hang from the castration wound, this is an emergency (Figure 19.1). It can happen several days after castration but most commonly occurs within the first few

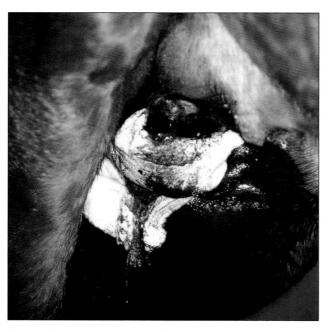

Figure 19.1 An emergency situation: loops of small intestine prolapsing through the castration wound

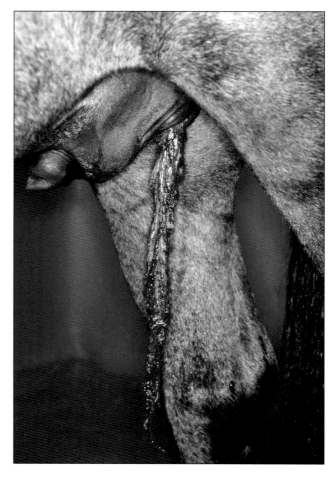

Figure 19.2 Omentum prolapsing from the castration wound

hours. Request immediate veterinary help and try to keep the gut off the floor using a clean sheet or towel tied in place. Provided the horse is not too shocked and the gut is not too badly damaged, the horse can sometimes be saved by immediate surgery under general anaesthesia.

Sometimes tissue known as **omentum** (a fold of peritoneum that contains fat, blood vessels and lymph nodes) will escape through the inguinal canal and hang from the wound (Figure 19.2). This is less serious and removal of the tissue may be all that is required.

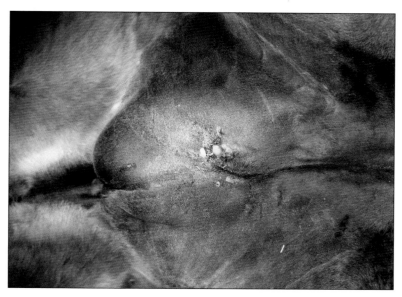

Figure 19.3 A discharging sinus from a scirrhous cord

INFECTION OF THE SPERMATIC CORD

Infection of the spermatic cord is known as **septic funiculitis**. The symptoms include pain, swelling and discharge in the scrotal region. The horse may appear lame and develop a temperature. Treatment includes antibiotics and opening the area up to re-establish drainage. A second operation to remove the diseased tissue may be necessary. A chronically infected stump is known as a **scirrhous cord**. Despite healing of the scrotal wound, granulation tissue and small abscesses develop on the stump of the spermatic cord. Discharging sinuses may develop and a hard swelling may be palpated through the skin (Figure 19.3). This can occur months or even years after the castration.

Treatment involves surgical excision of the infected tissue under general anaesthetic and a course of antibiotics.

HYDROCELE

An accumulation of fluid may form in the scrotum months or years after castration. The swelling can make the horse appear as though it is still entire (not castrated). The cyst is painless and treatment is not essential. It can be surgically removed under general anaesthetic but is usually left alone.

PERITONITIS

Mild inflammation of the peritoneum is not uncommon following castration but it becomes more serious when infection extends from the scrotal cavity into the abdomen. Signs include depression, pyrexia (the horse has a temperature), colicky signs and inappetance. Treatment includes antibiotics, non-steroidal anti-inflammatory drugs, fluid therapy and flushing of the abdominal cavity. The source of infection, e.g. an infected cord is removed. The condition can be fatal.

Points to remember

Castration will not necessarily eliminate stallion-like behaviour and between 20% and 30% of horses will continue to behave in this way. *Remember that the horse will remain fertile for a period of at least two weeks after the operation.* He should not be turned out with mares for six weeks.

Finally, it is important to be aware that although this is probably the commonest surgical procedure performed in the horse, it is relatively major and not without risk.

THE CRYPTORCHID HORSE (RIG)

When a male foal is developing in the mare's uterus, the testes form in the abdominal cavity close to the kidneys. In the last month of pregnancy, they normally migrate from the abdominal cavity down into the scrotum. Occasionally, one or both testicles may fail to descend or 'get lost' en route. This is called **cryptorchidism**. A **cryptorchid** horse has one or both testes retained in the abdomen or the inguinal region. Cryptorchid horses are also known as 'rigs'. The condition affects approximately 2–4% of 3–4-year-old colts.

The male hormone testosterone is produced by testicles whether they are in their normal position in the scrotum or somewhere else inside the horse's body. This means that rigs frequently display similar masculine behavioural characteristics to a normal stallion. Rigs may have a single undescended testicle (unilateral) or both may be retained (bilateral). The unilateral rig will have one descended testicle in the scrotum and one undescended testicle which is not visible or palpable from the outside (Figure 19.4). The bilateral rig on the other hand will have no testicles visible externally with both retained somewhere inside the body. Approximately 15% of rigs are bilateral.

If you have a horse with no visible testicles, this may be because:
- he is a true gelding (most likely)
- he is a bilateral rig with two retained testicles
- he is a unilateral rig and the one descended testicle has already been removed by incomplete castration (this is very poor practice which unfortunately still occasionally occurs)
- he does not have proper testes in the first place: monorchid (one testicle only) and anorchid (no testicles) horses are recorded, but this is so rare that it is barely worth considering.

How to spot a rig

There are normally clues from the horse's behaviour, with signs such as:

- demonstrating aggressive behaviour
- interest in mares
- attempting to cover mares in season
- stallion-like appearance, e.g. a well-developed crest.

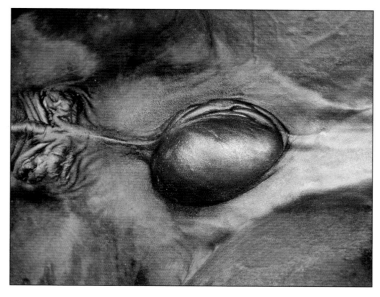

Figure 19.4 A unilateral cryptorchid with only one testicle visible

Although retained testicles produce normal amounts of male hormone, they are incapable of producing sperm due to the body heat of the horse. Thus a bilateral rig is likely to be infertile, whilst the unilateral rig is usually fertile since the descended testicle will be functioning normally. There are stallions that have bred successfully as unilateral rigs, but this is controversial. Most vets advise against it because cryptorchidism is an inherited trait and so by breeding from them, there is a considerable chance of producing more defective progeny. One USA study that looked at more than 5000 cryptorchid horses noted an increased incidence in some breeds. The highest incidence was found in Percherons, American Saddlebred horses, Quarter horses, and ponies and crossbred horses. However, in the Thoroughbred, Standardbred, Morgan, Tennessee Walking Horse and Arabian, the incidence was less than would have been expected statistically. This may have been a reflection of breeding policy.

Diagnosis

If the castration history of a particular animal is unknown and its behaviour gives cause for concern, a blood test can be used to determine whether a testicle is present.

- If the horse is over 3 years, the serum levels of **oestrone sulphate** are much higher in a horse with testicular tissue
- In younger horses, the testosterone levels are measured before and after an intravenous injection of human chorionic gonadotrophin (hCG). The **testosterone** level will rise 2-3 times in a horse with testicular tissue and remain unaffected in geldings
- Ultrasonography of the inguinal region and caudal abdomen can be helpful in the diagnosis of cryptorchidism and location of the retained testicle.

WHERE IS THE MISSING TESTICLE?

As stated, in the embryonic foal the testicles start to form inside the abdomen close to the kidneys. As the pregnancy progresses, the testicles grow and exit the abdomen through a slit-like passage in the muscles of the body wall (the inguinal canal) into the scrotum. At birth, both testicles are usually already descended and the inguinal canal becomes narrower so they cannot slip back into the abdomen. The majority of foals have testicles in the scrotum by the time they are 1 month old.

If a testicle is retained in the inguinal region, there is a chance that it will descend further as the horse matures. Descent often occurs between 1 and 2 years of age because the enlargement of the testicle that occurs at puberty may result in it dropping due to the increased size and weight. However, the body heat of the horse may prevent the retained testicle from enlarging. Unless a vet explores the area surgically, it can be extremely difficult to feel accurately the position of the misplaced testicle. Many colts do not like being handled in this area so sedation may be necessary.

The left testicle is slightly larger than the right testicle and is more likely to be retained in the abdomen. A retained right testicle is more likely to be found in the inguinal region.

Castration

When the horse is found to have no palpable testicles or just a single one, there are two possible courses of action.

- In young animals castration may be postponed in the hope that an inguinal testicle will descend over the next few months.
- Surgery may be performed to remove a retained testicle. If the location of the missing testicle is unknown, castration of a rig should be performed in a proper equine operating theatre rather than in the field as exploration of the abdomen may be necessary. This can be major surgery, particularly if the testicle is difficult to find.

In a unilateral cryptorchid (where the second testis is present in the scrotum), the retained testis is always removed first to ensure there are no problems finding it. A single scrotal testis is never removed on its own. This reduces the possibility of a rig being sold on as a 'gelding' at a later date to an unsuspecting purchaser.

Various surgical techniques are used depending on the location of the testicle and the surgeon's particular preference and expertise. If possible, it is desirable to avoid a full abdominal exploration under general anaesthesia as the risk of complications is higher and the recovery period is longer. Laparoscopic surgery, which involves a keyhole approach, may now be a better approach for abdominal rigs. In many cases, laparoscopy can be performed on the standing, sedated animal, with the advantage of much smaller wounds and faster recovery. However, it requires the appropriate equipment and surgical expertise. If the missing testicle is visualised with a laparoscope or ultrasonography, it can save a lot of the time that is sometimes spent searching the abdomen.

Prognosis

The prognosis is generally good. However, if the abdomen of a horse has to be thoroughly searched in order to find the testis, adhesions may develop and lead to subsequent bouts of colic.

Breeding

A cryptorchid animal should not be used for breeding as the condition is hereditary. In the past, if a colt was wanted for showing, racing or to stand at stud, hormone treatments were tried to encourage the testicle to descend. However, this treatment is not effective and should be discouraged as breeding from such an animal would only perpetuate the condition.

The false rig

Male horses that have been castrated but continue to exhibit undesirable masculine behaviour such as rounding up and mounting of mares are known as false rigs. This behaviour used to be attributed to the production of hormones from tissue inadvertently left behind during the castration process. This, however, is very uncommon.

The behaviour is much more likely to be the result of normal sexual experiences that occurred before castration. It often occurs when a new horse is introduced into a stable group or if a horse is sold and moves to a new environment.

A blood test taken before and after injection of hCG can be used to reassure the owner that the problem is a behavioural one. A decision can then be made on the suitability of the horse for the owner concerned.

INTRODUCTION TO BREEDING

There are three important questions that anyone considering breeding from a particular mare should ask.

- **Is she suitable for breeding?** Traits such as conformation and temperament are highly heritable and should be important considerations when selecting the mare and stallion. Mares should be selected for quality of type or performance and not simply because they are no longer suitable for any other purpose. Those with serious conformational defects should not be bred from as soundness is very important.
- **Are suitable facilities available?** Consideration must also be given to the facilities required. You will need a foaling box and suitably fenced good-quality pasture. Ideally the field should be shared with another mare and foal.
- **Can I afford it?** Stud fees, livery charges and routine and unexpected veterinary bills can add up to a substantial sum and there is no guarantee that a healthy foal will be produced or that the foal will mature into a quality horse.

General information

Most mares have a 21-day oestrous cycle. This is divided into:

- oestrus (average 5 days)
- dioestrus (14–16 days).

The cycles begin at puberty (approximately 18 months) and continue throughout the mare's life.

OESTRUS

The mare is receptive to the stallion and is said to be 'in season' (Figure 19.5).

Typical signs of oestrus include:

- adopting a urinating stance with the tail raised and passing small squirts of urine (Figure 19.6)
- opening and closing the vulval lips; this is known as 'winking' (Figure 19.7).

During this time one or more follicles in the ovaries increases in size and ruptures to release an egg (ovulation). The mare normally ovulates approximately 24 hours before the end of oestrus. The maturation of the follicle can be monitored by the vet on successive rectal and ultrasound examinations.

DIOESTRUS

The mare is no longer receptive and may behave aggressively towards the stallion. She is likely to put her ears back, swish her tail and may squeal or lash out (Figure 19.8).

Control of the oestrous cycle

The mare has a seasonal breeding period which is influenced by factors such as daylight length, temperature and nutrition. In the cold winter months, most mares stop having oestrous

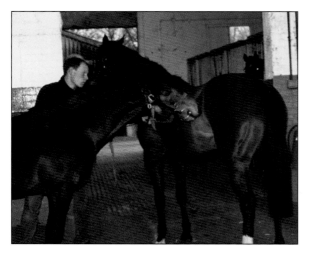

Figure 19.5 At stud mares are 'teased' by the stallion to see if they are in season

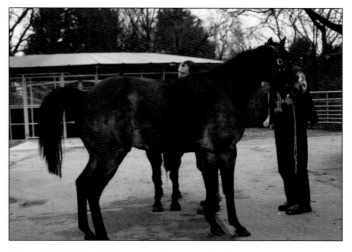

Figure 19.6 Typical stance of a receptive in-season mare

cycles and their ovaries become small and inactive. In February and March when they begin cycling, some mares have prolonged periods of oestrous behaviour but fail to ovulate. There is considerable individual variation between mares. Artifical lighting is sometimes used prior to the breeding season to encourage early return to oestrus.

The oestrous cycle is under hormonal control. When problems arise, oestrus or ovulation can sometimes be induced with hormone treatments.

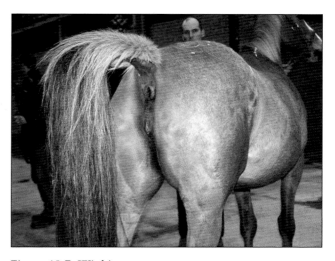

Figure 19.7 Winking

Gestation length

The gestation (pregnancy) length is 11 months (340 days), but considerable variation occurs with a range of 320–360 days and sometimes even longer.

Stallion selection

The choice of stallion should be made after consideration of the following factors.

- Conformation.
- Soundness and freedom from hereditary conditions.
- Performance records – achievements during his working career.
- Temperament – ideally calm and kind.
- Size.
- Fertility record.
- Cost and terms of the stud fee.
- Distance.
- Availability of artificial insemination (and success thereof).

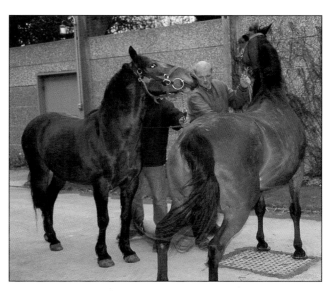

Figure 19.8 This mare is not receptive to the stallion

It is worth travelling to view the selected stallion. If at all possible, ask to see some of his offspring.

Veterinary care of the brood mare

The vet is usually consulted at several stages of the breeding programme, e.g:

- gynaecological examination prior to covering
- pregnancy diagnosis
- pre-foaling vaccination
- post-foaling checks.

Pre-breeding checks

The purpose of the examination is to check for any problems that could affect the mare's ability to conceive or carry the foal to full term. Ideally the checks should be made early in the season so any problems can be detected and treated.

HISTORY

The vet will want to know her:

- name and age
- breed
- previous breeding history
- health problems including lameness
- vaccination status
- body condition.

GYNAECOLOGICAL EXAMINATION (Figure 19.9)

This includes:

- taking a swab from the clitoral fossa and sinuses
- inspection of the vulva, vagina and cervix (Figure 19.10)
- taking a swab from the uterus for bacterial culture and examination of the cells under the microscope (Figure 19.11)
- rectal palpation and ultrasonographic examination of the uterus and ovaries (Figure 19.12) to check for any abnormalities and assess the stage of her oestrus cycle.

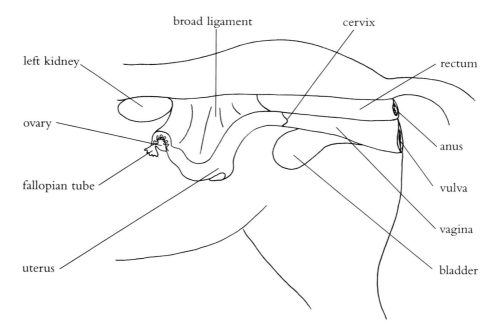

Figure 19.9 The reproductive tract of the mare

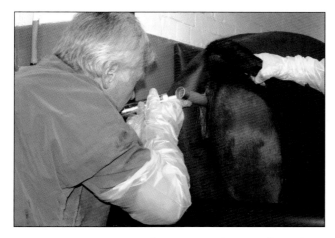

Figure 19.10 Inspecting the vagina and cervix through a speculum

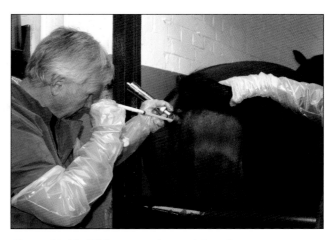

Figure 19.11 Taking an endometrial swab

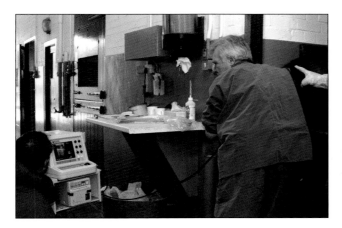

Figure 19.12 Ultrasonographic examination of the uterus and ovaries

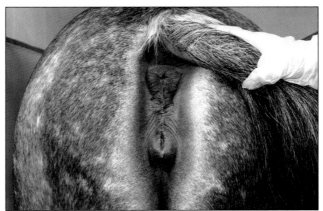

Figure 19.13 A forward-sloping vulva may aspirate air and become contaminated by faeces; this mare has had a Caslick's operation to prevent this

Preparation

If purpose-built stocks are not available, the mare should be examined in a stable. She must be adequately restrained by a competent handler and it is helpful if her tail is bandaged. The vet will require:

- a bucket of clean, warm water
- an assistant to hold the tail out of the way
- a power supply for the scanner.

On occasions it is necessary to apply a twitch or sedate the mare for the examination.

Assessment of the vulva

The vulva is checked for any signs of a discharge. The vulval lips should be vertical and meet together in the midline, forming a firm seal. If the vulva slopes forwards, the seal is

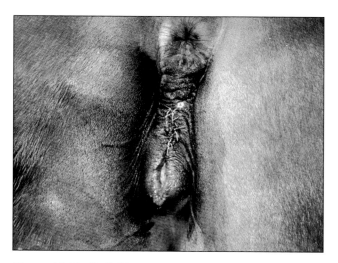

Figure 19.14 Caslick's operation

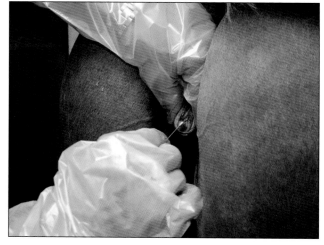

Figure 19.15 Taking a clitoral swab

easily broken and air may be sucked into the vagina as the mare moves (Figure 19.13). Aspiration of air and contamination by faeces can lead to inflammation of the vagina, cervix and the lining of the uterus, with resultant infertility.

If the vulval conformation is poor, a **Caslick's operation** may be carried out. This involves suturing the upper part of the vulval lips together under local anaesthetic (Figure 19.14). This must be opened before the mare foals or she will tear during foaling. It can be cut open at the start of second stage labour or it may be done by the vet a few days prior to foaling.

SWABS AND SMEARS

Swabs are taken to check for inflammation or infection of the reproductive tract. An infected (dirty) mare will not conceive, so covering her is a waste of time and money. More importantly, a mare with venereal disease will infect the stallion and any mares he subsequently covers. Maiden mares are included in this regime. There are two types of swab.

Clitoral swab

A clitoral swab is taken at the start of the breeding season. It can be taken at any stage of the oestrous cycle. A narrow-tipped swab is introduced into the clitoral sinuses and clitoral fossa (Figure 19.15). It is then cultured for bacteria that produce venereal disease. These include *Tayorella equigenitalis,* the organism responsible for contagious equine metritis (CEM), *Klebsiella pneumoniae* and *Pseudomonas aeruginosa.* The CEM culture takes 7 days.

Endometrial swab and smear

The endometrium is the inner lining of the uterus. An endometrial swab and smear can only be taken when the mare is in season and the cervix is relaxed. This is usually done early in oestrus so the mare can be covered in the same oestrus if the results are satisfactory. Using a sterile speculum, a sterile swab is passed through the cervix into the uterus. Following withdrawal it is cultured for 48 hours to see if any bacteria grow. A second swab is then inserted into the uterus and gently rubbed against the endometrium before being withdrawn and rolled onto a microscope slide. The slide is examined for the presence of endometrial cells and neutrophils. The presence of increased numbers of neutrophils and a positive culture of bacteria is indicative of inflammation of the endometrium, known as **endometritis**.

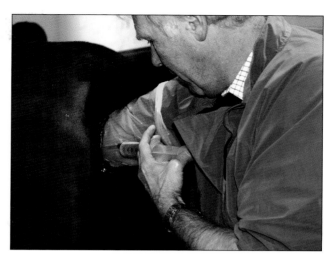

Figure 19.16 Infusing antibiotics into the uterus to treat a mare for endometritis

TREATMENT OF ENDOMETRITIS

When the laboratory results show the mare is suffering from endometritis, she is likely to be treated with infusions of sterile saline and antibiotics into the uterus for a period of 3–5 days (Figure 19.16).

A second swab and smear must be taken early in the following oestrus. If the treatment has been successful and there is no evidence of endometritis, the mare can be covered.

ENDOMETRIAL BIOPSY

If the mare fails to conceive, or the swabs and smears reveal persistent or recurrent infection or inflammation, an endometrial biopsy may be taken. This is done during dioestrus.

Biopsy forceps are passed through the cervix and a small piece of endometrium is removed and sent to a laboratory for histology (examination of the tissue under the microscope). This reveals the extent of any inflammatory or degenerative changes in the endometrium. Treatment can then be recommended and a prognosis for successful breeding given. A second biopsy is taken approximately 1 month later to assess the results of treatment.

ENDOMETRIAL ENDOSCOPY

Examination of the endometrium with an endoscope can provide the vet with valuable information such as the presence of cysts and damage sustained during previous pregnancies. The normal endometrium is smooth and pink in appearance. An inflamed endometrium may appear very haemorrhagic and have adhesions which obstruct the passage of the endoscope.

The control and treatment of venereal disease

Contagious equine metritis (CEM) caused by *Tayorella equigenitalis* is a notifiable disease in the UK. Any occurrence must be reported to the Divisional Veterinary Manager of DEFRA.

CLINICAL SIGNS

Most stallions carrying the disease show no outward signs. Mares may have a grey, mucoid vulval discharge or they can also be symptomless carriers of the disease.

TRANSMISSION

The disease is transmitted:

- during mating and artificial insemination
- during teasing
- on hands or equipment if hygiene standards are poor.

DIAGNOSIS

Diagnosis is confirmed if the organism is grown on swabs from:

- the clitoral fossa and sinuses, the endometrium or vaginal discharge of mares
- the urethra, urethral fossa, penile sheath and pre-ejaculatory fluid from stallions.

The swabs must be sent to an approved laboratory.

TREATMENT

Stallions are treated by thorough cleaning of the penis with an approved antiseptic solution and application of an antibiotic ointment for 5–7 days following removal of all accumulated smegma.

Mares with endometritis are treated with intrauterine infusions of antibiotic, thorough cleaning of the clitoral region and topical antibiotic treatment. With stubborn infections that are difficult to clear, surgical removal of the clitoris may be performed.

Freedom from infection in mares is confirmed by 3 negative clitoral swabs taken at intervals of at least 7 days and 3 negative endometrial swabs taken during successive oestrous periods.

Stallions require 3 sets of negative swabs taken at intervals of at least 7 days before they can be confirmed free of infection. In addition, the first 3 mares mated or inseminated by the stallion should have clitoral swabs taken 3 times at intervals of at least 7 days, starting 2 days after mating or insemination. These must be negative.

CONTROL

If a case is confirmed, there is a Code of Practice published by the Horserace Betting Levy Board (HBLB) (www.hblb.org.uk) that must be strictly adhered to. This includes:

- stopping all breeding activity immediately
- isolation and swabbing of infected horses
- swabbing of at-risk contacts
- notification of owners of mares who have left the premises, are booked to the stallion or have been inseminated with semen
- testing of stored semen
- foaling of pregnant mares that have been exposed to the infection in isolation; the placenta must be burned and both filly and colt foals swabbed.

Breeding should not be resumed until the premises are confirmed as free from the disease.

PREVENTION

The disease can be prevented by strict adherence to the recommendations for swabbing in the HBLB Code of Practice. The swabs should be taken from mares and stallions after 1st January of the year in which breeding activity is planned. Additional swabs are taken from stallions in the middle of the breeding season.

Blood test for equine viral arteritis (EVA)

A blood test should also be taken to test the mare for EVA prior to breeding and the stallion should be confirmed as clear before the mare visits him. It takes some time for the results of both the CEM swabs and the EVA blood tests to be confirmed and so it is advisable to have them taken at least 10 days before the mare goes to stud.

NATURAL COVERING

Once all of the pre-breeding checks have been carried out, then provided no problems have been detected, the mare is ready to be mated or 'covered'. Regular veterinary examinations may be performed to ensure this is done at the optimum time. Mating may take place:

- with the mares running free in a paddock with the stallion, or
- by supervised breeding in-hand.

The former is sometimes used on pony studs where the number of visiting mares is relatively small. The main advantage is that the reduced amount of supervision considerably reduces the costs. However, one of the main disadvantages is the increased risk of injury (from kicks and bites) to the mares or the stallion. The value of many stud animals today is too high to take any unnecessary risks and so most commercial studs practise breeding in-hand.

Breeding in-hand
LOCATION

The covering procedure involves the stallion being led to the mare that is presented to him when she is in full oestrus - a separate teaser stallion may be used to establish this. Mating normally occurs in a specially designated covering area with plenty of space and a non-slip floor. A rubber floor keeps dust levels to a minimum and can be thoroughly cleaned. The floor surface may be designed with a step or a slope to assist a stallion that is covering a mare that is larger or smaller than him.

SAFETY

Safety is an important consideration. Handlers of both the mare and the stallion should wear hard hats and gloves and be prepared for the animal to strike out or bite at any time. Both the stallion and the mare should be bridled and the mare should wear special covering boots made of felt or leather on her hind feet to reduce the risk of the stallion being seriously injured if she kicks. Some stallions bite the mare's neck during mating. If he is particularly aggressive, the mare may wear a protective neck cover.

HYGIENE

Prior to covering, the external genitalia of the mare will be washed with warm water to remove any faecal contamination. Her tail is normally bandaged to prevent the stallion's penis contacting the hairs. Assistants likely to have any contact with the external genitalia of either the mare or the stallion must wear clean, disposable gloves.

MATING

The mare is normally taken into the covering area first and held so she can see the stallion approaching. The stallion is then led to the mare from behind her on her left side, approaching at an angle of approximately 45 degrees. He will normally sniff and tease the mare for a short period before mounting her. As he mounts, the tail may be held out of the way by an experienced handler standing on the mare's right side. If necessary, the penis can be guided into the mare. Mating usually last for about 1 minute, but this varies between individual stallions. When the stallion ejaculates, his tail will be seen to move up and down and a pulse of fluid can be felt along the base of the penis by the handler holding the mare's tail. Following ejaculation, the stallion should be allowed to dismount slowly and then be backed away. The penis is then washed with clean warm water.

THE TIMING OF COVERING

Covering should occur at the optimum time to maximize the chances of conception. Mares are routinely teased every other day prior to mating to establish when she comes into oestrus. On average, the oestrous period lasts for 5 days and ovulation will take place 24 hours before the end of oestrus. The aim on most studs is to cover the mare 24 hours prior to ovulation and to cover them just the once. Regular veterinary examination is helpful to establish the optimum time. On the day after mating, the mare should ideally be re-examined by the vet to check whether she has ovulated and that there is no fluid in the uterus (see page 590).

TEASING

Following a successful mating and confirmation that the mare has ovulated, teasing is recommenced and carried out every other day from about day 14 after covering. If she does not return to oestrus by day 16–17 after covering, she will be presented to the vet for scanning to determine whether she is in foal.

ARTIFICIAL INSEMINATION (AI)

Artificial insemination is becoming increasingly popular for non-Thoroughbred breeds. It is currently not permitted for registry in the Thoroughbred Stud Book and it is worth checking that full registration of any other breed you select to breed by AI is permissible.

The semen is collected into an artificial vagina and subsequently inseminated into the mare. The semen may be utilized fresh, chilled or frozen.

Procedure

- The mare has all the routine pre-breeding checks including swabs and smears. At this time an assessment of the likely success of the procedure and the expense is made and discussed.
- The stallion is screened for venereal bacterial pathogens and equine arteritis virus. The sperm quality is assessed. The sperm of individual stallions may differ in its ability to survive processing and transport. Chilled sperm can survive between 12 and 72 hours and frozen sperm may remain viable for several years.
- The mare is closely monitored prior to insemination so that she is inseminated as close to ovulation as possible, ideally 12–24 hours before. Serial rectal and ultrasonographic examinations are performed. The mare may be injected with hormones to induce ovulation at a specific time.
- The appearance and motility of fresh or chilled semen is examined under a microscope before insemination to ensure that it is of good quality. The appearance of the sperm and its ability to swim progressively is checked.
- For the insemination, the mare should ideally be restrained in stocks.
- The tail is bandaged or wrapped in a plastic sleeve. The vulva and surrounding skin are carefully cleaned and rinsed with clean, warm water, then dried with a clean paper towel.
- The semen is deposited into the uterus using a warmed, sterile catheter. In some cases, if the mare is susceptible to endometritis or has fluid in her uterus, the semen is placed

at the site where the fallopian tube enters the uterus using an endoscope. This may also be done if the sperm quality is poor.

- The mare is re-examined later to check that ovulation has occurred. The timing of this examination depends on whether chilled or frozen semen was used. If the mare has not ovulated, a second insemination may be necessary.
- If the mare conceives, the embryo will migrate from the fallopian tube into the uterus 5 days after ovulation. Any excessive accumulation of fluid in the uterus or inflammation following insemination will reduce the chance of a successful pregnancy. A post-insemination examination is usually performed and if intrauterine fluid is identified, treatment will be undertaken to remove it. This may involve repeat injections of oxytocin if the cervix is relaxed or infusion of 1–2 litres of warm sterile saline into the uterus. The saline stimulates contraction of the uterus and expulsion of the fluid (Figure 19.17).

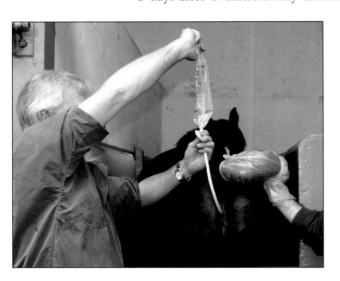

Figure 19.17 Infusing the uterus with warm sterile saline

The advantages of AI

- The semen from a single stallion can be used to inseminate more mares than a stallion could cover naturally.
- Transporting the semen means that mares and foals do not have to travel long distances to unfamiliar surroundings.
- There is no risk of injury to the mare or stallion from kicks and bites.
- Fewer bacteria enter the uterus than with natural service.
- In expert hands it can increase the chance of conception, especially in mares susceptible to endometritis.
- Frozen or chilled semen can be moved internationally.
- There is regular monitoring of semen quality and excellent disease control.

The disadvantages of AI

- AI can be costly. The mare needs frequent examinations by an experienced stud vet.
- The fertility rates can be disappointing.
- A high concentration of sperm in a small volume of fluid can cause endometritis in some mares.
- Thoroughbreds produced by AI cannot be registered as Thoroughbreds. Only natural covering is permitted.

EMBRYO TRANSFER

Embryo transfer involves collection of a fertilized embryo from one mare (the donor) and transplanting it into another mare (the recipient) on day 7 or 8 after fertilization has occurred. This method of breeding is becoming popular for top-class competition mares, allowing them to continue competing with minimal disruption to their competition programmes. In this manner they can produce more foals than would be possible with natural breeding. It is also useful for valuable mares that are no longer able to maintain pregnancy due to infertility as a result of endometrial degeneration or damage to the cervix. The Jockey Club does not permit embryo transfer in Thoroughbred mares.

Mare selection

Donor mares should have normal breeding cycles and be in good health. **Recipient mares** should be young (3–10 years), a similar size to the donor mare and have no history of reproductive problems. A previous successful pregnancy is an advantage. Both mares are thoroughly screened for any potential problems at the outset. If finances permit, it can be helpful to have more than one recipient mare available. A minimum of two mares is generally recommended.

Mare preparation

The oestrous cycles of the donor and recipient mares are synchronized using hormone injections. Ovulation is synchronized as far as possible. The recipient mare should ovulate from 1 day before to 2 days after the donor mare. The maturation of the follicle of the donor mare is monitored and when ovulation is imminent, the mare is mated or inseminated and injected with an ovulation-inducing hormone. The mare is then monitored by ultrasound examination to confirm that ovulation has occurred. Blood samples may also be taken to check that the progesterone concentrations are rising.

Embryo recovery

This is carried out on day 7 following ovulation. At this stage the embryo is in the uterus and can move around freely. Following careful preparation of the mare to reduce the risk of bacterial contamination, a sterile embryo-flushing catheter is introduced into the uterus. A special embryo flushing medium is allowed to flow into the uterus by gravity. An inflatable cuff prevents the fluid or catheter escaping from the uterus. The fluid is then drained from the uterus by gravity, passing through an embryo filter. This process is then repeated and the fluid in the filter is examined under the microscope for the presence of an embryo.

Embryo transfer

If a healthy embryo is retrieved, it is transplanted into the recipient mare. This can be done in the following ways.

- **Non-surgically** The embryo is transferred through the cervix of the recipient mare using a special insemination pipette and gently squirted into one of the uterine horns. The mare is treated prophylactically with antibiotics. Alternatively, the embryo may be transplanted in a semen straw with an insemination gun.
- **Surgically** The embryo is implanted into the uterine horn through a flank laparotomy in the standing, sedated mare. The embryo is introduced into the uterus through a large, blunt needle. Following closure of the abdomen, the mare is treated with antibiotics, non-steroidal anti-inflammatory drugs to control pain and is box rested for up to a week.

In the past, surgical transfer resulted in higher pregnancy rates (reports vary between 55% and 90%) than non-surgical transfer (22–50%). However, improved methods of non-surgical embryo transfer in experienced hands are now resulting in pregnancy rates of 85%.

CARE OF THE BROODMARE FOLLOWING COVERING OR INSEMINATION

Pregnancy diagnosis in the mare
There are a number of procedures used to confirm that a mare is in foal.

RECTAL PALPATION
This can be done at any stage from day 14 to 15 after ovulation (16 to 17 after covering) onwards. The vet assesses the tone, size and position of the uterus which change as the pregnancy advances. The foal may be felt from around mid-pregnancy. The vet may inspect the cervix which is usually whiter and much more tightly closed than the cervix of a non-pregnant mare. The rectal findings during early pregnancy are not always conclusive and cannot eliminate the possibility of twin conceptuses.

ULTRASOUND SCANNING
This is the most commonly used method for pregnancy diagnosis and the assessment of early foetal growth. It is performed from day 14 to 15 after ovulation (16 to 17 after covering) onwards. It is the most reliable method of detecting unwanted twin pregnancies. To rule out the possibility of twins, the mare is scanned at least twice in the early stages of pregnancy.

The procedure
To scan a mare during early pregnancy, an internal examination of the mare is required. To ensure this is done safely for both the vet and the mare, it is important that the mare is

properly restrained. Stocks are ideal for this purpose. Electricity is required to power the scanner and there must be a suitable area out of sunlight to view the scanner screen. To perform the scan, the vet will remove the faeces from the rectum and introduce the probe. This is then advanced until it lies over the uterus. It is moved from side to side, passing over the uterine horns and the ovaries. An image is seen on the screen. If the mare is pregnant, the embryonic vesicle appears as a distinct black sphere on the screen. When mares are examined as early as day 14–15 after ovulation, they are checked again a few days later. The embryo itself can be seen as a white speck within the circular black area between days 18 and 21 after ovulation. Even at this early stage, the pulsation of the heart is often visible. By day 26, the embryo is clearly visible as it lifts away from the wall of the vesicle and protrudes into the lumen.

A third examination is ideally carried out around day 28 and before day 35 (Figure 19.18) to ensure that the mare is still pregnant and to make certain that a twin has not been missed. The optimum time for determining the gender of a foal in utero is between 55 and 65 days.

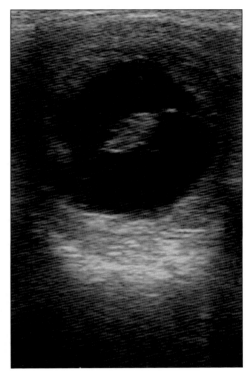

Figure 19.18 A 30 day embryo

BLOOD TESTS
Equine chorionic gonadotrophin (eCG)
From days 45 to 90, a blood sample may be taken and tested for the presence of eCG. This is produced by structures called endometrial cups which form when foetal cells invade the endometrium. The test is around 90% accurate. Occasionally a mare produces a false negative result, but inaccuracies more commonly involve false positives. This is because eCG continues to be produced if the foetus dies.

Oestrone sulphate
Oestrone sulphate is produced by the foetus and can be detected in the serum of pregnant mares from day 120. The levels fall in the last few weeks of pregnancy.

URINE TESTS
Oestrogens produced by the placenta and the foetus are present in the mare's urine from 150 days to full term.

Management of the in-foal mare
Once the pregnant mare is back at home, she will still require the following.
- Daily inspection.

- Regular hoof care.
- Appropriate feeding.
- Regular worming.
- Dental care.
- Vaccination. An influenza and tetanus booster 3–6 weeks before foaling gives the foal maximum protection. If the mare is to be vaccinated against equine herpesvirus, this should be done in the 5th, 7th and 9th months of pregnancy. Vaccination of mares to protect their foals from diarrhoea caused by equine rotavirus is carried out in the 8th, 9th and 10th months of pregnancy.
- Exercise. This depends on many factors such as the size, age, condition and fitness of the mare and the weight of the rider. Strenuous exercise should be discontinued from the 6th month of gestation. The brood mare should be turned out each day.

Pregnancy failure
FAILURE TO CONCEIVE AND EARLY EMBRYONIC LOSS
This can be due to the following.

- **Genetic factors**, e.g. chromosomal abnormalities. Defects may occur if mating and fertilization do not take place at the optimum time and either the sperm or the egg is 'aged' (beginning to deteriorate in quality).
- **Environmental factors**: malnutrition of the mare and overfeeding or underfeeding in the period after mating can adversely affect her fertility. Any illness resulting in a high temperature or prolonged colic can cause embryonic death.
- **Uterine factors**: any problem with the previous pregnancy such as a difficult birth or retained placenta can adversely affect the uterine environment in a subsequent pregnancy. Pregnancies established at the foal heat have a reduced viability. The presence of endometrial cysts can sometimes affect embryonic development as can the presence of fluid retained in the uterus after mating. All mares experience a transient uterine inflammation after mating but this usually resolves within 48 hours. In older mares the inflammation may last for a longer time, and the embryo cannot survive under these conditions.
- **Twin pregnancies** (see below).

Early embryonic loss may be predicted from the appearance on the ultrasound scan. The signs include:

- an embryonic vesicle that is smaller than expected for its age
- a vesicle with no embryo visible after the time when it should be seen
- an embryo that is smaller than expected for its dates.

TWINNING
Nearly all twin pregnancies result from double ovulations. These may occur close together

or several days apart within a single oestrous period. The incidence of double ovulations differs between breeds and increases with the age of the mare. Thoroughbred mares are reported to have a 15–25% occurrence of double ovulations with up to 15% incidence of twins.

Twinning is a serious source of loss to the breeding industry. Various reports suggest that between 53% and 73% of affected mares will abort and of all the mares with twin pregnancies, only 16–25% of mares will give birth to single or twin foals. The cause of embryonic loss is the inability of the

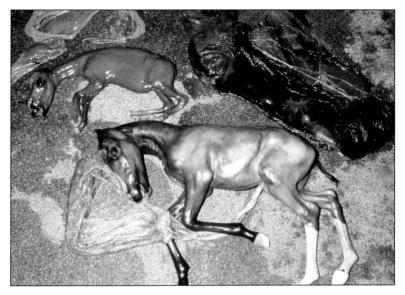

Figure 19.19 Aborted twins

endometrium to provide adequate nutrition for both embryos (Figure 19.19). Twins located in the same horn are likely to die earlier in the pregnancy because the vesicles are in contact with each other rather than with the lining of the uterus and their nutrition is reduced.

Diagnosis

- In early pregnancy, twinning is diagnosed by routine ultrasound examination *per rectum*.
- In late pregnancy, the presence of twins can sometimes be detected by scanning through the abdominal wall.

Subsequent action

Following the diagnosis of a twin pregnancy, there are 3 possible courses of action.

1 Do nothing in the hope that one embryo will die naturally. The mare is checked at day 35 and if 2 foetuses are still present, she can be injected with prostaglandins to abort the pregnancy.

2 Try to eliminate one of the foetuses manually. If this is done before the embryos attach to the uterus (i.e. before approximately 15–16 days post ovulation), the success rate can be up to 90%. The smallest vesicle is gently manipulated until it reaches the tip of one uterine horn and compressed until it is felt to 'pop'. If the foetuses are located in the same horn and have already become fixed to the endometrium, squeezing one is more likely to result in the death of both of them. If the twins are discovered after 40 days of gestation, very experienced stud vets may attempt to eliminate one of them by guiding a sterile needle through the wall of the vagina and into the foetal sac under ultrasound guidance.

3   Abort the pregnancy and start again. This is only possible up to 35 days when the endometrial cups develop. After 35 days, the pregnancy can be aborted but the mare is unlikely to return to fertile oestrus within the same breeding season owing to continued production of hormones by the endometrial cups.

Abortion of twins

Undetected twin pregnancies often end in abortion. If this occurs late in pregnancy, there is a possibility of problems during delivery which can lead to loss of the mare. Twins that are born alive are usually underweight and need a great deal of care. It is common for one or both of them to die within a few days of birth. Those that survive are less likely to achieve a high level of performance than single foals.

Abortion

The incidence of abortion in the last third of pregnancy is relatively low. However, even with the best of care, some mares will not carry their foals to term.

POSSIBLE CAUSES OF ABORTION

These include the following.

*   A twisted or abnormally long umbilical cord which restricts the circulation between the foetus and placenta. The average cord length is 70 cm (28 in) but some are up to 110 cm (43 in); it is thought that a longer cord is more likely to become tangled around the foetal limbs or compressed (Figure 19.20).
*   Infection: bacterial, fungal or viral (EHV-1, EVA).
*   Twins: the placenta is rarely able to nourish two foals to full term.
*   Maternal stress, e.g:
    *   malnutrition
    *   pain
    *   colic
    *   endotoxaemia, e.g. from serious types of colic
    *   a high temperature
    *   emotional disturbance from weaning or management changes
    *   transport
    *   general anaesthesia
    *   surgery.

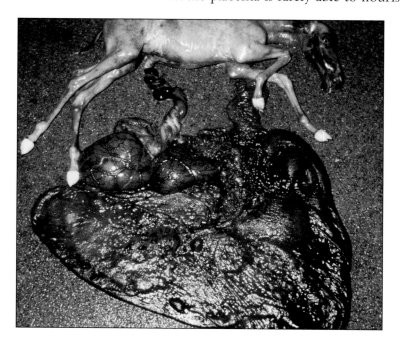

Figure 19.20 Abortion caused by a twisted cord

- Developmental abnormalities in the foal or foetal membranes.
- Uterine torsion.

Prompt veterinary attention is necessary in many of these cases as the life of the mare is also at risk.

Problems of late pregnancy
ABDOMINAL WALL OR PREPUBIC TENDON RUPTURE

In late pregnancy, the body wall is occasionally weakened by the combined weight of the foetus plus the membranes and fluids, to the extent that it tears. The muscles themselves may tear or the prepubic tendon which attaches them to the front of the pelvis can partially or completely rupture. The signs include an area of oedema (swelling) up to 10–15 cm (4–6 in) thick, extending along the ventral midline in front of the udder (Figure 19.21). The mare is often uncomfortable; she may show colicky signs and resent the area being touched. The udder may appear to have moved forwards.

The treatment is restricted exercise and non-steroidal anti-inflammatory drugs. A well-padded abdominal support bandage may be applied. Some mares are able to foal unassisted, but the abdominal wall is often too weak to push the foal out. An assisted delivery or caesarean section may be required, so the birth should be supervised. It may be possible to repair the defect surgically but this can be very difficult. Further pregnancy puts the welfare of the mare at risk.

MARE RUNNING MILK

If the mare runs milk prior to foaling, an alternate source of colostrum must be available (see page 603).

Preparation for foaling

If the mare is not foaling at home, she should ideally be moved to the foaling premises 4–6 weeks before she is due to foal. This gives her time to settle in and to acquire immunity to disease-producing organisms in the new environment. She will produce protective antibodies which are passed onto the foal in the colostrum.

For an average-sized mare, the foaling box should measure

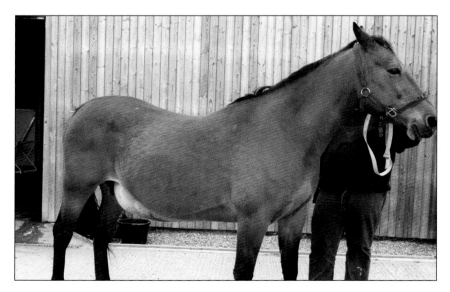

Figure 19.21 Prepubic tendon rupture

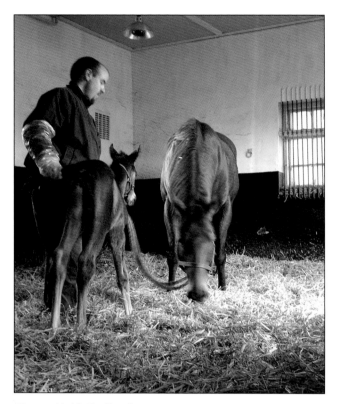

Figure 19.22 Foaling box

4.5 m x 4.5 m (13 ft x 13 ft). A clean, deep bed of good quality straw should be provided (Figure 19.22). Shavings are not suitable as they can block the nostrils of a newborn foal. A power point and a means of providing a sick foal with warmth should be available.

MAMMARY DEVELOPMENT

The udder of the mare begins to enlarge approximately 4 weeks before foaling. Most of the development takes place in the last two weeks when both the udder and the ventral abdomen can become oedematous (Figure 19.23). Drops of dried colostrum accumulate as waxy deposits on the teats 1–4 days before foaling (Figure 19.24).

These signs should not be taken as a reliable indication that foaling is imminent. Some mares show very little change until the last few hours while others run milk for days or weeks before foaling.

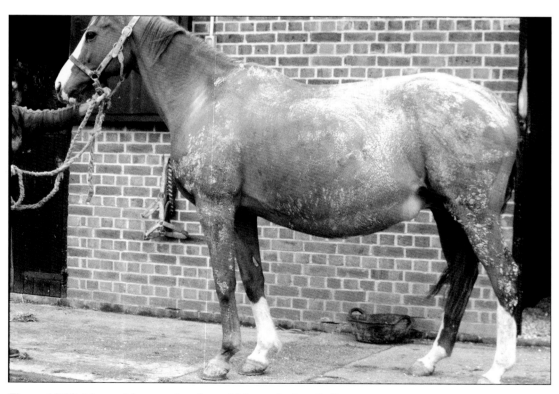

Figure 19.23 Mare with ventral oedema 24 hours before foaling

CHANGE IN MAMMARY SECRETIONS

The composition of the mammary secretions changes as the mare approaches parturition (foaling). If there is a particular need to know when foaling is imminent, the secretions can be tested. Milk strip test kits are available for measuring the electrolyte concentrations in the mammary secretions and may provide a guide to the maturity of the foetus and its readiness for birth.

VULVAL RELAXATION

Shortly before birth, the vulva lengthens and appears slightly swollen (Figure 19.25).

Foaling

The gestation (pregnancy) length of the mare is 11 months (340 days), but this can range between 320 and 360 days. As the foaling date approaches, the mare should be kept under close observation, including at night. However, this should be done calmly and discreetly to ensure that the mare is not unsettled. The observer should be familiar with the course of a normal foaling and call the vet if a problem occurs. Many studs use closed circuit cameras so the mare can be watched without being disturbed. Special foaling alarms are available.

FIRST-STAGE LABOUR

During first-stage labour, the mare experiences discomfort from uterine contractions. The signs include:

- restlessness
- sweating
- pawing the ground
- looking round at the flanks
- milk may drip or spurt from the teats.

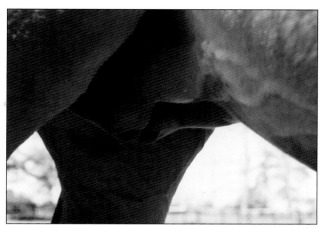
Figure 19.24 An udder 24 hours before foaling

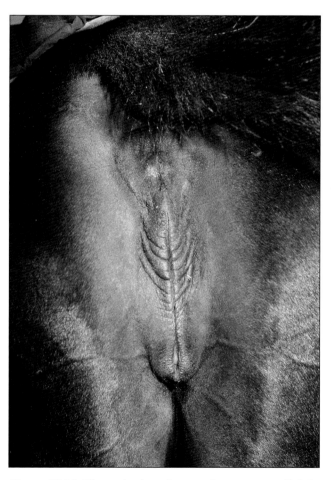
Figure 19.25 The vulva lengthens and may appear slightly swollen shortly before foaling

The periods of discomfort are separated by periods of calm. Maiden mares may roll or become quite distressed. The length of first-stage labour is extremely variable.

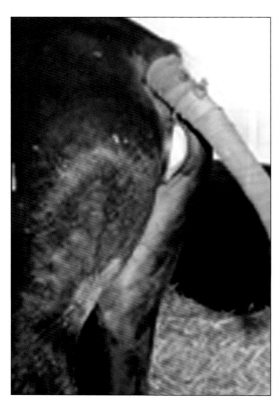

Figure 19.26 The amnion appears between the vulval lips

SECOND-STAGE LABOUR

Second-stage labour lasts for an average of 20 minutes. It begins when the placenta ruptures and a large quantity of clear, pale yellowish fluid is released. Most mares then lie on their sides and begin to strain. If the mare has a sutured vulva which has not already been opened, it must be cut at this stage.

After 5–10 minutes a white membrane called the **amnion** appears between the vulval lips (Figure 19.26). In a normal foaling the front feet are delivered first, followed closely by the muzzle. The mare continues to strain vigorously until the foal's hips have been delivered (Figures 19.27a–e). She will then stop straining but stay lying down for up to 20 minutes. *Do not disturb her,* especially for the first few minutes after foaling as blood is still passing from the placenta to the foal. It is quite normal for the foal's hind limbs to remain inside the vagina and unless the amnion is obstructing the foal's nostrils, no interference is necessary.

The umbilical cord breaks when the mare stands or the foal struggles to its feet. The foal's navel should then be dressed with an iodine dressing or antibiotic preparation recommended by your vet.

THIRD-STAGE LABOUR

The placenta is normally expelled within 1 hour of the foal being born. The mare may go down again and experience colicky pain as it is delivered. If the placenta has not been delivered within 3 hours, notify your vet.

Induction of parturition

Mares are rarely induced to foal as the normal gestation period varies from 320 to 360 days. The foal matures in the last 2–3 days of gestation and there is no 100% reliable method of determining if this has occurred. Artificial induction before foetal maturation takes place considerably decreases the foal's survival chances. The procedure may be considered in:

- mares with prepubic tendon rupture
- cases where foaling problems are anticipated
- cases where the mare or foal is considered to be at risk if the pregnancy continues.

Oxytocin is most commonly used to induce parturition.

Complications of induction include:

- the birth of weak or premature foals

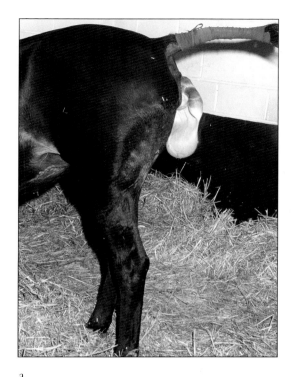

a

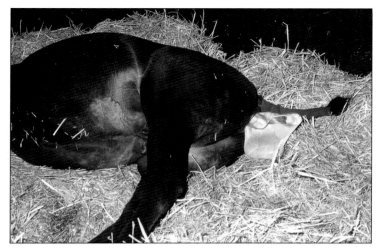

b

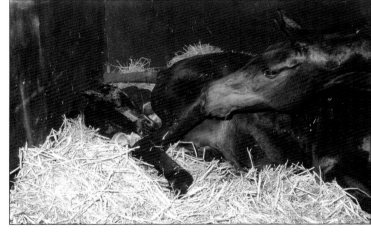

d

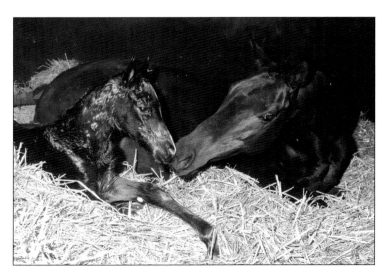

c

Figures 19.27a–e Normal foaling: a) the front feet begin to show, one slightly in advance of the other; b) the mare lies down and begins to strain vigorously; c) the foal's shoulders are being delivered; d) the new arrival; e) the mare remains lying down for some time after foaling, reaching round to lick and nuzzle her foal

e

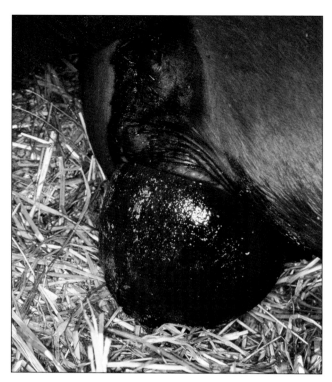

Figure 19.28 The appearance of the red allantochorion at the vulval lips is abnormal; placental separation has started and the membrane should be broken and the foal delivered as quickly as possible as it is being deprived of oxygen

- premature placental separation: a thick red membrane (the **allantochorion**) appears at the vulval lips instead of the white amnion (Figure 19.28)
- foaling difficulties
- retained placental membranes.

Post-foaling complications in the mare

There are a number of possible post-foaling complications which require immediate veterinary attention. These include the following.

- **Uterine tears** These are more likely to occur if there are foaling problems and the delivery has to be assisted. Occasionally they can occur during an apparently normal delivery due to a foetal foot perforating the uterus.
- **Prolapse of the uterus** This is uncommon, but more likely to occur if the mare had problems giving birth or if the membranes are retained. It tends to occur within the first few hours after birth.
- **Rupture of a major vessel** The incidence of severe haemorrhage from rupture of a uterine artery increases with the age of the mare. The mare often sweats and shows signs of extreme pain. The mucous membranes quickly become pale and the condition is often fatal.
- **Rupture of the caecum** This may occur due to the high abdominal pressures experienced during foaling.

All of these conditions are emergencies carrying a high risk of mare mortality. Fortunately their incidence is relatively uncommon. Retention of foetal membranes, however (see page 604), occurs in 2–10% of all foalings.

Post-foaling checks

Following the safe delivery of a foal, the following checks should be made.

THE FOAL

Most foals are on their feet within an hour of birth (Figure 19.29). The foal should search for the teats and suck vigorously within 2 hours of birth (Figures 19.30a and b). Most foals then suck 5–7 times per hour in the first few days. Veterinary attention should be sought if:

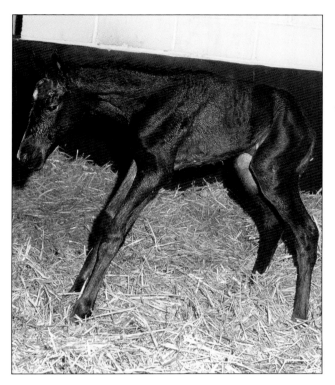

Figure 19.29 First steps: most foals are on their feet within 1 hour of birth

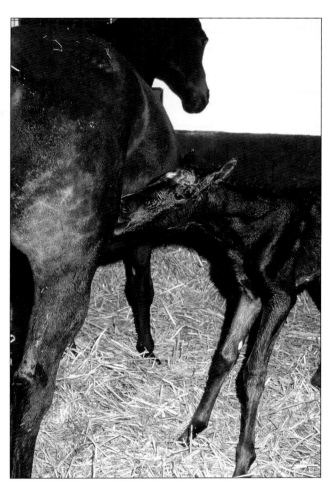

- the foal gives any immediate cause for concern
- it is not standing within 2 hours
- it shows little or no inclination to suck within the first 2 hours following birth.

THE IMPORTANCE OF COLOSTRUM

Colostrum is the thick, yellow liquid in the udder when the foal is born. It contains antibodies that provide protection against infection and must be sucked by the foal within the first few hours of life. If the mare runs milk prior to foaling, this essential protection is lost. Arrangements must be made to find an alternative source of colostrum. Contact your vet for advice. The quality of the colostrum may be checked by your vet using an instrument called a refractometer.

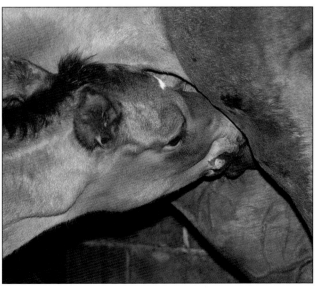

Figures 19.30a and b First feed: a) the foal instinctively searches for the teats; b) the foal should suckle within 2 hours of birth

VETERINARY NEWBORN FOAL CHECKS

A veterinary check of the newborn foal is recommended. Any problems and weaknesses can then be dealt with at once. The vet may give the foal tetanus antitoxin and antibiotic injections and take a blood sample from the foal to measure the IgG levels. This test is used to check whether the foal has received sufficient immunity from the colostrum. The foal's IgG level should ideally be 8 g/litre or above. A level of between 4 and 8 g/litre indicates partial failure of passive transfer (FPT) of immunity and below 4 g/litre means there is total failure. If FPT is diagnosed within the first 12 hours of life, the foal may be given good-quality colostrum. If the foal is more than 12 hours old or no colostrum is available, blood may be taken from the mare and the plasma component given to the foal as a slow intravenous transfusion.

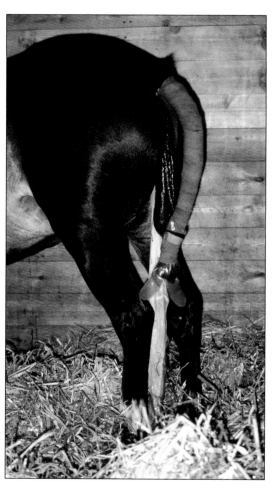

Figure 19.31 Retained placenta

THE PLACENTA

If the foetal membranes have not been expelled within 3 hours of birth, they are considered to be retained (Figure 19.31). This is most likely following abortion, difficulties foaling, twinning or when the mare has a caesarean section. It is important to spread the membranes out to check that they are complete (Figure 19.32). Even a small retained piece can result in serious complications. Bacterial multiplication within the uterus can quickly lead to septicaemia and endotoxaemia, with a potentially fatal result. Severe laminitis is a possible sequel.

If the membranes are retained, the first line of treatment is to give the mare small doses of oxytocin by injection at regular intervals. Any membranes hanging from the mare are tied up above her hocks to prevent them from becoming torn and contaminated. Gentle walking exercise may be helpful. If this fails to work or the mare had an assisted delivery, the uterus can be infused with sterile saline. This often promotes expulsion of the membranes, together with any uterine contaminants.

Manual removal may be attempted by your vet who will take great care not to tear the placenta and leave a piece inside the mare. Excessive pulling on the membranes increases the risk of uterine prolapse. After 2 days, the attachment weakens and in some cases, manual removal can be accomplished safely.

If the mare retains her membranes longer than 6 hours, the vet will usually administer systemic antibiotics and flunixin meglumine to control bacterial growth and combat

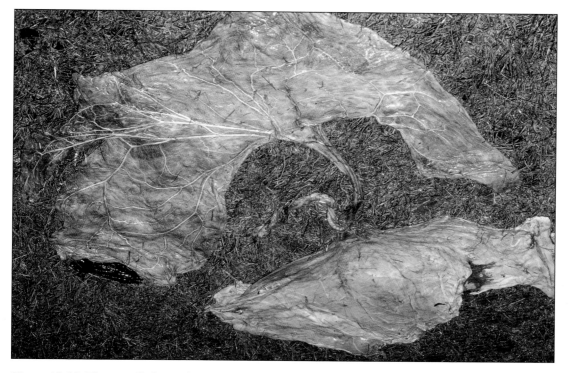

Figure 19.32 The expelled membranes should be laid out to check that they are complete

endotoxaemia. If she develops a temperature and becomes obviously ill, the uterus is flushed and intravenous fluids are administered. Frog supports may be applied in some cases because of the risk of laminitis with possible rotation and/or sinking of the pedal bone.

Summary

- Within 1 hour the foal should stand.
- Within 2 hours the foal should suckle.
- Within 3 hours the placenta should be passed. It this has not occurred within 6 hours, it is potentially a serious problem.

20
ENDOCRINE DISORDERS

EQUINE CUSHING'S DISEASE (ECD)

Equine Cushing's disease is a syndrome caused either by enlargement (hyperplasia) or a benign tumour (adenoma) of the pars intermedia of the anterior lobe of the pituitary gland which is situated at the base of the brain (Figure 20.1). These cause increased production of adrenocortitrophic hormone (ACTH) which is released into the bloodstream and stimulates the adrenal glands to produce cortisol. The condition develops slowly and the symptoms which develop due to the raised cortisol levels and pressure on adjacent parts of the brain are slowly progressive.

In a normal horse, secretion of hormones from the pars intermedia is controlled by a neurotransmitter called dopamine which is released by nerve endings in the hypothalamus. The disease is usually seen in older animals, generally over 15 years of age. For reasons that are currently unknown, aged horses and ponies affected by Cushing's syndrome have less dopamine production, allowing overactivity of the pars intermedia of the pituitary gland. The pars intermedia enlarges and occasionally an adenoma forms. Ponies appear to be more susceptible than horses and the disease also occurs in donkeys.

Clinical signs
These include:
- delayed shedding of a long and uneven hair coat
- growing a long curly coat of coarse hair that is not shed in summer (Figures 20.2a, b and c)
- poor temperature control and increased sweating
- lethargy
- drinking more than usual
- passing more urine than normal
- a good appetite but loss of condition
- loss of muscle tissue along the top line giving the horse a sway-backed appearance

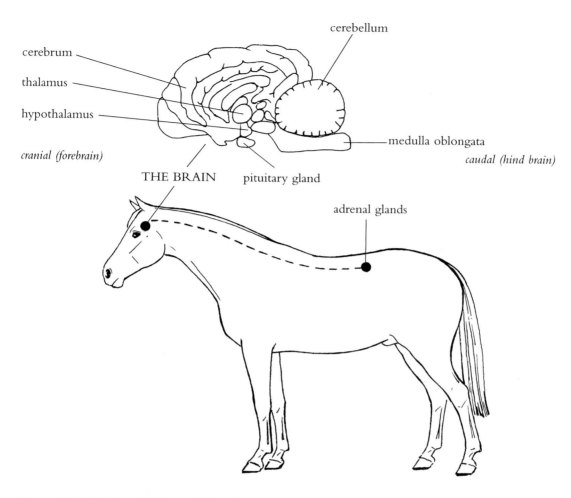

Figure 20.1 The horse's brain and the adrenal glands; it is the overproduction of cortisol by the adrenal glands as a result of pituitary gland enlargement or a tumour that is responsible for many of the symptoms which typify Cushing's disease

- a rather pendulous abdomen due to weakness and wasting of the abdominal muscles (the animal appears pot-bellied)
- recurrent attacks of laminitis
- poor healing and increased susceptibility to parasitic disease and infection, e.g. dental, skin and foot infections
- abnormal fat deposits above or around the eye.

In the early stages of the disease, affected horses and ponies are usually bright and appear to feel well in themselves. As the disease progresses, they may be affected by:
- progressive muscle weakness
- laminitis
- blindness (rare)
- seizures (rare).

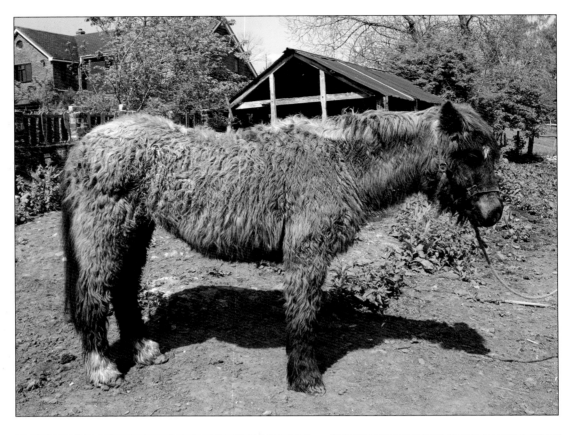

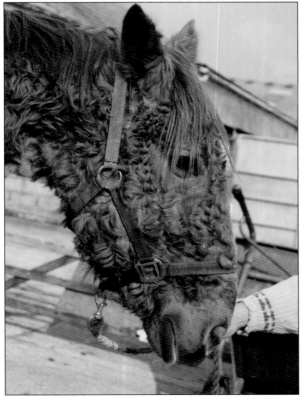

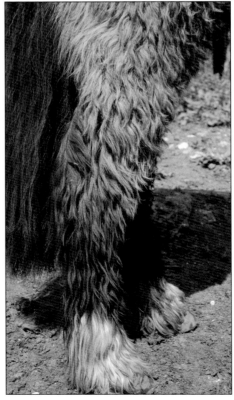

Diagnosis

Diagnosis is usually made on the history and clinical signs and a number of laboratory tests are used to aid confirmation of the diagnosis. Commonly used tests include the following.

- The low-dose dexamethasone suppression test. In this test a low dose of the corticosteroid dexamethasone is injected intramuscularly. A blood sample is taken immediately before and between 18 and 24 hours after injection and the cortisol levels of the two samples are measured. The administration of dexamethasone leads to suppression of cortisol output in normal horses, but has less effect on those with Cushing's disease. This is the most sensitive and accurate test for diagnosing Cushing's disease. There is some concern that this test could trigger laminitis in cushingoid horses; this very rarely occurs.

- Measurement of ACTH, cortisol, insulin and glucose levels in the blood first thing in the morning after the horse has been stabled and not given any food overnight. However, while ACTH measurements may be useful, cortisol and glucose measurements are less reliable. Insulin levels are raised in horses and ponies with ECD, but increased levels also occur in obese laminitic animals without ECD.

Haematology is not generally useful in the diagnosis of Cushing's syndrome. There may be a raised white cell count due to chronic infection.

Treatment
MANAGEMENT

The following management changes can significantly improve the horse's quality of life.

- Clipping the coat to reduce the sweating and aid thermoregulation.
- Providing shelter once it has been clipped.
- Modifying the diet to reduce the occurrence of laminitis while maintaining adequate protein and micronutrient (vitamin and mineral) levels. The diet should be based on forage and fibre feeds, avoiding cereals high in starch and sugars.
- Regular worming, vaccination, dental checks and hoof care.

MEDICATION

Treatment is expensive and must be given for the rest of the horse's life. There are four different medications currently in use.

- Pergolide (acts by increasing production of dopamine).
- Bromocriptine (increases dopamine production).
- Trilostane (acts by inhibiting steroid synthesis).
- Cyproheptadine (inhibits ACTH production from the pars intermedia).

Figures 20.2a, b and c The three photos show the distinctive curly coat associated with Cushing's disease

An improvement in the coat and a reduction in drinking and urination are usually seen within 3 weeks of starting medication. Treatment does not completely halt the progression of the disease but it can lessen the clinical signs and improve the animal's quality of life. Advanced cases are less likely to respond to treatment.

A trial is in progress to assess the effects of plant extract of *Vitex agnus castus* (Chasteberry, Monk's Pepper) on horses and ponies with Cushing's disease.

Prognosis

The disease cannot be cured. It often develops slowly over a period of several years. Treatment may extend or improve the horse's quality of life but medication is expensive and once started must be maintained. Many affected horses and ponies are able to live comfortably with good management for at least a couple of years. Ultimately, recurrent bouts of laminitis or infection are likely to necessitate euthanasia.

Cushing's disease is still not fully understood and is the subject of current research. Your vet will be able to inform you of any new developments in our understanding and treatment of this disease.

EQUINE METABOLIC SYNDROME (EMS) (PERIPHERAL CUSHINGOID SYNDROME)

Equine metabolic syndrome (EMS) is a complex and as yet poorly understood condition that is seen mainly in ponies and donkeys. It occurs in animals that are overfed and have insufficient exercise. The condition is most commonly seen in animals of 6 years of age and older.

Clinical signs

These include the following.

- The accumulation of large deposits of fat on the crest of the neck, over the shoulders and loins, at the head of the tail, in front of the udder or sheath and in the abdomen.
- Lethargy.
- Susceptibility to laminitis which may be insidious in onset. Chronic changes, e.g. divergent growth lines and widening of the white line may occur in the absence of obvious pain or lameness. Rotation and remodelling of the pedal bone may be seen on radiographs.
- Abnormal oestrus cycles in mares.

How does the disease occur?

When ponies have plenty to eat and large deposits of fat build up within the abdomen, the fat cells begin to secrete a number of hormones known as **adipokines**. These hormones which include cortisol affect the metabolism of the animal so they become resistant to the effects of insulin. Insulin is a hormone secreted by the pancreas. Following a feed, it helps to keep the blood sugar levels stable by assisting tissues such as muscle and the liver to take glucose up from the blood. If a horse is insulin resistant, the serum levels of glucose become abnormally high. This stimulates the production of more insulin, thus the insulin resistant pony has high blood levels of both glucose and insulin.

In the wild, animals such as Shetland ponies are thought to experience a short-term insulin resistance in order to cope with the harsh winters. During the summer, when food is plentiful, the animals build up body fat and gradually enter a state of insulin resistance. As food becomes scarce during the winter, the ponies benefit because the limited circulating glucose remains available for the brain and the lining of blood vessels that rely on it as an energy source, rather than being taken up by muscles. As the ponies lose weight and fat towards the spring, they become responsive to insulin again.

If, however, these ponies do not lose weight due to an abundant supply of food all year round, they enter a state of chronic insulin resistance with high circulating levels of glucose and insulin. The altered hormone balance and chronically high serum glucose levels cause constriction of the blood vessels to the feet and other harmful changes, e.g. an increased tendency for blood clots to form, which contribute to the development of laminitis.

Diagnosis

There is no specific test for EMS. However, when blood tests show a mild to moderate increase in serum glucose and high serum insulin levels after overnight fasting this supports a diagnosis made on the clinical signs. The results have to be interpreted with care as the stress response to painful conditions such as laminitis includes raised cortisol, insulin and glucose levels. Thus the test is only useful if the horse is pain free at the time it is performed (otherwise it is not possible to tell whether the high insulin and glucose caused the laminitis or is a response to it). Your vet may suggest further tests, e.g. an oral or intravenous glucose tolerance test to support the diagnosis.

Treatment

The most important treatments are dietary management and exercise.

- Affected animals should be fed on a mixture of hay and straw together with non-molassed sugar beet and small amounts of alfalfa. These feeds are low in calories and high in digestible fibre. Soaking the hay will further reduce the carbohydrates. Your vet will advise you on how much to feed, depending on the animal's body-weight and general health.
- A vitamin and mineral supplement should be added. Antioxidants such as vitamins C and E are beneficial.
- Titbits such as apples and carrots should be avoided or given in small amounts as an occasional treat. Once the pony has the disease, their access to grass should be severely restricted. The pony should only be allowed onto a bare paddock.

- If at all possible, the animal's exercise level should be increased as this is known to increase insulin sensitivity. This is not possible if they have laminitis.
- A number of medical treatments, e.g. trilostane, are used with variable results.
- Supplementation with chromium, magnesium and vanadium is currently being investigated.

Prevention

This is a syndrome that has resulted from domestication of the horse and intensive management of pastures which may have been grown for dairy cows, not ponies. It is possible to buy special grass seed mixes that do not produce lush growth and are much safer for overweight or laminitic horses and ponies. The use of fertilisers should be minimized.

With small ponies, cobs and donkeys one should be aware of the risks and aim to manage the animal's weight. Remember, the disease can be prevented by sensible dietary management.

21
EYE INJURY AND DISEASE

INTRODUCTION

The eyes of a horse are relatively prominent on either side of the head and are therefore susceptible to injury (Figure 21.1). If any abnormality is seen, *consult your vet at once* because early diagnosis and treatment assist healing and minimize the risk of serious complications. A painful eye should be regarded as an emergency.

Examination of an injured eye

If a horse is in obvious discomfort with its eyelids tightly closed, *do not* force them open. By trying to do so you could inadvertently apply sufficient pressure to rupture a severely damaged eye.

Leave the examination to the vet who can use topical anaesthesia, nerve blocks and sedatives to relax the horse and alleviate the discomfort. Once the pain is removed, the horse may open its eye and be more amenable to examination. The upper eyelid can then easily be lifted to view the structures underneath.

In addition to looking for external injuries, the vet will also check the internal structures of the eye (Figure 21.2) with a pen torch and an ophthalmoscope. This part of the examination needs to be carried out in a darkened box. Drops may be instilled into the eye to dilate (open) the pupil so the inside of the eye can be seen in more detail. The vet may carry out a number of other tests depending on the problem being investigated.

Some of the common eye injuries and diseases will now be considered.

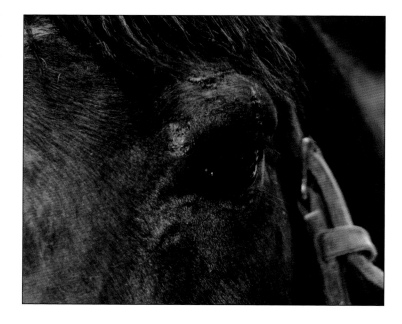

Figure 21.1 A bruised and swollen upper eyelid

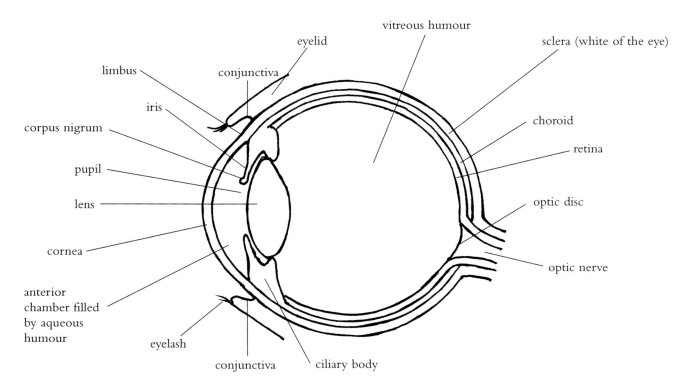

Figure 21.2 Vertical section through a horse's eye

TORN EYELIDS (Figure 21.3)

These require prompt and careful suturing. General anaesthesia may be required to achieve a good repair. If left to heal on their own, the eyelid margins are likely to distort and cause chronic corneal irritation and disease. Failure to treat this type of injury immediately may result in the additional complication of infection or corneal damage due to unaccustomed drying and exposure while the horse is unable to blink normally.

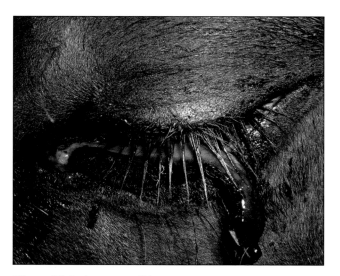

Figure 21.3 A torn eyelid

CORNEAL INJURIES

The cornea is the thick layer of transparent tissue (like a window) at the front of the eye. It is very susceptible to injury from thorns, twigs and barbed wire. Corneal injuries are prone to secondary infection by bacteria and fungi which can cause the development of deep, non-healing **ulcers** or

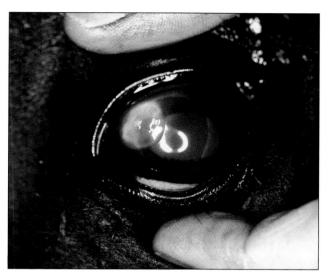
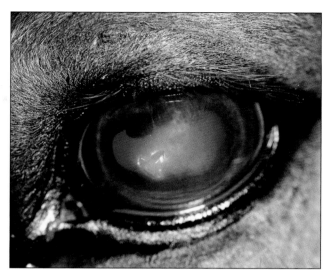

Figures 21.4a and b a) corneal ulcer; b) corneal abscess: a green dye has been applied to the eye

abscesses (Figures 21.4a and b). Inflammation of the cornea is known as **keratitis**. It can be caused by direct injury, chemical irritants, bacterial, fungal or viral infection.

Clinical signs

The clinical signs will include some of the following.

- Pain. The horse often keeps its eyelids tightly closed (Figure 21.5). This is known as blepharospasm.
- Photophobia. The horse squints and avoids bright light, being much more comfortable in a darkened environment.
- Profuse tear production. If secondary bacterial infection develops, the discharge becomes purulent.
- Cloudy, grey-white areas of oedema in the cornea (Figure 21.6).
- Irregularities on the normally smooth corneal surface. These can be small superficial lesions or more serious, deep ulcers (Figure 21.7).
- Foreign bodies embedded in the cornea.
- Blood vessels growing in from the corneal margin.
- The conjunctiva may be inflamed.

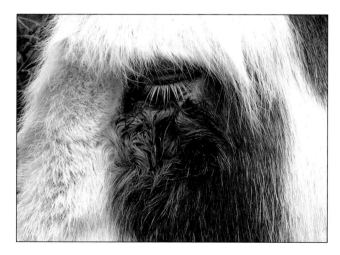

Diagnosis

Diagnosis is made following a thorough examination of the eye. Some corneal injuries are readily observed but very tiny ulcers or abrasions show up more

Figure 21.5 This donkey is keeping its injured eye tightly closed

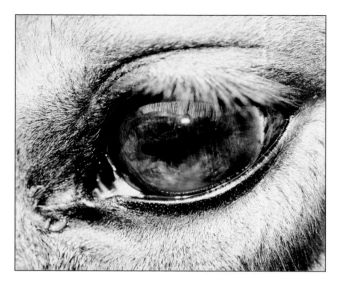

Figure 21.6 Corneal oedema

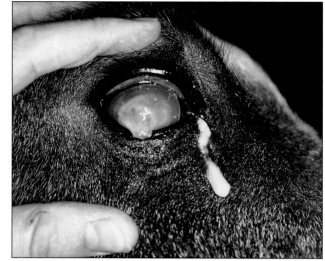

Figure 21.7 A deep melting ulcer

clearly following the application of various coloured dyes which stain them green or pink (Figure 21.8). The appearance of the lesion can be suggestive of the cause but swabs, scrapings or biopsies are necessary for confirmation of the diagnosis with deep or non-healing ulcers. The material can be examined under the microscope to detect the presence and type of bacteria or fungi. Antibiotic sensitivity testing is performed following culture of any bacteria.

Treatment

Topical medication is applied as directed by the vet. The type of medication depends on the nature of the lesion. In straightforward cases a minor injury will resolve following a few days of the appropriate antibiotic drops or ointment. However, other cases require aggressive and intensive therapy. Unfortunately some ulcers are very slow to heal and can be a source of much frustration to both the owner and the treating vet. Treatment may include the following.

- Removal of any foreign material.
- Topical antibacterial, antifungal or antiviral drugs.
- Topical anticollagenases in cases where bacterial infections are causing the cornea to liquefy or 'melt'.
- Topical non-steroidal anti-inflammatory drops or ointment.
- Topical atropine to dilate the pupil and prevent the iris adhering to the lens. This can happen if the iris is inflamed and the pupil is tightly constricted.
- Antibiotics or an antifungal drug may be injected underneath the conjunctiva from where they are slowly released.
- Systemic non-steroidal anti-inflammatory medication is often used to reduce the pain and settle the inflammation within the eye. Flunixin meglumine (Finadyne™) is the drug of choice.

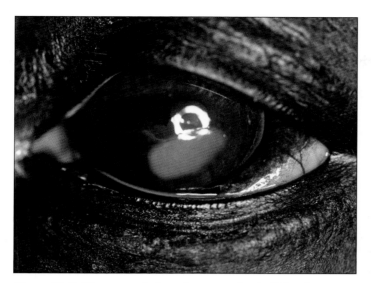

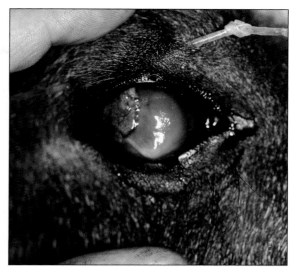

Figure 21.8 The corneal ulcer shows up clearly following application of a coloured dye (flourescein)

Figure 21.9 Pedicle graft: a flap of conjunctiva has been sutured over the ulcer

- In some cases, surgery is indicated. With superficial ulcers that fail to heal, the damaged epithelium is removed (debrided) so healing can begin.
- If the ulceration is severe, a pedicle of conjunctiva may be sutured over the debrided area of cornea (Figure 21.9).
- The third eyelid may be sutured across the cornea for protection or the eyelids may be temporarily sutured together.
- Another option for some corneal conditions is the use of an equine contact lens to act as a bandage over the damaged eye.

Warning

Never treat a painful eye with drops or ointment that was not specifically prescribed for the horse following a veterinary examination. Some ointments contain corticosteroids which delay healing and leave the eye vulnerable to serious secondary infections. The eye may never recover from inappropriate treatment and have to be removed.

Stable management

The horse should be kept in a darkened box and the environment should be as dust-free as possible. Soaked hay should be fed from the floor.

Prognosis

Superficial injuries that are correctly treated and managed usually heal within a few days. The prognosis for bacterial and fungal infections of the cornea is guarded. Deep ulcers take much longer to heal and may leave a scar. In some cases the infection perforates the cornea resulting in collapse of the eye. In this situation the prognosis for the eye is hopeless and it must be surgically removed (enucleated).

CONJUNCTIVITIS

Conjunctivitis is inflammation of the conjunctiva. The conjunctiva is the moist, pink mucous membrane that lines the eyelids and covers the third eyelid. It also attaches to the sclera (white part) of the eye. The healthy conjunctiva is moist and salmon pink in appearance. Conjunctivitis is the commonest disease of the horse's eye.

Causes

There are numerous causes of conjunctivitis. They include:

- bacterial infections
- systemic viral disease, e.g. equine viral arteritis, equine herpesvirus, equine influenza
- physical irritants, e.g. wind, dust, flies, chemical irritants, bright sunlight
- allergy, e.g. to pollen
- trauma
- foreign bodies
- eyelid deformities or tumours
- parasites, e.g. *Habronema, Onchocerca*
- conjunctival tumours, e.g. squamous cell carcinoma.

Conjunctivitis can also occur secondary to other eye diseases, e.g. keratitis and uveitis.

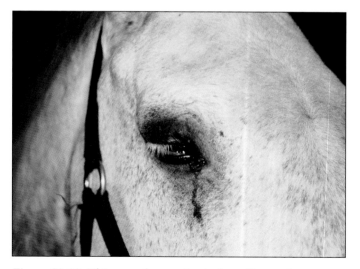

Figure 21.10 This pony has conjuctival swelling and tear overflow, and the eye is nearly closed because of the pain

Clinical signs

The condition may affect one or both eyes depending on the cause. The symptoms usually include:

- pain
- a tendency to keep the eye half closed
- conjunctival swelling due to oedema
- increased tear production; the tears often overflow and run down the horse's cheeks especially if the nasolacrimal ducts become blocked as a result of the conjunctivitis (Figure 21.10)
- a thick yellow discharge if bacterial infection is present (Figure 21.11)

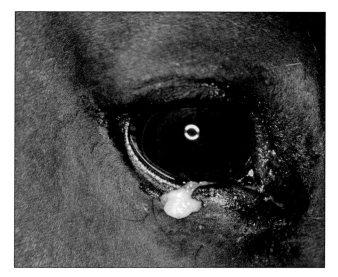

Figure 21.11 With conjunctivitis, the discharge may become thick and yellow

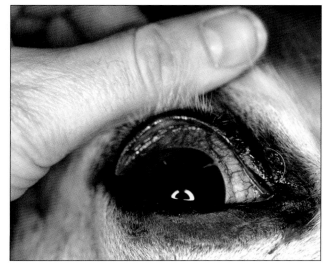

Figure 21.12 Inflamed conjunctiva

- inflammation of the conjunctiva which appears red with numerous small blood vessels clearly visible (Figure 21.12)
- possible development of follicles of lymphoid tissue.

Diagnosis

The diagnosis is made on the clinical signs. If the horse is obviously suffering from a respiratory virus, then that is likely to be the cause. In other cases, the conjunctival sac is thoroughly explored to rule out the presence of a tumour or foreign body. Swabs may be taken for bacterial culture and sensitivity. Scrapings or biopsies may be taken for examination of the cells and tissues where considered necessary. A coloured dye is often used to exclude the possibility of a corneal injury.

Treatment

The treatment depends on the cause of the conjunctivitis.

Viral infections tend to resolve spontaneously as the horse recovers from the virus.

Bacterial infections require topical antibiotics several times a day.

Allergic conjunctivitis responds to topical corticosteroids and removing the horse from the source of the problem if it can be identified.

Parasitic disease requires systemic treatment with moxidectin or ivermectin.

Habronema **lesions** are surgically removed.

Foreign bodies are removed and any resultant infection or inflammation is treated.

Tumours are identified from the biopsy results and treatment depends on their type.

In all cases, protection from physical irritants such as dust, wind and flies is an important part of the treatment. Flushing of the nasolacrimal duct is beneficial if it is partially or totally obstructed.

CATARACTS

A cataract is any opacity of the lens or its capsule. It may be small and non-progressive, causing little, if any, impairment of vision. Other cataracts are progressive. They affect the horse's sight and eventually lead to blindness.

Causes
Cataracts may be:
- congenital (i.e. present at birth), possibly due to problems such as infection, poor nutrition or exposure to toxins while the foal was developing in the uterus (Figure 21.13a)
- hereditary: in some breeds these may be present at birth or develop by three years of age
- acquired as a result of injury or disease (Figure 21.13b),
- the result of ageing changes
- unilateral (affecting one eye) or bilateral (both eyes).

Clinical signs
Horses with small, non-progressive cataracts show no clinical signs. Many of these are only discovered when the horse is vetted for a prospective purchaser. Where cataracts are causing a progressive loss of sight, the signs include:

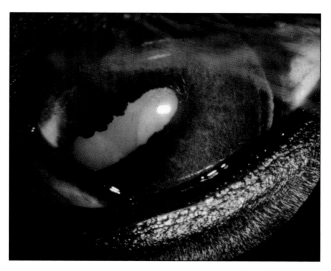

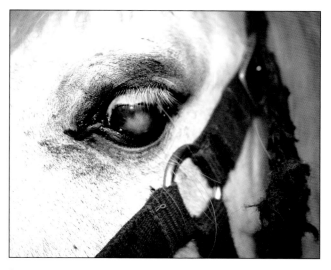

a   b

Figure 21.13a and b a) A congenital cataract in a Clydesdale foal; b) This pony has a dense cataract and corneal changes due to recurrent uveitis; the eye has also become smaller

- stumbling
- walking into objects
- an abnormal number of facial injuries
- an alteration in head carriage
- sudden shying
- uncharacteristic anxiety and jumpiness
- a greyish-white colour in the normally clear lens.

Diagnosis

Diagnosis is made by examination of the eye with an ophthalmoscope. Advanced cataracts can be seen with the naked eye as the lens becomes opaque. Certain types of cataracts are more likely to be progressive than others. Progression can only be confirmed by serial examinations over a period of time.

Treatment

There is no medical treatment that will reduce the lens opacity or halt the progression of cataracts. In carefully selected cases, e.g. some young foals with congenital cataracts, surgical removal may restore vision. Artificial lenses have now been developed for horses and it is hoped that with improved instruments, lens replacement will become a possibility for selected cases in the future.

Prognosis

The prognosis is good for small, non-progressive cataracts that have little effect on the horse's vision. With progressive cataracts the prognosis is poor. When the cataract occurs secondary to inflammatory changes within the eye, e.g. recurrent uveitis, the prognosis is guarded. Animals with hereditary cataracts should not be used for breeding.

EQUINE UVEITIS

When a horse has uveitis, the iris, ciliary body and the choroid (collectively known as the uveal tract), become inflamed.

Causes

Uveitis can occur as a result of:
- bacterial or viral infection
- a blow to the head
- injuries to, or penetrations of, the cornea
- tumours within the eye
- parasites, e.g. *Toxoplasma*, larvae of *Onchocerca cervicalis*.

In some cases the condition may arise due to a reaction of the immune system to bacteria, viruses or parasites. Alternatively, uveitis can be an autoimmune disease whereby an immune response is mounted against the horse's own tissues.

The treatment in every case is aimed at controlling the pain and preserving the horse's vision by preventing long-term damage to the eye.

EQUINE RECURRENT UVEITIS

Equine recurrent uveitis is a serious disease that can affect one or both eyes. It is also known as **periodic ophthalmia** and **moon blindness**. The name 'recurrent uveitis' arose because the disease has intermittent acute flare-ups between apparently 'normal' periods. It is now believed that in many horses the inflammation is continuous and persists at a low level between the acute flare-ups. This is known as equine persistent uveitis. The severity of clinical signs differs between different cases and between attacks. Fortunately the disease is not very common in the UK.

Causes

Equine recurrent uveitis is a syndrome that has a number of different causes. In some countries including Germany and the USA, it is associated with infection by *Leptospira spp.* bacteria. It may also be triggered by any of the causes listed on page 621. In many cases, there is no obvious cause. The condition is still poorly understood but is thought to be mediated by the immune system.

Clinical signs

These can develop very quickly over a period of hours.

They may include:

- pain
- a tightly closed eye
- increased discomfort in bright light (known as photophobia)
- increased tear production
- cloudiness of the cornea (due to corneal oedema)
- constriction of the pupil (known as miosis)
- a dark and dull appearance of the iris which never regains its former colour
- a red conjunctiva and sclera due to engorgement of tiny blood vessels
- swelling of the eyelid
- a hazy appearance of the aqueous humour
- a slight decrease in the pressure within the eyeball
- some affected horses feel very miserable and depressed.

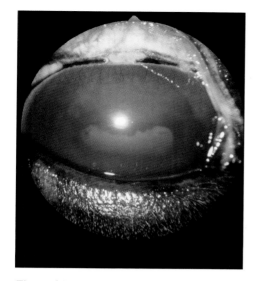

Figure 21.14 Acute equine recurrent uveitis: note the cloudiness of the cornea, constricted pupil and small blood vessels growing in from the corneal margin

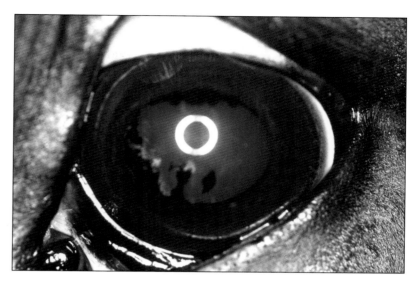

Figure 21.15 This horse with equine recurrent uveitis is in a quiescent phase between acute flare-ups; the iris is uniformly dull in colour and pigmented deposits can be seen on the anterior lens capsule

After a few days:

- small blood vessels may be seen in the cornea
- a collection of white blood cells and protein may be seen in the anterior chamber (hypopyon).

(Figures 21.14 and 21.15.)

Diagnosis

Diagnosis is made on the clinical signs. The vet will want to know about any previous health or eye problems the horse has experienced. Sedation and nerve blocks may be necessary for safe and thorough examination of the eye. Blood tests may be taken at the start of the condition and again two weeks later to look for antibodies to *Leptospira spp*.

Treatment

Treatment should be aggressive and immediate if the damage occurring within the eye is to be minimized. It is likely to include the following.

- Atropine drops are administered hourly until the pupil dilates (opens). This is necessary as the inflamed iris can become stuck to the front of the lens while the pupil is constricted.
- Corticosteroids may be given topically and/or by injection to reduce the inflammation. In some cases they are injected underneath the conjunctiva. Corticosteroids are not given if the cornea is ulcerated or active infection is present.
- Systemic non-steroidal anti-inflammatory drugs (NSAIDs) are used to help control the pain and inflammation. The drug of choice is flunixin meglumine. Once the inflammation is under control, treatment may be continued with phenylbutazone.

- Cyclosporine A, an immunosuppressive drug is now being used in the treatment of recurrent uveitis. It is not well absorbed when applied to the cornea so implants have been developed. These are placed in the eye through a small incision and they release the drug slowly for 5 years. The results so far are encouraging with reports of fewer attacks and those attacks that do occur are less severe than previous episodes.
- Antibiotics may be administered topically and systemically if there is damage to the cornea or bacterial infection is present.

Management

- The horse should be kept in a darkened box as light increases the pain, especially when the pupil has been dilated with atropine. The darkness encourages the pupil to dilate naturally.
- The food and bedding should be kept as dust free as possible to minimize further irritation of the eye and the risk of fungal infection. Hay should be soaked and fed from the floor.
- Ocular discharge should be regularly cleaned off the cheeks. Vaseline may be applied to prevent the skin becoming sore.
- Protective blinkers may prevent the horse rubbing its eye(s) and causing further damage (Figure 21.16)
- The horse should not be worked.

The course of the disease

The inflammation usually lasts for 7–10 days. The interval between episodes may be weeks, months or years. In many cases the inflammation never really subsides, just quietly persists. These horses may benefit from long-term or permanent medication provided there is no reason why this is inadvisable for a particular animal.

With each attack, further degenerative changes occur within the eye. The changes include the following.

- There is a gradual reduction in intra-ocular pressure and the eyeball becomes smaller.
- Retinal degeneration and cataract formation cause a progressive loss of sight.
- In some cases, the iris does not dilate fully despite the administration of atropine. The pupil margin becomes irregular in outline as parts of the iris remain attached to the lens. Pigmented deposits can be seen on the anterior lens capsule.
  (Figure 21.17.)

Prognosis

In general, the prognosis is guarded to poor. It depends on the cause, the frequency and severity of episodes and how promptly the treatment is given. Early recognition of the signs is very important. Once the diagnosis is established, the vet may leave emergency treatment with you for subsequent episodes. However, it is important that the horse is

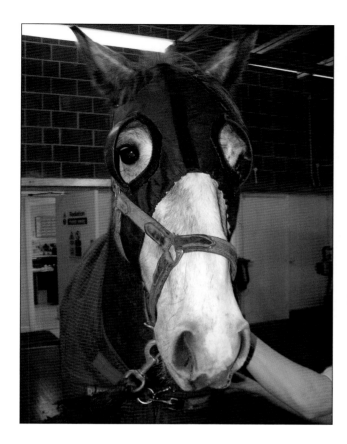

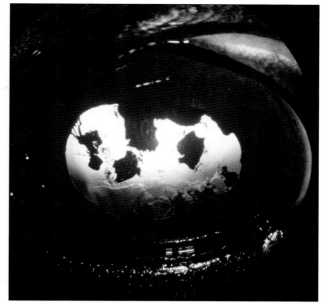

Figure 21.16 Protective blinkers (left)

Figure 21.17 Chronic uveitis: following recurrent episodes of the disease, the pupil is an irregular shape and there are multiple pigmented deposits on the anterior lens capsule (above)

examined promptly by the vet every time to check that there is no other injury to the eye.

The disease is unpredictable and a source of severe misery and discomfort. If the inflammation is not adequately controlled by the medication and the horse is in permanent discomfort, the eye can be removed.

THE PARTIALLY-SIGHTED HORSE

Sight may be lost because of a cataract or other eye conditions such as glaucoma or severe recurrent uveitis. It may also be lost following a serious injury or if the eye has to be removed to prevent the spread of a tumour (Figures 21.18 and 21.19). These horses require careful management to minimize the potential for hurting themselves or their handlers. For example:

- partially-sighted horses should be approached and handled with particular care so that they are not startled
- they should not be tied near projecting objects
- the field should be checked for low branches or obstacles that could cause injury
- affected horses may feel more comfortable turned out with a single companion rather than as part of a large group.

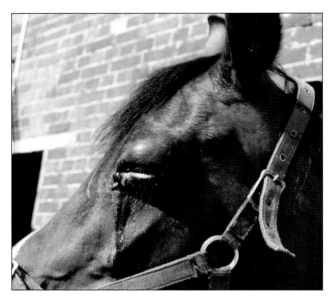

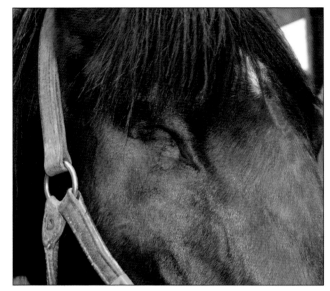

Figure 21.18 Ruptured eye immediately prior to surgery

Figure 21.19 This mare is now retired to stud following removal of one eye

The horse may find it easier to adjust if the loss of sight is gradual rather than sudden. Provided they are of a sensible disposition, one-eyed horses are capable of many activities.

> **Warning**
> When there is loss of vision or complete blindness in one eye, the other eye must be regularly checked for any sign of disease.

MEDICATING THE EYE

There are 3 routinely used methods of administering drugs to horses needing medical treatment for eye conditions.

1   Topical. Drops, gels or ointments are applied directly onto the cornea or into the conjunctival sac.
2   Systemic. Drugs are given orally or by intramuscular or intravenous injection.
3   Subconjunctival injection. A small volume of medication such as antibiotic or cortico-steroid may be injected into the conjunctiva. This ensures high therapeutic levels of the drug in the cornea and the front of the eye. It can be used as an adjunct to topical therapy or occasionally as an alternative if the latter is difficult.

How to apply eye ointment or drops
The treatment of many eye injuries and diseases involves frequent application of drops, gels or ointments. This is not always easy if the eye is sore and the horse is uncooperative.

Inexpert or careless technique can frighten the horse and cause further damage. The following tips may help.

1   First wash your hands.

2   In cold weather, warm the ointment to body temperature as this makes it easier to apply.

3   If at all possible, have an assistant to hold the horse.

4   Gently wipe any discharge away using moist cotton wool.

5   Remove the top and hold the tube in your right hand (or the left hand if left-handed). Squeeze the tube until the ointment can be seen at the nozzle.

6   Position the hand so that it rests against the horse's cheek (Figure 21.20).

7   With the fingers and thumb of your other hand, gently evert (turn out) the lower eyelid. Do not apply unnecessary force or pressure to the eyeball.

8   Squeeze a line of ointment or the required number of drops into the exposed conjunctival sac. It is often easiest to apply it at the medial corner of the eye (Figure 21.21).

With your hand fixed against the horse's cheek, there is less danger of the nozzle poking the eye as your hand will follow any sudden movement of the horse's head.

HYGIENE GUIDELINES

- Always wash your hands before applying treatment.
- Ensure the nozzle of the tube or syringe is not contaminated with dirt or discharge.
- Use a separate tube for each horse to avoid cross infection.
- Throw away any partly used tubes when the condition has resolved. All medication must be used within a month of the tube being opened.

The use of ocular lavage systems

When frequent medication is needed over a period of time, the horse often becomes

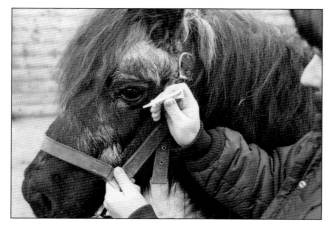

Figure 21.20 Rest your hand against the horse's cheek when applying eye ointment

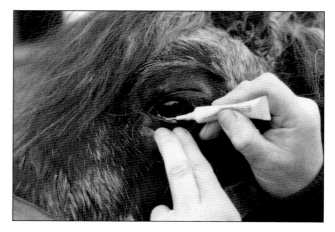

Figure 21.21 Evert the lower eyelid and squeeze the ointment into the conjuctival sac

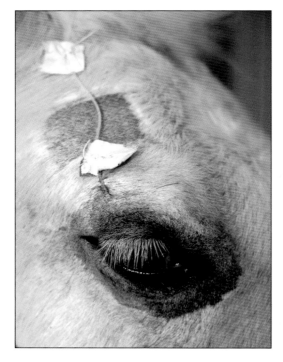

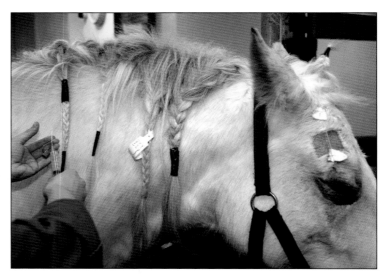

Figure 21.22 Subpalpebral lavage system: a catheter is passed through the eyelid and sutured in place (left)

Figure 21.23 Medication is introduced through a syringe, avoiding the need to handle the eye (above)

fractious and resentful. It is much easier for all concerned if a subpalpebral lavage or nasolacrimal duct irrigation system is fitted.

SUBPALPEBRAL LAVAGE SYSTEM

With this system, medication is administered through a purpose-designed catheter passed through the eyelid and sutured in place (Figure 21.22). The long, free end of the catheter is sutured at intervals as is passes backwards between the ears and along the neck. The medication can either be introduced through a syringe (Figure 21.23) or the end of the tube may be attached to a continuous drip or pump system.

INDWELLING NASOLACRIMAL CANNULA

The nasolacrimal duct runs from the inner corner of the eye to an opening on the floor of the nostril. Its function is to drain excess tear film from the eyes. With the horse sedated, the end of the cannula is passed through a small incision in

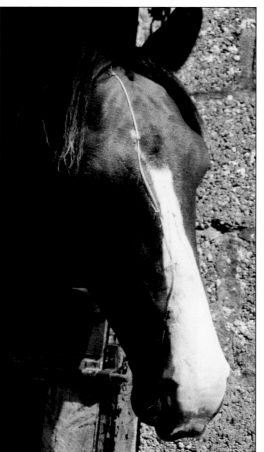

Figure 21.24 Indwelling nasolacrimal cannula

the skin of the false nostril. It is gently slid into the nasal opening of the duct and sutured in place. The remaining length of the tubing is sutured at intervals along the face and neck. Medication can then be introduced without any handling of the eye. (Figure 21.24.)

A head and neck cover made from comfortable stretch material can be used to prevent the tubing catching on projections and being pulled out. Both of these systems are usually well-tolerated by the horse.

Contact lenses

Contacts lenses are sometimes used to protect the cornea following an injury. They protect the cornea from dust and from drying out. Medicated lenses are sometimes used as a temporary, emergency treatment.

TUMOURS AFFECTING THE EYE

Sarcoids, squamous cell carcinomas and melanomas are the tumours that most commonly affect the eye and the surrounding tissues.

Diagnosis

It is important to make an accurate diagnosis so that the most appropriate treatment can be given. A diagnosis is made after consideration of the following.

- A thorough examination of the whole horse. For example, horses with sarcoids around their eyes often have them elsewhere on the body.
- Any predisposing factors, e.g. melanomas are common in grey horses and the incidence increases with the age of the horse. Horses with non-pigmented skin are susceptible to squamous cell carcinomas of the eyelid, conjunctiva and on the eye itself.
- The appearance of the tumour.
- The results of a biopsy sample.
- Ultrasonography can be helpful for determining the extent of tumours within and behind the eyeball.
- Squamous cell carcinomas often present with a characteristic cream-coloured ocular discharge. If a urine dipstick is used to test the tears of these horses, blood is sometimes detected.

Treatment

Most of the tumours that affect the horse's eye are slow growing. Unfortunately, they are often left until they have reached an advanced stage before veterinary attention is sought. The treatment options are determined by the type of tumour, its size and location. In each case the aim of treatment is to eliminate the tumour while preserving the eyelid and the function of the eye.

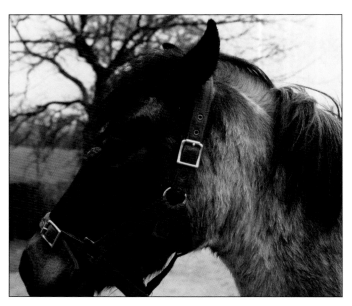

Figure 21.25 This pony's sarcoid was successfully treated with BCG vaccine injections

Treatment is also influenced by the facilities available as some treatments can only take place at specialist centres. The cost can be an important consideration.

The appearance and treatment of each of the commonest tumour types will now be considered in more detail.

Sarcoids

All 6 types of sarcoid, i.e. occult, verrucose, fibroblastic, nodular, mixed and malevolent (malignant) are found around the horse's eye. In this site they can be highly invasive and widespread, possibly due to the inoculation of tumour cells into adjacent sites by feeding flies. (Figure 21.25.)

TREATMENT OPTIONS

These include the following.

- Nodular and fibroblastic sarcoids around the eye often respond well to injections of the human BCG vaccine into the tumour. The injection is repeated after 1 week, then 2 weeks later, then 3 weeks later and so on, with the injection interval extended by 1 week each time until the lesion regresses. Between 3 and 7 injections are usually required. These injections stimulate the horse's immune system to reject the tumour tissue as part of the immune response to the vaccine. One drawback of the treatment is the risk of anaphylactic shock. The horse is usually pre-medicated to reduce this risk and kept under close observation following treatment.

- Injection into the lesion or topical application of chemotherapeutic agents.

- Radiation therapy is successfully used in the treatment of nodular and fibroblastic periocular sarcoids. Radioactive wires are implanted in the tissues. This destroys the tumour tissue and causes minimal scarring. However, the treatment may affect the pigment producing cells so the new skin and hair are white. Unfortunately this treatment is costly and carries significant health risks to the people carrying out the treatment. It is only available at specialist centres and is reserved for cases where other treatment has failed or is inappropriate.

- Do nothing, e.g. in cases where the tumour is widespread and malignant. Irradiation may be the only realistic treatment and as discussed above this is expensive and not widely available. Inappropriate interference may make the situation worse.

Squamous cell carcinomas

Squamous cell carcinomas may develop in several sites on and around the eye including the eyelids, conjunctiva, third eyelid, sclera and cornea. (Figure 21.26.) High levels of ultraviolet radiation from sunlight and non-pigmented skin predispose to this type of tumour which often resembles granulation tissue (proud flesh) in appearance. The tumour tissue is raised and slightly knobbly looking, pink in colour and may bleed easily. There may be a mucopurulent discharge from the affected eye.

The risk of developing squamous cell carcinomas can be reduced by keeping susceptible horses out of the sun or turning them out with protective masks Figure 21.27).

TREATMENT OPTIONS

These include the following.

- Chemotherapy. Topical 5-fluorouracil is applied to the tumour through a subpalpebral lavage system. The horse must be hospitalized during treatment periods as the drug is radioactive.
- Surgical excision. This is often combined with topical chemotherapy. If the tumour is large, the bulk of it is surgically removed prior to the commencement of chemotherapy.
- Irradiation.

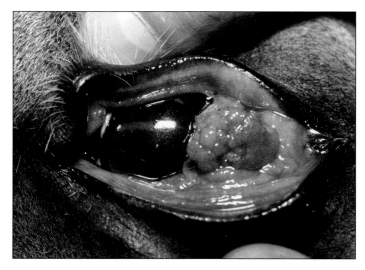

Figure 21.26 Squamous cell carcinoma

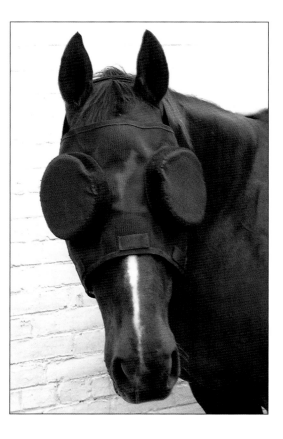

Figure 21.27 Protective mask

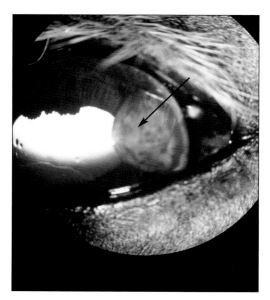

Figure 21.28 Iris melanoma

Melanomas

Melanomas can develop in the iris within the eye where they can be seen with the naked eye as pigmented masses (Figure 21.28). They also occur in the eyelids.

TREATMENT OPTIONS

These include the following.

- Monitoring the tumour and leaving it alone.
- Cimetidine. This is a drug that is given by mouth for a period of 3–6 months. The treatment is expensive and is not universally successful. However, a reduction in size or disappearance of the tumour occurs in some cases.
- Surgical removal of small tumours on the eyelids.
- Surgical removal of the eye if the tumour is causing discomfort or justifies this radical approach.

Prognosis

The prognosis for all tumours of the eye is guarded.

22
BEHAVIOUR PROBLEMS

STEREOTYPIC BEHAVIOUR

Stereotypic behaviour patterns include:
- crib-biting
- wind-sucking
- weaving
- box walking
- rug tearing
- self-mutilation.

In the past, these behaviour patterns have been referred to as stable vices and were attributed to boredom. They are now known to be caused by discomfort, frustration, stress and anxiety. The behaviour characteristically occurs when horses are disturbed, e.g. feeding time, rather than when they are resting quietly.

Stereotypies are repetitive behaviours that have no obvious purpose. However, performing the behaviour pattern has a calming influence on the horse by activation of specific neurophysiological pathways. Punishing the horse has no effect and physical restraints are frequently inhumane.

These behaviour patterns are not acquired by watching other horses perform them. If several horses in a particular yard are affected, this is likely to be because they are all subject to the same management system and routine. Isolation of an affected horse is detrimental to its welfare and only likely to make the problem worse.

The predisposition to develop stereotypic behaviour is hereditary. One study showed that in a particular set of environmental conditions, foals had a 25% chance of developing a stereotypy if neither the mare nor sire were affected. However, if either the mare or the sire showed stereotypic behaviour, this rose to 60%. If both were affected, the foal had almost 90% chance of developing a stereotypy. This often starts at weaning time, probably the result of stress, altered management and dietary factors.

Stereotypic behaviour has not been observed in wild horses; it is a response to the restrictions imposed by domestication.

Causes

Factors that precipitate stereotypic behaviour include:

- stress
- excitement
- frustration
- pain.

Typical situations that occur in stables on a daily basis and may trigger this behaviour include:

- feeding time, especially if the horses anticipate this and become agitated as the first feeds appear
- eating high concentrate, low roughage rations: recent research has shown this to be an important contributory factor as horses in the wild graze for many hours of the day
- stabling horses and denying them the opportunity to express normal behaviour patterns is a source of stress
- other horses in the yard going out on exercise or being turned out
- isolation from other horses
- the introduction of new horses to the stable or field
- any departure from the usual routine
- pain
- being sold.

CRIB-BITING AND WIND-SUCKING

Crib-biting and wind-sucking often occur together. The horse grasps a fixed object with its incisor teeth and contracts the muscles of the underside of the neck (Figure 22.1) This draws the larynx backwards and air is drawn into the upper oesophagus. Contrary to common belief, the air is not swallowed but is expelled. It is the movement of air that produces the characteristic gulping noise made by wind-suckers. Some horses crib without obvious wind-sucking; others can wind-suck without grasping a solid object.

Causes

Crib-biting is associated with:

- high grain and concentrate diets
- little turnout onto pasture
- restricted access to forage.

The above management practices lead to increased gastric acidity and the development of gastric ulcers. The acid is continually produced in the stomach whether the horse eats or not. A horse with restricted forage that has long periods without any food may produce insufficient alkaline saliva to buffer the acid. It may be that crib-biting increases saliva flow and decreases the discomfort caused by severe ulceration, but this has not been proven.

Regular suckling by foals reduces the gastric acidity. Foals often start to crib shortly after weaning. The removal of the opportunity to suckle together with the introduction of high-carbohydrate feeds combine to increase the stomach acidity. This and the stress of weaning may be the stimulus for the onset of crib-biting. Foals that are kept in at weaning are at higher risk than those turned out at pasture.

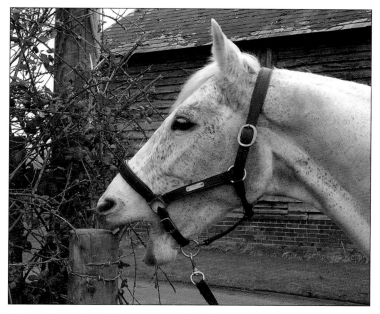

Figure 22.1 Crib-biting and wind-sucking

Clinical signs

In addition to the obvious behaviour pattern, affected horses may show:

- abnormal wear on the incisor teeth (Figure 22.2)
- poor appetite; these horses are often very picky feeders
- weight loss or failure to put on weight
- overdevelopment of the muscles running down the underside of the neck
- gastrointestinal problems, e.g. gastric ulceration.

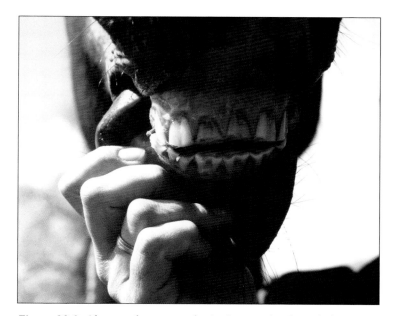

Figure 22.2 Abnormal wear on the incisor teeth of a crib-biter

Diagnosis

The diagnosis is made on the history and clinical signs. Take a video, it may be helpful to show it to your vet.

Treatment
MANAGEMENT

The aim of treatment should be to change the horse's management so that the horse no longer feels the need to perform this type of behaviour. Changes include the following.

- Turning the horse out to graze as much as possible.
- Avoid feeding concentrates wherever possible. If they must be fed, reduce the starch and sugar content.
- Put the feed into the horse's stable before bringing him in from the field. This reduces the period of intense anticipation and anxiety when a number of horses are fed together.
- Gradually increase the forage content of the diet. Ideally the horse should have access to forage at all times. If it needs to be restricted, the consumption can be slowed by using nets with small holes or by putting one hay net inside another.
- Make sure the horse is able to interact normally with other horses. The horse should be turned out with a small group of others with whom he feels safe and comfortable.
- Grilles can be placed in partitions between stables allowing visual contact with other horses. Partitions which allow physical contact between adjacent horses are beneficial provided the horse is happy with its neighbour. Anxious horses sometimes respond well to being moved to another stable with a new neighbour.
- Horses are social animals and should not be kept in isolation. Provision of a companion is important.
- A stable mirror can help in some cases.
- When a horse persists in cribbing and wind-sucking, it is a good idea to provide a suitable surface to reduce the wear on the teeth and the risk of splinters. A bar of wood, covered by rubber matting is ideal. It should be positioned close to the manger at chest height.

MEDICAL TREATMENT
- Where gastric ulceration is a problem, the use of drugs to treat the ulcers is recommended.
- Various drugs have been tried to influence the neurophysiological pathways involved in stereotypic behaviour. However, more work needs to be done.

TREATMENTS THAT PHYSICALLY PREVENT CRIBBING BEHAVIOUR
These practices do nothing to address the underlying problem and are not in the best interests of the horse. In some cases there are serious welfare implications. They include the following.
- Cribbing straps and collars (Figure 22.3).
- Unpleasant tasting substances spread onto surfaces used for cribbing.
- Electrifying the surfaces and fences.
- In the past, the muscles on the underside of the neck and their nerve supply were removed. The surgery is disfiguring and the results were variable. Again, it does nothing to address the cause of the behaviour and all of these treatments may increase the distress of the horse.

If some form of collar has to be used, it should be correctly fitted and removed at regular intervals. It should only be used as a temporary solution while management changes are being made.

Prevention

- Avoid sudden weaning. Gradual weaning is more natural and reduces the incidence of stereotypic behaviour. Foals should be kept at pasture with suitable companions and fed a suitable diet without excessively high levels of carbohydrate.
- Avoid diets and feeding practices that encourage gastric acidity.
- Avoid stabling horses for long periods.
- Provide suitable companions.

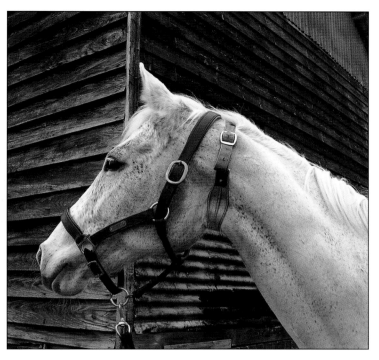

Figure 22.3 An anti-cribbing collar

WEAVING

A horse that repeatedly swings its head from side to side and rocks its weight from one front foot to the other is said to weave. This is usually a response to frustration and anxiety in a horse confined to the stable for long periods with limited social contact with other horses. Many horses perform this stereotypy when anticipating a feed, exercise or turnout. It often occurs if they are anxious when other horses are turned out or leave the yard for exercise.

This behaviour does not affect the performance of a horse but should be declared if the horse is sold. Abnormal wear patterns may develop on the shoes and it can be associated with weight loss.

Causes

- Long periods of confinement in a stable.
- Lack of close contact with other horses.

Factors such as insufficient forage may be a contributory factor in some cases.

Control

Control measures include:
- turning the horse out into a *large* paddock with a group of compatible companions;

they need sufficient room to express normal behaviour and move naturally at walk, trot and canter

- putting grilles in the partitions between adjacent boxes
- putting an extra 'top door' type window in the back wall of the stable
- using a specially designed and unbreakable stable mirror if the above options are not possible or do not prevent the behaviour; studies have shown this to be very effective at reducing weaving (Figure 22.4)
- providing ad-lib forage
- providing a companion, either another horse close by or a sheep, goat or chicken
- vary the stable routines so that the horse is less likely to become agitated in response to anticipation of a particular event.

The following are **not recommended**.

- V-shaped anti-weaving grilles on the stable door (Figure 22.5). These increase the horse's frustration and do nothing to address the cause. Many horses will just continue to weave inside the stable or toss their heads up and down through the grille instead.
- Isolating the horse from others in the mistaken belief that others will copy the behaviour. Further isolation increases the distress of a horse that is already struggling to cope with the management system imposed upon it.

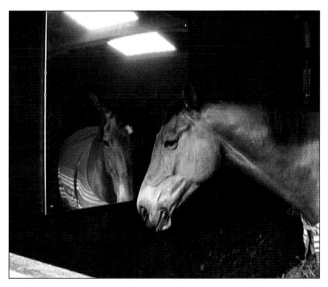

Figure 22.4 A stable mirror has a calming influence on some horses

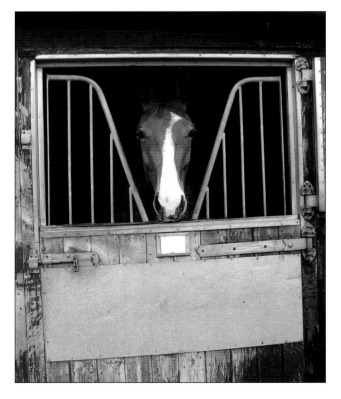

Figure 22.5 An anti-weaving grille

SELF-MUTILATION AND RUG CHEWING

Some stabled horses will bite or chew themselves or their rugs when confined to the stable for long periods of time. Stallions, in particular, may repeatedly lick or chew their chest, shoulder, flank or the inside of a forelimb. If the behaviour persists it can cause hair loss, white hairs or scarring. As the area heals, the skin may be itchy and this perpetuates the behaviour. These horses often squeal, buck or lash out in their stables.

Causes

These behaviours are associated with:

- long periods of confinement
- limited contact with other horses
- the feeding of high concentrate and grain rations
- restricted access to forage
- management or environmental changes
- proximity to a mare in season
- pain.

Other causes that need to be ruled out include the following.

- Parasitic infestation, e.g. ringworm, lice or chorioptic mange.
- Allergic skin conditions.
- Discomfort from the rugs. Most rugs are designed with the comfort of the horse in mind. However, they need to be fitted correctly and properly maintained. Applying layers of rugs may cause the underneath rug to move backwards and put uncomfortable pressure on the horse's chest, withers or shoulders. Alternatively, the horse may overheat. Rollers can also be uncomfortable or done up too tightly.

The horse should have a thorough veterinary examination to exclude these and any other unrecognized sources of pain and discomfort.

Treatment

The aim of treatment is to improve the horse's quality of life by enriching its environment and increasing its social interaction with other horses.

Management changes include:

- turning the horse out
- increasing the level of exercise
- providing ad-lib forage
- reducing the grain and concentrate in the diet
- allowing visual and social contact with other horses
- providing companionship, e.g. some racehorses are kept with a sheep, goat or chicken.

Any wounds or underlying conditions, e.g. gastric ulceration, should be treated. As a temporary solution the horse can have a bib fitted to the headcollar to prevent him chewing himself or his rugs (see Figure 3.29). However, this does not treat the underlying cause and wearing a headcollar for long hours can cause poll discomfort.

The welfare of stallions not used for breeding may be significantly improved by castration so that they can be turned out with other horses.

BOX WALKING

Some horses compulsively walk round their boxes for many hours of the day. This behaviour can lead to loss of condition and makes it almost impossible to keep the bedding fresh and clean.

In common with the stereotypic behaviour patterns already discussed, this is often a reaction to frustration and stress. Once the habit is established, it can be very difficult to break. Provision of toys or a stable companion may help, but turning the horse out with a companion is often the only solution.

AGGRESSION

There are a number of reasons why horses sometimes behave aggressively. Aggression can be a normal form of communication that occurs in the face of a perceived threat or it may occur as a result of frustration or pain. The spectrum of behaviour ranges from putting the ears back and presenting their rumps to lungeing forwards, biting and striking with a front foot. Whenever a horse exhibits persistently aggressive behaviour, an attempt should be made to identify the cause.

The veterinary investigation may include the following.

- A detailed history. The vet will want to know:
    - when the behaviour first started
    - details of the horse's management including feed, grazing, daily routine, contact with other horses and people
    - management prior to current ownership
    - the horse's medical history
    - details of any treatment already tried.
- A full clinical examination to identify any illness or source of pain. Aggression can be displayed by horses with:
    - chronic pain
    - hormone imbalance, e.g. mares with an ovarian granulosa cell tumour
    - severe liver disease

  – a brain tumour (rare)
  – infections such as rabies.
- Observation of the behaviour – a video may be helpful.
- A check of the saddle, bridle and rugs.

Some types of aggressive behaviour are 'normal', e.g. when a mare perceives the approach of a person or another horse to be a threat to her foal. In other cases, the horse will display mild aggression such as turning round with the ears back in an attempt to communicate discomfort, e.g. when approached with a badly fitting saddle.

Horses may display aggressive behaviour in their stables, simply because they are protective of their food or space or because they are unable to move away from the perceived threat. This may occur if the horse is managed in a way that prevents it from running freely with the opportunity to display normal equine behaviour. In these situations the horse may attack if their warning signs are ignored or inappropriately dealt with.

Treatment

Whatever the cause of the aggression, precautions should be taken to prevent anyone being hurt. If necessary, handlers should wear protective clothing including a hard hat, boots with steel toe-caps and body protectors. Nervous handlers are likely to make the situation worse by their own lack of confidence and jerky movements and so these horses need to be handled by experienced, confident people. Physical or verbal punishment aggravates the situation as it reinforces the horse's perception that the situation poses a danger.

It is important to try to pinpoint and remove the reason for the problem. Any systemic illness or painful condition should be treated. If the aggression is a learned response to a particular stimulus the following may be tried.

- Repetition of the stimulus many times without the associated unpleasant experience. For example, a horse may continue to object to being saddled despite being pain free and having a comfortable new saddle. In this situation, the new saddle may be placed on the back many times for example, during grooming without having the girths tightened or being mounted. This exercise should be done regularly at times when the horse is quiet and relaxed. As the horse becomes tolerant to the presence of the saddle, the girths may be attached. When this does not cause a problem, they can be done up loosely and then progressively tightened. Many horses will gradually come to accept that saddling is not unpleasant and stop showing aggressive behaviour. This is known as desensitization.
- Alternatively, a positive and pleasant experience can be introduced with the trigger for the aggressive behaviour. This is known as counter-conditioning.

This takes time and commitment from the owner and everyone who handles the horse. In some cases it may be advantageous to obtain the help of an equine behaviourist.

In every case, the management and environment should be carefully assessed to ensure that it is optimal for reducing frustration and anxiety. These horses need a suitable forage-based diet and time in the field to express their normal behavioural patterns.

If no cause can be found for the aggression and management and environmental changes make no difference, the assistance of a qualified equine behaviour specialist should be sought. If the aggressive behaviour still persists and the horse is a danger to itself, its handlers and other horses, euthanasia must be considered.

HORMONAL CAUSES OF BEHAVIOUR PROBLEMS

Behavioural problems in mares

Some mares become very temperamental when they are in season and on occasions this affects their usefulness as riding and competition horses. If this is a persistent problem, they should have a full clinical examination including a rectal palpation and ultrasound scan of their ovaries to rule out granulosa cell tumours (see next section) and other causes of bad behaviour such as pain.

Where no obvious cause is found and good management and handling are ineffective, the following treatment options can be considered.

- Dietary modification and use of one of the dietary supplements available.
- Administration of a progesterone-like drug, altrenogest (Equine Regumate™). This can be put in the feed or syringed directly into the mouth. It works by preventing follicle growth, oestrus and ovulation so the mare does not come into season. Long-term administration is expensive and there is a chance that it will reduce subsequent fertility by increasing the risk of endometritis (uterine infection). Some mares can take up to 6 months for their cycles to return to normal after the drug is withdrawn. In other cases, the behavioural problems return and the mare comes into oestrus shortly after the medication is stopped. Other medical treatments are sometimes used and should be discussed with your vet.
- Placing a sterile glass ball (like a large marble) in the uterus following ovulation. This causes continuous secretion of progesterone by the ovary and prevents the mare coming into oestrus. The effectiveness of this treatment varies from mare to mare, but is reported to be helpful in approximately 50% of cases. When the mare does come into season, the marble can be removed through the cervix.
- Removal of the ovaries. This is a major operation and is only carried out as a last resort for mares that are persistently unmanageable. It will not solve the problem if the ovaries are not the cause of the abnormal behaviour.

- Pregnancy. Many mares calm down if they are in foal and this option is sometimes used. Another possibility is to terminate the pregnancy after 35 days by manually compressing the conceptus. The mare will continue to secrete the hormones of pregnancy and may remain more placid for several months. This has been used in some racing Thoroughbreds.

In extreme cases, these mares can be dangerous and euthanasia should be considered.

Granulosa cell tumours

Granulosa cell tumours account for $2\frac{1}{2}$ –4% of equine cancers and are the commonest type of tumour affecting the ovary. They can grow to be very large (the record is 59 kg [130 1b]) but are usually detected much earlier when they are around the size of a grapefruit or football. They are normally benign. These tumours produce hormones which can cause a range of behavioural changes.

CLINICAL SIGNS

The behavioural changes include:
- stallion-like behaviour and aggression
- continuous oestrus (constantly in season)
- anoetrus (not coming into season at all).

Other, less common signs include:
- colic or low grade abdominal discomfort
- lameness.

Many of these tumours secrete the male hormone testosterone. Some mares develop cresty necks, become abnormally muscular and have an enlarged clitoris. They may attempt to mount other mares. A common reason for consulting the vet is because the owner wants to know why her normally sweet mare has become so unpredictable and aggressive. Affected mares are infertile and the tumours may be discovered in broodmares during a routine gynaecological examination.

DIAGNOSIS

The diagnosis is made on:
- rectal palpation: the enlarged ovary is hard and may have a smooth or knobbly surface
- ultrasonography: the enlarged ovary may have multiple cysts, a single large cyst or be a solid mass
- blood tests; these are not always diagnostic, but more than 50% of affected mares will have raised serum testosterone levels.

Typically, the opposite ovary is small and inactive.

TREATMENT

The treatment is surgical removal of the affected ovary. Small tumours may be removed using local anaesthetic, with the mare sedated and standing, often via laparoscopy. Larger tumours may require general anaesthesia for removal.

Following the surgery, the mare is given routine antibiotic cover and box rest with in-hand walking exercise for 4–6 weeks. Non-steroidal anti-inflammatory drugs are administered post-operative pain is common.

COMPLICATIONS

Wound swelling and breakdown are not uncommon following this operation.

PROGNOSIS

The prognosis is good. The mare's behaviour generally returns to normal within a few weeks of surgery. The remaining ovary usually starts to function normally between 2 and 18 months later. In a very small number of cases the tumour is found to be malignant and spreads to other organs of the body.

Behaviour problems in stallions and geldings

Information on these topics can be found in Chapter 19, The Cryptorchid Horse.

COPROPHAGIA

Coprophagia is the practice of eating faeces. This is normal behaviour for foals that may be observed to eat the mare's droppings. It may have a beneficial effect by introducing the foal to normal gut microorganisms.

In adult horses, the behaviour may be associated with a protein deficiency in the diet, so this should be checked. Affected animals will eat their own faeces or those of another horse. It can be reduced by prompt removal of the droppings from the stable and field. Where appropriate, dietary changes should be made.

PICA

Pica is the name given to ingestion of soil or other substances such as wood which are not part of the horse's normal diet. This behaviour often reflects a nutritional imbalance or a behaviour response to the environment in which it is kept.

Causes

These include:

- a mineral deficiency
- lack of fibre in the diet
- lack of environmental stimulation.

Horses with insufficient iron or phosphorus often eat soil and those with inadequate dietary fibre will chew wood. Many horses indulging in this type of behaviour are kept in poor conditions such as plots of overgrazed land with bare patches and very little grass. These horses often have limited space or opportunity to demonstrate normal equine behaviour.

Diagnosis

The diagnosis is made from the history or by observing the behaviour. The vet may check that the horse does not have any underlying disease of the digestive system that affects its ability to digest or absorb the food provided. The composition of the diet must be examined in detail. The horse sometimes requires a blood test to check that it is not anaemic.

Treatment

This may involve:
- providing a salt lick
- adding a vitamin and mineral supplement to the diet
- increasing the fibre content of the diet
- allowing the horse access to better quality pasture
- providing the horse with companions.

HEADSHAKING

'Headshaking' is a term used to describe a horse's behaviour when it repeatedly tosses its head in response to nasal or facial irritation or pain.

Clinical signs

An affected horse or pony may:
- flick its nose violently in a vertical direction
- toss its head up and down
- shake its head from side to side or in a rotary fashion
- flip its upper lip; in longstanding cases, the nasolabialis muscle which lifts the upper lip may become abnormally developed
- act as though a bee has flown up its nose
- sneeze and snort

- suddenly stop and rub its nose on the inside of the forelimb or on the rider's leg
- strike at its nose with a forelimb
- rub its nose on the ground while moving or on the stable wall at rest
- immerse its nose in water in an apparent attempt to relieve the discomfort.

The symptoms tend to be seasonal, occurring mainly in the spring and summer and regressing in the autumn and winter. Bright sunlight seems to trigger this behaviour; affected horses and ponies are often worse on warm, sunny days. Some are affected more on windy days, others are reported to improve. A number of horses develop the symptoms in the autumn and some will headshake all year round. There is a tendency for the headshaking period to become longer each year.

This behaviour is unpredictable and may unbalance or unseat the rider, making the affected animals dangerous to ride. It characteristically occurs at trot, usually within 10 minutes from the start of exercise, when the horse warms up. As exercise continues, the horse may become quite frantic in its attempts to rub its nose. The condition may be worse when the horse is excited. Some horses exhibit the behaviour at rest in the stable.

All types of horses and ponies can be affected. The average age of onset is between 7 and 9 years. Some studies have shown that geldings appear to be twice as likely to be affected as mares.

GRADING OF HEADSHAKING SYMPTOMS

Because the symptoms vary in severity from horse to horse and from one season to another, a grading system has been established.

Grade 1 The clinical signs are mild and intermittent, with twitching of the facial muscles. Affected horses are rideable.

Grade 2 The clinical signs are moderate. Symptoms are associated with specific conditions and affected horses are rideable with some difficulty.

Grade 3 Riding is possible but not enjoyable and the animal is difficult to control.

Grade 4 The horse is unrideable and uncontrollable.

Grade 5 The behaviour of the horse is very unpredictable and dangerous.

Causes

Contrary to previous theories, headshaking is not due to a simple allergy. The behaviour is usually a response to nasal irritation or facial neuralgia. In the majority of cases, it is considered to be due to hypersensitivity of a particular branch of the trigeminal nerve (the posterior ethmoid branch of the ophthalmic division) which supplies sensation to most of the nasal cavity. A small number have abnormal sensitivity of the muzzle due to irritation of the infra-orbital branch of the nerve. In a few horses, more than one sensory branch of the trigeminal nerve may be involved. In each case, it is thought that the nerve is somehow affected so the nasal cavity becomes irritated and pain fibres are activated. Human patients with trigeminal neuralgia complain of severe, sharp pains that may be intermittent or prolonged, often triggered by touch, chewing or cold wind. The condition can cause severe suffering. In horses, the nerve may be irritated by increased airflow and turbulence during exercise, together with irritants such as pollen and dust.

Unfortunately, it is often impossible to identify the specific cause of the nerve irritation and resultant headshaking. Investigation can be expensive and unrewarding. Many cases are described as **idiopathic**, which means that we do not know the cause. However, a number of conditions must be ruled out before a diagnosis of idiopathic headshaking is made. These include:

- the presence of ear mites
- inflammation of the outer, middle or inner ear, or irritation from a foreign body inside the ear
- sinusitis
- gutteral pouch disease
- dental problems, e.g. sharp teeth ulcerating the gums; pain from the bit impinging on the soft tissues, the wolf teeth or tushes; a tooth abscess or decay
- neck pain
- eye disease including inflammation, mobile iris cysts, retinal lesions
- a tumour within the nasal cavity or elsewhere on the head
- discomfort from poorly fitting tack, inappropriate bitting or bad riding
- any other obvious source of head irritation
- boredom from long periods in the stable.

Once these have been eliminated, other possible causes of nerve irritation include:

- nasal irritation due to a seasonal pollen allergy (allergic rhinitis)
- photosensitization of the nerves due to increase in light intensity – this has been recognized in man
- increased levels of ozone in the atmosphere when the sun shines
- increased air turbulence and blood flow through the nasal mucosa when the horse is exercised
- possible triggers such as a respiratory infection, e.g. strangles (uncommon).

Diagnosis and investigation

Headshaking is a symptom of many conditions, rather than a specific diagnosis in itself. The investigation to rule out many of the conditions listed above is likely to include:

- observation of the horse at rest and at exercise; if your horse only exhibits the signs intermittently, take a video for your vet to watch
- close inspection of the tack fitting

- palpation and observation of the head and neck
- dental inspection
- endoscopic examination of the upper respiratory tract including the gutteral pouches and also of the ear canals
- radiography of the head
- examination of the ears and eyes.

Idiopathic headshaking is suspected if no obvious cause is found and confirmed by a positive response to specific nerve blocks. In one recent study, most horses temporarily improved 90–100% when the posterior ethmoidal branches of the trigeminal nerve were numbed with local anaesthetic.

Management

- Some owners report an improvement if the horses are ridden indoors, or only on dull, wet days or at night. However, this imposes severe restrictions on the use of the horse.
- Careful attention should be paid to the comfort and fitting of the tack. Headpieces pressing on the back of the ears and buckles situated over the temporomandibular joint can cause chronic pain. Bitless bridles have been tried on affected horses, but they rarely improve the situation.
- Affected horses should be protected from fly irritation as much as possible.

Treatment

The best treatment is to determine the cause and eliminate it. However, in the majority of cases, this is not possible. As a first line of treatment, the following have been tried.

- Use of a nose net (Figure 22.6). This is reported to reduce the symptoms in 75% of cases, with 60% of horses improving by 50% or more, and 30% improving by 70% or more. The net may act as a crude filter and decrease the irritation from pollen, dust and midges or it may alter the way the air flows through the nostrils. By constantly touching the nose and stimulating the sensory nerve receptors, the net may reduce the sensitivity of the nose to factors that trigger the headshaking behaviour. A fly fringe attached to the noseband can also be effective.
- In one large study of 245 headshakers, trimming the horses' whiskers had no effect in the majority of cases. However, with some horses the nose nets only worked if the whiskers were trimmed so that they did not contact the net. Other horses were reported to have worse symptoms if long whiskers contacted the net.
- Coloured contact lenses were popular at one time, but they provide only temporary relief in a small number of horses.
- The use of masks which shield the eyes from direct sunlight appears to help some horses.
- A change of environment is sometimes helpful.

SURGICAL TREATMENT

Injection of an agent which causes the posterior ethmoid branches of the trigeminal nerve to cease to function is usually successful, but the effect only lasts for an average of 6–9 months. The procedure may be repeated but has to be carried out under general anaesthesia.

In the few cases that improve when local anaesthetic is injected around the infra-orbital nerve, neurectomy (cutting the nerve) may be considered. However, this causes loss of sensation to the nose and muzzle which cannot be good for a grazing animal. There are also reports of the cut end of the nerve becoming permanently inflamed, causing great distress to the animal and frantic rubbing of its muzzle.

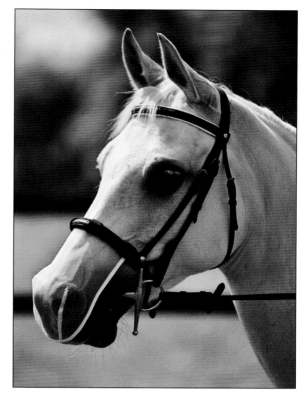

Figure 22.6 Pony with a nose net

In severe cases, a permanent tracheostomy (see page 443) may be performed as a last resort, so that the horse can breathe without drawing air thorough its nostrils.

MEDICAL TREATMENT

Various medical treatments have been used to treat the condition.

Cyproheptadine is a medicine used to treat vascular/cluster headaches in humans. It is not always successful in alleviating the symptoms of headshaking when used alone, but when combined with carbamazepine, a good success rate is reported.

Carbamazepine is a human anticonvulsant drug. It can alleviate the symptoms of headshaking without causing any side effects. However, horses quickly become tolerant to it, so the benefit is often only temporary. It may be used on its own as well as in combination with cyproheptadine.

Drugs such as antihistamines, non-steroidal anti-inflammatory drugs, corticosteroids, antibiotics and nasal decongestants are rarely effective.

COMPLEMENTARY THERAPIES

In most cases, complementary therapies including homeopathy, herbal supplements and acupuncture are not helpful.

Prognosis

Unless a specific cause can be determined and eliminated, the prognosis is guarded as there is no consistently effective treatment for headshaking.

Warning

If an animal shows mild signs of headshaking behaviour one year, it may be worse the following season. Since many of the horses and ponies show no symptoms during the winter months, they are often sold on to new homes at this time.

23
VETERINARY CARE OF THE DONKEY

ALEX THIEMANN
MA VetMB CertEP MRCVS

This chapter by Alex Thiemann MA VetMB Cert EP MRCVS is included to highlight some of the differences between horses and donkeys. It is an important aspect of their welfare that donkeys are not treated as small horses.

Alex Thiemann qualified from Cambridge Veterinary School in 1989. She spent 3 years in mixed practice, 6 years in equine practice and then joined The Donkey Sanctuary in 1998, where she is now Senior Clinician. In addition to working in the UK, Alex has also spent time at Donkey Sanctuary projects overseas including Kenya and Spain.

INTRODUCTION

Donkeys have had a close association with horses for a long time, but there are a number of differences between the two species which it is important to recognize.

In the UK donkeys are kept primarily as companion animals or for pleasure activities such as showing and driving (Figure 23.1). They are well suited to riding therapy and work with special-needs children and adults.

In developing countries donkeys form an important part of the economy (Figure 23.2). They are better suited to survival in harsher conditions than horses, but being low status animals they may suffer severe abuse.

DONKEY CLASSIFICATION AND CHARACTERISTICS

Classification

The domestic donkey (*Equus asinus*) has 62 chromosomes.

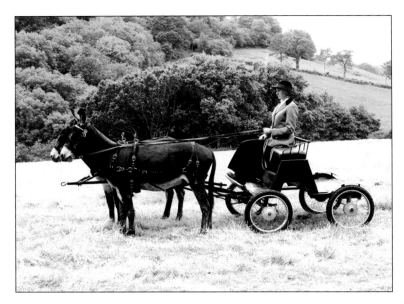 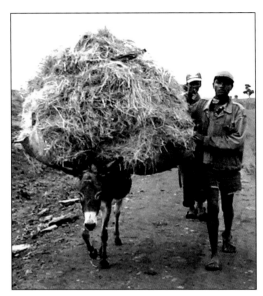

Figures 23.1 and 23.2 Donkeys in different parts of the world experience a wide range of lifestyles

The domestic horse (*Equus caballus*) has 64 chromosomes.

These species can interbreed but produce (generally) infertile hybrids: mules or hinnies with 63 chromosomes. A mule is the crossbred produced from a female horse (mare) mated with a donkey stallion. A hinny is the crossbred produced from a female donkey (jenny) mated with a horse stallion.

More exotic crossbreds may also be encountered, e.g. the zonkey: a donkey mated with a zebra; or the zoney: a pony mated with a zebra; both of which will have the intermediate characteristics of the species.

Physical characteristics

The size range for donkeys is as follows.

- The smallest is the Miniature breed, which must be less than 9 hh (91.44 cm or 36 in) at the withers.
- Most UK donkeys range from 9.2 to 11 hh (from 96.52 cm or 38 in to 111.76 cm or 44 in)
- The Spanish Andalucian donkey can be up to 15.2 hh (157.48 cm or 62 in) while the exceptionally thick-coated Poitou (a French breed) can be up to 15 hh (152.4 cm or 60 in)
- In the USA, donkeys are classified as Miniature, Standard and Mammoth. The Mammoth ass is over 13.3 hh (139.7 cm or 55 in) at the withers and was originally bred from the large Spanish and French donkey breeds. These large donkeys are traditionally used for ploughing and draught work. Today Mammoth donkeys are also

used for breeding large mules for pleasure riding, driving and showing. Mules are very popular animals in the USA.

Reproductive characteristics
THE JENNY

The female donkey is known as a jenny. The oestrus cycle length is approximately 23 days, with an oestrus period of approximately 7 days. Gestation length is quoted as being variable from 365 to 375 days, with live births being recorded from $10\frac{1}{2}$ to 14 months.

Ideally a jenny should not be bred until she is mature at approximately 3 years (Figure 23.3). Rectal palpation for pregnancy diagnosis may be slightly more difficult due to the smaller size and more sloping pelvis of the donkey. Blood and urine tests may be used for diagnosis of pregnancy in the donkey as in the horse.

The jenny is at increased risk of hyperlipaemia (see pages 501 and 658) during pregnancy and lactation due to her hormonal balance. It is important to monitor at-risk animals. If a jenny does become hyperlipaemic during pregnancy, it may be necessary to attempt induction or termination of pregnancy to save the jenny. However, this procedure is high risk. The variable gestation length means that it is hard to predict the foal's readiness for birth and the jenny may also die or suffer complications due to the stress of the procedure. Following birth, if there is any doubt that the foal has received adequate colostrum, the commercially available immunoglobulin test kits and the hyperimmune serum can be used in the donkey foal as in the horse.

Older jennies may suffer from a variety of uterine and ovarian problems. The

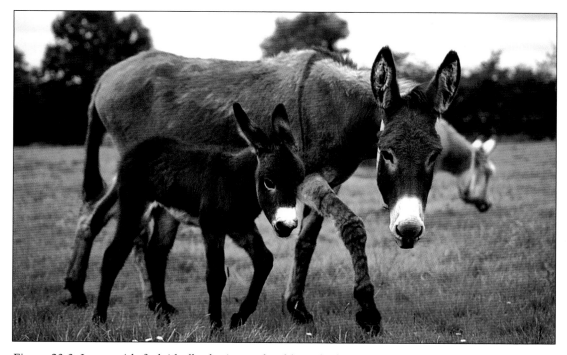

Figure 23.3 Jenny with foal: ideally the jenny should not be bred until she is mature at 3 years

examination of any off-colour jenny should include full examination of the reproductive tract. Encountered problems include:

- cystic, haemorrhagic, and neoplastic (cancerous) ovarian conditions which may present as vague abdominal discomfort with behavioural changes
- uterine infections and cancers.

In selected patients, surgical removal of the affected ovary and/or uterus may be beneficial.

THE JACK

The male donkey is known as a jack and may be sexually mature from approximately 1 year. In contrast to the horse, the jack does not generally require sheath cleaning, and squamous cell carcinoma of the penis is very rare. However sarcoids in the groin and on the sheath and penis are common problems and may be difficult to treat.

Castration

It is preferable to castrate youngsters at around 6 months of age, as learned sexual behaviours may not be removed by castration. Castration in the donkey is complicated by risk of haemorrhage and the need for ligation (tying off) of the major blood vessels, necessitating general anaesthesia.

There are a number of surgical techniques used and the vet will decide which is the most suitable for your donkey. His age, condition and general health will all be taken into account following a clinical examination. Excessive swelling after the operation may be a problem in donkeys owing to their sedentary nature, especially in older animals. Every effort must be made to encourage exercise and non-steroidal anti-inflammatory drugs (NSAIDs) will help to control the swelling and pain. Your vet will advise you of the most appropriate post-surgical management.

Cryptorchidism (rig) also occurs in the donkey. This is diagnosed from a human chorionic gonadotrophin (hCG) stimulation test as described for the horse.

Physiological characteristics

The normal body temperature is 37.1 °C, (98.8 °F) with a range from 36.2 to 37.8 °C, (97.2 to 100 °F). Donkeys are desert-adapted animals and studies have shown them to have a better ability to cope with heat and dehydration than horses, and to survive on poorer quality forage than the horse. However these studies have been done on heat-adapted donkeys and should not be used as an excuse for poor management of donkeys from cooler climates such as the UK.

BLOOD TESTS

The haematological and biochemical normal values for the donkey differ from those of the horse, so blood samples should ideally be submitted to a laboratory regularly dealing with samples from donkeys. The values from the Donkey Sanctuary are tabulated opposite.

Haematological Parameters		Median	5 percentile	95 percentile
White Blood Cell Count 10^9/l	Donkey	10.2	6.1	16.1
	Young Donkey	13.5	7.8	21.9
Neutrophils – %	Donkey	50.5	28	78
Neutrophil count – 10^9/l	Donkey	5.0	2.2	13.3
Lymphocytes – %	Donkey	43	17	65
Lymphocyte count – 10^9/l	Donkey	4.2	1.8	7.8
	Young Donkey	6.2	2.5	14.0
Eosinophils – %	Donkey	4	1	10
Eosinophil count – 10^9/l	Donkey	0.38	0.09	1.15
	Young Donkey	0.30	0	1.63
Basophils – %	Donkey	0	0	0.08
Basophil count – 10^9/l	Donkey	0	0	0.5
Monocytes – %	Donkey	1	0	5
Monocyte count – 10^9/l	Donkey	0.13	0	0.80
Total Red Blood Cell count – 10^{12}/l	Donkey	5.5	4	7.3
Packed Cell Volume – litre/litre	Donkey	0.33	0.25	0.38
	Young Donkey	0.34	0.27	0.43
Haemoglobin – g/dl	Donkey	11.6	9	15.3
Mean Corpuscular Volume – fl	Donkey	64	57	79
Mean Corpuscular Haem. – pg	Donkey	21.9	18.9	28.6
Mean Corpuscular Haem. Conc.– g/dl	Donkey	34.8	31.4	39.1
	Young Donkey	35	25.3	54.0
Biochemical Parameters		**Median**	**5 percentile**	**95 percentile**
Creatinine – µmol/l	Donkey	75	53	141
	Young Donkey	83	61	107
Creatine Phosphokinase – IU/l	Donkey	97	36	360
Total Bilirubin – µmol/l	Donkey	2.7	1.4	7.7
Urea – mmol/l	Donkey	3.9	1.9	7.6
Triglycerides – mmol/l	Donkey	1	0.2	4.3
	Young Donkey	0.7	0.2	2.0
Total Protein – g/l	Donkey	70	58	82
	Young Donkey	64	53	78
Albumin – g/l	Donkey	28	20	34
Total Globulins – g/l	Donkey	40	29	53
	Young Donkey	34	23	50
γ-Glutamyl Transferase – IU/l	Donkey	29	13	79
Glutamate Dehydrogenase – IU/l	Donkey	2.9	0.7	14.6
	Young Donkey	2.2	0.7	7.1
Aspartate aminotransferase – IU/l	Donkey	220	119	402
Alkaline Phosphatase – IU/l	Donkey	265	150	563
Glucose			3.1	5.0

Young Donkey = Donkey less than 2 years old.
N.B. Enzyme assays are run at 37 °C (CPK, GGT, GLDH, AAT, ALP)

Two significant differences are:

- the donkey's red cell count is significantly lower than that of the horse but the red cell volume is about twice the size, leading to an overall haemoglobin level (the oxygen carrying molecule), only slightly lower than that of the horse.
- The resting triglyceride level of the donkey (0.2–4.3mmol/l) is higher than that quoted for the horse (<0.35mm/l).

Other differences between the donkey and the horse
PHARMACOLOGICAL DIFFERENCES

There are a number of differences in metabolism between the donkey and the horse. Unfortunately the data is incomplete and only a limited number of drugs have been adequately researched. However, a number of non-steroidal anti-inflammatory drugs (NSAIDs) have been studied. Phenylbutazone, for example, is metabolized faster in the donkey, so higher doses or shorter dosing intervals are required, e.g. 2.2–4.4mg/kg by mouth twice daily. Flunixin meglumine is also metabolized faster than in the horse and should be given twice daily instead of once daily. However, carprofen appears to be more slowly metabolized in donkeys than horses and once daily dosing is required. It is important to remember that donkeys may be stoical in the event of pain and care should be taken to regularly reassess patients. A number of donkeys in the UK are geriatric and may have hepatic (liver) or renal (kidney) impairment and your vet will take this into consideration when prescribing these medicines.

ANATOMICAL VARIATIONS

Apart from the variation in conformation and relative sizes of the muscle groups there are a few anatomical features, which it is helpful to recognize.

- The nasolacrimal duct of the donkey opens high up, on the dorsal surface of the false nostril about 1.5 cm ($\frac{7}{10}$ in) from the nasal mucocutaneous junction.
- The nasopharyngeal recess at the back of the pharynx is deep and may be felt as a blind-ended pouch when stomach tubing.
- The male donkey usually has vestigial teats on the prepuce, which may cause confusion.
- The chestnuts are only found on the forelegs.
- The dorsal hoof walls in the donkey are more vertical than those of the horse, an angle of 55–60 degrees being usual.

BEHAVIOURAL DIFFERENCES

- Donkeys are not such 'flight animals' as horses and tend not to panic in unusual situations. This can be an advantage as recovery from anaesthesia is generally good.
- Donkeys are said to be stoical in the face of pain, and are much less demonstrative than horses. This factor can lead to delayed diagnosis and treatment when problems arise.

- Subtle behavioural signs must be recognized and acted upon in order not to miss clinically ill donkeys.
- Donkeys can become closely bonded to companions and suffer stress-related hyperlipaemia if separated.

Physical examination

A sick donkey is examined in exactly the same way as a sick horse. The examination may include the following.

- Taking the temperature and listening to the chest and abdomen with a stethoscope.
- A detailed history and close behavioural observation. Donkeys with hyperlipaemia may appear to eat and drink but not actually swallow the food; this is known as sham eating and drinking.
- Blood samples taken early in the examination can give an indication of lipid levels in the blood from their appearance before accurate lab results are available (see Figure 17.19).
- A dental examination with a Haussman's gag may be performed. Dental care of the donkey is frequently neglected especially in older animals, leading to sharp edges and large hooks causing soft tissue inflammation and infection which may predispose to choke and colic.
- Rectal examination of most standard-sized donkeys can be achieved (Figure 23.4); even a limited rectal examination will give information as to faecal consistency, mucosal quality, excess gas etc. If the donkey is very small and rectal examination is not practical, then abdominal ultrasound may be used as an alternative.
- External palpation (gentle pushing from the outside) of the ventral abdomen may be useful to detect anterior abdominal pain, e.g. in cases of pancreatitis (see page 659).
- A stomach tube can be passed in colic cases using a pony- or foal-sized nasogastric tube (Figure 23.5).
- Peritoneal taps may be difficult to obtain due to the very thick (up to 14 cm [5 $\frac{1}{2}$ in]) mid-line fat deposits.

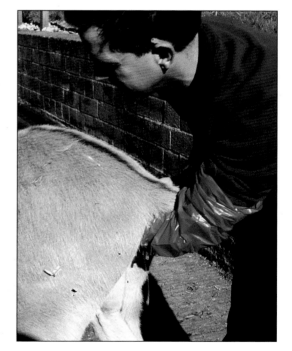

Figure 23.4 Rectal examination of most standard-sized donkeys can be achieved

> **Warning**
>
> It is important to take note of any change in a donkey's behaviour or demeanour as they are generally more stoical than horses. A donkey may just seem dull or slightly off colour when in fact it is seriously ill.

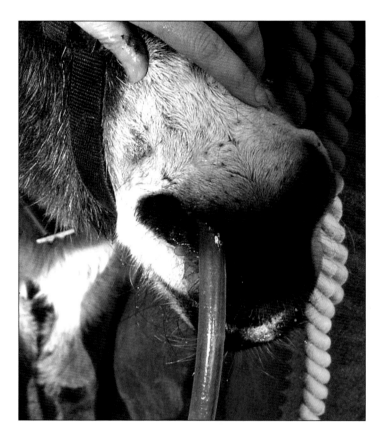

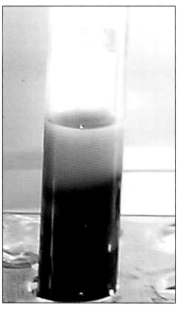

Figure 23.5 A stomach tube can be passed in a donkey in the same way as in a horse (left)

Figure 23.6 This blood sample has very high triglyceride levels (above)

Specific conditions and their management
HYPERLIPAEMIA

- See Chapter 17 for a full description of this condition.
- Donkeys are well known as high-risk subjects for this disease. Donkeys' resting triglyceride levels are significantly higher than those of ponies, and they are frequently obese, which predisposes them to insulin insensitivity and hyperlipaemia (Figure 23.6).
- Pregnant and lactating jennies are especially high risk.
- Any concurrent disease, which causes a degree of anorexia, is a risk for development of the disease. Care must be taken to monitor triglyceride levels in a variety of conditions, e.g. after dental extraction, or when the donkey is suffering from colic.
- Clinical signs include depression, anorexia, sham eating and drinking, elevated pulse and respiratory rates, reduced gut motility, dry mucus-covered faeces, congested mucous membranes, ataxia, and ventral oedema.
- Gastric ulceration may accompany anorexia, and so hyperlipaemic, anorexic donkeys are sometimes treated with gastric protectants, e.g. omeprazole, ranitidine, sucralfate.
- Pancreatitis may accompany hyperlipaemia; this can be detected by raised plasma amylase and lipase, and anterior abdominal pain that is poorly responsive to analgesia.
- The treatment protocol used at the Donkey Sanctuary is outlined below.

Plasma Triglyceride	Approach to Treatment	Prognosis
5–8 mmol/l	Encourage voluntary feeding of tempting, succulent foods. Grazing.	Values should return quickly to normal if feeding continues.
8–10 mmol/l	Nasogastric intubation with electrolytes, glucose and/or Ready brek® (breakfast cereal).	Good
10–15 mmol/l	Nasogastric intubation (as above), intravenous (i.v.) fluids if necessary.	Fair if results are reduced promptly. Treat seriously.
15–20 mmol/l	Nasogastric intubation (as above), and i.v. fluids.	Guarded
over 20 mmol/l	Nasogastric intubation (as above). Intensive i.v. fluids.	Poor

Additional therapy includes low dose NSAIDs, antibiotics and multivitamins. Feeding by nasogastric tube is not performed if there is intestinal stasis (the gut is not moving – known as ileus).

PANCREATITIS
- This is a little understood disease, which is encountered in the donkey in the acute and chronic forms.
- Acute cases may be found dead, or show signs of acute abdominal pain. Massively raised serum amylase and lipase are measured. The disease may be seen in association with hyperlipaemia.
- Chronic cases may present as dull animals with milder elevations of serum amylase and lipase. These cases may respond to aggressive fluid therapy combined with nonsteroidal anti-inflammatory drugs and antibiotics.
- Pancreatic neoplasia (cancer) has been found on post mortem of aged donkeys.

COLIC
Colic in the donkey may be difficult to detect due to the subtle behavioural signs. Many donkeys with colic show dullness and lack of appetite with increased time lying down, rather than the dramatic signs shown by horses. Suspected colic cases should receive a full examination including rectal evaluation. As mentioned above, a peritoneal tap may be difficult due to the thickness of the intra-abdominal fat.
- Impaction of the pelvic flexure is relatively common in donkeys with poor dentition

and in those stabled when box rest is required. The signs tend to be very low grade and this can lead to delayed diagnosis. The impacted mass may harden and damage the mucosal wall leading to a poor prognosis. Thus donkeys undergoing stable rest should have a semi-laxative diet and regular monitoring of faecal output.

- Concurrent hyperlipaemia accompanies many cases of colic so blood samples should be taken in any case of colic causing inappetance.
- Abdominal neoplasia can be a significant cause of mortality in geriatric animals; such cases may present as colic or show a wide range of other signs.
- If exploratory laparotomy is going to be attempted on surgical colic cases, the vet will measure triglycerides and pancreatic enzymes as the prognosis is as dependent on the medical health of the donkey as on the surgical skills of the veterinary team.

THE DULL DONKEY

The dull donkey is frequently a diagnostic challenge as no specific cause may be obvious to the owner. The chart below shows the results of a retrospective study over 1 year of dull donkeys at The Donkey Sanctuary. The range of causes is extremely wide and includes the potentially life-threatening conditions such as hyperlipaemia, liver disease and colic. For this reason you should call your vet promptly if your donkey is dull.

Differential diagnosis of dullness

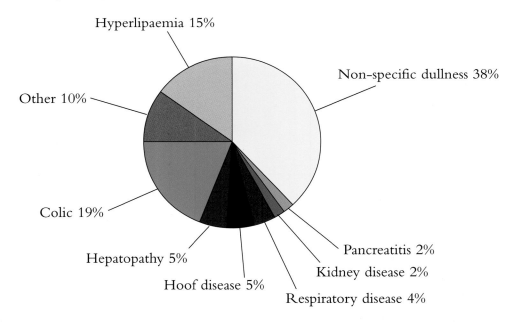

CUSHING'S DISEASE

This condition is recognized in donkeys and the presentation and clinical signs are similar to those in the horse. A long coat with delayed shedding and recurrent laminitis are the commonest clinical signs. The diagnostic and treatment protocols follow those recommended for the horse; there is no specific data currently available for the donkey (Figure 23.7).

RESPIRATORY DISEASE

The donkey suffers from a similar range of respiratory disorders as the horse. The following points should be noted.

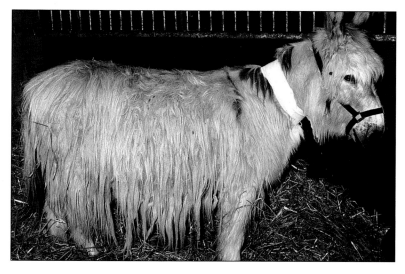

Figure 23.7 Donkey with Cushing's disease

- Herpesvirus infection. Donkeys can suffer from and carry the equine herpesvirus (EHV) and a related asinine herpesvirus (AHV). The range of clinical signs seen is as in the horse. Donkeys often live very sheltered lives and do not mix with a range of animals at shows etc., and so may have low exposure to infection and poor natural immunity. This means that a previously infected donkey that becomes sick or stressed may become an infective shedder of virus particles. Care should be taken to isolate newly acquired donkeys and take samples from those with signs of respiratory problems to minimize the spread of disease.

- Influenza virus infections are seen in donkeys. They are reported to suffer more serious clinical signs and to be at increased risk of developing secondary bacterial broncho-pneumonia than horses. Donkeys with influenza should be treated promptly with antibiotics and have serum triglycerides monitored to avoid hyperlipaemia. Vaccination against infection is strongly recommended.

- *Dictyocaulus arnfieldi*, the lungworm, is a parasite well adapted to the donkey host where it will grow to maturity and produce eggs, without producing clinical signs. In the past this has made the donkey a threat to horses grazing with them, which show more severe clinical signs. The anthelmintics ivermectin and moxidectin are both effective against lungworm at the standard dose rates, and so with good worming policies the donkey no longer poses a risk.

- Tracheal disease. Tracheal stenosis (narrowing) and collapse may be encountered especially in geriatric individuals. This may be due to a combination of age-related degeneration in the tracheal cartilage and chronic lower airway disease causing increased respiratory effort. The presentation is of a chronic cough with a characteristic 'honking' sound or acute respiratory distress. The area of collapse is frequently in the mid to distal tracheal region. Treatment is often unrewarding and aimed at limiting mucosal swelling and treating underlying lung disease.

- Chronic lung disease. Due to the non-athletic nature of most donkeys, early respiratory disease is often unnoticed. This can lead to an irreversible fibrosis of much of the lung, which is poorly responsive to available therapies. Such cases are best managed in a clean-air environment. Secondary infections may prove difficult to treat and carry a grave prognosis.

General anaesthesia

Donkeys generally make good surgical patients and do not panic on induction or recovery. The vet will make a careful pre-operative assessment to pick up subtle or low-grade problems. Pre-operative blood samples are useful in elderly patients.

Foot care

The donkey has a smaller and more upright hoof than the horse and the solar surface is more oval. Donkeys frequently suffer from neglected hooves and it is common to see laminitis and grossly overgrown hooves. Seedy toe, thrush and white line abscesses are common and are treated as in the horse. Donkeys are stoical in the event of foot pain and it is often surprising how severe the radiographic changes are in cases of chronic foot disease. As donkeys are usually kept for companionship rather than competition, some may be successfully treated despite chronic changes, as long as adequate pain relief can be provided.

- On radiographs of a normal donkey foot it is usual to see the middle distal $\frac{1}{4}$ to $\frac{1}{2}$ of the phalanx (P2) to be within the hoof capsule. An ongoing project at The Donkey Sanctuary has measured the distance from the coronary band to the top of the extensor process of the distal phalanx (P3) to be approximately 12 mm. This can make interpretation of lateral X-rays of laminitic hooves more difficult than in the horse, and other parameters such as the degree of rotation of the pedal bone and deviation from the dorsal hoof wall must be assessed.

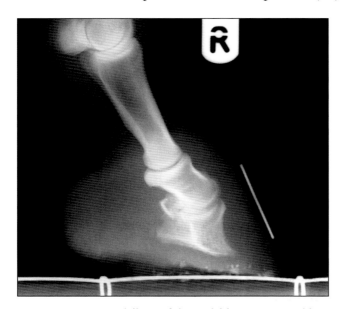

Figure 23.8 Remodelling of the pedal bone to resemble a 'Turkish slipper' in a donkey with chronic foot pain due to laminitis

- Frog supports are not indicated in donkeys with laminitis as the frog is usually recessed and may be further back in the hoof than in the horse. Comfortable pads are used instead.

- Donkeys are often kept on restricted diets to control obesity. These animals may benefit from a nutritional supplement designed to promote healthy hoof growth.

- Radiographs should be taken in cases of chronic foot pain; those showing severe pedal bone changes have a very poor prognosis. Typical changes include a 'Turkish slipper' appearance of the tip of P3 combined with demineralization and rotation (Figure 23.8).

- Plastic shoes may help provide temporary pain relief to donkeys with thin or dropped soles. Many farriers are more comfortable fitting these rather than nailing shoes to small donkey hooves.

- Overfeeding young donkeys is known to contribute to flexural deformity of the distal interphalangeal joint, which may require surgical treatment to correct.

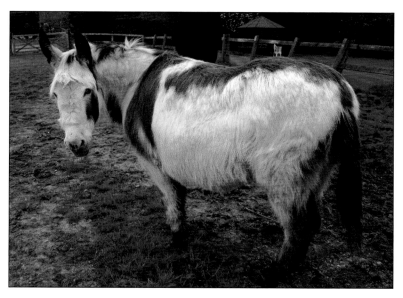
Figure 23.9 An overweight, elderly donkey

Obesity

Donkeys in the UK are often presented with severe obesity (Figure 23.9); this puts them at high risk from hyperlipaemia and laminitis and places strain on the heart, lungs and joints. It is difficult to diet obese donkeys without causing hyperlipaemia and before attempting a weight-loss programme, the donkey should have a full health check. Those with existing high triglycerides will need special monitoring. It is best to attempt weight loss extremely gradually and to measure feed intake which should be reduced to a dry matter intake of approximately 1.6% of body-weight per day, aiming for a weight loss of about 1 kg (2.2 lb) per week. Your vet will advise you on this. An exercise regime will help to increase weight loss. In cases where these measures are not effective, thyroid hormone function should be assessed.

Acknowledgement

Thank you to The Donkey Sanctuary.

The Donkey Sanctuary was founded by Dr Elisabeth D. Svendsen, MBE in 1969 and has taken over 11,000 donkeys into care since then. The aims of The Donkey Sanctuary are to prevent the sufferings of donkeys worldwide through the provision of high quality, professional advice, training and support on donkey welfare. In addition to the Sanctuaries in Devon and Southern Ireland, there is a donkey-fostering scheme, which provides homes for over 2000 donkeys. The Donkey Sanctuary also works with special needs children to provide riding therapy at special units throughout the country. Overseas there are projects to aid the health and welfare of donkeys in Ethiopia, Kenya, Mexico, India, Egypt and Spain.

24
VETERINARY PROCEDURES

THE PREPURCHASE EXAMINATION

If you are considering buying a horse, it is advisable to have it examined by a veterinary surgeon who specializes in horses before you proceed. With their specialist knowledge and equipment, vets are often able to detect problems that are not obvious to the owner or the prospective purchaser. The format of the examination is outlined in a Joint Memorandum prepared by the Royal College of Veterinary Surgeons and the British Veterinary Association. It is currently undergoing revision, which may result in warranties from the vendor being included. This would be part of the negotiations between buyer and seller and would not involve the vet directly. It would help to cover the areas such as previous history, allergies and vices that may not be detectable by the vet during the examination.

It is important to be aware that a prepurchase examination by a vet is essentially a risk assessment that tells you about the horse on that day, but cannot provide a guarantee for the future nor pick up certain subtle problems such as intermittent back pain or lameness if they are not present on the day of the examination.

Prepurchase examinations are carried out on behalf of a prospective purchaser. The examination is a very thorough one and on average takes 1–2 hours. If all is well, and the horse is considered suitable for the purpose intended, a Certificate of Veterinary Examination of a Horse on behalf of a Prospective Purchaser will be issued (Figure 24.1).

Arranging the examination

If this is to be your first horse and you do not know an equine vet or the horse in question is too far away for your own vet to examine, you will need to contact a suitable practice. Ask your own vet or local equine practice to recommend one. Your vet may be prepared to travel to see a horse or be able to recommend an equine veterinary colleague in the area.

Failing that, contact the vendor's vet and ask about other equine vets in the area. If the vendor's vet is willing to conduct the prepurchase examination, this provides a useful opportunity to check the horse's medical history as they are ethically bound to disclose all

**CERTIFICATE OF VETERINARY EXAMINATION
OF A HORSE ON BEHALF OF A PROSPECTIVE PURCHASER**

CERTIFICATE No:
V 42953

This is to certify that, at the request of (Name & Address) _____

_____

I have examined the horse described below, the property of (Name & Address) _____

_____

at (Place of Examination) _____ on (Time & Date) _____

IDENTIFICATION	
NAME of horse (or breeding)	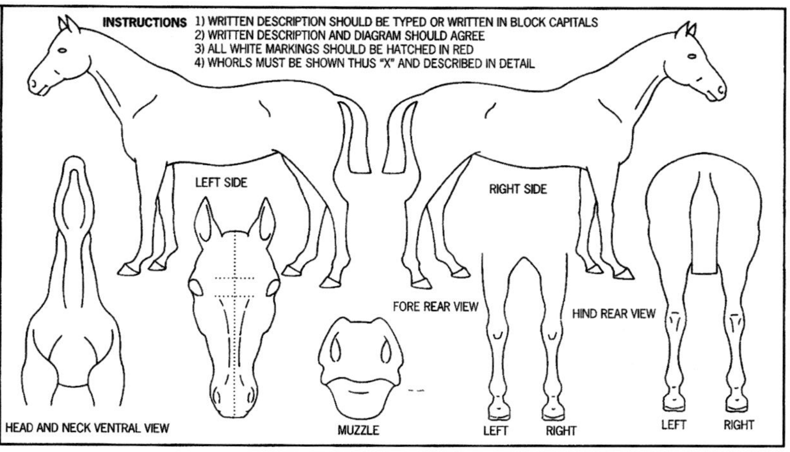 INSTRUCTIONS 1) WRITTEN DESCRIPTION SHOULD BE TYPED OR WRITTEN IN BLOCK CAPITALS 2) WRITTEN DESCRIPTION AND DIAGRAM SHOULD AGREE 3) ALL WHITE MARKINGS SHOULD BE HATCHED IN RED 4) WHORLS MUST BE SHOWN THUS "X" AND DESCRIBED IN DETAIL
BREED OR TYPE	LEFT SIDE RIGHT SIDE
COLOUR	
SEX	FORE REAR VIEW HIND REAR VIEW
AGE by documentation	
APPROX. AGE by dentition **(See Note 1 - overleaf)**	HEAD AND NECK VENTRAL VIEW MUZZLE LEFT RIGHT LEFT RIGHT

IDENTIFICATION

Head: _____

_____

Neck: _____

_____

Limbs: LF _____

RF _____

LH _____

RH _____

Body: _____

_____

Acquired marks/brands/microchip: _____

REPORT OF EXAMINATION (See Note 2): I find no clinically discoverable signs of disease, injury or physical abnormality other than those here recorded (or recorded on the attached sheet)

_____

_____

_____

_____ **Cont'd on attached sheet Yes/No**

Radiological or specialised techniques included in addition to the standard procedure _____

Report appended YES/NO   Blood taken and stored for testing for NSAIDs and other substances YES/NO   **WARRANTY (see Note3)**

THE OPINION (See Note 4): On the balance of probabilities the conditions set out above | ARE | ARE NOT | Delete clearly as appropriate

likely to prejudice this animal's use for _____

Owing to _____ stages _____ of the standard procedure were omitted **(See Note 5)**

Veterinary Surgeon's Signature _____ Date of Signature _____

Veterinary Surgeon's Name (in block capitals) _____

Address _____

_____ **NOTES - See overleaf**

Figure 24.1 The 5–stage examination certificate

relevant information provided the vendor consents to this. If the vendor does not agree, the vet cannot carry out the examination. However, many vets will not examine a horse for purchase if it belongs to one of their clients because of the potential conflict of interest. If you and the vendor both use the same vet, you may need to find someone else to carry out the examination. Discuss this with the vet and the vendor.

Briefing the vet

It is very important that the vet knows the intended use of the horse and the purchaser's level of experience. Without this information, the vet will be unable to offer an opinion on whether the horse is likely to fulfil the buyer's expectations. The vet will explain the procedure and also the scope and limitations of the examination. Wherever possible, the purchaser should attend the vetting. A great deal can be learned about the temperament of the horse during the examination. Any points raised by the vet can then be discussed before a decision is made.

Preparation for the vetting

It is important that the vendor understands the procedure and what the vet's requirements on the day will be. Consideration should be given to the following.

STABLING

The horse or pony should be stabled the night before the examination and not exercised prior to the vet's visit. This increases the likelihood of respiratory allergies or slight stiffness being detected.

GROOMING

The horse must be clean and dry but the feet should not be oiled. The horse should be well shod or the vetting may have to be postponed. Loose shoes and risen clenches can be a danger to the horse and it is not possible for the vet to assess soundness if the horse is presented with a shoe missing. It is false economy to avoid the expense of shoeing if the horse needs new shoes prior to the examination.

RIDER AND ASSISTANT

The vendor should provide a competent rider to exercise the horse. Alternatively, the purchaser can ride the horse so that nothing can be disguised. An assistant should be available to hold or lead the horse when required.

FACILITIES

Suitable facilities for exercise must be available. A firm, level surface is required for the trotting up. Waterlogged fields, hillsides and hard, rutted surfaces are unsuitable for stage 3 of the examination. A dark loosebox is needed for examination of the eyes. If necessary, the horse should be transported elsewhere. These arrangements need to be made beforehand to avoid wasting time.

The vetting procedure

The examination is carried out in 5 stages.

1 Preliminary examination.
2 Trotting up.
3 Strenuous exercise.
4 Period of rest.
5 A second trot up and foot examination.

The examination *does not include:*

- rectal palpation
- pregnancy diagnosis
- a full neurological examination
- an accurate height measurement which must be obtained separately under the Joint Measurement Board scheme
- radiography, endoscopy, ultrasonography, scintigraphy, ECG
- blood tests for underlying illness or drug administration
- performance warranty
- warranty of temperament and freedom from vices.

Additional examinations, e.g. radiography, endoscopy or ultrasonography, may be requested in advance by the purchaser or the vet may recommend them following the clinical examination. A blood sample is frequently taken at the time of the prepurchase examination. This blood can be screened immediately for non-steroidal anti-inflammatory drugs (NSAIDs), sedatives or other substances or stored in case a problem is detected shortly after purchase. The sample is stored for 6 months. There will be an extra charge for these procedures and tests and the vendor's permission must be obtained.

THE EXAMINATION

Stage 1 – preliminary examination

The horse is observed at rest in the stable. Its general condition and resting respiratory movements are noted. The horse is then methodically and thoroughly examined. The tests include the following.

- Listening to the horse's heart and lungs with a stethoscope. It is important to be as quiet as possible during this stage of the examination.
- Inspection of the teeth for an estimate of age. This is not always accurate or reliable due to individual variations and environmental conditions under which the horse has been kept. Horses over the age of 8 years are referred to as 'aged'. The teeth will also

be checked for alignment, abnormal wear, dental overgrowths, the presence of wolf teeth, sharp edges and any other abnormality.

- Examination of the eyes with a pen torch and ophthalmoscope.
- Checking the body and limbs. Hands are run over the horse's body and every part is carefully palpated and inspected for scars or abnormalities.
- Hoof conformation is noted and the feet are squeezed with hoof testers to check for any tenderness.
- The limbs are flexed to ensure there is no pain or restriction of movement.

During this time the vet will look around the stable to check for any evidence of crib-biting and that the horse's droppings are normal. Note will be taken of the type of bedding and whether the hay is soaked.

The horse is now taken outside and inspected in daylight. Conformation is assessed with the horse standing square on a hard, level surface.

Stage 2 – trotting up

This part of the examination must be carried out on a hard, level surface. The horse should wear a bridle if the examination is performed on a road.

- The horse is walked in a straight line away from the vet for approximately 30–40 m, then turned and walked back. The vet will observe the horse from in front, behind and from the side.
- This is repeated at trot. The handler should run beside the horse's shoulder and allow unrestricted movement of the horse's head. The vet is looking for any lameness or gait abnormalities.
- Flexion tests are usually performed. Each limb in turn is held in a flexed position for approximately 1 minute. The horse is asked to move off in trot. Stiffness or lameness is suggestive of joint disease or other problems.
- The horse is observed turning in small circles in either direction.
- The horse is asked to walk backwards.
- Next, the vet will observe the horse on the lunge on both soft and firm surfaces if possible. This includes small-diameter circles on a hard surface at trot.

If all is well up to this point, stage 3 is commenced.

Stage 3 – strenuous exercise

The amount of exercise depends on the age and fitness of the horse, its anticipated use and the facilities available. The aims of this part of the examination are:

- to make the horse breathe deeply and rapidly so any unusual breathing sounds are heard
- to increase the heart rate so abnormalities can be detected

- to work the horse sufficiently hard that undetected strains and injuries show up during the examination or as lameness or stiffness following a period of rest.

The horse is worked, but not exhausted. Individual examinations vary, but a riding horse is usually observed at walk and trot on a 20 m circle. A couple of 10 m circles are included at trot on both reins. The horse is then asked to canter for 5–10 minutes, passing close to the vet on each circuit. Any unusual respiratory noises are noted. The speed is then increased to a controlled gallop. The heart rate and rhythm and the rate and depth of breathing are recorded immediately the horse is pulled up. The horse is then untacked and returned to the stable.

Young, unbroken horses or tiny ponies may be lunged. Pregnant mares are excluded from this part of the examination.

Stage 4 – a period of rest

The horse is allowed to rest in the stable for up to 30 minutes. The slowing of the heart and respiratory rates are monitored. During this time, the vet will record the horse's details for identification purposes and check documentation such as the passport, vaccination certificate and breeding papers which should be made available. A blood sample may be taken at this point or at the end of the examination.

Stage 5 – second trot and foot examination

The horse is walked and trotted up as before. The horse is turned in a tight circle in both directions and asked to walk backwards for a few steps if this has not been done earlier. This is to check the horse's suppleness and for any gait abnormalities that could indicate a neurological problem, e.g. wobbler syndrome, stringhalt or shivering. If there are any concerns over the horse's feet, the vet may ask the vendor for permission to remove the shoes.

ADDITIONAL TESTS AND SPECIALIST OPINIONS

The vet may recommend further investigation to confirm or eliminate a possible problem at this stage. Some clients or their insurance companies request radiographs for high-value horses. However, the limitations of radiography have to be understood and accepted. For example, minor changes may be seen on radiographs of the navicular bone, but not all of these horses will go on to experience foot pain.

On occasions, the opinion of a specialist may be sought, e.g. a cardiologist to check out the significance of a heart murmur.

The veterinary report

Following the examination, if all is well the vet will issue a written report with the findings of the examination and discuss any abnormalities with you. You will receive an opinion on whether or not the horse is fit for its intended use at the time of the examination.

Written reports are not always supplied if the horse is not considered suitable for the purpose intended. A Certificate of Veterinary Inspection of a Horse Not Recommended for Purchase may be issued.

If any stages of the examination have been omitted, the vet's opinion will be based solely on the partial examination performed.

Insurance

Obtaining a 5-stage Certificate of Veterinary Examination of a Horse on behalf of a Prospective Purchaser is by no means a guarantee that the horse will be accepted for cover by your chosen insurance company. If this is essential, it is advisable to delay purchase until the insurance company has a copy of the certificate and agreed to the required cover.

Limited examinations

Prospective purchasers sometimes ask vets to carry out a limited examination involving only stages 1 and 2. Under these circumstances the purchaser is advised of the limitations of the examination and asked to sign a letter acknowledging this.

Summary

The prepurchase examination is a worthwhile investment as it may prevent you from spending a large sum of money on a horse that is unlikely to fulfil your requirements. As the examination is time-consuming, it is not cheap. You should ask your vet for an estimate of the cost before the examination is undertaken. Tell your vet of any particular concerns that you have before the visit and provide all available information such as performance records and videos.

Try to be as sure as possible that this is the right horse for you before the veterinary inspection. Ask the vendor or observe the following for yourself.

- Can the horse be caught easily?
- Does he load and travel without problems?
- Is he quiet to shoe?
- How does he behave in traffic?
- Is the horse good to clip?
- Has the horse had any behavioural problems that affect riding such as napping or headshaking?

It is advisable to ask some all-encompassing questions such as whether there is anything in the horse's temperament, physical health or past history that may affect your decision to purchase. Ask the vendor how long they have known the horse and had it under their personal care. Is the horse currently insured and are there any exclusions in place? Has the horse had any corrective farriery? Preparing these questions in advance will help to ensure that nothing is forgotten.

The answers to these questions can make a difference to the value and usefulness of the horse to you and include points that may not be shown up by a veterinary examination for purchase. Obtaining a warranty from the vendor on these issues together with aspects of medical history such as allergies including sweet itch or a stable cough is recommended.

ESTIMATING THE AGE OF A HORSE FROM ITS TEETH

Estimating the age of a horse from its teeth is not straightforward. The older the horse, the less accurate it becomes as a number of factors influence the wear on the teeth. These include the following.

- Environmental factors such as soil and pasture type. Horses grazing on sandy soils or rough pasture will wear their teeth more than those on good soil with young, lush grass.
- Management factors such as diet. Horses fed large amounts of concentrates and relatively little forage will wear their teeth differently from those spending long hours at grass.
- Behaviour such as crib-biting and wind-sucking which may cause abnormal wear of the incisor teeth.
- Developmental abnormalities such as parrot mouth where the teeth do not meet each other normally.

However, consideration of the following can be helpful.

Eruption times

In young horses, a reasonable estimate of age can be made by looking at the incisor teeth to determine which permanent teeth have erupted, i.e. have come through the gum, and whether or not they are in wear, i.e. the opposing teeth have erupted sufficiently to meet together.

However, this is still variable and not as reliable as accurate documentation of the horse's age. Suitable documents include Weatherby's passports and breeding papers.

Baby teeth	Eruption age	
Central incisors	Birth or first week	
Lateral incisors	4–6 weeks	
Corner incisors	6–9 months	
Cheek teeth	Present at birth or within first 2 weeks	
Adult teeth	Eruption age	In wear
Central incisor	$2\frac{1}{2}$ years	3 years
Lateral incisor	$3\frac{1}{2}$ years	4 years
Corner incisor	$4\frac{1}{2}$ years	5 years

Table to show the eruption times of the temporary and permanent incisors

Baby teeth	Eruption age
1st, 2nd and 3rd premolars	Birth to first 2 weeks
Adult teeth	**Eruption age**
Canine teeth or tushes	4–5 years
1st premolar or wolf tooth	5–9 months
2nd premolar or 1st cheek tooth	$2\frac{1}{2}$ years
3rd premolar or 2nd cheek tooth	3 years
4th premolar or 3rd cheek tooth	$3\frac{1}{2}$–4 years
1st molar or 4th cheek tooth	9–12 months
2nd molar or 5th cheek tooth	2–3 years
3rd molar or 6th cheek tooth	$3\frac{1}{2}$–4 years

Table to show the eruption times of the other teeth

DEFRA approved passports and vaccination certificates are not always reliable as they may only record information given to the vet at the time of completion and obtained by making an estimate from the appearance of the teeth.

Appearance

- The baby incisors tend to be whiter and smaller than the permanent teeth.
- The adult incisors tend to be larger and more square in shape, and are a yellowish or brownish colour.

The difference in appearance between temporary and permanent incisors is usually quite obvious but on occasions it can be difficult to decide from the appearance whether the horse is a 2-year-old with 6 temporary teeth or a 5-year-old with all its adult incisors. The general appearance and maturity of the horse can help make this decision as can the presence of canine teeth (tushes) in male animals which usually do not erupt until between the ages of 4 and 5 years. (See Figures 24.2 and 24.5.)

The angle of the incisors

When viewed from the side, the permanent incisor teeth in a young animal are relatively short and meet together in an upright, nearly vertical fashion. As the horse ages, the teeth become longer and more horizontal in appearance.

All of the features discussed below are extremely variable and cannot reliably be used to tell the age of a horse.

Hooks

Traditionally, horses were believed to develop a hook on the back edge of the upper corner incisor when they reached 7 years old. This occurs in some horses but is not a reliable sign.

The shape of the cutting surface of the incisors

Newly erupted incisors have an oval cutting surface (also known as the occlusal surface or table). As the horse ages, these become rounder and when the horse is in its teens they become triangular. As the horse ages further they tend to become rounder again.

The infundibulum and enamel ring

A newly erupted permanent incisor has an obvious depression called the infundibulum and this is surrounded by an enamel ring (Figure 24.6). As the incisors wear, the infundibulum becomes shallower and gradually disappears. As a rough guide, it disappears from the central incisors between 5 and 7 years, from the lateral incisors between 6 and 9 years and from the corners between 7 and 10 years. The enamel ring or 'mark' is eventually worn away when the horse is in its mid teens.

The dental star

The dental star is a brown mark that appears as a horizontal line on the occlusal surface of the central incisors as the horse reaches 6–7 years of age. It can be seen between the diminishing infundibulum and the outer (front) edge of the tooth (Figure 24.6). On average it develops in the lateral incisor between 7 and 9 years and the corner incisor between 8 and 10 years. The dental star changes shape and position as the horse becomes older, changing from a horizontal line near the edge of the tooth to a round mark in the centre.

Galvayne's groove

This is a dark-coloured groove which appears in the centre of the outer surface of the upper corner incisor tooth when the horse is 9–10 years. It extends half-way down the tooth by the time the horse is 15 and all the way down when it is 20 years old. By 25 years the groove is no longer visible in the upper half of the tooth and it may have completely disappeared by 30 years. However, this is fairly unreliable. In some horses the groove is difficult to see and in others it covers different lengths of the tooth on opposite sides of the mouth.

Summary

It is possible to make a reasonable estimate of a horse's age from its teeth up until 5–6 years of age. Between 7 and 10 years it may be possible to estimate the age to within a year or two. Beyond 10 years of age, looking at the teeth is not a reliable way to tell the horse's age.

(Figures 24.2–24.14.)

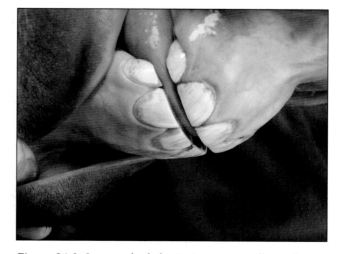

Figure 24.2 2 years: the baby incisors are smaller and whiter than the permanent teeth

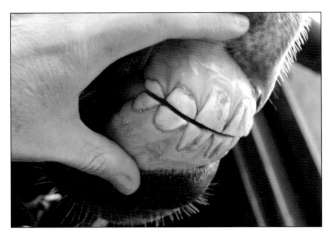

Figure 24.3 3 years: the central incisors are permanent; the lateral and corner incisors are baby teeth

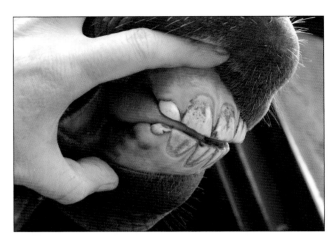

Figure 24.4 4 years: the central and lateral incisors are permanent but the corner incisors are still baby teeth

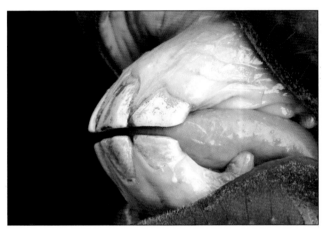

Figure 24.5 5 years: all of the permanent incisors have erupted and are in wear; the presence of tushes and the maturity of the horse help to differentiate these from 2-year-old teeth, with which they are sometimes confused

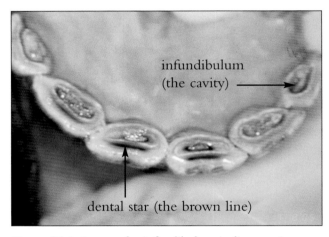

Figure 24.6 6 years: the infundibulum is disappearing from the central incisors; the dental star is present in the central incisors and one lateral incisor

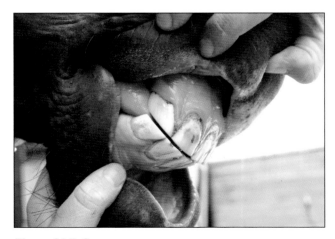

Figure 24.7 8 years

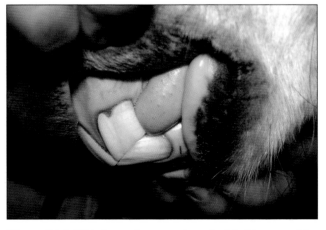

Figure 24.8 This horse is approximately 10–11 years old; Galvayne's groove is just appearing

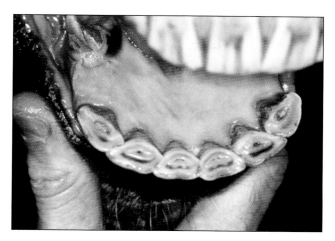

Figure 24.9 10 years: the infundibulum is disappearing from the corner incisors; the dental star is present in all the incisors

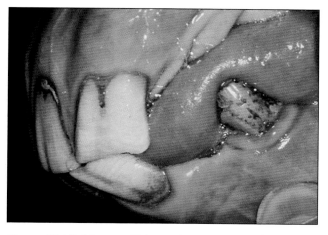

Figure 24.10 13 years: Galvayne's groove extends approximately one third of the way down the upper corner incisor teeth

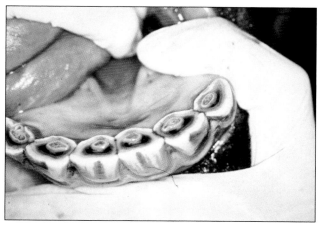

Figure 24.11 15 years: the tables are triangular, the infundibula are gone and the dental star is seen clearly in all the incisors

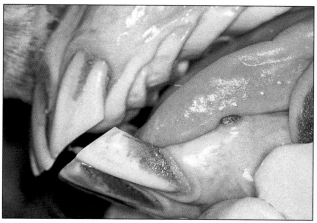

Figure 24.12 16 years: Galvayne's groove is present and extends just over half the length of the upper corner incisor

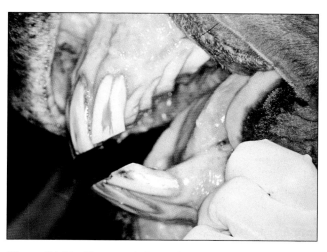

Figure 24.13 20 years: Galvayne's groove is present along the whole length of the upper corner incisor

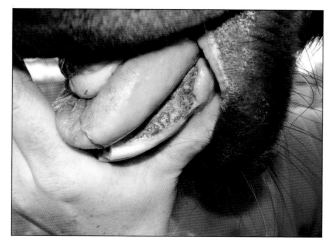

Figure 24.14 As the horse ages, the teeth become longer and more horizontal

BLOOD TESTS

Blood tests may be taken:

- as part of a routine health check
- to provide more information when the cause of a horse's illness is obscure
- to confirm or eliminate a clinical diagnosis.

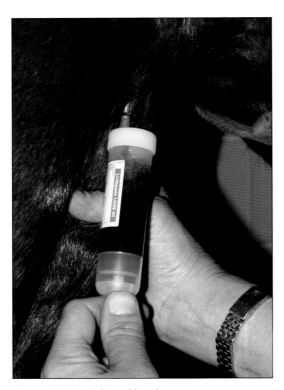

Figure 24.15 Taking blood

Taking blood samples

Blood is usually obtained from the jugular vein in the horse's neck (Figure 24.15). Samples for haematology must be collected when the horse is relaxed and before exercise. This is because when the horse is excited or exercised the spleen contracts and pushes a reserve pool of red blood cells into the circulation. The artificially high result could result in a mild anaemia being missed. Approximately 30% of the total red blood cells are stored in the spleen of the resting horse.

The components of blood

Blood is made up of the following.

RED BLOOD CELLS

These are also known as **erythrocytes** or **red blood corpuscles**. They give blood its red colour. The cells contain a pigment called **haemoglobin**. This combines with oxygen in the lungs and transports it to the tissues. Carbon dioxide is transported in the opposite direction.

WHITE BLOOD CELLS

These cells are also known as **leucocytes**; they defend the body against infection. There are five different types:

- neutrophils (also called polymorphs)
- lymphocytes
- eosinophils
- monocytes
- basophils.

PLATELETS

Platelets play an important part in the clotting mechanism of blood.

All the above components are suspended in a fluid known as **plasma**.

Haematology

Haematology is the study of blood. It includes the following measurements.

PCV – PACKED CELL VOLUME

This is the percentage volume of whole blood that is taken up by the red blood cells.

RBC – RED BLOOD CELL COUNT

This is a measure of the number of red cells in the circulation. It is measured as the number of red blood cells x 10^{12} per litre of blood.

Hb – HAEMOGLOBIN

This is a measure of the amount of oxygen-carrying pigment in the blood. It is measured in grams per decilitre ($\frac{1}{10}$ litre).

MCV – MEAN CORPUSCULAR VOLUME

This is the average volume of the red blood cells.

MCHC – MEAN CORPUSCULAR HAEMOGLOBIN CONCENTRATION

This is a measure of the concentration of haemoglobin in the red blood cells.

MCH – MEAN CORPUSCULAR HAEMOGLOBIN

This is also a measure of haemoglobin content in the red blood cells.

WBC – WHITE BLOOD CELL COUNT

Total and differential white cell counts are recorded (see page 678).

Interpretation of test results

Each laboratory has its own normal range. If serial blood tests are used to monitor the health of an individual horse, the blood should always be sent to the same laboratory.

RED CELL VALUES

A low RBC, PCV or Hb, indicate that the horse is anaemic. Higher-than-normal values are suggestive of excitement, dehydration or toxic shock. The type of animal and its level of fitness are considered when the results are interpreted. For example, a PCV of 30 is acceptable for a child's pony at grass but would be considered abnormally low for a racehorse in training.

PLATELETS

An increased number of platelets in the blood is known as **thrombocytosis**; this can occur with excitement, persistent or chronic haemorrhage, chronic infection or inflammation. A lower than normal platelet count is called **thrombocytopenia**; this can occur with a number of conditions including severe haemorrhage.

WHITE CELL VALUES

The **total white cell count** is affected by alterations in the numbers of the individual cell types. It can be a useful indicator of the presence of infection. A low total white cell count is known as a **leucopenia**. A raised total white cell count is a **leukocytosis**. As a general rule, the following apply.

- A persistently low white cell count is associated with chronic or recurrent viral infection.
- A low white cell count is often seen in the early stages of a bacterial infection. Over the next few days, a raised total white cell count develops.
- Serious infections such as peritonitis often result in a very low total white cell count.

Useful information can also be obtained by looking at any change in value of the individual white cell types when compared to their normal range.

NEUTROPHILS

Neutrophil numbers rise in response to bacterial infection. They are able to migrate from the small blood vessels into connective tissue where they engulf and kill bacteria. In severe, overwhelming bacterial infections and acute viral infections, their numbers in the circulation may be low.

LYMPHOCYTES

These cells are important for recognizing antigens such as viruses, bacteria and fungi. They stimulate antibody production. Their numbers may decrease in response to a viral infection.

EOSINOPHILS

Eosinophils may rise in response to allergic or parasitic conditions. Their numbers are lowered by administration of corticosteroids or in horses with Cushing's disease.

MONOCYTES

The numbers increase in the presence of inflammation from tissue damage or infection. They migrate from the blood into the tissues and become transformed into large macrophages which engulf and digest bacteria, viruses and dead tissue.

BASOPHILS

The numbers of basophils in equine blood are very small. They are involved in allergic and parasitic conditions.

Biochemistry

Biochemical tests are carried out on serum or plasma. Plasma is the fluid part of whole blood and it contains fibrinogen. Serum is the liquid component of clotted blood. It does not contain fibrinogen as this has been used up in the clotting process. These tests provide a great deal of information about what is happening in different parts of the horse's body. Variations from the normal range can point to problems in specific organs, and so they can be a valuable aid to diagnosis. They also play a part in the routine monitoring of performance horses and may be helpful in making training and management decisions.

The following biochemical tests can be performed.

TOTAL PROTEIN

This is the sum of the albumin and globulin components of the blood.

Albumin

This is raised if the horse is dehydrated, toxic or excited. Albumin levels are low with malnutrition, gut damage, liver or kidney disease

Globulin

The globulin can be separated into several fractions by a procedure called protein electrophoresis. Increases in the different fractions indicate the following.

Alpha 2 (α2) – occurs with tissue damage.

Beta 1 (β1) – indicates an antibody response to migrating strongyle larvae.

Beta 2 (β2) – liver damage.

Gamma globulins (γ) – antibody response to viral or bacterial infection.

IgG

This test is used to measure the level of immunity the foal receives from the maternal colostrum. It is usually performed on the second day after the foal is born. The results show whether the foal needs treatment. Levels of more than 8g/l are satisfactory. Levels between 4 and 8g/l indicate partial failure of colostral immunity. Levels of less than 4g/l indicate total failure of passive transfer (FPT) of immunoglobulins to the foal via the colostrum.

PLASMA FIBRINOGEN

This protein is raised where tissue damage is present, e.g. chronic infections, internal abscesses and parasitic disease.

SERUM AMYLOID A

This is another protein that increases with infection and inflammation.

PLASMA VISCOSITY

This increases with raised protein levels, and so rises with inflammation and tissue damage.

ALKALINE PHOSPHATASE (SAP)

Levels of SAP are raised with:

- chronic liver disease
- abnormal bone metabolism
- intestinal problems.

As this test is not specific, the results are used in conjunction with the clinical findings and other blood tests to pinpoint the problem.

INTESTINAL PHOSPHATASE

This is raised with intestinal damage.

LACTATE DEHYDROGENASE (LDH)

This rises in response to a number of diseases. It can be divided into 5 components which indicate different disease processes:

LD1 – haemolysis (breakdown of red blood cells), heart muscle damage

LD2 – damaged heart muscle

LD3 – is not specific enough to be useful

LD4 – intestinal damage

LD5 – liver or skeletal muscle damage.

L-GAMMA GLUTAMYLTRANSFERASE (GGT)

GGT is raised with:

- chronic liver cirrhosis
- cholangiohepatitis

For reasons that are not fully understood, elevations of this enzyme are sometimes seen in apparently healthy horses in training.

GLUTAMATE DEHYDROGENASE (GLDH)

GLDH levels are raised with acute liver damage or intestinal disease.

BILE ACIDS

These are raised if the liver is not functioning properly: the higher the level, the worse the prognosis for recovery.

BILIRUBIN

Levels may be raised with liver disease, massive internal haemorrhage or if large numbers of red blood cells are being broken down.

BROMOSULPHALEIN (BSP) CLEARANCE

This is a test used to check liver function. A dye is injected into the bloodstream and blood samples are taken at set times afterwards. The rate of clearance of the dye from the blood is compared with results obtained from healthy horses.

ASPARTATE AMINOTRANSFERASE (AST)

Levels are raised with:

- acute liver damage
- acute muscle damage.

Levels are highest 24–48 hours after an episode of muscle damage. They gradually return to normal over the next 10–21 days and are a good indicator of muscle recovery.

CREATINE KINASE (CK)

CK is raised with acute muscle damage; the levels peak at 6–12 hours and return to normal after 3–4 days if no further damage occurs.

TROPONIN

This is used to monitor damage to heart muscle.

UREA

Urea is raised if the kidneys are not functioning normally.

CREATININE

This is also raised with kidney pathology.

TRIGLYCERIDES

Fat is stored in the body as triglycerides. These are raised in horses with hyperlipaemia and if there is a problem with the metabolism of fats.

GLUCOSE

Horses and ponies with Cushing's disease often have abnormally high blood glucose levels. Glucose levels are measured in certain tests to see if the gut absorption is normal.

AMYLASE

Amylase is raised with pancreatitis, but this is rarely seen in horses.

ELECTROLYTES AND MINERALS

In order for the body to function properly, electrolytes such as calcium, phosphorus, magnesium, sodium, chloride and potassium must be present in the correct quantities and ratios. Imbalances may be seen in horses with diarrhoea, exhaustion from overexertion or suffering from exertional rhabdomyolysis.

FRACTIONAL EXCRETION

Tests involve taking urine and blood samples at the same time or within two hours of each other. Additional information about the electrolyte status of the horse is obtained from these tests which may be helpful in identifying the need for dietary supplementation.

MAMMARY SECRETIONS

The levels of protein, calcium, magnesium, sodium and potassium in the mammary secretions of a pregnant mare provide a guide to the maturity of the foal and how close to foaling the mare is. This can be useful if for any reason induction of labour or caesarean section is being considered.

BLOOD GASES

Blood gases are measured in cases of respiratory and intestinal abnormality. They are only used in equine hospitals with on-site laboratories as they have to be analysed soon after collection.

Many blood tests are not specific so they are used as an aid to diagnosis in conjunction with the clinical findings from the examination of the horse.

RESTRAINT OF THE HORSE

Most horses tolerate a wide variety of treatments when held in a headcollar by a quiet, competent handler. However, in situations where a horse is frightened or in pain, additional restraint may be necessary to ensure:

- the optimum treatment
- the safety of everyone present.

The following methods can be used:

- confinement to a restricted space
- using a bridle or a chifney bit
- holding a leg up
- using a twitch
- sedation
- general anaesthesia.

Using a stable or holding pen

Some horses try to move away from a person cleaning a wound or administering a treatment. When confined in a stable, the animal will usually move against the wall and then stand quietly and accept the procedure. Using a stable eliminates interference from other horses and ponies.

Use of a bridle or chifney bit

If the horse is strong, excitable or aggressive, using a bridle or chifney bit may help to increase the degree of control.

Holding a leg up

Lifting a forelimb makes it more difficult (but not impossible) for a horse to kick out. When you are attending to a hind limb injury on a sensitive horse, the forelimb on the same side should be lifted by an assistant. If you are both on the same side, the handler can pull the horse's head towards you if it lashes out. The quarters will then swing in the opposite direction. When dealing with a forelimb, the opposite forelimb should be lifted.

Using a twitch

The twitch is often used when the aforementioned methods of restraint have proved inadequate. In many cases it enables the treatment to proceed without further problems. However, if it is used for any length of time one needs to consider whether it is appropriate or humane; sedation may be a better option. There are several methods of twitching a horse and several types of twitch.

ROPE TWITCH

A twitch can be made from a piece of cotton rope or plaited baler twine looped through the end of a length of broom handle. Stand to one side of the horse and put your hand

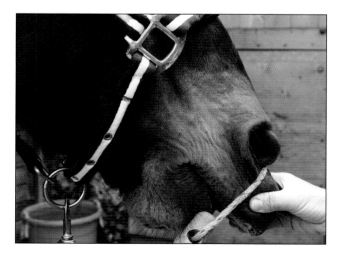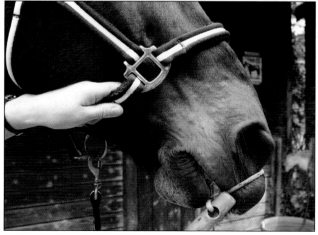

Figure 24.16a and b Applying a rope twitch: a) the rope loop is placed over the horse's lip; b) the rope is tightened around the lip and muzzle

684 THE VETERINARY CARE OF THE HORSE

halfway through the loop of rope and grasp the horse's upper lip gently and firmly (Figure 24.16a). Slide the loop forwards over your fingers so it is positioned around the grasped lip. Twist the handle so the rope tightens around the muzzle. Continue twisting until the rope is sufficiently tight that it does not slip off if the horse moves its head (Figure 24.16b). The handle should then be held by an assistant as a twitched horse may suddenly take exception to it, necessitating prompt removal.

Application of the twitch usually causes the horse to go into a sleepy, trance-like state. The head drops and the eyes may close. The horse becomes less sensitive to painful stimuli. This may be due to the release of endorphins from the brain or because the twitch is painful. The twitch should not be left on for more than 15 minutes. Once it has been removed, the muzzle should be rubbed gently to restore the circulation.

Warning

Some horses will not tolerate the twitch at all and others will only stay calm for a short period of time. If the horse rears or strikes out, remove the twitch at once. If you lose your grasp on the twitch, the horse may swing its head violently with the twitch still attached to the muzzle and this can be dangerous for you and the horse.

When using a twitch, keep the stable door closed but not bolted. It is very important for handlers to be able to leave the box quickly when dealing with a fractious horse.

CHAIN TWITCHES

These are used by some vets. They are harsher, but have the advantage of falling off immediately if the handler releases their grasp.

NECK OR HAND TWITCH

In some horses, simply grasping the muzzle or a fold of skin on the side of the neck is an effective method of restraint (Figure 24.17). The neck skin may be gently twisted if necessary.

EAR TWITCH

Gently grasping the ear of a horse and twisting it slightly or pulling it downwards is another method of restraint that is sometimes used. However it is not generally recommended as poor technique can make a horse head shy.

HUMANE TWITCH

The humane twitch (Figure 24.18) is an aluminium tool applied over the horse's muzzle. The ends are squeezed together and fixed in a closed position with the attached cord. It works in a similar fashion to the rope twitch, but is easier to apply to some horses. The disadvantage is the shorter length of the handle if the horse raises its head.

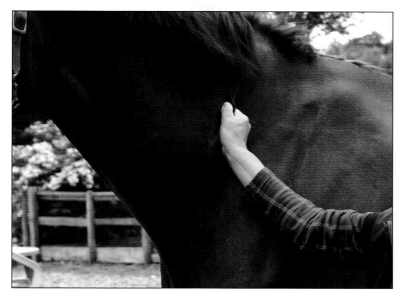

Figure 24.17 Neck twitch

Figure 24.18 Humane twitch

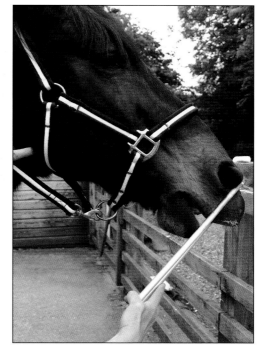

CHAIN SHANK

This is sometimes used on a horse that cannot be twitched. However, it should only be used by experienced handlers because incorrect use can cause severe injury to the horse. The first part of the lead rope is made of a metal chain. This can be attached to the headcollar and passed over the nose or through the mouth or across the upper gums. The latter two are an extremely severe form of restraint.

In every case, the restraint is used for the minimum possible time.

Sedation

Where physical methods of restraint have failed or are considered inappropriate or undesirable, the vet will administer a sedative. A number of sedative drugs are available. These may be used singly or in various combinations, depending on the degree of sedation required. Some also have analgesic or muscle relaxant properties.

In any situation the degree of sedation depends on:
- the drugs used
- the dose
- the temperament of the horse
- the horse's level of excitement at the time the drug is administered; sedatives work most effectively when given to a relaxed horse in a quiet environment.

ADMINISTRATION

Sedatives are usually given by intravenous or intramuscular injection. Acepromazine (ACP) is also available in oral gel or tablet forms.

Examples of situations requiring sedation include:

- treatment of painful wounds
- minor surgical procedures, e.g. suturing a wound
- taking radiographs or performing ultrasound scans if the horse is nervous and likely to damage itself or the equipment
- teeth rasping and clipping of head-shy horses
- turning a horse out after a prolonged period of box rest.

General anaesthesia

In situations where it is essential for the horse to remain completely still, the horse may have to be given a general anaesthetic.

EQUINE GENERAL ANAESTHESIA
Karen Coumbe MA VetMB CertEP MRCVS

A horse may require a general anaesthetic for a routine planned procedure such as castration or for an emergency such as urgent colic surgery. When you are told your horse needs surgery, there is a tendency to focus on the operation itself and forget the anaesthetic. It is easy to take anaesthesia for granted as an integral part of the procedure. For every horse, it is essential to consider the anaesthetic risks when making the decision whether or not to proceed with surgery. A recent detailed survey on equine anaesthesia reviewed more than forty thousand anaesthetics. This investigated the perioperative deaths: those during, and within seven days of, general anaesthesia. This study revealed an overall death rate of 1.6%. If the horses that were already ill with colic were excluded, the death rate was still approximately 1%; 1 death in 100 horses is frightening in comparison with the perioperative mortality rate in man, which is 1 in 10,000. In companion animals (cats and dogs) it is about 1 in 700. This means that there is a significant risk of any horse dying under any anaesthetic.

Although 1% might almost be an acceptable anaesthetic death rate for horses that were ill, it is alarming when it applies to normal healthy horses undergoing surgery for routine procedures. For this reason it is important that any anaesthesia and surgery is only ever performed when it is genuinely justifiable rather than, for example, simply removing blemishes for cosmetic reasons. If it is not going to truly benefit the horse, you need to ask whether it is worth doing. Your vet should be able to advise you.

There are several reasons why horses are difficult to anaesthetize. Unlike people, horses are not already lying down quietly counting to ten when the anaesthetic is administered.

Care has to be taken to ensure that they do not harm themselves as they collapse or when they struggle to stand after surgery. Modern anaesthetic techniques help, as do the well-padded 'knock down' and 'recovery' boxes available at many equine hospitals, which are designed to reduce injury. Where it is imperative that a horse stands up with particular care, for instance after a delicate fracture repair, vets may use a system of ropes attached to its head and tail and have experienced helpers controlling the horse and supporting it as it stands. In the United States there are some very sophisticated systems to encourage steady recoveries; for instance, floating the horse in a rubber ring in a water tank.

Unfortunately the horse's large size complicates anaesthesia. They are extremely heavy, especially when they have to lie still under anaesthetic for any length of time. The muscles on their underside can be damaged by their body-weight. When horses are positioned on their backs during an operation, the large stomach and hind gut squash the lungs and make it more difficult for the horse to inhale enough oxygen with each breath. Their large hearts beat slowly anyway and under anaesthesia the heart can all too easily stop altogether. Cardiac arrest was the commonest cause of anaesthetic death in the survey of perioperative equine fatalities.

Many more sophisticated operations are performed on horses these days, yet the anaesthetic risk has remained about the same. The advances in surgery require more complex and potentially challenging anaesthesia, but the number of anaesthetic deaths has not increased because there has been an enormous increase in the knowledge, equipment and medications available to anaesthetize horses safely. Vets now are able to successfully perform much more complicated procedures, such as colic surgery and fracture repairs.

What you should do if your horse needs a general anaesthetic

In an emergency there will be no opportunity to plan ahead, but for a routine operation you should do the following.

- Notify your insurers first. Always discuss the details of any operation with your insurers since you need their agreement to proceed. Some companies request an extra premium to cover the extra risk. In an emergency, the insurers should be notified as soon as it is possible to do so.

- Arrange for the shoes to be removed before any surgery, so that the horse is less likely to damage itself when lying down or standing after the anaesthetic.

- Check with your vet about starving the horse before surgery. Many vets routinely starve a horse overnight and sometimes longer for certain operations.

- Arrange for the operation to be performed in the safest possible place. In order to carry out major surgery, the horse should be admitted to an equine hospital where full theatre facilities and vets with specialist skills in both anaesthesia and surgery are available. This reduces the risks involved with an anaesthetic, and if problems do occur, more equipment and expertise is readily available. Some surgery is done in the field, particularly relatively routine procedures such as castration, in which case ensure there is a clean, empty paddock available. Check with your vet in advance exactly what will be required. Nowadays many equine practices have good hospital facilities available and therefore it is foolhardy to carry out major surgery in the field.

What an equine general anaesthetic involves

The planning phase This vital phase may include giving painkillers and any other necessary treatments in advance of surgery. A thorough check-up is carried out to detect any potential dangers. The anaesthetic regime can then be modified to suit that horse or, if necessary, the operation postponed until the horse is fit enough to be anaesthetized. In addition, the horse's temperament can be assessed. Frequently the neck is clipped and a catheter inserted into the jugular vein to provide a pain-free route for giving the anaesthetic injections and for intravenous fluid therapy. The area for surgery may also be clipped to save time later.

Pre-anaesthetic stage This often includes giving the horse a 'pre-med' injection as a tranquillizer, which reduces anxiety and provides protection for the horse's heart once anaesthetized. The horse is then groomed, the feet washed and the tail bandaged.

Induction or start of anaesthesia Ideally the anaesthetic is induced (or started) in a padded box, so that the horse lies down gently onto a soft surface. Initially the horse is heavily sedated and then several minutes later an anaesthetic injection is given to render the horse unconscious.

Maintenance of anaesthesia Once the horse is lying down, an endotracheal tube (a long hollow tube) is passed through the mouth, via the larynx (throat) and down into the windpipe. A cuff is blown up around the tube so that the horse only breathes the gases supplied via the anaesthetic machine. This is a mixture of oxygen and the anaesthetic gas that keeps the horse 'asleep'. Sometimes cocktails of intravenous anaesthetic drips are used instead of the horse breathing in anaesthetic gases.

An overhead hoist may be used to move the horse from the padded box into the theatre – some patients may weigh up to 1000 kg (2,200 lb) (Figure 24.19). The horse is then carefully positioned on the operating table, either on its side or back depending on the surgery to be performed. Positioning is very important, especially for operations lasting several hours, in order to avoid a complication known as post-anaesthetic myopathy, when the horse's muscles become swollen and painful as a result of poor blood supply whilst being compressed by the horse's weight during the operation. For some horses, this can be a serious and distressing problem.

During any operation the horse is constantly monitored so that the depth of the anaesthetic is known (Figure 24.20). The eye reflexes are noted and the rate and character

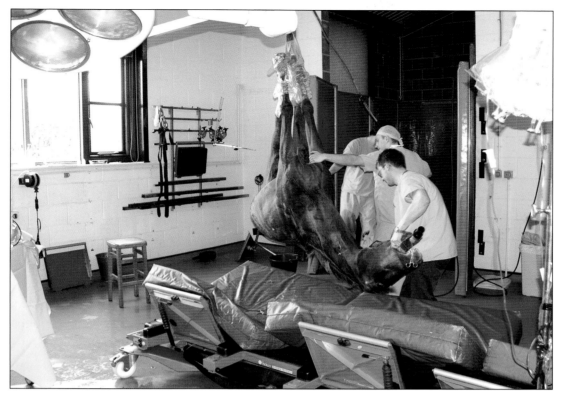

Figure 24.19 An overhead hoist is used to carefully manoeuvre the horse into position

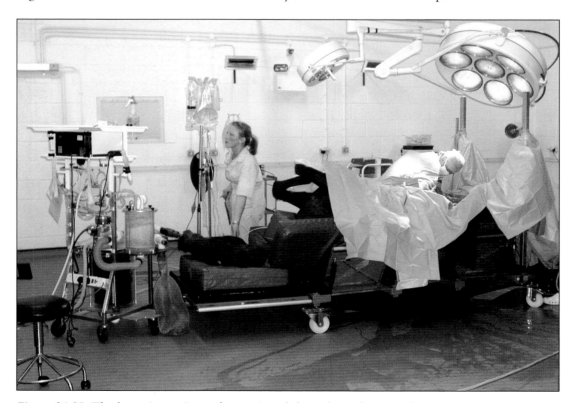

Figure 24.20 The horse is continuously monitored throughout the operation

of breathing are recorded. Sometimes it is necessary to control the horse's breathing via a ventilator. Sophisticated monitoring equipment records the horse's heart rate and rhythm and other vital signs. A catheter may be placed in an artery to monitor blood pressure and if it drops, specific extra treatment is given. Low blood pressure during surgery can result in major complications.

Recovery Once the operation is finished the horse is hoisted back into a padded recovery room. Usually the horses are left alone to slowly come round in a darkened, quiet environment whilst being watched carefully from a safe distance. Sometimes it is necessary to give further sedative drugs to make the recovery smoother. Excitable horses that try to stand up before they are co-ordinated enough to do so, may require this. The recovery phase of the anaesthetic is a risky time when complications can occur. Occasionally a horse may fracture a leg whilst trying to stand. As the horse comes round from the anaesthetic its movements are unpredictable and it is dangerous for people to be in with them. It is not until the horse is safely standing up that an operation has been successfully completed.

Summary

It is important to arrange for the operation to be performed in the safest possible place with experienced knowledgeable personnel in charge. The ideal anaesthetic prevents pain and stress for the horse before, during and after surgery. Some procedures can be performed with the horses standing under heavy sedation and by using local anaesthesia, but in many cases a general anaesthetic is essential for successful surgery to be performed. Pain relief is crucial throughout any procedure, as an unstressed pain-free patient will heal faster.

THE ADMINISTRATION OF VETERINARY MEDICINES TO HORSES

There are a number of ways that medicines can be given to a horse:
- orally (by mouth)
- by stomach tube
- by intravenous, intramuscular or subcutaneous injection
- topically
- by inhalation
- as an enema
- by intrauterine administration.

As a rule, your vet will make the procedure as efficient and easy as possible for all concerned. However, there are a number of factors that have to be taken into consideration. These include the following.

- The urgency of the situation. If a horse has an overwhelming infection or is in severe pain, then wherever possible the required treatment will be injected intravenously. In this way, high levels of the medication are attained in the circulation in the shortest possible time.

- Available forms of the medication. Some treatments are only suitable for intramuscular injection, e.g. thick antibiotic suspensions. Other products, e.g. the sedative acepromazine, are available as tablets and oral gel, as well as an injectable form suitable for intravenous or intramuscular administration.

- The temperament of the horse. Some patients are very difficult to inject and so, if at all possible, these animals will be given medicine in their food.

- The willingness of the horse to eat the medication. It is important that the horse receives the full dose of any medication administered, so fussy feeders may be injected if they dislike the taste.

- The location of the problem. Small skin wounds often heal without the need for systemic medication and topical applications may be all that are required. Sometimes the drugs need to be delivered directly to the site of infection, e.g. into the uterus of a mare with endometritis or onto the cornea of a horse with a corneal ulcer.

The oral route

These medicines can be given in the following ways.

- Mixed with the feed. Carrots, apples or molasses can be added to increase palatability. If the horse obviously dislikes the taste, then mixing the medicine with a small amount of palatable concentrate and feeding it first, sometimes works. The horse can then enjoy the rest of his meal. If the horse still will not eat it, then the medication can be mixed with apple sauce or peppermint flavouring and given using an empty, washed-out worming syringe or purpose-designed oral dosing syringe.

- As a paste. Wormers, some antibiotics and anti-inflammatory drugs, electrolytes, vitamin and mineral preparations come in syringes so the paste can be administered onto the back of the tongue (see page 50 for administration tips).

Stomach tube

A stomach tube is useful for administering large volumes of fluid or medicine directly into the lower part of the oesophagus or the stomach. This may be necessary if the horse is dehydrated or has an intestinal impaction. The warmed, flexible tube is passed up the nostrils into the pharynx and is swallowed by the horse so that it passes into the oesophagus (gullet). The vet will carry out several checks to ensure the tube is in the oesophagus and not in the trachea. A funnel is attached to the end of the stomach tube and the fluids drain into the stomach. Alternatively, the fluids may be pumped into the horse with a stomach pump. This procedure must only be carried out by a vet because if the fluids accidentally enter the windpipe and lungs, the horse will develop pneumonia or experience immediate drowning and death.

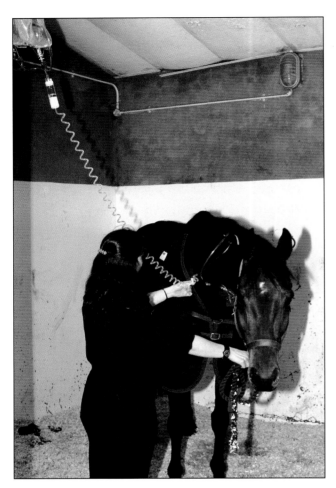

Figure 24.21 Large volumes of fluids may be administered intravenously

Injections

Intravenous injections are given if:

- the effect of the medication is needed as quickly as possible
- the drug is irritant to the tissues if given by any other route
- large volumes are necessary, e.g. when fluids are administered to a toxic or dehydrated horse (Figure 24.21).

If the horse is hospitalized and needs regular medication, an in-dwelling catheter may be positioned in the jugular vein. This is readily accessible and prevents soreness and resentment from frequent injections.

Intramuscular injections are often used to administer vaccines and antibiotics. In certain circumstances, the vet may leave a course of treatment for you to give to your horse. The technique is described in detail in the next chapter.

Subcutaneous injections are used to give medicines just under the skin. They are less commonly used for horses than in dogs and cats, but tetanus antitoxin may be administered in this way.

All injections must be given with clean hands, using sterile syringes and needles into a clean horse, to reduce the risk of infection.

Topical application

Creams, ointments, powders and antibacterial or antifungal washes are often applied directly onto wounds, when only a local effect is needed. The cornea (front) of the eye, for example, is often treated topically if damaged or diseased.

Inhalation

A number of drugs used to treat respiratory disease are administered using special inhalation devices. This ensures that the treatment is delivered directly to its target site, i.e. the lungs.

Enemas

Newborn foals experiencing constipation due to retention of the meconium are often treated with enemas. This is something that should only be done by a vet or a correctly trained and experienced person.

Intrauterine administration

Mares suffering from uterine inflammation (endometritis) are often treated by the infusion of antibiotics and sterile saline directly into the uterus. The skin around the vulva and anus is washed and the vet will use a gloved and lubricated hand to insert the end of a sterile catheter through the cervix into the uterus. Antibiotic washes are syringed through the catheter into the uterus. On occasions, in-dwelling catheters are stitched in place for the duration of the treatment. Larger volumes of fluid may be lavaged in and out of the uterus to eliminate infection and inflammation.

ISOLATION

It is sometimes necessary to isolate an individual horse or a group of animals away from other horses on the premises. This is usually owing to an outbreak of an infectious disease such as strangles or while an infection such as herpesvirus is suspected and being investigated.

'Isolation' in the strictest sense, means a completely separate unit with its own staff. Items such as protective clothing, tools and equipment are only used on that unit and not taken anywhere else. The stables should be steam cleaned and disinfected between each occupant.

Ideally, the following guidelines are adhered to.

Premises

- The isolation unit should be a separate, enclosed building of sound, permanent construction, which is capable of being cleaned and disinfected effectively.
- It should ideally be at least 100 m (330 ft) away from buildings, fields, bridleways and roads used by other horses.
- Adequate supplies of fresh, clean water should be available for drinking water and cleaning purposes.
- Enough food and bedding for the whole of the isolation period must be stored within the facility before isolation commences.
- All equipment used for grooming, cleaning and feeding must only be used within the isolation facility.
- Protective clothing should be available at the entrance to the facility. It should not be removed from the premises.
- The isolation unit should have its own muck heap.

Procedures

- Before the unit is used, all of the equipment and tools should be disinfected with an approved disinfectant (ask your vet or look on the DEFRA website www.defra.gov.uk).
- People caring for the isolated horses must not come into contact with any other horses during the isolation period.
- The isolation period will be advised by the vet. No horse should be allowed to leave until the last horse to enter the facility has completed the isolation period.
- Only authorized people should enter the unit.
- The unit must be securely locked when no staff are present, to prevent unauthorized entry to the unit.
- The attending vet will give advice on special procedures necessary for dealing with a particular disease.

The above procedures are possible with a purpose-built or specially adapted isolation unit. However, where facilities are unexpectedly needed on smaller equine establishments, the attending vet will give advice and make recommendations that can be achieved with the facilities available. The above guidelines should be adhered to as much as possible.

When there is no separate isolation unit, the following steps should be taken.

- Infectious horses should be moved to a separate area of the premises if possible.
- The person looking after the sick horses should not have contact with the other horses. If there are not enough people to achieve this, the healthy horses should be attended to first.
- Protective clothing should be worn when working with the infected horses. This should remain in the isolation area.
- An approved disinfectant (as advised by your vet) should be used for cleaning boots and all equipment, feed bowls, rugs, headcollars etc.
- Great care should be taken to avoid inadvertent transmission of the infection to healthy horses. Take special care not to get discharges or infected fluids on your clothes, hands or hair.

It is sensible for any equine yard with new horses entering on a regular basis to consider some form of isolation policy for new arrivals as it is common for these horses to bring new infections with them.

EUTHANASIA

Having a horse put to sleep is something that unfortunately many horse owners will have to face at some time. Euthanasia is a method of providing a humane and painless death. It may be done as an emergency procedure or planned in advance.

The most common reasons for euthanasia include:

- prevention of suffering, e.g. with an incurable and painful disease or following a serious injury
- ending the life of an old horse or pony
- economic considerations, e.g. when the horse is no longer capable of being ridden or fulfilling the activities for which it was purchased and keeping it in retirement is financially prohibitive.

How is it carried out?

There are two methods of euthanasia commonly used.

LETHAL INJECTION

The horse is given an overdose of anaesthetic-type drugs. An intravenous catheter is usually placed in the jugular vein and the horse may be given a sedative. Once the sedative has taken effect, the lethal injection is administered. The horse will collapse and quickly become unconscious. Death occurs shortly afterwards. Sometimes the horse will gasp once or twice which can be disconcerting if you are not expecting it.

SHOOTING

One of 2 methods will be used.

1 *Free-bullet humane slaughtering pistol*

    This method of euthanasia results in instant death of the horse. Again, a sedative may be given first. The muzzle of the gun is placed on the horse's forehead. The horse will fall down instantly with its legs extended and blood may pour from the nose. With this method there are involuntary movements of the horse's legs and occasional gasps for a short period of time after the horse is dead. The muscles then relax. The horse will be brain dead although the heart may continue to beat for a few minutes.

2 *Captive bolt stunner*

    The horse is stunned and becomes unconscious by the firing of a retractable bolt into the brain. This is followed by a procedure known as pithing whereby the brain is destroyed by insertion of a rod through the bolt hole. This method can be used in situations where it is not safe to use a free bullet.

Who can perform euthanasia?

The following people may carry out the procedure:

- your vet
- a hunt kennelman
- a knackerman
- a licensed horse slaughterer.

Only the vet can administer a lethal injection. The hunt kennelman and knackerman can be booked in advance and will sometimes attend in an emergency or collect a horse that has died.

In order for the horse to be slaughtered for human consumption at a licensed abattoir, it *must be fit to travel and accompanied by its passport*. The horse must not have received any medication for the previous six months. Some medicines, e.g. phenylbutazone, are not permitted at any time if the horse is to be slaughtered for human consumption. Appointments need to be booked in advance.

Disposal of the carcass

The options for disposal of the carcass are limited and depend on the method of euthanasia and the health of the horse when it died. Your own vet will advise you on the options available.

CREMATION

There are many companies that now offer a collection and cremation service. This option is costly but available regardless of the method of euthanasia. The ashes may be returned in a special casket if requested.

INCINERATION

This is offered commercially and is also available at some hunt kennels. It is usually cheaper than cremation.

HUNT KENNELS

Provided the horse was not put down by lethal injection or was not suffering from a disease making it unsuitable for consumption, many hunts will use the carcass as food for the hounds. However, this may change following recent legislation banning hunting with dogs. DEFRA has proposed an alternative carcass collection service to replace the valuable service provided by hunt kennels.

BURIAL

You need to check with your local Trading Standards Office whether this is permitted. The European Union Regulations do not allow burial of pet horses as they consider the horse to be a food animal. At the time of writing, DEFRA does allow burial of pet horses at the discretion of the local authority. Each case is considered on an individual basis.

Advance considerations

Having any animal put down is a distressing experience, so it is a good idea to plan ahead in order to avoid rushed decisions under difficult circumstances. If you have any questions or worries, discuss it with your vet who will be accustomed to helping with these difficult situations.

WHEN IS THE RIGHT TIME?

Most people 'just know' when the time has come for their horse to be put to sleep. The most important consideration is your horse's quality of life. If it is suffering from a disease which affects its quality of life or is experiencing chronic pain from which there is no hope of recovery, then it is time to make the decision and prevent further suffering. If you need to discuss it with anyone, consult your vet.

SHOULD I BE THERE?

Rest assured that everyone concerned will want your horse's last minutes to be peaceful. The people involved are professionals who care about animals and are used to dealing with this sensitive task. If you are able to be calm and relaxed during the procedure, then your presence is likely to be reassuring for your horse. If you are visibly distressed, then it may be better to ask a trusted friend to do this for you. Your vet may require you or someone on your behalf to sign a consent form. In a yard with several horses, it is essential that someone is present who can advise the vet which horse is to be put down.

WHICH METHOD SHOULD I CHOOSE?

If the euthanasia is planned in advance, the choice may be determined by personal preference. However, there are situations when one method is more appropriate than another, so be guided by your vet at the time. The welfare of the horse and the safety of the people around must be the first consideration.

WHERE SHOULD IT TAKE PLACE?

The selected location should be safe for people and other animals in the vicinity. In some emergency situations the horse cannot be moved but under normal circumstances you do have a choice. It is not possible to predict which way the horse will fall so there should be plenty of space. The selected site should be accessible to a vehicle for removal of the body. If advance arrangements have not been made for collection at the time of euthanasia, the site should be away from public view. If you have neighbours nearby, try to warn them first. The other owners in a livery yard should also be warned.

Many people choose to have elderly or ill horses quietly put to sleep at home. The horse is in familiar surroundings and does not experience any stress from travelling. However, if the horse is happy to travel, some people prefer to take them to the hunt kennels or to an equine hospital where they can be unloaded and euthanased on arrival. Death is instantaneous and without the horse having any premonition.

NOTIFICATION OF THE INSURANCE COMPANY

If the horse is insured for loss of use and a claim is going to be made, the insurance company must be notified in advance. With the exception of an emergency situation, the permission of the insurers is needed otherwise the claim may be invalidated.

If a horse is destroyed on humane grounds, it must meet certain criteria to satisfy the requirements of a mortality insurance policy. The British Equine Veterinary Association guidelines state that euthanasia should be carried out if '…*the insured horse sustains an injury or manifests an illness or disease that is so severe as to warrant immediate destruction to relieve incurable and excessive pain and that no other options of treatment are available to that horse at that time*'. The insurers should be notified as soon as possible. They will require a veterinary certificate confirming the identity of the horse and the reason why it was destroyed. They may also ask for a post mortem.

LEGAL CONSIDERATIONS

In the event of your horse being found in a situation where it is suffering in a way that requires urgent euthanasia and you cannot be contacted, the vet has the authority to carry out the task with the consent of a police officer under current legislation.

25

FURTHER ADVICE
AND PRACTICAL TIPS

INSURANCE

Insurance is a competitive business. Most equine magazines have several advertisements and each company is trying to attract your custom. However, equine insurance companies are under increased financial pressure due to the sophisticated (and consequently expensive) diagnostic techniques such as scintigraphy and magnetic resonance imaging that are now increasingly available. Before taking out an insurance policy it is very important that you are fully aware of the extent and limitations of the selected policy.

Do I need insurance?

There is no legal requirement to insure your horse, but at the very least it is advisable to have Public Liability cover. This insures against claims and legal costs arising from damage or injuries caused by your horse. Recent cases in the press have highlighted this need. In one example, a couple of ponies escaped from a well-fenced field and caused an accident resulting in serious injury to the driver of a car. Despite the owners having taken all reasonable precautions to keep their animals secure, they were faced with an enormous compensation bill. Public Liability insurance is included in membership of organizations such as the Pony Club, the British Horse Society (Gold membership), British Eventing, British Dressage and the British Show Jumping Association.

Veterinary fee cover is another area where insurance is recommended. With new developments in medicine, surgery and anaesthesia, the costs of successful treatment can escalate. It is hard for the vet as well as the owner of a horse if a particular treatment cannot be carried out due to economic restraints. Around 75% of horses now survive colic surgery, but the cost can run into several thousands of pounds which is prohibitive for many owners.

The decision on whether or not to insure your horse and the type of cover needed must be made after weighing the risks against the costs.

Types of insurance cover

The various options include the following.

PUBLIC LIABILITY

See above.

DEATH FROM INJURY OR ILLNESS

This is known as **all risks mortality insurance** and covers payment up to the sum insured (or market value if less) if your horse dies from an accident or illness or is humanely destroyed by your vet. The British Equine Veterinary Association and the insurance industry have established a very strict set of criteria that need to be fulfilled for a humane destruction claim to be justified. The insured horse must 'sustain an injury or manifest an illness or disease that is so severe as to warrant *immediate destruction* to relieve *incurable and excessive pain* and that *no other treatment options* are available to the horse at the time'.

To give a few examples, the following situations would qualify.

- A horse with a severe, irreparable fracture where the bone is in many pieces.
- A horse with severe spinal injuries that cannot stand.
- A horse in severe shock from a ruptured gut.

However, the policy *would not cover* the following situations.

- A horse with colic that the attending vet believes to have a good prognosis if surgery is carried out promptly and suitable facilities are available.
- The pony with advanced and progressive liver disease that has become thin and depressed.
- An advanced eventer sustaining a serious career-ending injury that renders it unsuitable for further competitive work.
- A racehorse that breaks down, i.e. develops a tendon injury to a superficial digital flexor tendon that will prevent it from ever racing again, but does not stop it being turned out to grass after a suitable period of box rest.

It is very important to understand that these conditions *do not qualify for humane destruction*. This can seem harsh especially in cases such as the pony that has liver disease and no hope of recovery. In these cases, the owner may elect to have the animal euthanased rather than pay for surgery or let the horse continue to lead a miserable life, but the terms of the insurance should have been understood at the outset. It goes without saying that leaving the animal to deteriorate to a point where it does qualify for humane destruction is a serious welfare issue that your vet will not support.

When a horse or pony is destroyed on humane grounds, your insurance company should be notified as soon as possible as they may require a post mortem examination. Your vet will be asked to write a report giving the details and confirming the horse's identity.

Inevitably there is always the potential for differences of opinion. This is why it is essential to discuss destruction of the horse with the insurers *before* the event whenever possible. In certain circumstances your vet may obtain a second opinion from a professional colleague.

PERMANENT LOSS OF USE

Permanent loss of use means that the horse is rendered *permanently incapable* of fulfilling the function for which it is insured. This cannot be

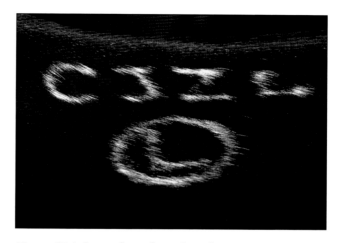

Figure 25.1 Loss-of-use freeze brand

claimed until the horse has been given the appropriate treatment for the condition and sufficient time has elapsed to be certain there is no chance of recovery. The premium for this type of cover is considerably more expensive than for a mortality policy. In the event of a successful claim, the insurance company will usually pay 100% of the sum insured or the market value if this is less. In some cases, the owner may elect to keep the horse in retirement and accept a reduced sum. The horse is likely to be freeze branded with an 'L' inside a circle to show that it has already been the subject of such a claim (Figure 25.1). Again, the insurance company must be notified prior to euthanasia being carried out. They may wish to send their own vet or consult a veterinary specialist to assess the horse first.

VETERINARY FEES

Policies differ in the amount of cover they provide. You need to check the following.

- The maximum amount that can be claimed per incident.
- If there is an upper limit to the amount claimed in any year.
- Whether the policy covers complementary therapies such as acupuncture and homeopathy and treatments such as physiotherapy and remedial shoeing.
- The 'excess' for each claim. This is the amount of each claim that you have to pay yourself and it varies between insurance companies. If two unrelated conditions are diagnosed at the same time, you are likely to have to pay two excess fees. With some companies it is possible to have a reduced premium if a voluntary high excess of several hundreds of pounds is accepted. This helps the owner who wants to be protected only in the event of a very high vet's bill, e.g. following a serious accident or colic surgery. It is sometimes referred to as 'catastrophe fee cover'.
- The length of time that the insurance company will pay for the treatment of a long-term problem. This is normally one year after the horse first developed the condition.

DISPOSAL COSTS

This is the cost of removing and disposing of your horse's body following death or euthanasia.

LOSS BY THEFT OR STRAYING INCLUDING RECOVERY FEES

The insurance company will pay the market value of the horse if it cannot be found plus a contribution towards the cost of trying to recover it.

HIRE OF A HORSE

Some policies offer a fixed amount towards the hire of a replacement horse if your own is incapacitated.

The following are also included on most policies.
- Personal accident.
- Dental treatment.
- Saddlery and tack.
- Loss of entry fees.
- Stable insurance cover.

In general, the more comprehensive the cover selected, the higher the premium. It is advisable to select the type of cover you require and obtain quotes from several companies. Before making a decision, read the small print and check the details carefully.

Applying for insurance cover

The insurance company requires assurance that the horse is in good health at the inception of the policy. You will be asked to sign a declaration of health or if the horse is above a certain value or being covered for loss of use, a 5-stage vetting certificate may be required. In some cases X-rays of the feet or particular joints (usually fetlocks, knees and hocks) will be requested.

Warning
- Always answer the questions truthfully or a claim may be declared invalid at a later date. Failure to disclose a fact that seems irrelevant at the time may jeopardize an expensive future claim. For example, if your horse has a mild bout of spasmodic colic due to escaping into the lush pasture next door and gorging himself, you should notify the insurance company even if you are not making a claim. Failure to do so may mean they refuse to pay the fees for an unrelated surgical colic later on.

- The fact that your horse has a 5-stage prepurchase examination certificate, does not guarantee that it will be accepted for cover by an insurance company. It may be wise to defer purchase until the insurance company has agreed to cover the horse.
- If a problem is decided to have existed before the insurance cover was taken out, the insurers are likely to refuse to pay for treatment. If, for example, you purchase a horse with a small sarcoid on its thigh, the risk of it becoming a problem later on is one you must weigh up when making the decision to buy the horse. Sarcoids are very unpredictable in their behaviour so any costs incurred will be your responsibility and not that of the insurance company. Another example would be the horse with poor hoof conformation and foot balance that is sound at the time of purchase. The vet's fees are unlikely to be covered if the horse develops chronic foot pain in the next few months.

Points to consider when taking out an insurance policy
THE TYPE OF COVER

In addition to the choices discussed above, the cost varies with the value and proposed use of the horse. The higher the value of the horse and the riskier the activities it is used for, the greater the premium. A horse used for light hacking is on average less likely to become injured during the course of its work than a three-day-event horse.

DISCOUNTS

A number of companies offer discounts for freeze-marked horses and owners insuring more than one horse.

DATE THE COVER COMMENCES

This is very important as most policies exclude illness and disease occurring within the first 14 days of insurance cover. It is very important to obtain accident and public liability cover from the time you take over ownership of the horse.

REPUTATION OF THE INSURANCE COMPANY

Some insurance companies are helpful and quick to process claims whereas others can take considerably longer. It is worth asking other horse owners for their experiences.

Making a claim

As soon as the horse becomes ill or is injured, the insurance company must be notified. This applies even if you do not have cover for veterinary fees or if the injury is minor and unlikely to exceed the policy excess. Many insurance companies can now be contacted 7 days a week.

This ensures that in the event of an apparently simple case becoming more serious, the insurers can be certain the horse has received appropriate veterinary treatment from the start.

It may be helpful to record details of the vet's visits, telephone conversations with the insurance company and to keep copies of letters sent in a safe place for future reference.

A claim form is sent for completion by the owner and the attending vet. The vet will fill in details concerning the diagnosis, treatment and costs involved. This may incur a small charge that cannot be claimed back from the insurance company.

At the end of treatment, a veterinary certificate may be required to confirm that the horse has made a full recovery and is back in full work.

Changes within the insurance industry

In order to bring the UK insurance industry in line with Europe, recent changes have been introduced. Responsibility for the regulation of veterinary insurance products has been transferred to the Financial Services Authority (FSA). The new guidelines may affect the way in which your vet is allowed to handle your claim. For example, your vet is still able to provide you with information to help you complete the claims form, but may no longer be allowed to help you negotiate settlement of the claim or query a rejected claim. Your vet will explain the changes that apply to your individual circumstances.

Exclusions
WHAT IS NOT INCLUDED?

There are certain procedures that the insurance company will not pay for. These include:
- castration and any of the complications associated with this routine procedure
- removal of wolf teeth
- treatment to help a mare conceive.

In many cases they will not pay for:
- hospitalization; some insurance companies exclude this and consider the fees to be part of a horse's daily living expenses
- transport to a veterinary hospital
- post mortem examinations, unless specifically requested.

Some policies require an additional premium if the horse needs a general anaesthetic. This should be organized in advance wherever possible.

EXCLUSIONS FOLLOWING A CLAIM

Once the insurance company has paid out for a particular injury or disease, this is likely to be excluded from future cover. For example, it is reasonable for tendon injuries to be excluded following a severe strain of the superficial digital flexor tendon. However, it is not reasonable for the whole of the injured leg to be excluded from any future unrelated claims. The horse may cut itself in the field and this should be covered. Equally, the owner of a horse with navicular disease should be able to claim for accidents such as a nail penetration of the foot.

If you think an exclusion is too broad, speak to the insurance company and discuss the situation. In some cases, exclusions may be lifted after the horse has fully recovered from a disease.

Fraudulent claims

Unfortunately, there are people who insure horses for vet's fees, knowing full well that the horse has a problem. This is not only dishonest, but ultimately it leads to inflated premiums for everyone else.

Complaints

If you feel that an insurance claim has not been satisfactorily dealt with, you should consult the insurance ombudsman.

SECOND OPINIONS AND REFERRALS

In some circumstances, either you or your vet may decide that a second opinion would be of value to help treat your horse or pony. As the owner of a horse, you can ask for a second opinion or referral at any time. A **second opinion** means seeking another opinion to confirm the diagnosis. A **referral** involves sending the horse to another practice for diagnosis and possibly treatment. In each case, the horse continues to be the patient of the original vet.

Second opinions and referrals are routine in equine practice. Over the past 20 years there have been major advances in diagnostic imaging, surgical techniques and medical treatment. Much of the equipment is prohibitively expensive and beyond the means of many practices. It also requires specialist training and experience for optimal results. Thus, horses are often referred when sophisticated equipment, operated by a vet who is experienced in the particular field, is required to make a diagnosis or provide the best treatment.

When obtaining a second opinion, it is very important that the correct procedure is followed. Your vet will make all the arrangements and provide an up-to-date case history. This will include a description of the horse's clinical signs, the results of any tests performed and details of any medication given. Any X-rays or scans will also be provided.

Never ask a second vet to examine your horse without providing all of the history and letting them know that another vet is involved. The Guide to Professional Conduct for veterinary surgeons states that a vet should not knowingly take over a colleague's case without informing the vet in question and obtaining a clinical history. Apart from the professional courtesy, these rules are made for the welfare of the patient. In the absence of the case history, tests may be unnecessarily repeated or incompatible treatment given. Your vet is unlikely to be offended if you ask for a second opinion. However, he or she is likely to be annoyed if they find out that another vet has unknowingly examined the horse, without all the relevant information.

With the development of new technology and the rapid increase in veterinary knowledge, it is likely that in the future, many more equine vets will undertake specialist postgraduate training in a particular field. Whilst most conditions can be treated at home by your own vet, referral to a centre of excellence for specialist treatment of some conditions is likely to become increasingly common.

BOX REST

Box rest means confining the horse to a stable. This may be for a few days to a few weeks or even months, depending on the severity of the injury or illness. Horses may require several weeks of confinement following colic surgery whereas some orthopaedic injuries will require box rest for many months.

Objective

The purpose is to prevent uncontrolled exercise and allow an injury to heal. Stabling reduces the risk of further damage occurring. With a programme of care and rest, many horses with minor strains and sprains make a full recovery.

Management
CHANGE OF ROUTINE

Many owners worry that their horse will become distressed by the change in routine. However, most horses settle quite quickly. If the horse is particularly anxious, a mild tranquilliser such as acepromazine (ACP) can be helpful for the first few days.

COMPANIONSHIP

Horses are social animals and most prefer being kept with other horses. If possible, try to stable the horse where he can see others. Animals such as sheep and goats can make good companions. If the horse has to be kept on his own, spend some time each day grooming and talking to him. Some horses are comforted if they can see their own reflection in a stable mirror.

It is a good idea to consider your own situation and the horse's temperament. Horses, like people, are individuals. Some are happier left undisturbed in a quiet corner, while others enjoy watching the activities of a busy yard. If you feel unable to cope with the situation for any reason, consider sending the horse to a well-run livery yard for the duration of the enforced rest.

FEEDING

The horse will need less food than when he was working. Whenever possible, good quality forage should be offered ad lib. This helps to retain normal gut movement and reduce boredom. In the case of a laminitic pony or overweight animal, however, the forage may be restricted. Soaking hay for half an hour helps to reduce the amount of dust and fungal spores inhaled by the horse.

There are a number of low-energy, high-fibre concentrates formulated specifically for horses on box rest. Small feeds give the horse something to look forward to during the day and ensure he receives enough vitamins and minerals. Carrots and apples can be added as a treat. Alternatively, the use of a plastic ball that releases horse and pony cubes through a small hole as it is pushed around can help to keep the horse occupied. However, this does not work well on a deep bed, nor does it help weight control.

Whenever a horse is confined more than normal, or the diet is changed, it is important to check that he is still producing droppings regularly and not becoming constipated. Laxative feeds including occasional bran mashes may be helpful.

DRINKING WATER

Fresh drinking water should always be available. Buckets should be emptied and refilled each day or more often if they become contaminated. Make sure the horse drinks enough and is comfortable with automatic drinkers if these are the only source of water. In freezing weather, taking the chill off the water may encourage the horse to drink more.

VENTILATION

Special attention should be paid to the ventilation of the box so the horse has plenty of fresh air, without standing in a draught. Poor circulation of air, dusty forage and dirty bedding can make the atmosphere very unhealthy. An allergic cough is the last thing an injured horse needs while he is confined to the box.

BEDDING

The horse needs a dry, comfortable bed. This should be kept scrupulously clean to minimize odours, mould growth and the risk of thrush infection. The type of bedding recommended differs with the condition being treated. Laminitic ponies are best on a deep bed of shavings but these are unsuitable for a horse with an open wound which cannot be bandaged. Deep straw or paper beds are comfortable, but they wind round the limbs of horses that are severely lame or have large dressings, making movement even more difficult. Horses that eat their straw beds are best kept on wood shavings, paper or cardboard. Many horses will eat their beds if they are bored and this can lead to digestive problems such as impactions. It is always advisable to monitor the output of droppings in horses that are kept in for any length of time.

Whatever material is used, there should be enough for the horse to lie down in comfort and for the urine to be absorbed. Rubber matting can be used with any of the bedding types.

CARE OF THE FEET
The feet should be picked out daily and carefully inspected for the first signs of thrush. Regular trimming by the farrier is just as important as when the horse was in work.

EXERCISE AND REHABILITATION
The purpose of box rest is to control the horse's exercise and prevent violent, uncontrolled movements which could exacerbate the injury. Do not be tempted to turn the horse out, for even a short period, it is just too risky. As the horse begins to recover, your vet may recommend that you start to walk him out in hand. Always use a bridle and lunge rein to minimize the chance of the horse getting away from you. Sometimes ACP is necessary to start with if he is very excited.

Turning out after a period of box rest
Special care should be taken when turning a horse out for the first time after a period of box rest. The following steps are advised.

- Wherever possible, use a suitable paddock with good fencing and a reasonable covering of grass. Avoid hilly, uneven or stony ground.
- Choose a quiet time of day.
- Do not give the horse a feed beforehand so that it will be inclined to graze rather than gallop.
- It is advisable to walk the horse for 20–30 minutes prior to turnout so his muscles are thoroughly warmed up. This reduces the risk of a spontaneous fracture occurring as a result of explosive leaping and bucking movements.
- If considered necessary, ask your vet to come and give an injection of sedative.
- Walk the horse to the field wearing a bridle. Take him to a safe area that is not too close to the gate, trough, fences etc. If possible, allow him to graze in hand for a few minutes. When he is relaxed, gently slip the bridle off and quietly move away. Be prepared for him to suddenly buck or kick in excitement.
- Leave the horse by itself or with a sensible companion. Check on him throughout the day.

IDENTIFICATION OF HORSES

Freeze marking

Freeze marking is one method of giving your horse a clear and permanent identification mark (Figure 25.2). The characters (letters and numbers) are marked on the left side of the saddle region or the left shoulder, using a very cold instrument. The pigment cells in the skin are killed and the new hair growth is white. Grey and coloured horses are identified using the same technique but a bald mark is created on the shoulder. The initial fee charged for freeze marking covers your horse while it remains in your ownership.

THE PROCEDURE

The horse should be held in a stable or enclosed space by an experienced adult. The area to be marked is clipped and cleaned with alcohol. The cold markers are held in place for 15–45 seconds. The procedure may give an uncomfortable sensation while the chilled markers are applied.

Within minutes, the area begins to swell. This usually persists for 24 hours. Over the next few weeks the dead skin and hair fall away. The mark becomes bald and may look rather pink. In time, this will be covered with white hair. The freeze mark takes 3–4 months to develop.

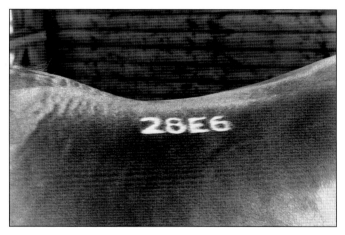

Figure 25.2 A freeze mark

AFTERCARE

The horse can be turned out immediately afterwards. It does not matter if the horse rolls or gets muddy as the skin is not broken. A 4–7 day period with no ridden exercise is recommended, although some horses can remain sensitive for up to 3 weeks. It therefore makes sense to plan the procedure for a time when an enforced rest is convenient. The horse may be lunged during this time. Rollers should also be avoided in the recovery period. A thick numnah is recommended while the freeze mark is forming.

Horses marked on the shoulder can usually be ridden after 2 days.

ADVANTAGES

- Horse thieves are less likely to steal a freeze-marked animal.
- If the animal is stolen, it can be readily identified.
- The freeze-mark company liaise with the police and co-ordinate the search for a stolen horse. Ports, horse sales and slaughter houses are notified. The service is provided 24 hours a day, 365 days of the year.
- Some insurance companies offer a reduction in premium if the horse is freeze-marked.

DISADVANTAGES

- Freeze marking is not recommended until a horse is 12 months old.
- Some horse thieves have their own equipment and alter the marks.
- In the winter, a horse with a thick coat may need the area clipped for the mark to be read.
- Some owners consider the mark to be a blemish and think it spoils the appearance of the horse.

LOSS-OF-USE MARK

When a horse is the subject of a loss-of-use claim, it is marked with an 'L' inside a circle on the instructions of the insurance company. This prevents the horse from being fraudulently sold on at a later date. If the horse does not already have a freeze mark, it will be given a 4-digit reference number.

THE MICROMARK

Horses that have been microchipped can be freeze marked with a small horseshoe-shaped mark. This is to alert thieves to the fact that the horse is traceable. The freeze mark is 35 mm ($1\frac{1}{2}$ in) wide.

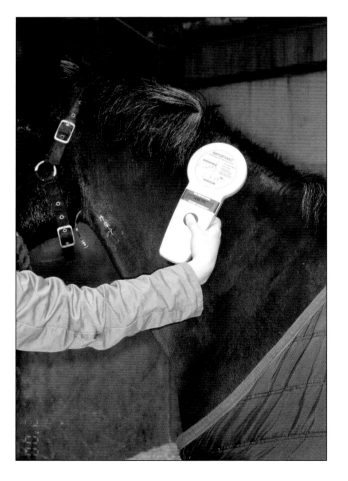

Microchipping

Horses may be implanted with a small microchip as a permanent method of identification. The site is beneath the crest in the middle third of the neck on the horse's left side. The area is clipped and swabbed, then the microchip is introduced through a wide-bore needle. The procedure is very quick and most horses tolerate it without complaint. Whilst the implant is less visible it cannot be tampered with. The chip is read with a portable scanner (Figure 25.3).

If the horse goes missing, its details are passed on to a nationwide network of contacts including the police, vets, sale rings, ports, abattoirs and Trading Standards Officers.

Brands

Many Warmblood horses have their own distinguishing brands.

Figure 25.3 Scanning a horse for a microchip

THE CONTROL OF FLY IRRITATION

During the UK summer, flies can cause a great deal of irritation to grazing animals whilst in other countries they are a problem all year round. In addition to making the horse itchy and sore, they can spread disease from one animal to another. They are a particular nuisance for mares with foals as they feed on the soft skin around the udder. A few examples include the following

Midges (*Culicoides spp.*), active at dawn and dusk, will bite horses (and people) and cause sweet itch in susceptible animals. They are an intermediate host of *Onchocerca cervicalis*.

Stable flies (*Stomoxys calcitrans*) breed in wet, soiled bedding. They feed on the horse's blood and their painful bite can leave a raised lump with a small scab. They can act as an intermediate host for *Habronema microstoma*.

House flies (*Musca domestica*) breed in muck heaps and feed on the manure. They do not bite the horse but are a source of irritation as they cluster in groups around the eyes, nostrils and sheath and feed on liquid discharges. They are intermediate

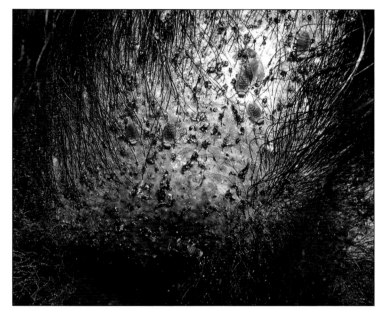

Figure 25.4 Flies feeding inside a horse's ear

hosts for *Habronema muscae* and carry bacteria on their hairy legs and feet. These flies can introduce infection into wounds and cause conjunctivitis.

Black flies (*Simulium spp.*) particularly like to feed on the parts of the horses' body with little hair, e.g. inside the ears (Figure 25.4) and on the ventral midline in front of the udder and sheath.

Horse flies (*Tabanus spp.*) suck blood from the neck, legs and underside of the horse. Their bite is very painful and causes raised wheals. Horses will often become anxious and gallop around the field trying to escape from them.

Bots (*Gasterophilus spp.*) irritate the horse as they lay their eggs.

Total fly control is virtually impossible, although some success is achieved with the following measures.

Shelter

Provision of a cool, clean shelter is the most effective method of fly control. During hot weather, horses benefit from being stabled by day and turned out at night. The shelter should

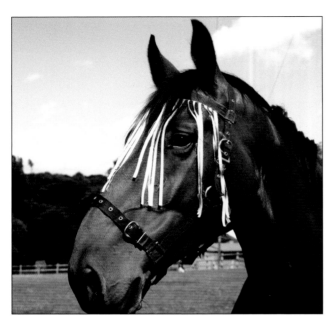

Figure 25.5 Fly fringe

be situated as far as possible from fly breeding grounds such as stagnant water and the muck heap. Screening the door and windows with a fine mesh may help to protect the horse from *Culicoides* midges. Some yards use fans in their barns to blow the flies away. Where there is no shelter available, the horse should have access to some shade.

A companion

Turning horses out in pairs is helpful as they can stand head to tail and flick the flies from each other with their tails.

A summer sheet or fly rug

These protect a large area of the horse from biting flies both in the field and when stabled. Boett® Blankets are very effective for horses and ponies suffering from sweet itch.

Fly fringes and protective face and ear covers

A fly fringe attached to the headcollar helps to deter flies from feeding around the eyes (Figure 25.5). The disadvantage is that the horse has to wear a headcollar which could possibly become caught on gateposts etc.

Protective face and ear covers give excellent protection (Figures 25.6a and b). They

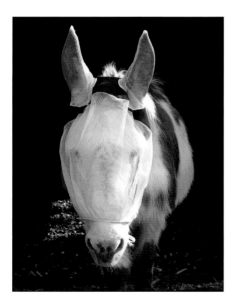

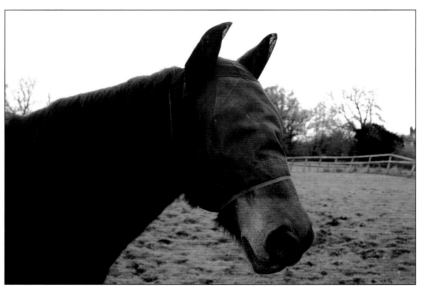

Figures 25.6a and b There are many designs of protective face and ear covers; choose the type that is most comfortable and suitable for your horse: a) donkey wearing a fly net; b) horse wearing a fly mask, which has a detachable nose piece (not shown)

should be made of a light, cool material and be a comfortable fit. Horses should be checked regularly as flies sometimes become trapped inside them. They may not be suitable for every situation. There is a concern that some designs restrict the horses' vision which could lead to an accident where playful youngsters are kept together in a group. Some horses are suspicious and frightened of the masks to begin with. If this is likely, it is sensible to try it on the horse when it is relaxed in the stable.

There is a view that there are more paddock injuries in horses with fly masks as they cannot see each other's faces and expressions. The counter argument is that unprotected horses become agitated trying to escape the fly nuisance.

Good hygiene

Excellent stable hygiene and frequent removal of the muck heap will help to reduce the number of flies.

The use of fly repellents and creams

Fly repellents can be purchased from vets, saddlers and agricultural merchants. The instructions should be followed carefully. *Do not* be tempted to transfer liquid repellents into spray bottles as inhaling the preparation may be harmful. It is advisable to test the product on a small area of sensitive skin, e.g. the inside of the horse's thigh, before treating the whole horse.

Insecticidal or barrier creams, e.g. Sudocream® or petroleum jelly (Vaseline®)can be applied to the inside of the horse's ears and the areas with only sparse hair cover on the ventral midline around the udder and sheath. Deposits of cream should not be allowed to build up inside the ears or enter the ear canal.

Insecticidal bands or tags can be attached to the headcollar or tied into the mane and insecticidal wound powders may be applied to small cuts and grazes.

Treatment

Occasionally, specific treatment is required for problems caused by flies. These include:
- ivermectin to treat *Habronema*, *Onchocerca* and *Gasterophilus*
- antibiotic (+/– corticosteroid) eye ointments for conjunctival infection or inflammation; discharge should be regularly cleaned away with warm water and cotton wool
- corticosteroids or antihistamines for severe skin reactions.

HOW TO GIVE AN INTRAMUSCULAR INJECTION

Whenever possible, injections are administered by the vet. However, when the horse needs a course of treatment, antibiotics are sometimes left for the owner or carer to inject into the

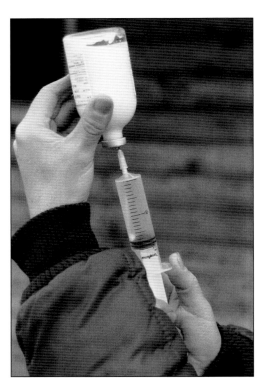

Figure 25.7 Filling the syringe

muscle. Intravenous injections should always be given by the vet.

When injecting a horse, good hygiene and cleanliness are essential. If the contents of the bottle, the syringe or the needle become contaminated, discard them immediately.

Preparing the horse

The horse should be:

- clean and dry; never inject a horse through a wet, muddy coat
- adequately restrained; whenever possible, ask someone to hold the horse.

Filling the syringe

- First, wash your hands.
- Check the contents of the bottle and read the instructions.
- Shake the bottle thoroughly.
- Wipe the rubber stopper of the bottle with a piece of cotton wool soaked in surgical or methylated spirit.
- Snap off the end of the needle case and attach the sterile needle, still covered by the needle cap, onto a sterile syringe. Remove the needle cover. *If you drop the needle or accidentally touch it at any stage, discard it and use a new one.*
- If the drug to be injected is a thick suspension, give it a final shake. Draw a volume of air into the syringe that is equivalent to the dose of medication to be given.
- Hold the bottle upside down and push the needle through the rubber stopper. Inject the air slowly into the bottle. Now check that the tip of the needle is below the fluid level and withdraw the plunger (Figure 25.7).
- Withdraw a little more treatment than is required. With the syringe still in the upright position, return the excess to the bottle. This normally removes any air bubbles.
- Withdraw the needle from the bottle and replace the needle cap.
- If any of the medication spills onto your hands, wash it off immediately.

Common difficulties

A CONSIDERABLE VOLUME OF AIR ENTERS THE SYRINGE WITH THE MEDICATION WHEN THE PLUNGER IS WITHDRAWN

There are 2 likely explanations for this.

1   The tip of the needle is intermittently protruding above the fluid level in the bottle.
2   Air is being drawn in at the join between the needle and the syringe. Tightening the connection eliminates the problem.

To eliminate bubbles of air from the syringe, hold it in the vertical position with the needle uppermost. Withdraw the plunger and draw a little air into the syringe. Now flick the syringe smartly with your finger nail. Repeat this until the air bubbles have all burst. Depress the plunger to exclude the air from the syringe.

WITHDRAWING THE DRUG IS DIFFICULT AND REQUIRES A VERY STRONG PULL ON THE PLUNGER

This is especially common with thick antibiotic suspensions when they have become chilled. Unless the medicine has to be kept in the fridge, store it in the house at room temperature.

Injection technique
SELECTING THE SITE

There are 3 sites routinely used for intramuscular injections:

1   the gluteal muscles of the hindquarters
2   the muscles at the front of the chest
3   the neck muscles.

When a large volume of antibiotic is injected daily, the horse may begin to feel bruised and sore. A stiff neck can make a horse feel very miserable and prevent him from lowering his head to graze. If the temperament of the horse permits, a better place to inject him is in the large gluteal muscle mass of the hindquarters or the chest. The injection can be given on alternate sides each time.

Injecting into the gluteals

*   Ask an assistant to hold the horse and to stand on the same side as you.
*   Stand to one side of the horse, just in front of the quarters.
*   Stroke the horse and talk to him.
*   Remove the capped needle from the prepared syringe.
*   Grasp the hub of the needle and remove it from the cap. Hold the hub firmly between your thumb and first two fingers.
*   Still holding the needle, tap the horse with the side of your hand close to the injection site. After several taps, insert the needle perpendicular to the skin to its full depth. Tapping the horse first makes it less likely that it will be startled when the needle is inserted.
*   *Check that no blood fills or drips from the hub of the needle.* If it does, remove the needle and start again.
*   Attach the filled syringe. Pull back on the plunger to check that no blood is drawn into the syringe before proceeding any further.
*   Depress the plunger to give the injection. Considerable pressure may be required to

inject thick antibiotic suspensions. In order to prevent the needle and syringe being forced apart, hold the joint between them with the thumb and forefinger of the other hand.

- Withdraw the needle. Do not be alarmed if there is a trickle of blood from the injection site.
- Avoid the temptation to pat the horse at the injection site immediately afterwards as it may be tender.

Always complete a course of antibiotics, even if the horse appears to be better.

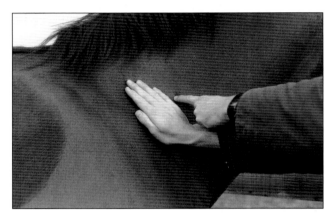

Figure 25.8 The recommended site for an intramuscular injection into a horse's neck

Injecting into the neck (method 1)
This may be the easiest site if you have not injected a horse before.

- The site for injection is a hand's breadth in front of and halfway along the front of the scapula. This should be approximately in the middle of a line drawn from the crest to the underside of the neck (Figure 25.8).
- Tap the horse as described above and insert the needle in a horizontal direction to its full depth. Proceed with the injection. (Figures 25.9a–d.)

Injecting into the neck (method 2)
This technique is particularly useful for young and fractious animals.

- Leave the needle attached to the filled syringe and remove the cap.
- With the left hand, grasp a fold of skin close to the injection site (Figure 25.10a).
- Gently, but deliberately, slide the needle through the skin and deep into the muscle.
- Draw the plunger back to check that no blood is drawn into the syringe and proceed with the injection (Figure 25.10b).

Injecting into the chest
This site is good for repeated injections, especially if it is not safe to inject the gluteals. It has the advantage that if the injection site swells, it is less debilitating than at other sites. The area to inject is in the muscle on either side of the breastbone (Figure 25.11). Your vet will show you the best place. The needle is inserted by tapping the horse as described previously, then inserting it in a horizontal direction.

Injecting foals
Young foals should not be injected in the neck as any subsequent stiffness will discourage

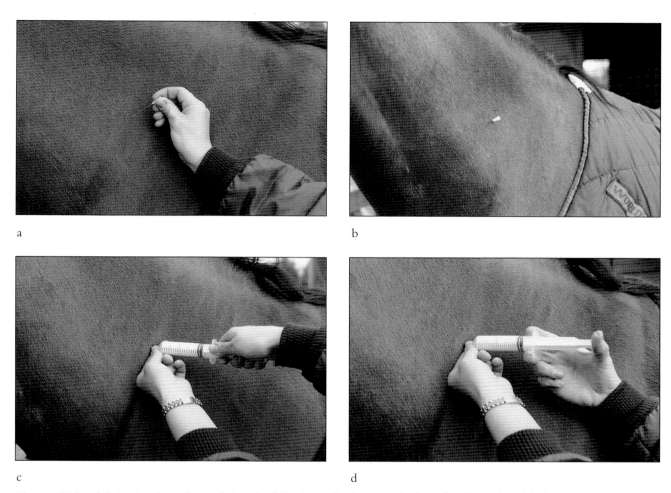

Figures 25.9a–d Injecting into the neck (method 1): a) tap the horse with the side of your hand before inserting the needle; b) check that no blood fills or drips from the hub of the needle before attaching the syringe; c) attach the syringe and pull back the plunger to check that no blood enters the syringe; d) proceed with the injection

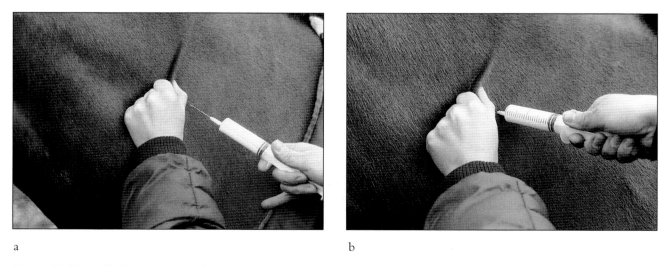

Figure 25.10a and b Injecting into the neck (method 2): a) grasp a fold of skin and slide the needle through the skin deep into the muscle; b) pull the plunger back to check no blood is withdrawn into the syringe and proceed with the injection

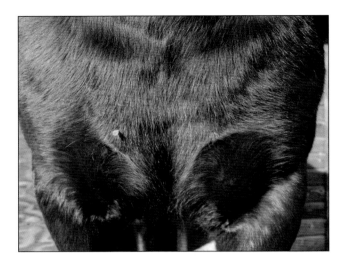

them from suckling. The muscles of the rump or the back of the thigh are the most commonly used sites. They must be free from faecal contamination. Expert restraint is absolutely essential.

Figure 25.11 A needle has been inserted at the site for injecting into the chest

Possible complications
THE NEEDLE DROPS INTO THE BED AND CANNOT BE FOUND

Hypodermic needles in the bedding are a potential danger to people and horses. The bedding must be removed and searched with care until the needle is found.

THE HORSE IS UNCOOPERATIVE

Use further restraint, e.g. a twitch. Prepare the injection first so the twitch is only on for a short time. If the horse is still difficult and you feel you are unlikely to be successful, do not continue. Allow the horse to relax and seek experienced help.

BLOOD APPEARS IN THE HUB OF THE NEEDLE OR THE SYRINGE WHEN THE PLUNGER IS WITHDRAWN

Do not inject the treatment. Some substances such as antibiotic suspensions are lethal if accidentally injected into the bloodstream. Remove the needle and start again.

THE HORSE DEVELOPS A STIFF NECK

Raise the feed bowl and water bucket from the ground so the horse can still eat and drink. Hot fomentations may help to ease the stiffness. Inform your vet who may prescribe a non-steroidal anti-inflammatory drug such as phenylbutazone to reduce the inflammation and discomfort.

THE HORSE DEVELOPS A SWELLING IN ITS BRISKET

This is usually due to bruising or a haematoma and will subside in a few days.

AN ABSCESS FORMS AT THE INJECTION SITE

This may be due to non-sterile technique, but can also occur in spite of careful technique and preparation. Contact your vet.

Disposal of needles and syringes

Never throw used needles and syringes into the dustbin. Return them to the vet's surgery. Partially used bottles of treatment can be stored for a short period of time, provided the contents are sterile. Do not use them to treat another horse without prior consultation with your vet.

THE STORAGE OF MEDICINES

All medicines should be stored correctly and safely.

Guidelines for storing medicines

- Medicines and dressings should be stored so they remain clean and dry. A sealed tin or box within a cupboard is ideal.
- They should not be exposed to extremes of temperature. If possible, the storage area should be relatively cool. Medicines should be kept out of direct sunlight and away from radiators.
- Some medicines need to be kept in the fridge. This will be clearly stated on the label.
- All medicines should be kept out of reach of children and animals, and so are best stored in a locked cupboard.
- Each medicine must be labelled with:
  - the name and address of the veterinary practice
  - the name and address of the client
  - the date the treatment was dispensed
  - the name of the medication
  - the correct dose
  - the method of administration
  - the duration of treatment
  - the name of the horse for which the treatment is prescribed.

Disposal of medicines

Some medicines cannot be stored once the container has been opened. Unfinished bottles and tubes must be disposed of safely. Contact your vet for advice or take them to the surgery.

Discard out-of-date medicines and dressings. The expiry date is usually printed on the packaging or container.

Hygiene

Take care not to contaminate tubs of ointment that are used over a period of time. Wash your hands thoroughly each time ointment is used.

VETERINARY RECORDS

A written record should be kept of all treatment, including routine worming and vaccinations that each horse receives. These records should be stored where they are readily to hand. When horses are kept at livery, the person running the yard should have access to this information.

It is advisable for owners of livery yards to obtain *written permission* to call the vet out to any horse left in their care. This ensures prompt veterinary attention if an emergency occurs and the owner cannot be contacted. It can also prevent disputes over responsibility for fees incurred.

PASSPORTS

Why do we need passports?

Every horse and donkey in the UK is now required to have a passport of its own. (Horse Passports Regulations 2004). This is because in Europe the horse is classed as a food-producing animal. As members of the European Union, we have to comply with their food-safety laws. These have been made to protect humans from residues of medicines given to food-producing animals.

The law states that a maximum residue limit (MRL) must be established for each medicine. This is the maximum level of drug residue left in the animal tissue at the time of slaughter that is considered to be acceptable. Each medication must also have an established withdrawal period. This is the length of time before slaughter during which the drug must not be used.

Problems arise because the testing of these medicines to establish the required data is very expensive. Since equine medicines make up only a small section of the market, the cost of testing is unlikely to be recovered by the sales of the products. If the testing and continued production becomes uneconomic for the pharmaceutical company concerned, these medicines will no longer be available for the horse. This has serious welfare implications.

The introduction of passports allows the continued use of medicines such as phenylbutazone for which no MRLs are available, provided the horse never enters the human food chain. In each passport, there is a declaration the owner can sign which states that the horse identified is *not* intended for human consumption. The horse is identified by a completed silhouette diagram and a written description. Once this declaration has been signed, it cannot be changed. The horse can then be treated with any prescibed medication and it does not need to be entered in the passport.

If the horse *is* intended for human consumption, the owner must sign the appropriate declaration in the passport. Any medicines administered are recorded in the passport and there must be a 6-month interval between the medicine being administered and presentation for slaughter. Certain medicines including acepromazine (ACP) and phenylbutazone *cannot* be given. Since February 2005, no horse will have been accepted for slaughter for human consumption without a passport with the appropriate signed declaration.

Since February 2005, a horse without a passport cannot be:

- sold
- taken to competitions
- exported
- used for breeding
- slaughtered for human consumption.

Whenever a horse is sold, the passport must accompany it and then be returned to the passport-issuing authority so the change of ownership can be recorded.

DRUGS AND THE COMPETITION HORSE

The International Equestrian Federation (FEI: Federation Equestre Internationale) has a Code of Conduct and comprehensive list of Veterinary Regulations that are designed to ensure the wellbeing of horses participating in equestrian sports under their jurisdiction. The Jockey Club and other organizations have their own regulations, all of which are aimed at ensuring adequate care and management of the horse while at competitions.

Prohibited substances

The FEI has drawn up a list of prohibited substances which give good overall guidelines. This is to ensure that horses compete on their individual merits and their performance is not improved by the use of medication. It is intended to protect the horse as well as to ensure that the competition is fair. Horses should only compete if they are fit and healthy. Serious injury could result from competing horses treated with any medication that might mask existing injury or disease.

The list of prohibited substances includes any preparations that are capable of acting on one or more mammalian body systems including:

- the nervous system
- the cardiovascular system

- the respiratory system
- the digestive system other than certain specified substances for the oral treatment of gastric ulceration[1]
- the urinary system
- the reproductive system[2]
- the musculoskeletal system
- the skin (e.g. hypersensitising agents)
- the blood system
- the immune system other than licensed vaccines
- the endocrine system.

These include:
- antipyretics, analgesics and anti-inflammatory substances
- cytotoxic substances
- endocrine secretions and their synthetic counterparts
- masking agents.

Threshold substances

There are other substances that are permitted, provided the concentration in the tissues, body fluids or excreta does not exceed a particular threshold. Thresholds are established for:
- substances naturally occurring in the horse
- substances arising from plants traditionally grazed and harvested as equine feed
- substances in equine feed arising from contamination during cultivation, processing or treatment, storage or transportation.

These include:
- available carbon dioxide
- dimethyl sulphoxide
- hydrocortisone
- nandrolone
- salicylic acid
- testosterone (geldings)
- testosterone (fillies and mares)
- theobromine.

[1] Oral treatment with ranitidine, cimetidine and omeprazole is permitted by the FEI at the time of writing and does not require the use of a medication form.

[2] The FEI currently permits the use of Regumate™ (altrenogest) for treatment of mares with behavioural problems related to oestrus. This must be used at the manufacturer's recommended dose for the treatment of mares only following completion of Medication Form 2 (see page 724).

The rules for prohibited and threshold substances are reviewed annually. Competitors should be familiar with the up-to-date rules which can be found on the FEI website (www.horsesport.org). The acceptable levels of the individual threshold substances are also listed here.

Desensitization and hypersensitization of limbs

- Horses are not allowed to compete under FEI rules if any part of their limbs has been desensitzsed by neurectomy (denerving).
- The use of anything that makes the limbs more sensitive to touch is considered to be an abuse of the horse. Random bandage checks may be carried out.

Precautions

Every year, embarrassing and distressing incidents are reported when horses awarded medals at major international competitions are later stripped of their titles owing to positive tests. Sometimes this is due to accidental contamination, e.g. mistakenly using a feed bucket that has been used to give medicine to another horse. Another example is treating a small wound with a cream, forgetting that it may contain a prohibited substance. These mistakes can be avoided by ensuring that the following checks are made.

- Both you and anyone else responsible for the care of the horse must be aware of the current rules.
- Your vet must be informed of the next competition date before the horse is given any medication including sedatives.
- All feedstuffs and supplements must be free from banned substances. Feeds for competition horses should be certified 'free of prohibited substances'. Problems have arisen with caffeine, theobromine and theophylline. Competition riders often keep back samples of each batch of feed so they can be tested if there is a positive result.
- Horses receiving medication must have their own clearly marked feed buckets and utensils for mixing feeds. One medicine in particular is anecdotally said to cause problems through contamination of equipment or the environment: isoxuprine, which is used for the treatment of navicular syndrome and laminitis, has been detected in tests of horses that have not knowingly been given the drug. It is recommended that competition horses are not put in the stables of horses that have received the drug for any period of time without thorough cleaning first.
- Particular care must be taken with herbal preparations as many of these contain prohibited substances.

The selection of horses for testing

Horses may be subject to:
- obligatory testing, e.g. all winners of major events
- random testing

- spot testing: this will be done if the performance or demeanour of a particular horse gives rise to suspicion.

If your horse is selected for testing, it is recommended that you or someone appointed by you stays in attendance throughout the whole procedure.

The treatment of horses while under FEI regulations
PROHIBITED SUBSTANCES

Occasionally a horse will sustain a minor injury that requires treatment with a prohibited substance, but does not render him unfit for competition. Prior to any treatment, the vet looking after the horse must contact the Veterinary Commission/Delegate to discuss the individual case. Provided the horse is still considered fit to compete and not to have an unfair advantage as a result of the treatment, it may proceed. A form for the Authorisation of Emergency Treatment (Medication Form 1) is completed and signed by the treating vet, the Veterinary Commission/Delegate and the President of the Ground Jury. An example would be the use of a minimal amount of local anaesthetic to suture a small skin laceration. This rule applies even if the horse had been officially withdrawn from the competition, but the signature of the Ground Jury President is not required.

If a horse needs treatment during transportation to the event, e.g. due to mild spasmodic colic, the attending vet must provide a signed statement describing the reason for treatment, the substance, the dose, route and exact time of administration. On arrival at the event, the Veterinary Commission/Delegate must be informed. The case will be considered and a decision made as to whether the horse can compete with retrospective completion of Medication Form 1.

DECLARATION OF ALTERNATIVE TREATMENT

If a competitor wishes the horse to have acupuncture, chiropractic or physiotherapy treatment (including the use of lasers, ultrasound, magnetic blankets, massage etc.) at an event, prior written permission must be obtained from the Veterinary Commission/Delegate and have the approval of the team or treating vet. Medication Form 2, Declaration of Alternative Treatment is used.

AUTHORIZATION FOR MEDICATION THAT IS NOT PROHIBITED

Substances that are not on the prohibited list include:
- rehydration fluids
- electrolytes
- oxygen
- antibiotics (with the exception of procaine penicillin)

- wormers (with the exception of levamisole)
- some treatments for gastric ulcers, i.e. ranitidine, cimetidine and omeprazole.

These substances still need the approval of the Veterinary Commission/Delegate prior to use and Medication Form 3 must be completed before treatment.

Clearance times for drugs

The majority of medications are eliminated from the horse's system and are not detectable after 8 days. However, there is *no guarantee* that a drug will not be detectable after this period. The clearance time is affected by factors such as dose, the route of administration, the diet, concurrent administration of other drugs and the individual horse's metabolism. Some medications may remain in the system and be detectable for a longer period.

Medication of any sort should therefore be avoided when a competition date approaches. If treatment is unavoidable, consult your vet about the withdrawal time of the particular drug and the advisability of competing.

Alarming developments

The FEI have recently found several cases where horses have tested positive for anti-psychotic drugs. These include reserpine, fluphenazine and guanabenz. They are being given to modify the behaviour of excitable horses to make them more relaxed and co-operative. Quite apart from the fact that this is a serious breach of the rules, some of the drugs have potentially dangerous side-effects including lowering of the heart rate and blood pressure as well as sedation. It is likely that if the horse is mildly sedated, it may not respond as expected in any challenging situation. Use of these drugs therefore subjects both the horses and riders to unknown risks.

The future

Drug detection is becomingly increasingly more sensitive and sophisticated. The laboratories can detect trace amounts of a wide range of medications and the list is constantly being updated.

In addition, random drug testing can be carried out at any competition, not only international events.

Rules for individual equestrian sports

The FEI rules have been discussed in some detail. However, the rules vary between the governing bodies of the individual disciplines. For example, the use of phenylbutazone is currently allowed by the British Show Jumping Association and the polo governing body. It is important for competitors to be familiar with the current rules for their own sport.

TRANSPORTING YOUR HORSE

Most of us who own horses will need to transport them at some stage. Whether this is to a show, for a ride in the countryside or to a veterinary hospital for investigations and treatment, the experience can quickly become a miserable one if problems are encountered during loading or on the journey itself.

In most cases, these problems can be avoided by taking the time to familiarize the horse with the lorry or trailer and making sure that the first few experiences are positive ones. If the horse is forced into a trailer in a stressful situation, it is hardly surprising that he will resist it next time. The following tips may help.

In advance

- If you are planning a journey with a youngster or inexperienced horse, park the trailer or lorry in the yard a few days before so they are used to its presence. Offer the horse a small feed close to the vehicle each day or from a bucket on the bottom of the ramp. Do this in quiet, relaxed surroundings so the horse has no sudden frights.
- Familiarize your horse with the clothing he will be wearing for the journey, e.g. travelling boots or bandages, tail guard, poll guard (Figure 25.12), rug etc. Some horses sweat during the journey so the rug should be of a breathable material that wicks the moisture away from the coat. Take a spare rug for the return journey. Unclipped horses do not usually require rugs to travel. However, a cooler rug should be taken to prevent them becoming chilled on arrival if they do sweat up.
- Make sure your horse is fit and well for this experience. Travelling sick horses should be avoided especially if they have any kind of respiratory disease as this increases the risk of pleuropneumonia (also known as transit or shipping fever, see page 420). The saying 'sick horse on, sicker horse off' applies to every horse that travels. The only justifiable exception is when horses are travelled to an equine hospital for treatment.

The vehicle

- Check that everything is in good condition and working order.
- The vehicle should be parked in a safe location, i.e. inside the yard, not on the road. If possible, parking it against a wall may be helpful.
- Make sure the vehicle is light and airy with all the doors open. This will be more attractive to a horse than a dark, enclosed space.
- Make sure the ramp is down properly so it does not move when the horse steps on it. The ramp should be covered with a non-slip material and have horizontal battens sited at intervals to prevent the horse slipping. The angle of the ramp should not exceed 25 degrees.
- Each horse should be separated by a well-padded partition. Partitions that do not reach

the floor but have a sheet of rubber hanging down from them allow horses to adopt a wider stance which helps them to adjust their balance.

- Check the suitability of the vehicle for the size of the horse. A tall horse needs enough headroom and a small pony in a trailer needs a breast bar adjusted to the correct height.
- The floor should be covered with non-slip matting and if desired a light covering of dust-extracted shavings.
- The ventilation should be adequate but not draughty. In warm weather, all the vents should be left open.

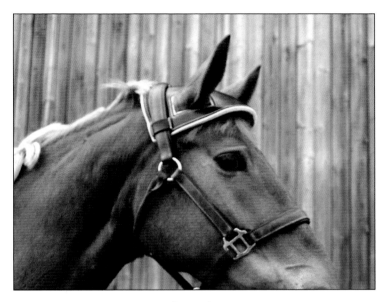

Figure 25.12 A protective poll guard

On the day

- Stay calm and relaxed. If you are worried, your horse will sense this.
- Allow plenty of time. It is sensible to plan your horse's first loading or travelling experience as a practice, rather than having to meet a deadline.
- Load up the car and the trailer (or lorry) first so you are ready to leave once the horse is on board.
- Make sure you have someone to help you secure the partition or breech strap and lift the ramp slowly and gently once the horse is inside.
- Choose a quiet moment, i.e. *not* when a group of other horses is leaving the yard.
- Load a quiet, experienced traveller first as a companion for the journey.

Loading

- Have the horse restrained in a good headcollar, halter or bridle. Wear gloves to protect your hands in case he pulls back.
- Focus the horse's attention on walking forwards and lead him purposefully towards the vehicle. If he stops at the bottom of the ramp or halfway up to look inside, allow him to do so for a short period of time. Try to keep his attention in front of him. Food or treats such as mints can be used to encourage and reward him. Make a fuss of him when he walks inside. Have an assistant ready to secure the breech strap or close the partition.
- Tie the horse so that he has the freedom to raise and lower his head and look round. It is very important for the horse to be able to lower his head to allow respiratory secretions to drain.
- Allow a little time before starting the engine and driving off. Offer a small net of

soaked hay or haylage to focus his attention while you make the final preparations.

- If travelling a single horse, load him on the right-hand side of the trailer, i.e. away from the camber of the road.

The journey

- Every time the vehicle starts and stops or turns a corner, the horse has to brace himself to maintain his balance. This is why the support of the breast bar, partition or ramp are so important for his comfort and why he should be tied in a fashion that allows him to make these adjustments.
- Acceleration and deceleration should be done slowly and steadily as should negotiating corners, winding lanes and roundabouts.
- Sudden braking should be avoided. Try to anticipate lack of consideration from other road users who may well pull out in front of you.
- If at all possible, make the first journey a short trip to somewhere the horse will enjoy, or just travel a short distance and come home again.
- The continual need to rebalance is tiring for the horse. If a long journey is necessary, plan 15 minute rests every 2 hours. During this time you can check your horse, offer him water and stretch your own legs.
- On long journeys, your horse should be given the opportunity to urinate. If the floor does not have drainage holes, sufficient shavings should be available to absorb this. Male horses need to be allowed to stretch out to perform.
- If the journey takes longer than a day, the horses should be unloaded and stabled overnight. Plenty of fresh water should be offered as some horses become dehydrated on long journeys. It is also important for a horse to get his head down to drain any fluid from the airways.

Air hygiene

A humid atmosphere full of fungal spores and ammonia fumes from soiled bedding material is very unhealthy for any horse. If you are undertaking a long journey it is essential that the vehicle has adequate ventilation. Using good quality hay and soaking it before the journey will significantly reduce the number of fungal spores that are inhaled.

Horses that are known to have an allergy to hay should not be travelled with dry hay or share a vehicle with other horses eating it. These horses may be offered haylage as an alternative. Remember that mouldy old bedding is also a source of fungal spores.

In a trailer, the top doors above the rear ramp should be left open so the horse has fresh air and can look around. It may be necessary to close them for a short period if the rain is driving in and soaking the horse or you are stuck in abnormally heavy traffic and the horse is very unsettled by the proximity of large vehicles (e.g. lorries with air brakes) behind.

If it is possible to muck out safely during a long journey, this will help with air hygiene. Special absorptive products are available to help minimize ammonia smells from urine on the floor.

Just in case

It is wise to prepare for the unexpected such as a breakdown, flat tyre or traffic jam. Take an extra hay net, fresh water and a bucket with you in case of unscheduled delays. It is a sensible precaution to have a bridle on board just in case you have to unload the horse for any reason.

A mobile phone and the numbers of breakdown associations could be invaluable.

At the end of the journey

When you arrive at your destination, open up the top doors of the trailer or the ramp of the lorry so the horse can see his new surroundings. Do not hurry his exit from the lorry or trailer. Let him look around and take it slowly, he may be stiff from the journey.

Legislation

There are several laws that lay down specific rules for horses being transported long distances. They are designed to look after the welfare of animals in transit. The standards stipulate the minimum care that must be given to animals transported for commercial purposes including the length of rest periods and the provision of food and water. All horses in transit should be accompanied by their passports and any other important documentation.

Commercial transport

If your horse is being transported by a commercial transport company, they should take care of everything for you and provide an experienced driver and groom to accompany the horse. For international travel, the horse will need a certificate from the vet stating that they have examined the horse and found it fit to travel. The vehicle should be regularly cleaned with a disinfectant that kills viruses and bacteria in accordance with guidelines issued by the Horserace Betting Levy Board.

Sedation

As a general rule, sedation should be avoided apart from emergency situations. The horse is less able to balance itself or control its body temperature. Some horses sweat profusely when they are sedated. This is an issue you may need to discuss with your vet in relation to a particular horse.

FURTHER READING

Care and Management of the Older Horse, Heather Scott Parsons, J. A. Allen

The Complete Equine Emergency Bible, Karen Coumbe MA VetMB CertEP MRCVS and Karen Bush, David & Charles

Equine Veterinary Nursing Manual, editor Karen Coumbe MA VetMB CertEP MRCVS, Blackwell Science

Equine Behaviour, A guide for veterinarians and equine scientists, Paul McGreevy BVSc, PhD, Saunders

Farewell, Making the Right Decision, Humane Slaughter Association and Council of Justice to Animals

First Aid for Horses, Karen Coumbe MA VetMB CertEP MRCVS, J. A. Allen

Hands-on Healing for Pets, Margrit Coates MNFSH MBRCP, Rider

Healing for Horses, Margrit Coates MNFSH MBRCP, Rider

Horse Anatomy, A pictorial approach to equine structure, Peter Goody BSc MSc(Ed) PhD, J. A. Allen

The Horse from Conception to Maturity, Peter Rossdale OBE PhD MA DESM FRCVS with Melanie Bailey, J. A. Allen

Horses Talking, Margrit Coates MNFSH MBRCP, Rider

The Injury-free Horse, Amanda Sutton, David & Charles

The Injured Horse, Amanda Sutton, David & Charles

Saddle Fitting (an Allen Photographic Guide), Kay Humphries, J. A. Allen

Veterinary Acupuncture, Ancient Art to Modern Medicine, 2nd edition, Allen M. Schoen DVM, MS, Mosby

Veterinary Notes for Horse Owners, 18th edition, Captain M. Horace Hayes FRCVS, Ebury Press

USEFUL WEBSITES

Association of British Veterinary Acupuncturists (ABVA) www.abva.co.uk
Association of Chartered Physiotherapists in Animal Physiotherapy
    www.acpat.org.uk
British Association of Equine Dental Technicians www.equinedentistry.org.uk
British Equine Veterinary Association www.beva.org.uk
British Veterinary Dental Association www.BVDA.co.uk
DEFRA website www.defra.gov.uk
Farriers Registration Council www.farrier-reg.gov.uk
FEI website www.horsesport.org
Horserace Betting Levy Board www.hblb.org.uk
Humane Slaughter Association www.hsa.org.uk
The Laminitis Trust www.laminitisclinic.org
National Federation of Spiritual Healers (NFSH) www.NFSH.org.uk
The National Sweet Itch Centre www.sweet-itch.co.uk
The Royal College of Veterinary Surgeons www.rcvs.org.uk
Sue Devereux's website: www.equineacupuncture.co.uk

INDEX

prepurchase examination 667
red blood cells 676
worm infestation 44
blood vessels
'bursting' *see* exercise-induced pulmonary haemorrhage
dilation in feet 158
skin 517, 518
Boett® Blanket 531
bog spavin 255–6
bone cysts 289–90
bone fusion (ankylosis) 226, 232
bone infection 285–8
bone marrow 457, 458
bone scan *see* scintigraphy
bone spavin 227–33
boots, poultices/dressings 78
Borrelia burgdorferi 243, 538
bots 42–3, 711
anthelmintic agents 47
botulism antitoxin 318
botulism (forage poisoning) 316–19
'bowed' tendon 189
bowel disease, infiltrative/inflammatory 486
box rest 706–8
box walking 640
bracken 513
brain, MRI scans 112
bran 134
bran poultice 75
brands 710
breakover 148–9, 231
breathing 443
breeding 579–605
artificial insemination 589–90
choice of stallion 581
costs 579
donkeys 653–4
embryo transfer 591–2
from cryptorchid 577, 579
natural covering 587–9
oestrous cycle 579–81
suitability of mare 579
testing for EVA 404–5
bridle
in dorsal displacement of soft palate 445
fitting 648
restraint of horse 683
British Association of Equine Dental Technicians (BAEDT) 31
British Equine Veterinary Association (BEVA) 31, 36, 700
euthanasia guidelines 698
British Horse Society, Welfare Department 401
British Show Jumping Association 725
British Veterinary Dental Association (BVDA) 31, 36
'broken down' 187
broken knees 248–50
'broken-winded' 427
bromocriptine 609
bromosulphalein (BSP) clearance 681
bronchi 391, 392
bronchioles 392, 427
bronchoalveolar lavage (BAL) 395–6, 421
bronchodilators 431–2, 434
bronchospasm 427
broodmare
care of in-foal 593–4
EHV infection 400–2
mammary secretions 599, 682
pregnancy diagnosis 592–3
reproductive tract 582
signs of foaling 597–9
signs of oestrus 580

stress during pregnancy 596
suitability for breeding 579
vaccinations 24, 25, 316, 594
venereal diseases 586–7
veterinary care 581–6
Brucella abortus 265
burial, carcass 696–7
bursae 262–5
acquired 262–5
atlantal 322
bicipital 262
congenital 262
navicular 120–1, 132, 133, 170, 174, 196, 262, 265
supraspinous 262, 322
bursitis 262–3
acute 263
chronic 263–5
septic 265
bursoscopy 117
'bute' *see* phenylbutazone
'bute' test 374
buttercups 513–14

caecum, rupture 602
calcium 134, 236, 296, 298
canine teeth 26, 33
canker 141–2
cannon bones
asymmetric growth 279–81
sore shins 268–70
capillaries 447, 457, 517
lungs 391, 392
capillary refill time 450, 476
capped elbow 264
capped hock 263–4
carbamazepine 649
carcass, disposal 696–7
cardiac arrhythmias 448, 454–6
cardiac cycle 449
carpal valgus 279–81
carprofen 222
carpus *see* knee joint
cartilage
foot 91, 121, 179–80
hyaline 212–13
ossification 179–80, 235
transplants 226
cartilage cell transplants 226
Caslick's operation 583, 584
castration 571–6
see also gelding
cataracts 620–1
cations, dietary 296
cellulitis 73–4, 462
CEM *see* contagious equine metritis
Certificate of Veterinary Examination (for purchase) 664, 665
cervical vertebrae 320–2
stenosis in wobbler syndrome 306–10
chain shank 685
chasteberry 161, 610
check ligament, inferior 188
strain 197–8
chemotherapy
eye tumours 531, 630
melanomas 566–7
sarcoids 563
chest, intramuscular injections 716
chest drain 421, 422
Chinese medicine 373
chiropractic 334, 379–84
conditions suitable for treatment 383–4